ESSENTIALS OF ADULT AMBULATORY CARE

ESSENTIALS OF ADULT AMBULATORY CARE

Editor

LISA M. RUCKER, M.D.

Assistant Professor of Medicine
Albert Einstein College of Medicine
Bronx Municipal Hospital Center
Bronx, New York

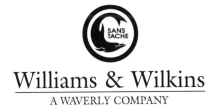

Williams & Wilkins

A WAVERLY COMPANY

BALTIMORE • PHILADELPHIA • LONDON • PARIS • BANGKOK
HONG KONG • MUNICH • SYDNEY • TOKYO • WROCLAW

Editor: Jane Velker
Managing Editor: Crystal Taylor
Production Coordinator: Cindy Park
Copy Editor: Therese Grundl
Illustration Planner: Cindy Park
Cover Designer: Maria Karkucinski
Typesetter: Bi-Comp
Printer: Port City Press
Digitized Illustrations: Bi-Comp
Binder: Port City Press

351 West Camden Street
Baltimore, Maryland 21201-2436 USA

Rose Tree Corporate Center
1400 North Providence Road
Building II, Suite 5025
Media, Pennsylvania 19063-2043 USA

Accurate indications, adverse reactions and dosage schedules for drugs are provided in this book, but it is possible that they may change. The reader is urged to review the package information data of the manufacturers of the medications mentioned.

Printed in the United States of America

First Edition, 1997

Library of Congress Cataloging-in-Publication Data

Essentials of adult ambulatory care / editor, Lisa M. Rucker. — 1st
  ed.
        p. cm.
    Includes bibliographical references and index.
    ISBN 0-683-07456-3
    1. Ambulatory medical care. I. Rucker, Lisa M.
    [DNLM: 1. Ambulatory Care—handbooks.   WB 39 E775 1997]
  RC46.E878   1997
  616—dc20
  DNLM/DLC
  for Library of Congress   96-28283
                                                             CIP

The publishers have made every effort to trace the copyright holders for borrowed material. If they have inadvertently overlooked any, they will be pleased to make the necessary arrangements at the first opportunity.

To purchase additional copies of this book, call our customer service department at **(800) 638-0672** or fax orders to **(800) 447-8438.** For other book services, including chapter reprints and large quantity sales, ask for the Special Sales department.

Canadian customers should call **(800) 268-4178,** or fax **(905) 470-6780.** For all other calls originating outside of the United States, please call **(410) 528-4223** or fax us at **(410) 528-8550.**

Visit Williams & Wilkins on the Internet: **http://www.wwilkins.com** or contact our customer service department at **custserv@wwilkins.com.** Williams & Wilkins customer service representatives are available from 8:30 am to 6:00 pm, EST, Monday through Friday, for telephone access.

97 98 99
1 2 3 4 5 6 7 8 9 10

For the students who teach me,
the husband who supports me,
and the daughter who delights me.

PREFACE

While teaching the adult ambulatory care clerkship at Albert Einstein College of Medicine, my colleagues and I searched for a concise, soft-cover textbook, which we could recommend to our students. It became apparent that none existed; therefore, we decided to write *Essentials of Adult Ambulatory Care.*

We wanted to write a text specifically for students taking a clerkship or elective in ambulatory or primary care medicine. In that most care occurs in outpatient clinics of hospitals, free-standing practices, and in the patient's own home, we wanted to focus the text on patient care in these settings. My colleagues and I examined our practices at the Bronx Municipal Hospital Center and compiled a list of the most common issues and problems encountered in the medical clinic. We then considered what our students need to know about approach to the patient, differential diagnosis, and patient management, based on fundamental medical concepts. The result is *Essentials of Adult Ambulatory Care*, which bridges the student's knowledge of pathophysiology and the problems encountered in clinical practice.

Essentials of Adult Ambulatory Care is designed to be a portable text, which can be used as a quick reference during a routine day in clinic. It focuses on common adult ambulatory problems, emphasizing history taking, the basic physical examination, and indications for ordering laboratory tests to form a concise, logical differential diagnosis.

This text is divided into three sections. Section I, "Practice of Adult Ambulatory Medicine," includes an overview of each issue discussed, the indications for ambulatory, versus bed, treatment, and the principles, or guidelines, for care. Chapters in the second section, "Approach to Patients," address approaches to patients with common complaints (e.g., issues associated with aging, HIV infection, substance abuse) by presenting the scope of the issue, including pitfalls and distinct patient needs, pathophysiology, and guidelines for care. These chapters include illustrative cases with self-assessment questions and answers. Section III, "Evaluation and Management of Common Problems in Adult Ambulatory Care," discusses common problems encountered in ambulatory settings. These chapters follow a consistent organization: introduction, pathophysiologic correlation, clinical and laboratory evaluation (including history, physical examination, and laboratory evaluation), differential diagnosis, management, illustrative cases with self-assessment questions and answers, and suggested readings.

The relative emphasis on differential diagnosis versus management in the common problems chapters varies, depending on the subject matter. For example, for common conditions such as chest pain, hypertension, and diabetes, the management sections are more detailed than the management sections for less common problems. Illustrations, photographs, tables, flowcharts, and decision-making trees are included throughout to encourage the development of diagnostic skills.

I thank my contributing authors for their work on *Essentials of Adult Ambulatory Care*. I believe we have achieved our goal of creating a useful, concise yet comprehensive, and timely text for medical, nurse practitioner, and physician assistant students studying ambulatory or primary care medicine.

ACKNOWLEDGMENTS

I thank Dr. Cynthia Chong who helped greatly to formulate the initial plan and outline of this book.

I also thank Ms. Joanne Ciuti for her untiring efforts to organize and perfect each chapter, her secretarial support, and her cheerfulness.

CONTRIBUTORS

DAVID ACKMAN, M.D.
New York State Department of Health
Albany, New York

ANGELA ASTUTO, M.D.
Instructor of Medicine
Jacobi Medical Center
Adult Primary Care
Bronx, New York

MATTHEW A. BERGER, M.D.
Associate Professor of Medicine
Department of Medicine
Albert Einstein College of Medicine
Bronx, New York

ROBERT L. BRAHAM, M.D.
Associate Professor of Medicine
Medical Director
Director of Ambulatory Care
Jacobi Medical Center
Bronx, New York

PAMELA CHARNEY, M.D.
Director, General Internal Medicine–Women's
Health Track
Associate Professor of Internal Medicine
Assistant Professor of Obstetrics and Gynecology
Jacobi Medical Center
Albert Einstein College of Medicine
Bronx, New York

CYNTHIA M. CHONG, M.D.
Assistant Professor of Medicine
Department of Medicine
Albert Einstein College of Medicine
Bronx, New York

MARGARET P. CHOU, M.D.
Attending Physician
University Hospital
Boston University School of Medicine
Boston, Massachusetts

JOSEPH CONIGLIARO, M.D., M.P.H.
Assistant Professor of Medicine
Department of Internal Medicine
University of Pittsburgh
Director, Health Improvement Clinic
Pittsburgh VA Medical Center
Pittsburgh, Pennsylvania

ROSEMARIE CONIGLIARO, M.D.
Assistant Professor of Medicine
Department of Medicine
Division of General Internal Medicine
University of Pittsburgh
Pittsburgh, Pennsylvania

CHARLOTTE DEUTSCH, M.S., F.N.P., C.S
Family Nurse Practitioner
Columbia Presbyterian Medical Center

SUSAN DRESDNER, M.D.
Instructor of Medicine
Adult Primary Care
Jacobi Medical Center
Bronx, New York

LEANNE FORMAN, M.D.
Orlando, Florida

ELIZABETH JENNY-AVITAL, M.D.
Assistant Professor of Medicine
Department of Medicine
Division of Infectious Diseases
Albert Einstein College of Medicine
Bronx, New York

RHAZIB KHAUND, M.D.
Chief Resident
Miriam Hospital
Brown Affiliate Hospital

LORI A. LEMBERG, M.D.
Instructor in Medicine
Department of Internal Medicine
Jacobi Medical Center
Albert Einstein College of Medicine
Bronx, New York

ANDREW S. LUSTBADER, M.D.
Department of Psychiatry
Yale University
New Haven, Connecticut

PAUL MARANTZ, M.D., M.P.H.
Associate Professor of Epidemiology and Social
Medicine
Associate Professor of Internal Medicine
Albert Einstein College of Medicine
Bronx, New York

THOMAS McGINN, M.D.
Assistant Firm Leader
Department of Medicine
Montefiore Medical Center
Bronx, New York

LINDA McLAUGHLIN, M.D.
Instructor of Medicine
Adult Primary Care
Jacobi Medical Center
Bronx, New York

B. ROBERT MEYER, M.D.
Associate Professor of Medicine
Director of Medicine
Jacobi Medical Center
Albert Einstein College of Medicine
Bronx, New York

CAROLE MORGAN, Ph.D.
Assistant Professor
Epidemiology and Social Medicine
Albert Einstein College of Medicine
Bronx, New York

CHRISTINE L. OMAN, M.D.
Center for Women's Health
Virginia Mason Medical Center
Seattle, Washington

DAISY M. OTERO, M.D.
Department of Internal Medicine
Montefiore Medical Center
Clinical Instructor
Department of Family Medicine
Albert Einstein College of Medicine
Bronx, New York

SHARON PARISH, M.D.
Assistant Firm Leader
Montefiore Medical Center
Department of Medicine
Bronx, New York

RAFAEL PELAYO, M.D.
Clinical Instructor
Department of Psychiatry & Neurology
Stanford University Medical Center
Stanford, California

STELLA PIERRE, M.D.
Instructor of Medicine
Adult Primary Care
Jacobi Medical Center
Bronx, New York

PERRY PONG, M.D.
Assistant Director
Department of Medicine
Albert Einstein College of Medicine
Bronx, New York

LISA M. RUCKER, M.D.
Assistant Professor of Medicine
Albert Einstein College of Medicine
Jacobi Medical Center
Bronx, New York

DIANE SIELDECKI, M.D.
Harvard Pilgrim Health Care of New England
Providence, Rhode Island

MARGARET SMIRNOFF, R.N., M.P.H.
Coordinator
Tuberculosis Elimination Program
Mount Sinai Medical Center
New York, New York

JAMES K. STULMAN, M.D.
Clinical Instructor
Department of Medicine
Montefiore Medical Center
Bronx, New York

LUZ S. VASQUEZ, M.D.
Assistant Clinical Professor of Medicine
Yale School of Medicine
New Haven, Connecticut
Medical Attending
Primary Care Practice
West Haven Veterans Administration Hospital
West Haven, Connecticut

FABIO VOLTERRA, M.D.
Medicine, Hematology/Oncology
Bronx, New York

KATHLEEN WARD, M.D.
Assistant Professor of Medicine
Director, Adult Primary Care
Jacobi Medical Center
Albert Einstein College of Medicine

ELEANOR WEINSTEIN, M.D.
Assistant Professor of Medicine
Department of Medicine
Albert Einstein College of Medicine
Bronx, New York

KIN M. YUEN, M.D.
Clinical Instructor
Department of Internal Medicine
Stanford University Medical Center
Stanford, California

CONTENTS

Section I

PRACTICE OF ADULT AMBULATORY MEDICINE

chapter 1

ADULT AMBULATORY CARE: AN INTRODUCTION
Cynthia Chong and Lisa Rucker

Governmental and insurance reimbursement practices have shifted the care of chronically ill patients and those recovering from severe disease from the hospital to the office. The ambulatory care clinician, often practicing in both settings, has to master new strategies to effectively manage the care of sick outpatients. Clinicians are once again becoming familiar with house calls and are pioneering the delivery of specialized treatments, e.g., administration of in-home intravenous antibiotics, that until recently were confined to the hospital.

Care of adults in the outpatient setting is complex. The clinician must keep current with a tremendous amount of information, e.g., changes in diagnostic modalities and up-to-date recommendations for screening and treatment regimens. More than ever the clinician must focus on prevention or early detection of disease and its complications. He or she must practice affordable cost-contained care and be easily accessible to patients.

INTERDISCIPLINARY CARE

Ambulatory clinicians are increasingly part of a network of care. This network is usually multidisciplinary with the ambulatory clinician directing referrals and maintaining the patient's interests. Referrals include those to specialists, home care, physical therapists, social services, mental health workers, and dietitians. It is essential for the ambulatory clinician to elicit preferences, financial constraints, as well as explain the referral to the patient. The ambulatory care clinician then has the background to discuss diagnostic tests and treatment recommendations made by colleagues. At times, the conversation with a colleague may provide key information to make more useful recommendations. It is essential that ambulatory care clinicians have a picture of how these other services may assist patients and maintain clear lines of communication. Relationships between referring clinicians may be decided by multidisciplinary practices, locale, or a shared notion regarding how to provide patient-centered care.

Ambulatory clinicians are involved in certifying patients for various government or insurance benefits, medical supplies, employment, and education. These can affect the patient's life in different degrees; at times they are perfunctory (e.g., school physical) and occasionally are areas of contention (e.g., excuse from jury duty). Although in cases of contention every attempt should be made to represent the patient's interests, clinicians should trust their own judgment.

PROVIDER-PATIENT RELATIONSHIP

The relationship between the provider and the patient is ever evolving. The provider-patient relationship is less likely to be as patronizing as in the past. Depending on the patient's expectations and the provider's flexibility, the relationship may range from openly collegial to a mixture of collegial and patronizing to entirely patronizing.

Some clinicians form a partnership as a coach and teacher with their ambulatory patients to perform treatment strategies effectively. In this approach, clinicians coach patients to do what will be good for them. Not unlike sports, the clinician-coach provides information, explanations, and suggestions regarding how to reach an end. The patient executes. Coaching strategies include breaking processes down so they can be easily envisioned and performed, using language that is easily understood, explaining the goals and techniques, allowing for mistakes, and stating the importance of practice.

Regardless of the nature of the relationship, the provider tries to understand each patient as an individual within the context of health and sociocultural position. The provider's knowledge helps him or her to better teach, assess, and motivate the patient. In a successful relationship the provider and patient share the responsibility for the patient's health care.

Ambulatory patients, as opposed to those who are admitted to a hospital, decide they need a clinician. They choose to begin, continue, or terminate a relationship with a clinician. They have not relinquished their decision-making role to an emergency room provider or hospital team. Thus they set the tone for and participate in their own care. The importance of the patient in a patient-clinician partnership in care cannot be understated. Consider the length of an office visit compared with the time the patient is on his own. The individual patient's environment, including home, family, friends, beliefs, employment, and finances, must be accounted for in any therapeutic plan. Unlike the hospital setting, the patient largely monitors medications, testing, and physical signs. The ability of the clinician to listen for and understand patient cues contributes to a successful partnership.

The costs of health care have skyrocketed. Many citizens have limited access to care when they are sick because the prices are high. Even the financial costs of routine preventative health care are burdensome. Cost considerations limit testing and treatment options and may influence the provider-patient relationship.

HISTORY AND PHYSICAL EXAMINATION

The ambulatory history and physical examination are different from what is performed inpatient. Ambulatory patients differ from hospital-based patients in an important way: they do not arrive with a diagnostic label invoking pathology of an organ system by which to categorize them and direct their care. Ambulatory patients seek care for a broad array of issues: staying well, planning for the future, medical conditions, emotional needs, and other requirements. Examples of why patients seek ambulatory care include immunizations, physical exams, hypertension management, rashes, psychological counseling, and forms for benefits. Sometimes the reasons for a visit are unclear; patients may feel the need to frame a visit with an organ system complaint distinct from their underlying concerns. It

follows that the approach to ambulatory patients must be different.

Patients who are satisfied with their professional care are likely to follow treatment plans and use medical services appropriately. An approach that is centered on the patient's needs is useful to enhance satisfaction. The patient's needs may be biological, social, or psychological. The patient's background will provide information about the patient and explain why the patient has chosen to visit a clinician and lay the foundation for a therapeutic plan.

History-taking is a logical place to begin. The usual approach to the medical history is to gather all information as quickly as possible to develop a treatment plan that can be immediately implemented for an acutely ill patient. This may occasionally be useful in the ambulatory setting, but more often it is not. Alternatively the approach should allow the patient to unfold a story that relates the events leading to the visit. The exhaustive history is truncated in the outpatient setting. The review of systems is often condensed to "Is anything else bothering you?" Validation occurs when the clinician restates the patient's concerns and their effects. This allows the patient to know he or she was heard and that the concerns are valid. The clinician can say, "I see how worried you are about that pain." or "I can understand how the shortness of breath stopped you from going on." It also gives the patient the opportunity to correct or expand the clinician's understanding of the concerns. Validation sets the stage for creating strategies to help the patient cope with and resolve concerns.

The ambulatory patient's physical exam begins when the provider first meets the patient and listens to the story. Gait, appearance, speech, cognitive skills, memory, affect, body habitus, and gross motor function can be assessed at this stage. When the formal physical exam begins, ambulatory clinicians should include simple functional assessments of vision using newsprint or a pocket Snellen eye chart, hearing using a ticking mechanical watch, and motor skills by observing aspects of dressing. Breast examination, pap testing, and hemocult testing are necessary but need not be performed during the first visit unless it is an area of concern. Careful attention should be given to areas of patient concern (e.g., cardiac exam in a patient with chest pains) or to confirm suspicions raised by the story.

Follow-up examinations focus on the problematic organ system identified by history or previous diagnosis. Much of the physical examination has been shown to be otherwise superfluous. However, mastery of history and examination skills is growing more important because the ambulatory provider is practicing under more stringent time constraints than in the past several decades.

GOAL

The goal of care is to help the patient achieve the greatest level of health possible. Ambulatory settings are appropriate for promoting "wellness" as distinct from treating "illness." The strategy of primary prevention is intervention to prevent disease, thus preserving "wellness." Primary prevention is largely "low tech" and underemphasized in clinical teaching. However, economists tout the overall savings by primary prevention in direct medical costs (e.g., treating illnesses) as well as indirect costs (e.g., value of lost work days). Of course, the monetary value of feeling well is immeasurable!

One first step in promoting wellness is avoiding an unnecessary label of illness. Ambulatory clinicians can reframe concerns that do not reflect illnesses in nonmedical terms. These terms would not lessen the importance of the concerns but would move the discussion away from illness to wellness. For example, a clinician who sees a patient with loss of weight and energy could reassure the patient that these are understandable, normal, and are part of healing when the unexpected death of his spouse is revealed as an aside. Reframing the patient's concerns reassures the patient and shifts the discussion away from illness (weight loss) to wellness (grieving). The clinician avoids both an unnecessary medical workup and the "sick" role.

Encouraging healthy lifestyles is another primary prevention strategy. Smoking cessation, low fat/high fiber diets, exercise, stress reduction, weight loss, substance abuse cessation, and safer sex practices are only a fraction of possible lifestyle changes. The impact is greatest if the lifestyle change proposed relates to concerns expressed by the patient. A patient concerned that chest pains may indicate heart disease would likely be receptive to changing to a low cholesterol diet. Success is enhanced by limiting advice to one or two changes, setting achievable targets, readdressing the desired changes in subsequent visits, and involving other professionals, e.g., a dietitian. Advice should be practical and focused. Global remarks such as "low fat" should be refined to "limit eggs to twice weekly and steamed vegetables are great."

Public health regulations are usually outside the focus of ambulatory clinicians. However, use of automobile seat belts can be encouraged in the ambulatory setting. Immunizations are the most "high tech" of the primary prevention strategies and will be discussed in a later chapter.

REWARDS

Adult ambulatory medicine offers many rewards for the provider. The work is intellectually satisfying, economically profitable, and socially worthwhile. The practitioner has the unique opportunity to develop a long term relationship with the patient. He or she shares the sadness of illness but also the joys of recovery and of life itself. The greatest reward for high quality care is the knowledge of a job well done and the pleasure and privilege of caring for the patient.

chapter 2

CLINICAL REASONING
Robert L. Braham

Although the general approach to diagnostic and therapeutic decision making for ambulatory patients is the same as that for hospitalized patients, the emphasis is often different, and the process is usually more subtle and complex. Students often perceive this process to be "softer" in the ambulatory setting for acutely ill patients because of several factors. These include the subtlety of clinical clues (e.g., a sad expression on the patient's face) and the low technology approach to some clinical situations (e.g., information on smoking cessation given to a patient as the only outcome of an initial visit). Even more importantly, students are confused and put off by the sometimes conflicting recommendations suggested by different mentors and teachers in similar clinical situations and the willingness of experienced mentors to adopt a "wait and see" attitude and to solicit the patient's opinions rather than to quickly make *the* diagnosis and determine *the* treatment plan. The intent of this chapter is to give students and trainees the tools to understand these differences and an appreciation that science and intellectual concerns are equally important in making decisions in the ambulatory setting.

All visits to providers occur for a reason. In most cases, the reason may be obvious: the patient has dysuria or is required to have a preemployment physical examination. Not uncommonly, the reason is not so obvious. Patients may come for an examination "just to see if everything is okay" and mention nothing about the abdominal pain they fear is due to a malignancy (or only mention in passing on the way out the door, "I read in the newspaper that they have a new test for prostate cancer"). In all cases, the clinical reasoning process addresses the questions of diagnosis in relation to interventions that could be made to reassure the patient, treat an illness, or determine a prognosis.

The general concepts to remember follow.

- The world of clinical medicine is an uncertain place. Rarely does the clinician know that the patient absolutely does (probability = 1.0) or does not (probability = 0) have the disease of interest.

  In most clinical situations, providers (and patients) can live with uncertainty. Treatment error is always a possibility, but the need for diagnostic certainty depends on the penalty for being wrong. Dr. Alvan Feinstein has written that this quality of clinical "chagrin" is what motivates most clinical decision making (see Feinstein listed under "Suggested Readings").

- One should obtain additional clinical information only if it could change what is done for the patient. This means that experienced clinicians often adopt "wait and see" attitudes, live with uncertainty, and forgo extensive diagnostic evaluations for many clinical presentations until a clearer picture emerges or the patient gets better.

- A clinician constructs a differential diagnosis by balancing the probabilities of a disease or condition with the penalty for being wrong for certain diagnoses ("ruling them out") even if they are unlikely. Dr. Walsh McDermott has written that in the overwhelming majority of clinical encounters, the difference between a mediocre and superb clinician (and his or her clinical reasoning) has no effect on the patient's future well-being. The trick for the learner and clinician is to determine which encounters are in this crucial minority and act accordingly.

To illustrate these principles, examine the general clinical reasoning employed in three relatively common clinical scenarios.

- A 45-year-old man comes to the clinic for the first time for a "checkup." History and physical are unrevealing except that he says he has trouble reading the newspaper unless he holds it fairly far from his eyes. He has no risk factors for coronary artery disease. He has no other visual symptoms, and his eyes are normal on exam except for presbyopia. The consensus of the medical literature at present suggests that he should have his cholesterol measured and be referred for evaluation for reading glasses, but no other diagnostic tests or therapeutic interventions are clearly indicated.
- Two different patients come to the emergency department on consecutive nights with 8 hours of pleuritic chest pain. The clinicians are concerned about the possibility of pulmonary embolus in both cases. Within 4 hours it is determined that both have mild arterial hypoxemia and indeterminate perfusion lung scans. The first patient, who is a 35-year-old healthy woman who had a recent lengthy airplane trip, is treated with heparin overnight without further testing. The second patient is an 85-year-old man with hemoccult positive stool and a hemoglobin of 10. The clinician demands that a pulmonary arteriogram be performed before administering heparin.
- A 22-year-old woman comes into the urgent care center with 24 hours of dysuria. She has no known allergies and had one urinary tract infection 4 years ago. She is afebrile, looks well, and has no costovertebral angle tenderness. Her urine shows 20 white cells per high powered field and many Gram-negative bacteria. The clinician prescribes 3 days of trimethoprim/sulfamethoxasole but *does not* culture her urine. The patient is told to take her temperature at home and call if she develops a fever or if her symptoms do not resolve over 3 days. The clinician notes to have her called by a staff member in 10 days to verify she is asymptomatic.

Sound clinical judgment involves at least a general knowledge of the predictive value (see "Glossary") of normal and abnormal laboratory results and an appreciation of the most cost-effective way to use testing to make diagnostic or therapeutic decisions. Because there are no tests with 100% sensitivity and 100% specificity, in general the test with a high sensitivity is preferred as a screening test, and a test with high specificity should be cho-sen as a confirmatory test. The cut off point for normality is a critical question in routine clinical situations. In general, normality and abnormality are defined in operational terms. This means that a clinical observation or test that prompts further investigation or treatment is considered abnormal.

Most clinical data are dimensional; they can be measured quantitatively (e.g., weight or serum cholesterol). Although the simplest approach to dimensional data is that of "statistical normality" in which the normal range is defined as two standard deviations from the mean, this is rarely clinically useful. In a purely Gaussian distribution two standard deviations from the mean would encompass 95% of the observations. Clinical data are rarely of a Gaussian distribution, and this approach would mean that by definition 5% of "normal" patients would be abnormal, and a battery of 20 tests in a normal person would only have a 36% (0.95^{20}) chance of being completely normal.

In addition, this would leave the clinician in the ridiculous position of telling the 45-year-old man who finds it impossible to read the newspaper that this is normal for people his age and therefore that nothing should be done. When reviewing the cholesterol results the clinician will prescribe diet or drug therapy on the basis of risks and benefits defined in ways that are particular to the patient—not the average 45-year-old American man.

The choice of a cutoff point also has an effect on the sensitivity and specificity of a test. A cutoff of 1 mm of ST segment depression on the electrocardiogram will make an exercise tolerance test more sensitive but less specific for the diagnosis of coronary artery disease than a cutoff of 2 mm. This effect of a change in cutoff point has also been evidenced by a change in the criteria for the diagnosis of diabetes mellitus to decrease sensitivity and increase specificity by raising the blood sugar levels necessary for making a diagnosis of diabetes mellitus (Diabetes 1979;28:1039). The effect of doing this was to prevent the overdiagnosis of diabetes mellitus because the early detection of prediabetes was found to confer more harm than benefit.

Another important statistical concept in analyzing dimensional data is "regression to the mean." This phenomenon describes the fact that in biological systems with inherent variability, the "grand total" mean of past experience is a better guide to future measurements than one current value. For example, patients initially found to have a low serum potassium level on one measurement will on average be found to have a higher serum potassium level on second measurement.

Table 2.1.
Incremental Gain Expected from Exercise Tolerance Test in Confirming or Excluding Coronary Heart Disease According to Prior Estimates of Likelihood of Disease

Prior estimate of likelihood of disease	Test positive		Test negative	
	Predictive value	Incremental gain	Predictive value	Incremental gain
90	97	7	29	19
80	92	12	48	28
70	88	18	61	31
60	82	22	71	31
50	75	25	79	29
40	67	27	85	25
30	57	27	90	20
20	43	21	94	14
10	25	15	97	7

Values expressed in %; >1 mm change assumed to be 80% sensitive and 74% specific.
Adapted from Griner PF, Panzer RJ, Greenland P. Clinical diagnosis and the laboratory. Chicago: Year Book, 1986:21.

A clinician usually is concerned with predictive values rather than sensitivity or specificity (see "Glossary"); i.e., given a positive test, what is the probability that disease is present, and given a negative test, what is the probability that disease is not present? These post test probabilities can only be computed if the clinician can give an estimate of the pretest probability of the disease in the patient or population under study. The formal method for computing the predictive value of a test is detailed in chapter 9 of the book *Medical Decision Making* by Sox et al. (see Suggested Readings). In brief, when the pretest likelihood of disease is high, a positive result tends to confirm, but an unexpected negative result is not particularly helpful in eliminating the possibility of disease. When pretest likelihood disease is low, a normal result tends to exclude but an unexpectedly positive result is not particularly helpful in confirming the disease. The greatest utility for a test occurs when the pretest estimates are intermediate, neither very high nor very low. Thus, a patient with classic angina who might have a pretest likelihood of ischemic heart disease of 90% would have a posttest probability of 97% after a positive exercise tolerance test and a posttest probability of ischemic heart disease of 71% after a negative exercise tolerance test (positive predictive value = 97%; negative predictive value = 29%) (Table 2.1). A positive exercise tolerance test in a young person with no particular risk factors whose pretest likelihood is 10% would have a posttest probability of isch-

emic heart disease of only 25% and a probability of 3% with a negative exercise tolerance test.

In practice, clinicians have an intuitive feel for the probability of a disease in a specific patient (even if not an exact number) and a feel for three "thresholds" of probability that are important in deciding whether to (a) do nothing further, (b) test more before initiating therapy, or (c) proceed and treat on the basis of the information already available. The first of the three thresholds is the probability below which the clinician would neither test nor treat the patient—the testing threshold. The 45-year-old asymptomatic man with no risk factors for coronary artery disease falls below this threshold, and the clinician neither orders an exercise tolerance test nor treats him for coronary artery disease (keep reading to understand why).

The next landmark, the treatment threshold refers to the probability at which one should be indifferent between giving and withholding treatment. The optimal choice is to withhold treatment when the estimated probability of disease is smaller than the treatment threshold and to administer treatment when the probability is greater than this threshold. The level of this threshold is determined by the risks and benefits of the specific treatment. The 85-year-old man has a higher treatment threshold for anticoagulation (one has to be surer of the diagnosis) because the risk of anticoagulation is higher than in the young woman.

The last landmark is the test treatment threshold, which refers to the level of probability over which a patient ought to be treated without any

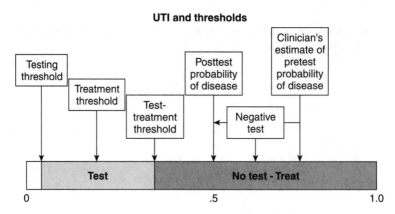

Figure 2.1. Probability of disease and the three thresholds of probability. UTI, urinary tract infection.

future testing. The 22-year-old woman exceeded this probability and was treated without a urine culture.

These general principles are illustrated in Figure 2.1. The clinician should do a diagnostic test if the result will cause the probability of the disease to cross over the treatment threshold probability. The actual levels of the thresholds and the widths of the bars depend on the risks and benefits of testing and treating, but the same principle applies in all clinical decision making. If the clinician's estimate of the pretest probability of a bacterial urinary tract infection in the young woman is 75% and he or she would treat anyone with a probability over 20%, there would be no reason to culture before initiating treatment because the patient's probability of 75% exceeds the test treatment threshold.

Last, if two diagnostic strategies are equally efficacious in making a diagnosis, the one that has the lowest "cost" is preferred. Cost is defined in terms of dollars and patient risk and inconvenience The methodology of cost effectiveness and its related discipline cost benefit analysis can be quite complex, but in many clinical situations (see "Suggested Readings") a consensus has emerged.

In summary, clinical reasoning requires "hard" quantitative understanding of probabilities, costs (dangers and dollars), and benefits in all clinical settings but often more so in an ambulatory setting. If one thinks of a spectrum in which one end is a patient with a "suspicious" breast lesion on mammogram, the decision about the next step is relatively straightforward—biopsy. It is much less clear what to do with a patient with multiple complaints who presents to a clinic without classic signs and symptoms for a clinical syndrome. For a great number of experienced clinicians, dealing with this challenge is extremely rewarding. The authors hope as the student readers proceed, they will share the excitement with those who have gone before them.

GLOSSARY OF TERMS

cost benefit analysis economic analysis in which a single or multiple interventions are measured in positive or negative financial terms; it is derived from industry ("Is it worth putting another Kmart in this town?") and is generally felt to be more rigorous by economists and intensely disliked by physicians and medical journal reviewers; its units of measurement by definition must be positive or negative financial return; because the usual "positives" are earning power after intervention and medical costs are negatives, any program aimed at low or nonearners (elderly, poor, women, disabled) may be shown to be unprofitable (joint replacement in elderly is a classic example of a program with a huge negative "bottom line").

cost effectiveness analysis economic analysis in which alternative interventions are measured in terms of cost and benefit; the simplest example is two antibiotic regimens, both of which eradicate the urinary tract infection in 99% of cases, but one is half the cost of the other and is thus twice as cost effective; a more complex example is two screening regimens for colorectal cancer, one that leads to more colonoscopies and therefore both monetary costs and costs of adverse effects; the usual comparison unit in this sort of analysis is dollars per unit time (e.g., survival measured in years). Cost effectiveness analyses are common in the medical literature.

cutoff point arbitrary value used to separate positive from negative results for any given test or procedure.

false negative rate 100 − sensitivity (percent) = probability that test or procedure result will be negative when the disease is present.

false positive rate   100 − specificity (percent) = probability that test or procedure result will be positive when the disease is not present.

negative predictive value   probability that the disease is not present when the test or procedure is negative.

positive predictive value   probability that the disease is present when the test or procedure is positive.

sensitivity   probability that a test or procedure result will be positive when the disease is present.

specificity   probability that the test or procedure result will be negative when the disease is not present.

test-treatment threshold   probability of disease at which the decision is between testing and treating empirically.

testing threshold   probability of disease at which the decision is between (*a*) not testing and not treating or (*b*) testing and using the result to determine whether to treat.

treatment threshold   probability of disease at which the decision is a tossup between treating and not treating the patient.

true negative rate   specificity (percent).

true positive rate   sensitivity (percent).

SUGGESTED READINGS

Feinstein AR. The "chagrin factor"—a qualitative decision analysis. Arch Intern Med 1985;145:1257–1259.

Griner PF, Mayewski RJ, Mushlin AI, Greenland P. Selection and interpretation of diagnostic tests and procedures. Ann Intern Med 1981;94:559–600.

Griner PF, Panzer RJ, Greenland P. Clinical diagnosis and the laboratory. Chicago: Year Book, 1986:1–35.

Kassirer JP. Diagnostic reasoning. Ann Intern Med 1989;110:893–900.

McDermott W. Education and general medical care. Ann Intern Med 1982;96:512–517.

Sackett DL, Haynes RB, Guyatt GH, Tugwell P. Clinical epidemiology. Boston: Little Brown, 1991:3–18.

Sox HC ed. Common diagnostic tests: uses and interpretations. Philadelphia: American College of Physicians, 1987.

Sox HC, Blatt M, Higgins M, Marton K. Medical decision making. Boston: Butterworth, 1988.

chapter 3

STAYING HEALTHY
Kathleen Ward

When did keeping people healthy emerge as an important task of medicine? Modern medicine developed around treating the sick. But promoting health is not a new approach. Public health at the turn of the century focused on correcting conditions that caused disease and therefore would prevent disease in the future. In 1923, the American Medical Association published *Periodic Health Examination: A Manual for Physicians,* which was last updated in 1947. After World War II and the development of antibiotics, however, medicine in the United States turned toward treating disease rather than preventing it.

Recently the promotion and maintenance of health have again captured national attention. Interestingly, disease prevention has emerged as the dominant concept within these areas. The terms health promotion and disease prevention overlap and are often used interchangeably, but slightly different perspectives are meant. Although interrelated, their relationship can be viewed as that of a more inclusive category (health promotion) containing a more specific category (disease prevention).

The brevity of this chapter is not meant to mirror the role health promotion activities will inevitably play in modern medicine. Understanding what promotes and maintains health is complex, as are developing and implementing effective methods to do so. Although the store of knowledge is not as large as one would like, it continually grows.

As a description of the goal of health promotion, the World Health Organization definition of health is appropriate: "Health is not merely the absence of disease but a state of physical, mental, and social well-being." Health promotion is the integrating framework in this chapter. Topics include immunizations, screening tests, and counseling strategies. Respective recommendations are presented in Tables 3.1–3.3.

IMMUNIZATIONS

A history of immunizations and medical conditions should be obtained from all patients before appropriate recommendations about immunizations can be given. For adults immunizations against influenza, pneumococcus, hepatitis B, and diphtheria-tetanus are usually considered. In addition to these four, rubella or measles-mumps-rubella vaccine is considered for young adults. Recommendations for vaccination change frequently. The Centers for Disease Control and Prevention and state or local health departments have the most current information.

Influenza Vaccine

The influenza vaccine provides coverage against influenza A and B viruses that are predominantly circulating in the current season. The changing antigenic picture of influenza virus necessitates annual immunizations. Statistics reveal a 40% reduction in clinical illness and an 80% reduction in death in the elderly who have received the vaccine. The vaccine is given in the fall to provide adequate time for immunity to develop before the beginning of the influenza season in December. Persons who have a known allergy to eggs or egg proteins should not receive the vaccine. Those individuals for whom vaccination is recommended include patients older than 65, patients younger than 65 with chronic medical conditions, and health care workers.

Pneumococcal Vaccine

The 23-valent pneumococcal vaccine contains capsular material from 88% of the *Streptococcus pneumoniae* that cause bacteremia in the United States. In every age group, the vaccine has a proven efficacy of 60% for all included serotypes. Even though the vaccine is given only once, patients who have

13

Table 3.1.
Immunizations

	Age 18–40	Age 41–65	Age >65
Influenza (annual)	a	a	all
Pneumococcal vaccine (one time only)	a,b,d	a,b,d	all
Hepatitis B	c	c	c
Tetanus-diphtheria	every 10 years	every 10 years	every 10 years
Measles-mumps-rubella	born after 1956 without evidence of immunity		
Rubella	women of childbearing age without evidence of immunity	women of childbearing age without evidence of immunity	

[a]Recommended for those with chronic medical conditions.
[b]Recommended for those who are immunocompromised (e.g., asplenia, sickle cell anemia, lymphoma, multiple myeloma, chronic renal failure, nephrotic syndrome, or HIV disease).
[c]Recommended for those at high risk for HBV disease (e.g., health care workers or patients exposed to blood products, hemodialysis patients, homosexual-bisexual males, intravenous drug users).
[d]Revaccination of high risk patients (those with chronic renal failure, immunodeficiency, transplants) should be considered every 6 years.

Table 3.2.
Physical Exam and Screening Tests

	Age 18–40	Age 40–50	Age 50–65	Age 65–75	Age 75–85
Blood pressure	every clinical encounter	every clinical encounter	every clinical encounter	every clinical encounter	every clinical encounter
Height	every 5 years	every 5 years	every 5 years	annual	annual
Weight	every 5 years	annual	annual	annual	annual
Clinical breast exam		annual	annual	annual	annual
Mammogram		d	annual	annual	at discretion of clinician
Rectal exam		annual	annual	annual	at discretion of clinician
Pap smear	every 3 years after negative tests[a]	every 3 years after negative tests[a]	every 3 years after negative tests[a]	b	b
Fecal occult blood test		after age 45, annual	annual	annual	annual
Cholesterol	every 5 years[c]	every 5 years	annual	annual	annual

[a]Annually for high risk groups (e.g., early age of sexual activity, multiple sexual partners, low socioeconomic status).
[b]Screening can be stopped if three negative tests obtained.
[c]Fractionate if level >240 or 200–240 with risk factor.
[d]Consider annually or every 2–3 years for first degree relatives of a woman with breast cancer.

received the obsolete 14-valent vaccine should receive the 23-valent vaccine. Individuals for whom the vaccine is recommended include all patients older than 65, patients younger than 65 who have chronic medical conditions, and immunocompromised patients (e.g., persons diagnosed with asplenia, sickle-cell anemia, lymphoma, multiple myeloma, chronic renal failure, nephrotic syndrome, or human immunodeficiency virus (HIV) disease).

Table 3.3.
History and Counseling

	Age 18–40	Age 40–50	Age 50–65	Age 65–75	Age >85

Medical history
  Allergies
  Immunizations
  Alcohol use
  Other substance abuse
	every 5 years	every 5 years	every 5 years	annual	annual

Sexual history	every encounter				
Tobacco use	every encounter				

Counseling
  Nutrition
  Tobacco use
  Exercise
	annual	annual	annual	annual	annual

Safety
  Seat belts
  Child safety seats
  Alcohol and drugs
  Driving
  Smoke detectors
  Firearms in the home
	annual	annual	annual	annual	annual

Safer sex (sexually transmitted diseases)	every encounter				

Hepatitis B Vaccine

Hepatitis B virus vaccine is available as a recombinant-derived vaccine. Plasma-derived vaccine is no longer distributed in the United States. Hepatitis B vaccine is up to 95% effective in preventing hepatitis B infection. Decreased antibody response is found in patients with HIV disease, those on hemodialysis, and in patients older than 50. Antibody levels decrease over time; 50% of those vaccinated have low or undetectable antibody levels, but those with normal immune systems continue to be protected. The vaccine is recommended for all infants and those individuals at high risk of hepatitis B infection. High risk individuals include health care workers frequently exposed to blood or blood products, hemophiliacs or other recipients of certain blood products, hemodialysis patients, sexually active homosexual or bisexual males, intravenous drug users, household or sexual contacts of hepatitis B-positive patients, and patients with multiple sexual partners or those who have been treated for sexually transmitted diseases.

Tetanus and Diphtheria

The most common types of toxoid for adult immunization against tetanus are tetanus-diphtheria toxoid and tetanus toxoid. It is recommended that tetanus-diphtheria toxoid be used for adults because of the prevalence of low diphtheria antibody levels in adults. It is recommended that all adults receive a tetanus-diphtheria toxoid booster every 10 years. An alternative approach is to give one tetanus-diphtheria toxoid booster at age 50. Adults who have not received a primary series should receive the three primary vaccinations and then a booster every 10 years. It is not recommended that individuals receive a booster vaccination more frequently than every 10 years because of the risk of developing high tetanus antibody levels that can lead to an Arthus hypersensitivity reaction.

Measles-Mumps-Rubella

Individuals born after 1956 should receive immunization with measles-mumps-rubella if they lack evidence of immunity. Immunity is defined as receipt of live vaccine after the first birthday, clinician-diagnosed measles or mumps, or laboratory evidence of immunity. Those vaccinated against measles between 1963 and 1967 may have received inactivated vaccine and should receive one dose of the live vaccine.

Rubella

Women of childbearing age should be screened for immunity to rubella, either by documented history of rubella vaccine or serologic antibody testing. Rubella vaccine produces antibody response in 95–98% of recipients. History of illness is not sufficient

Table 3.4.
Health Screening—Choosing a Condition

- Condition must have a significant effect on the quality and length of life.
- Acceptable methods of treatment must be available.
- Condition must have an asymptomatic period during which detection and treatment significantly reduce morbidity or mortality.
- Treatment in the asymptomatic phase must yield a therapeutic result superior to that obtained by delaying treatment until symptoms appear.
- Tests to detect the condition in the asymptomatic period must be acceptable to patients and available at a reasonable cost.
- Incidence of the condition must be sufficient to justify the cost and/or risk of screening.

Adapted from Frame PS, Carlson SJ. A critical review of periodic health screening using specific screening criteria. Part 1: selected diseases of respiratory, cardiovascular, and central nervous systems. J Fam Practice 1975;2:29–36.

evidence of immunity. Because of the possible risk of congenital rubella syndrome, women receiving the vaccine should agree not to become pregnant for 3 months.

SCREENING

The criteria listed in Table 3.4 were developed to select conditions for which screening is appropriate. Before screening is planned, the conditions that are prevalent in the population must be known. If the criteria for screening are not met, the value of screening is uncertain.

The specific diseases for which screening is recommended are reviewed in this section. These diseases are believed to fit within the criteria noted in Table 3.4. A complete presentation and discussion of conditions not covered here can be found in the sources listed under "Suggested Readings."

Hypertension

Hypertension affects 50 million Americans and is a leading risk factor for coronary artery disease (CAD), stroke, and renal disease. Blood pressure should be measured at all clinical encounters. The most common interval recommended is every 1–2 years in those who are normotensive and annually in those with a diastolic blood pressure of 85–89 mmHg. Blood pressure should be measured using the Guidelines for Sphygmomanometry. Please see the chapter on hypertension.

Cholesterol

Elevated blood cholesterol is one of the three modifiable risk factors for CAD, which is the leading cause of death in the United States. Hypertension and smoking are the other two modifiable risk factors. Epidemiologic studies have shown that cholesterol lipoprotein subfractions are significant in CAD, with low density lipoprotein cholesterol directly and high density lipoprotein cholesterol inversely associated with the incidence of CAD.

The measurement of serum cholesterol can vary in an individual and between laboratories; therefore one measurement should not be relied upon to make a decision about therapeutic alternatives. Most recommendations suggest that cholesterol screening should begin in young adulthood. The appropriate interval for screening is determined by initial serum cholesterol values and the presence of other risk factors for CAD but should be approximately every 5 years. Cholesterol should be fractionated for individuals with total cholesterol levels greater than 240 mg/dl or for those with a total cholesterol of 200–239 mg/dl with two or more risk factors for CAD. Risk factors for CAD are male gender, smoking, hypertension, obesity, diabetes, and premature CAD in a first degree relative.

Breast Cancer

Breast cancer is the most common type of cancer among women, with an estimated 180,000 new cases and 46,000 deaths in 1994. Early detection improves mortality from breast cancer. The major risk factors for breast cancer are age over 50, personal history of breast cancer, and a first degree relative with breast cancer. Other factors identified as associated with some increased risk of breast cancer include nulliparity, first pregnancy after age 30, menarche before age 12, menopause after age 50, obesity, high socioeconomic status, and personal history of endometrial or ovarian cancer.

Women aged 50 or older should undergo annual screening with clinical breast examination and mammography. The age at which to stop screening is not as clear, but age 75 is a cutoff according to some sources. Women between 40 and 50 should have an annual clinical breast examination. Annual mammography in this age group should be reserved for patients at highest risk for breast cancer, especially those patients with a first-degree relative with premenopausal breast cancer. There is no evidence that annual mammography in women at average risk yields significant benefit. Although the evidence does not support specifically recommending breast self-examination, there is little evidence to warrant changing current practices about annual breast self-examination beginning at age 35. Breast self-examination may contribute to ongoing awareness of the need for screening. Mastery of breast self-examination while in the 30s should increase proficiency in this technique as the patient ages.

Cervical Cancer

The incidence of invasive cervical cancer has been reduced 70% by screening. Screening is done by obtaining a Papanicolaou (Pap) smear of the cervix. A properly collected Pap smear has a sensitivity of 50–90% and a specificity of 90%. The natural history of cervical cancer suggests the time from development of precancerous lesions to invasive carcinoma is 8–9 years; thus all early stage malignancies initially missed can be detected by repeat testing. Pap smear screening should begin when sexual activity begins or by approximately age 18–20.

Recommendations about the appropriate interval for Pap smears vary, but most sources suggest that after three consecutive negative tests screening can take place every 3 years. Annual Pap smears are recommended for women with risk factors for cervical cancer (e.g., multiple sexual partners, sexual intercourse at an early age, and low socioeconomic status). The age at which to discontinue Pap smears is unclear, but generally at age 65 they can be discontinued if screening Pap smears have been negative. It is probably prudent for women age 60–65 who have never been screened to have three negative smears before stopping screening. Proper technique in collecting the Pap smear is important as well as using laboratories with adequate quality control measures.

Prostate Cancer

The natural history of prostate cancer, especially stages A and B, is not well understood, and the benefit of early treatment in terms of reduced mortality has not been shown. There is little evidence that screening by digital rectal examination reduces mortality from prostate cancer. The sensitivity of digital rectal examination is limited because many tumors are out of the reach of the examining finger, and stage A tumors are by definition nonpalpable. There is no evidence that serum prostatic-specific antigen or transrectal ultrasonography should be used as screening tests in asymptomatic men.

Colorectal Cancer

Screening for colorectal cancer remains controversial regarding what tests to perform and at what

Table 3.5.
Fecal Occult Blood Testing Technique

- Advise patient to avoid the following several days before and during collections:
  Red meat (beef, lamb), processed meats, liver
  Melons, radishes, turnips, horseradish
  Excess vitamin C foods (citrus fruits and juices)
  Vitamin C tablets greater than 250 mg
  Aspirin, nonsteroidal anti-inflammatory drugs
  Use of iodine-containing solutions to the anal area
- Two separate samples from different sections of three consecutive bowel movements should be applied in a thin film to guaiac-impregnated cards
- Guaiac-impregnated cards should be processed, optimally within 6 days of collection
- Rehydration with one drop of water before application of developer
- Miscellaneous
  Dietary iron *does not* cause false-positive results
  Even one positive window is a positive and needs follow-up
  Cards should *not* be mailed to clinicians in regular paper envelopes

age and how often. However, it is not disputed that early detection reduces mortality. Most invasive colorectal cancer develops from adenomatous polyps that progress over the course of a decade. People at increased risk for colorectal cancer should be screened, including those with familial polyposis, familial cancer syndromes, colorectal cancer in a first-degree relative, a personal history of adenomatous polyps, inflammatory bowel disease, or endometrial, ovarian, or breast cancer.

Annual digital rectal examination beginning at age 40 is recommended by the major authorities, but there is no evidence to support this procedure. Less than 10% of colorectal cancer will be found by digital rectal examination, the majority being rectal cancer. The cost and the risk are low, and as with breast self-examination, it may present the opportunity to review risk factors and provide counseling.

The evidence to recommend fecal occult blood testing is not strong. This is related to problems with the test itself. The sensitivity of fecal occult blood testing in low risk patients is 25%. The sensitivity can be improved to 30–40% by rehydration of cards, but this is at the cost of reduced specificity. It is probably prudent to offer fecal occult blood testing to all individuals beginning at age 45. Proper collection, summarized in Table 3.5, should be emphasized. Patients at higher risk should be offered more invasive screening tests as indicated by their personal history.

Sigmoidoscopy has a specificity of nearly 100% and a sensitivity that is dependent on the length of the instrument and skill of the examiner. A 35-cm flexible sigmoidoscope reaches 45–50% of cancers compared with a 60-cm flexible sigmoidoscope that reaches 50–60% of cancers. There is insufficient evidence to recommend screening sigmoidoscopy in low risk, asymptomatic individuals. It seems prudent to recommend periodic screening sigmoidoscopy for individuals at higher risk. The interval for screening would be determined by risk and initial findings.

Genetic Screening

Screening has moved, for certain conditions, to the molecular level. Much genetic screening to date has focused on conditions that affect not the individual being screened but their progeny (e.g., cystic fibrosis, sickle cell anemia, Tay-Sachs disease). Recently genes have been identified that are associated with the development in adulthood of both uncommon disorders (e.g., Huntington's disease and Alzheimer's disease) and certain common cancers, notably breast and colon cancer. Individuals inheriting these altered genes are at higher risk for developing the diseases in question than those without these alterations although the amount of increased risk varies among diseases. Colon cancer genes (MSH2 and MLH1 that can predispose individuals to hereditary nonpolyposis colon cancer) and breast cancer "susceptibility" genes (BRCA1 and BRCA2) have been cloned, and commercial tests soon will be available. Germline mutations of the p53 gene, a tumor suppressor gene, have been implicated in a range of cancers, and active research is underway to map the complexity of p53 mutations.

Genetic screening offers the ultimate "advanced notice" of a disease. The value to the individual of predictive presymptomatic genetic screening for a disease that has no current treatment or cure is controversial. Issues of ethics and psychological morbidity must be considered as affordable genetic screening tests come into wide use.

COUNSELING STRATEGIES

Little evidence exists for the efficacy of counseling, but it is recommended because behavior changes may be more valuable to health than many screening tests offered to patients. Assessment of patients' understanding of the relationship between behavior and health is an important first step because knowledge alone is frequently not a sufficient stimulus for change. Patients value and are eager for information about maintaining their health. Counseling that utilizes a combination of strategies (e.g., individual counseling, written and audiovisual materials, community resources) that is appropriate for the average patient's level of comprehension should be given to all patients because the potential benefits are great and the cost and risk of the intervention are low. Counseling, no matter how brief, is better than no counseling.

Nutrition

Patients should be counseled and provided with information about nutrition. Specifically, information should be included about maintaining ideal body weight to avoid obesity (defined as more than 20% above desirable body weight). Obesity can predispose to glucose intolerance, hypertension, and other diseases and can hinder mobility, limit the ability to gain information from the physical examination, and prohibit certain diagnostic studies (e.g., cardiac catheterization and other radiologic studies). In addition to maintaining ideal body weight, counseling should focus on limiting dietary fat to only 30% of total calories with 10% of total calories from saturated fat. Whole grain foods, vegetables, and fruits are high in complex carbohydrates and fiber and should be encouraged. Counseling about sodium restriction and calcium supplementation should be given to those patients at risk for hypertension and to adult women, respectively. Utilization of other trained professionals (e.g., nurses or dietitians) is encouraged if the clinician's ability to give specific dietary counseling is limited by time and/or skills. The primary provider should periodically assess the diet and encourage compliance with the recommendations even if others do the specific counseling.

Tobacco Use

Smoking cessation counseling should be offered to all patients who smoke cigarettes, cigars, or pipes. Counseling against the use of smokeless tobacco should also be given. Those who do not smoke should be advised not to start. A brief unambiguous statement on the need to stop using tobacco is the most effective clinician message. Nicotine gum and nicotine patches should be used only in conjunction with smoking cessation counseling or other types of behavior modification.

Exercise

The Centers for Disease Control and Prevention recommend that adults exercise. Patients should receive counseling to encourage regular physical activity. The type of activity should be tailored to the individual, taking into account health status and personal environment. The benefits of exercise include preventing obesity, enhanced cardiovascular fitness, enhanced bone mass in women, and improved sense of well-being. The clinician should provide or have information about developing an exercise program. Patients should be encouraged to begin a regular exercise program with progression, as appropriate, to achieve cardiovascular fitness. At least 30 minutes of exercise three times per week that produces an increase in heart rate to 70% of maximum predicted heart rate is sufficient aerobic exercise. (Maximum predicted heart rate equals 220 − age). Regular encouragement to exercise, as with all counseling, will reinforce the importance of this activity.

Safety

Safety can be defined as preventing injuries and/or the risk of injury. Patients should be counseled about several areas of safety. Although there is mixed evidence of effectiveness of this counseling, it is worthy of implementation because of the burden of suffering that is associated with unsafe activities and behaviors. Counseling should focus on areas that pertain to the individual and his or her environment. Questions regarding operation of a motor vehicle, the type of home, who lives with the patient, and alcohol and drug use are important when taking a history about safety issues. All patients should be counseled to always use seat belts; children should also use seat belts or specific child safety restraints. Patients should not drive nor should they ride with a driver who is under the influence of alcohol or illicit drugs. Patients should be advised not to participate in activities that require accurate reflexes and attention (e.g., operating power tools or firearms, boating, and swimming) when under the influence of alcohol. Patients should be advised to install and maintain smoke detectors in their home. Also, the danger of keeping firearms in the home should be discussed and the practice discouraged. More family members and friends are killed than intruders when guns are kept in the home.

Safer Sex

Counseling about safe sexual practices should be offered to all patients. Sexually transmitted diseases, especially HIV disease, are the focus of this counseling. Effective counseling requires that a complete sexual history be taken, including related behaviors (e.g., intravenous drug use) that would indicate risk for sexually transmitted diseases.

Patients should receive information about the transmission of sexually transmitted diseases and effective strategies such as abstinence, a monogamous sexual relationship with an uninfected partner, and the use of latex condoms with each act of intercourse. The risks of anal intercourse should be presented if applicable. Specific condom information regarding type, correct application, use of lubricants/spermicides, and correct removal should be given. Screening tests for gonorrhea, chlamydia, syphilis, hepatitis B, and HIV are recommended for high risk patients. High risk patients include those with multiple sexual partners, prior history of sexually transmitted disease, those who practice anal intercourse, prostitutes and their sexual partners, use of illicit drugs, and inmates of detention centers.

Advance Directives

Sometimes in the course of a serious illness a patient loses the ability to reason or communicate. Some patients have definite ideas about what types of lifesaving or life prolonging procedures they would desire if they were in such a scenario. An advance directive, a document listing what the patient does or does not want performed, can be used to assure that the patient's wishes are known and to guide future care.

Advance directives should be discussed with each patient. The outpatient provider should try to elicit preferences while the patient is healthy or at least stable. Preferences should be written, signed by the patient, and witnessed.

SUGGESTED READINGS

ACP Task Force on Adult Immunization and Infectious Diseases Society of America. Guide for adult immunization, 3rd ed. 1994.

Clinicians' handbook of preventive services. Washington DC: Department of Health and Human Services, 1994.

U.S. Preventive Services Task Force. Guide to clinical preventive services, 2nd ed. Baltimore: Williams & Wilkins, 1996.

chapter 4

PRINCIPLES OF PHARMACOLOGY FOR THE AMBULATORY PATIENT

B. Robert Meyer

Drugs are in many ways the medical practitioner's scalpel. They are the major tools for effective treatment. How carefully and precisely these tools are used is a primary factor in the ability to help patients. An early clinical pharmacologist observed almost a century ago:

> The day has come when something more is demanded of the practitioner or physician consultant than a diagnosis . . . Our obligation will not be satisfied until general principles (of drug treatment) have been fitted to the particular patient. The *what* may be the easiest determined; the *how much*, the *when*, and *under what precautions* must be fully stated.
>
> *Wilcox. The Teaching of Therapeutics (1903), quoted in Reference 1.*

These observations are more true than ever today. Unparalleled advances in diagnostic sophistication in the last decade have been matched by a revolutionary increase in the number of therapeutic options available to clinicians. If the promise of better health for patients offered by the increasingly sophisticated diagnostic and therapeutic options is to be realized, the utilization of these options must be directed by clinicians increasingly sophisticated in the science of therapeutics.

This chapter will focus on the following points:

- A basic review of critical concepts of pharmacokinetics: including bioavailability, half-life, clearance, volume of distribution, and loading doses;
- A review of the role of therapeutic drug monitoring in the context of ambulatory care;
- A review of practical issues surrounding prescribing drugs: the use of generics and the problem of patient compliance with medications.

PHARMACOLOGY IN THE UNITED STATES

The Food and Drug Administration (FDA) approves between 20 and 30 new drugs for use in the United States each year. In addition to these new chemical compounds, several times that number of new formulations or new delivery systems for existing drugs are introduced each year. As each of these new products is introduced, it is accompanied by trumpeting of its unique value by the pharmaceutical company that created it and brought it to market. These pharmaceutical companies are often the major (or sole) source of information for the clinician about a new drug or formulation.

Clinicians who graduated from medical school in the 1970s took their last course in pharmacology before the introduction of calcium channel blockers, angiotensin-converting enzyme inhibitors, second or third generation cephalosporins, and a host of other compounds. These clinicians actually find that most drugs prescribed are entities about which they have no formal education. In this context there is no substitute for the intelligent, critical, and somewhat skeptical clinician. The medical provider must be continually alert to the need for critical assessment of the potential benefits of a new drug. The potential dangers of any new form of therapy, and the need for continuing observation and gathering of information about the safety and efficacy of new drugs, are not totally appreciated even after approval by the FDA. The clinician ought to rely for clinically relevant current pharmacologic information on relatively unbiased publications prepared by independent sources. These include such sources as "The Medical Letter," the "AMA Drug Evaluations Manual," or the "AHFS Drug Information Annual."

The typical course of enthusiasm for any new drug therapy is described in Figure 4.1 (2). An

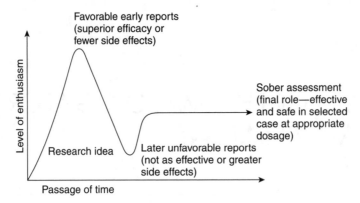

Figure 4.1. Effect of time on enthusiasm and use of new drugs (from Sjoqvist F, Burga O, Orme LE. In Speight TM, ed. Avery's drug treatment: principles and practice of clinical pharmacology and therapeutics. Baltimore: Williams & Wilkins, 1987).

initial idea is followed by enthusiasm and development. Early success is followed by further enthusiasm and a tendency to overestimate the importance of the new drug. This is then followed by a period of skepticism and a tendency to downgrade the importance of the new therapy. Only with time does a mature and reasoned assessment of the true role of a new drug emerge. Clinicians should remember this pattern and strive not to ride too high on the initial wave of enthusiasm nor sink too far into the trough of depression that may follow. Medical providers operate in a society in which the use of therapeutic drugs is common and expected more so than any other place in the world. Approximately two-thirds of all office visits to a physician end with a prescription of a drug (3). According to one estimate, in the 1980s approximately 1.5 billion prescriptions were written annually in the United States, which is about six prescriptions per citizen per year (4). On average, physicians in the United States are approximately four to five times more likely to prescribe a drug to treat a patient with a given condition than their counterparts in Scotland. It is doubtful that Americans are four to five times healthier than the Scots as a result of drug therapy.

In some settings, the provision of a prescription is the expected conclusion of an office visit. Many clinicians who observe their own behavior will note that writing the prescription may be used to signal the patient that the office visit is ending. As the prescription pad is pulled out of the drawer, the patient sees that the visit is concluding and then prepares to leave. The patient may also feel (and

the provider reinforces this) that he or she is *getting something* for the visit.

PHARMACOKINETICS

Pharmacokinetics is the science that describes in a quantitative manner the course of absorption, distribution, metabolism, and clearance of drugs by the body. It can be a useful tool for the prediction of drug dosing regimens, avoidance of drug toxicity, and the assessment of drug efficacy. An understanding of pharmacokinetics is essential for prescribing drugs.

Absorption and Bioavailability

All drugs are absorbed into the body from their site of administration. The process of absorption is complicated, and the course, magnitude, and efficiency of the absorptive process are critical to proper dosing of a drug. The most efficient and rapid absorption of drugs is from an intravenous infusion in which the efficiency is 100% and the absorption immediate. For many drugs, subcutaneous administration and occasionally intramuscular administration are nearly as efficient and almost as rapid. For all other routes of administration (e.g., oral, transdermal, rectal, intranasal, or others) the efficiency of absorption is less than 100%, and the rate of absorption is significantly slower.

In the case of oral administration, oral *bioavailability* is a function not only of absorption across the mucosa of the gastrointestinal tract but also the first-pass metabolism of the drug by the liver. First-pass refers to hepatic metabolism that occurs before the drug enters the systemic circulation. The amount of a drug absorbed from the gastrointestinal tract is the oral bioavailability of a drug. The practicing clinician can make a reasonable estimate of bioavailability by simply comparing the dose of a drug when given parenterally to that when given by the alternative route. For example, propranolol is often given orally in doses of 10–120 mg at a time. When given parenterally the typical dose is 1–2 mg! Clearly, propranolol has poor oral bioavailability. In contrast, the usual doses of parenteral and oral phenytoin are identical, suggesting efficient oral absorption. Occasionally clinicians have ignored the lesser absorption of the oral compared with the parenteral form. Oral digoxin has a bioavailability that is significantly less than 100%. When differences in bioavailability are overlooked (e.g., when a patient who was maintained on 0.25 mg intravenous digoxin daily in the hospital is then placed on an oral dose of 0.25 mg outpatient) the true dose of digoxin received by the patient is decreased by approximately 20%.

Clearance

Clearance is the term used to quantitatively describe the removal of a drug (or any substance) from the body. Plasma clearance is usually the most useful type of clearance to describe. The plasma clearance of a drug is described as the amount of plasma that is cleared of a drug in a unit of time. This clearance is the result of the metabolic activity of the liver and the filtration capacity of the kidney. The clinician does not need to recall the value of the plasma clearance but should be aware of the mechanism of clearance. Because clearance is only one determinant of half-life, it is really better to recall a drug's half-life for dosing. The important thing to recall about a drug's clearance is the relative contribution of the liver and the kidney to the process so that appropriate dosage adjustments can be made if they are not functioning properly.

Half-Life

The half-life of a drug is the time it takes for the plasma concentration (amount of drug in the blood) to decrease by 50%. By tradition, drugs are administered with a frequency based on their half-lives. Thus drugs with 6-hour half-lives are given every 6 hours. Although it is not always the most convenient and effective means of administering a particular drug, it remains a reasonably useful predictor of the frequency of dosing necessary to minimize the occurrence of toxicity. It is also useful for pre-

Table 4.1.
Some Representative Pharmacokinetic Data on Selected Drugs

Drug	Clearance (ml/min)	Half-life (hr)
Acetaminophen	250–450	1.3–3.0
Amitriptyline	700–1000	9–25
Atenolol	180	6–7
Captopril	1000	1.5
Clonidine	140–300	12–16
Digoxin	75	34–44
Famotidine	400	2.5–4
Furosemide	130–210	1–2
Glipizide	1400–2600	3–4.7
Glyburide	91	1.4–1.8
Haloperidol	625–1025	10–20
Ibuprofen	40–70	1.8–2.0
Imipramine	750–1300	8–16
Isosorbide dinitrate	3100	4
Morphine SO_4	560–2400	1–7
Nifedipine	450–750	4–5.5
Nitroglycerin	5500–7100	0.3–0.5
Propranolol	625–1100	3.4–6
Ranitidine	650–800	1.7–3.2
Vancomycin	65	4–6
Verapamil	500–2600	2.7–4.8
Warfarin	3	12–72

Adapted from Melmon and Morelli, 1992.

dicting the appropriate adjustment of dose when necessary. Thus if the half-life of a drug is doubled, it is reasonable to either increase the interval between doses by a factor of two or decrease the size of each dose by 50%. A quick look at Table 4.1 will show the variability in half-life among different drugs.

Volume of Distribution

Volume of distribution is often misunderstood. In essence it is a mathematical term that is used to relate the two preceding concepts. If a body clears 50 ml/min of drug A, and it takes 180 min to clear 50% of the drug ($T_{1/2}$), then how many milliliters of drug A must there be to clear? The important point to remember is that "volume" here is not a definable physical parameter but a conceptual reality that identifies how much of the drug is actually in the serum and is being "cleared" in those "ml/min" terms.

Relationship of $T_{1/2}$, Volume of Distribution, and Clearance

$T_{1/2} = 0.693$ volume of distribution/clearance

All preceding terms are related by this equation.

Again, the precise equation need not be recalled. However, the equation clarifies how the volume of distribution and clearance can interact to alter half-life. In cases where the drug is in ascites or excessive adipose tissue, the volume of distribution changes (volume to be cleared increases), and even though the clearance is unaltered, a drug's half-life will be changed. In other circumstances, a change in clearance may be associated with a change in volume of distribution, and the two changes may either cancel each other or magnify each other.

THERAPEUTIC DRUG MONITORING

The ability to rapidly, cheaply, and accurately measure the amount of drug in the serum of a patient at a particular time is now a reality. Automated systems are available in most labs that make this a potentially routine clinical tool. For certain compounds the measurement of serum drug concentrations is a useful tool for optimizing drug therapy. Perhaps the biggest mistake in the use of drug levels is the belief that they provide a definitive answer and direction for therapy. Sometimes this is true. However, it is wise to remember that it should *always* be the patient's clinician who assesses the efficacy or toxicity of therapy. It should *never* be the laboratory technician performing a drug assay. Although the clinician can obtain useful assistance from the laboratory, the clinical picture should always guide interpretation of the results. Therapeutic drug monitoring is useful when there is a known and consistent relationship between serum concentrations of a drug and clinical effects. Then therapeutic drug monitoring may be useful if any of the following apply.

- The clinician cannot determine whether a patient has complied with therapy and wishes to know whether the patient has actually taken the drug in question.
- The drug is for the treatment of a condition where a failure of therapy would have serious consequences and there is no way to easily predict the occurrence of treatment failure. A classic example is the use of phenytoin levels in the guidance of therapy for a seizure disorder. This may also apply in some situations in which antiarrhythmic therapy is given.
- The drug has a known toxicity that is predictably related to serum concentrations of drug and is either dangerous, significantly unpleasant, or irreversible. A classic example is

Table 4.2.
Some Drugs for Which Serum Drug Levels Are Useful

Drug	Therapeutic Level
Acetaminophen	10–20 mg/L
Carbamazepine	4–12 mg/L
Digoxin	0.75–2.0 mg/L
Lithium carbonate	0.4–1.4 mg/L
Phenobarbital	10–20 mg/L
Phenytoin	10–20 mg/L
Procainamide	4–8 mg/L
Theophylline	10–20 mg/L
Valproic acid	50–100 mg/L

the use of phenytoin levels as a guide to dosing.

A listing of some drugs for which therapeutic drug monitoring may be useful, together with commonly used target serum concentrations, can be found in Table 4.2.

LOADING DOSE

In certain situations clinicians are unwilling to wait the necessary time for the drug to accumulate to the concentration needed to achieve the desired effect. This circumstance usually occurs when the medical problem is urgent or emergent and/or where the time to achieve these levels with routine dosing is long. In general, steady state is achieved after four to five half-lives have elapsed. For a drug such as digoxin with a half-life of 33 hours or more, steady state concentrations will not be reached before 130 hours or more. If digoxin is urgently needed to control heart rate in a patient with angina and rapid atrial fibrillation, a loading dose of medication is indicated. This loading dose is *not* substantially affected by clearance (loading dose refers to filling, not emptying). Appropriate loading dose regimens have been worked out for most drugs in which they are needed. A practical reality of side effects sometimes determines the rate at which a loading dose can be administered.

WRITING THE PRESCRIPTION

Surprisingly, most clinicians are never actually taught how to write a prescription. They are often simply told what to write by a supervisor, and after repetition they learn what is involved. An articulation of the components of prescription writing is presented here and illustrated in Figure 4.2. Every prescription should include, in addition to the pa-

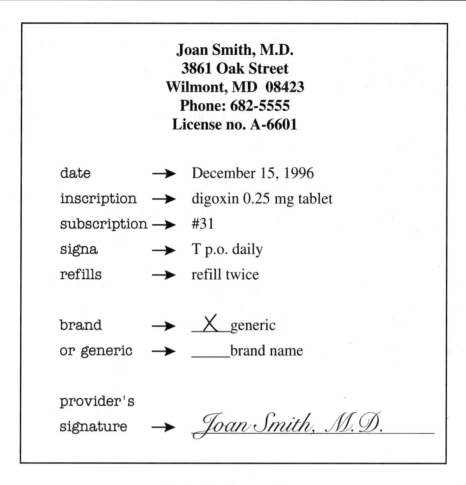

Joan Smith, M.D.
3861 Oak Street
Wilmont, MD 08423
Phone: 682-5555
License no. A-6601

date	→	December 15, 1996
inscription	→	digoxin 0.25 mg tablet
subscription	→	#31
signa	→	T p.o. daily
refills	→	refill twice
brand	→	__X__ generic
or generic	→	_____ brand name
provider's signature	→	*Joan Smith, M.D.*

Figure 4.2. The prescription.

tient's full name and address, the following elements: date, inscription, subscription, "signa," number of refills, and brand or generic instruction.

The physician must always remember that the most important part of any prescription is not the piece of paper on which it is written but the verbal communication between the provider and patient on why the medication is being given, what its expected benefits and potential dangers are, what precautions should be taken, and when the patient should call about a potential problem. The paper prescription should be a written reinforcement; it is not the actual communication of this information.

Date

The date is important because the need for renewal can be predicted and reviewed. If therapy is designed for a specific time, its end date can be known.

The difference between the date of writing and the date at which the prescription was actually filled by the patient is sometimes useful. Out-of-date prescriptions cannot be filled. Prescriptions should never be postdated.

Inscription

The inscription is the name of the drug to be prescribed. In this context either the approved generic name for the drug or the exact brand name should be written, together with the size of the tablet or capsule, concentration of a liquid dosage form, or other appropriate description of the strength of the preparation. Abbreviations should always be avoided. Although unlikely to occur, the confusion of "$MgSO_4$" (magnesium sulfate) and "MSO_4" (morphine sulfate) only has to occur once to cause tragedy. The number of other possibilities for confusion make the use of full written names essential. It is also traditional at this point to specify the nature of the dosage form. This may be tablets, capsules, extended release capsules, metered dose inhaler, suppository, transdermal patch, etc.

Subscription

The subscription instructs the pharmacist how much of the medication is to be dispensed. Most providers begin this section with the phrase "dispense" or a # sign. It is sometimes conventional to ask the pharmacist to dispense a "1 month's supply." This practice is to be discouraged. The clinician should usually calculate how much medication is appropriate to dispense. Sometimes it is not a bad idea to give the patient a few extra pills to account for the pill that is dropped on the floor or in the sink or otherwise lost. In other situations where the potential for abuse is present, it is best to calculate precisely how many pills the patient is to be given and to note this in the record. The provider can also use this portion of the prescription to instruct the pharmacist whether to dispense the medication in childproof containers, to premix a solution, to leave the solution unmixed, and so forth.

Signa

Signa means "label," and it is the instruction to the pharmacist about how the bottle should be labeled. In addition to prescribing dosing frequency and other directions (e.g., take medication with food or on an as needed basis) the label instructs the patient how to determine when to take the medication. Again the use of shortcuts should be discouraged. Writing the instructions in English rather than shorthand will avoid the uncommon, but nonetheless potentially serious, confusion of abbreviations such as "q.i.d.," "q.o.d.," or "q.d." In addition, if the provider wishes to emphasize the instructions to the patient, they should be repeated as faithfully and as detailed as is practical. The provider who takes the time to carefully write a prescription will emphasize to the patient that the means of taking the medication is important and worthy of careful attention. It is unrealistic to expect the patient to follow instructions seriously if they are scribbled so haphazardly or incompletely that the pharmacist and patient find them difficult to interpret.

Refills

The clinician indicates refills of medications when the length of therapy will exceed 1 month, the patient is tolerating the medication, it is at the appropriate dose, and the desired therapeutic effect is being achieved. Obviously the decision about how many refills to give (if any) must reflect all of these factors together with the patient's reliability, the ease with which the patient can return for follow-up, and the nature of the drug. Drugs with abuse potential are often limited by law to 1 month or less, with no possibility of renewal.

Brand or Generic

Every state in the nation has adopted laws designed to promote the use of generic drugs. Depending on the state, the exact procedures for instructing the pharmacist to dispense only the brand drug are established and should be reviewed. These regulations are often further modified by health care plans that see financial benefits to compelling the use of generics (see "Generic Drugs" for a discussion of the medical issues surrounding generic prescribing).

COMPLIANCE

The best and most effectively designed therapy cannot work if the patient does not take the medication as prescribed. As discussed above, the most important part of the prescription is the initial verbal communication that informs the patient why the clinician wishes to prescribe this medication, elicits the patient's reaction to the plan of care, and enlists the patient's participation in the therapeutic plan. Yet the problem of compliance remains difficult for the clinician.

When providers assess the results of a failed therapy, there is sometimes a tendency to blame compliance. It is not that the prescription or plan of care was bad, it is that the patient did not do what he or she was told. The clinician should guard against this understandable tendency to dodge partial responsibility. Providers are generally poor at assessing patient compliance. In studies of the accuracy of physician's assessments it has been noted that when all goes well and the patient improves or the desired endpoint is achieved, compliance tends to be overestimated. When therapy fails, the tendency is to underestimate the patient's compliance.

Patient's Lifestyle

Active human beings find compliance with even relatively simple and uncomplicated drug regimens to be a difficult challenge. This is particularly true when the patient feels well and is being asked to take the medication to treat an asymptomatic problem like mild to moderate hypertension, hyperlipidemia, or a healed deep venous thrombosis. In all cases, the provider should anticipate the difficulties the patient will face and discuss them with the patient. Patients who are starting a diuretic such as furosemide may want to start the medication on a day when they will be staying home. There is nothing more discouraging to compliance than being caught in rush hour 1 hour after taking the first dose of a powerful diuretic! When prescribing a medication, the patient's lifestyle should be considered. A business person who has working lunches will simply not want colleagues to observe a pill or other medication being taken immediately after a meal. A construction worker may not wish to use an asthma inhaler at the job despite the occurrence of symptoms in what might be a dusty environment.

Dosing Regimens

Despite these efforts at communication and anticipation of problems, patients still find it difficult to fully comply with a clinician's prescription. Most studies of compliance suggest that maximal ease of compliance is achieved with dosing regimens that are once or twice a day. More frequent dosing generally is difficult to incorporate into most lifestyles. Less frequent dosing (every other day or twice a week) becomes so infrequent that it is too easy to forget.

Formulation of Drug

A clinician who decides to prescribe a medication must also decide on the particular formulation. Improved pharmaceutical industry technology has led to various novel formulations beyond the traditional pill. Some are listed in Table 4.3.

TABLETS

The traditional tablet is a rather simple compounding of drug, starch filler (added for size and easy handling), and chemical dye (added for distinctive identification). This tablet was designed to rapidly and completely disintegrate after being swallowed. Today, this traditional tablet is becoming more the exception than the rule.

Various oral dosage systems have been developed. These systems are designed to remain relatively intact for extended periods after ingestion. Instead of rapidly releasing their contents into the lumen of the intestine, they release their contents

Table 4.3.
Some Different Drug Delivery Systems Available in the United States (Partial Listing Only)

Extended release oral formulations	Topical inhalational
Nifedipine	Corticosteroids
Verapamil	Beta-mimetics
Diltiazem morphine	Ipratroprium bromide
Theophylline	Chromolyn sodium
Procainamide	Depot injections
Levodopa-carbidopa	Haloperidol
Valproic acid	Leuprolide acetate
Transdermal patches	Medroxyprogesterone
Clonidine	Topical nasal application
Nitroglycerin	Vasopressin
Estrogen	Nitroglycerin
Scopolamine	
Fentanyl	

in a slow process that extends over 6–12 hours. These various systems are labeled "slow-release," "extended-release," "long-acting" or some other epithet. They often can change a drug from an every 4-, 6-, or 8-hour medication to an every 12- or 24-hour medication. These medications can be effective and may enhance compliance. However, they can be expensive. Compliance is low if the patient cannot afford to buy the medicine!

In addition to the barrier of cost, the extended release tablet is sometimes a problem if the patient develops a complication of therapy or a new medical problem that contraindicates the initial drug. With a traditional tablet, the drug is gone after a fairly short time. With an extended release preparation, the continued absorption of the drug cannot be stopped; absorption may last a full 24 hours.

TRANSDERMAL PATCHES

Transdermal patches can provide extended continuous delivery of various medications including nitroglycerin, estrogen, scopolamine, fentanyl, and clonidine. These systems are designed to adhere in showers and during the "wear and tear" of daily life. They can remain effective for 24 hours to 1 week with only one application. During their application they release medication into the skin in a continuous and predictable fashion. They also offer the unique opportunity of stopping therapy at any point by the simple removal of the patch from the skin.

DEPOT INJECTIONS

Although the details of different techniques for depot injection formulation may be quite different, one system is to develop multiple miniature encapsulations of drugs into microspheres. Each of these microspheres has an individual rate of dissolution and release of drug into surrounding tissue. By carefully formulating the mixture of these spheres, a preparation can be designed that slowly releases its contents into the tissue over a period of days to weeks. In this way, once daily injections can be replaced by weekly, monthly, or even annual injections. With one birth control preparation, Norplant, sustained release over 3–5 years has been achieved. Just as in the case of extended release tablets the convenience of single administration and improved compliance is obtained at the price of a longer commitment to treatment and some difficulty in reversal of therapy should this be indicated.

DRUG DISCRIMINATION BY THE PATIENT

An underappreciated problem in drug therapy is the ability of the patient to actually discriminate between different tablets. Even the best plans for therapy and careful instructions to patients may fail if the patient cannot identify which pill is which. Although pills are formulated with different colors it may well be that patients with visual or mental impairments continue to have difficulty in identifying the correct tablet. Elderly patients were asked by one set of investigators to identify two different white tablets placed next to each other. The patients could only correctly distinguish the two medications (Lasix 40 mg and Lanoxin 0.25 mg) 55% of the time (5). The clinician should therefore take considerable care to be sure that the patient can understand the directions for treatment and also actually physically carry them out. The use of weekly or daily pill dispenser systems can be helpful. Medications can be loaded into the dispensers by a nurse or family member, so the patient needs only to empty each container at the appropriate time.

GENERIC DRUGS

Cost

The motivation behind legislation designed to encourage the use of generic drugs is purely financial. Overall generic drugs are cheaper. After the expiration of patent protection of a drug product (typically 4–8 years after its initial introduction), the generic drug manufacturers are permitted to produce identical products for sale and distribution. An abbreviated process of FDA approval for these products allows generic manufacturers to provide the FDA with proof that their product has identical pharmacokinetic characteristics to the brand name and then to receive rapid approval for marketing. Generic drug makers (unencumbered by the costs of new drug development, extensive FDA review and approval, as well as large promotional and marketing expenses) can offer their generic versions of the brand name at lower wholesale costs to pharmacies. Unfortunately some of the cost savings associated with generics have gone to the pharmacies or health care plans that control the retail dispensing of drugs rather than the patient. As a result, the full financial benefits of generic prescribing have not been seen by consumers.

Quality

Are generics really equivalent? This is an almost impossible question to answer precisely. Based on the data provided to the FDA, they are. However, there is little or no data on the quality control of generic manufacturers. Unfortunately there have been problems noted in compliance with codes of ethics and professional standards by some generic companies. Is a particular product still as good when the company is making its 1,000,000th tablet as it was when they made their 100th? Absent a track record for an individual generic manufacturer and absent any knowledge about which generic version of the brand a particular pharmacy is dispensing at a given time, the answer is "hopefully, yes." In this context, the clinician who writes a prescription may well wish to write for brand name drugs when the issue of cost is not particularly important to the consumer. If a patient has a drug plan that does not force the generic, is willing to shop for the lowest brand price, or is simply willing to spend a little (or a lot) more, there is no reason not to prescribe the brand name drug.

Appropriate medical therapeutics can sometimes seem rather simple. This may often be the case. However, the truly rational and scientific therapy for patients is considerably more subtle and complex than it may initially appear. Clinicians must work to optimize treatment so that patients can fully benefit from the vastly improved therapeutic options now available.

REFERENCES

1. Nierenberg DW, Melmon KL. Introduction to clinical pharmacology. In Melmon KL, Morrelli MD, Hoffman MD, Nierenberg MD, eds. Melmon and Morrelli's clinical pharmacology: basic principles in therapeutics, 3rd ed. New York: McGraw-Hill, 1992.

2. Sjoqvist F, Burga O, Orme LE. In Speight TM, ed. Avery's drug treatment: principles and practice of clinical pharmacology and therapeutics. Baltimore: Williams & Wilkins, l987.
3. Soumerai S, Avorn J. Principles of educational outreach ("academic detailing") to improve clinical decision making. JAMA 1990;263:549–556.
4. Meyer BR. Improving medical education in therapeutics. Ann Intern Med 1988;108:145–147.
5. Hurd PD, Blevins J. Aging and the color of pills. N Engl J Med 1984;310:202.

SUGGESTED READINGS

Avorn J, Chen M, Hartley R. Scientific versus commercial sources of influence on drug prescribing behavior of physicians. Am J Med 1992;73:4–8.

Kroenke K. Polypharmacy: causes, consequences, and cure. Am J Med 1985;79:149–152.

Montanmat SC, Cusack BJ, Vestal RE. Management of drug therapy in the elderly. N Engl J Med 1989;321: 303–310.

Section II

APPROACH TO PATIENTS

chapter 5

SPECTRUM OF PATIENTS
Cynthia Chong and Pamela Charney

The provider-patient relationship can create common ground for communication and sharing. On an initial visit, both the patient and provider arrive at the threshold of their new relationship with several suitcases in hand. These suitcases contain many identities including age, personal definitions of family and community, gender, ethnicity, religion, and economic class as well as level of education. Some identities are readily visible. Others are revealed only after trust is established. Because an individual's response to his or her health is profoundly affected by perception and experience, it is important to know, acknowledge, and understand a patient's self-identity. Providers can bridge differences more effectively by expanding beyond their personal experiences and learning from individuals with other backgrounds.

During initial encounters, exploring the social dimensions of the patient's story provides a backdrop by which patient preferences can be better understood. Beginning the interaction with open-ended questions encourages the patient to include a personal definition of family and community. A great deal can be learned about the patient by listening to not only what is said but how it is said. Many elements of a social history are included in Table 5.1. Even if all the questions are reviewed on the first visit, this type of information often continues to unfold. As trust evolves, with further opportunities, patients often share more personal information.

Significant life cycle events for most patients include education, employment, family, formation of significant relationships, and the diagnosis of acute, chronic, or lethal medical conditions. All contain elements that are both similar and dissimilar to any provider's previous life experience. If the provider does not assume that the patient's world view is similar to his or her own, the relationship is more likely to be based on mutual understanding.

Self-identity begins with how one was raised within a community, region, and family. As time passes, self-identity is affected by life's events, often becomes more conscious, and may dramatically alter. Each individual's journey to self-definition is rich with experience. One of the clinician's most important roles is to be a witness for the patient through the process of self-definition and the evolution of his or her life story. In a long term clinician-patient relationship, the patient's perceptions, including how life's stresses were responded to, is part of what is shared. This sharing requires learning about an individual's community, culture, religion, family and family roles, sexual preference, economic status, education level, abilities, and disabilities.

PATIENT'S COMMUNITY

A community is any group of individuals with similar qualities or interests who define themselves as unique. Identity can be common geographical location, ethnic or racial background, or sexual preference. Interests can include religion or spirituality, music, or hobbies. Within each medical practice certain communities are more represented than others. When providers change locations, especially geographic areas, exposure to different communities follows.

Communities within a neighborhood can provide important social networks, services, and resources for patients and their families. It becomes easier to make referrals for patients when clinicians are acquainted with local services. Ideally, providers should also be concerned with community health as well as the health of the individuals seen in their practice. Some community health problems can best be approached by community focused preventive measures, e.g., decreasing violence or substance abuse.

Table 5.1.
Elements of the Social History Addressing Identity

How do you identify yourself (community, race, religion)?
Whom do you live with?
What is your relationship to those with whom you live?
Are you sexually active: with women, men, or both?
Describe who is in your family now.
Do you have any children?
Describe your family of origin.
Are you religious? If so what religion?
What school level did you complete?
Can you read the newspaper?
What is your occupation?

Some communities are defined by sexual behavior. Gay and lesbian individuals may choose to belong to a homosexual community for mutual support and acceptance. Although the proportion of the population self-identified as gay and lesbian is controversial, a recent survey of gay and lesbian physicians revealed that even physicians were hesitant to acknowledge their sexual preference to their caregivers. The physicians surveyed reported multiple episodes of harassment and suboptimal care because of homophobia. This supports the observation that clinicians' attitudes affect the care patients receive. In the social history, detailed questioning about sexual partners informs the patient that the clinician is willing to comprehend the diversity in sexual behavior. The Parents and Friends of Lesbians and Gays (PFLAG), a national organization dedicated to improving acceptance of gay and lesbian individuals, and the Gay and Lesbian Medical Association (GLMA) are excellent resources.

Religious communities often have specific views on the care of the physical and mental as well as spiritual aspects of life. These views guide choices and practices that may be distinct or may introduce dilemmas. These ideas become especially important when patients are adjusting to a new diagnosis, choosing treatment options, or discussing advanced directives. For example, many Jehovah's Witness patients would risk death rather than accept a blood transfusion; divorce may be difficult or impossible for Pentacostals or Catholics even in abusive relationships; artificial contraception is not accepted by many religions. The provider must remember that there is diversity in each religion as well as among religions. Individual perspectives must be ascertained and patient autonomy preserved when directing care. Clarification and docu-

mentation of these and similar issues facilitate comprehensive, respectful care.

Clinicians' own religious beliefs can also affect their ability to provide care. Professional responsibilities at times conflict with personal feelings. It can be a challenge to be nonjudgmental and consider all options when the clinician's religion suggests only one correct response. Clinicians have a responsibility to acknowledge to the patient that their perspective is influenced by religious beliefs. When this occurs, the patient might obtain care elsewhere.

RACIAL AND CULTURAL DETERMINANTS OF HEALTH

The 1992 census indicated there were 254 million residents of the United States. Admittedly, undercounts of undocumented aliens, minorities, and various urban municipalities probably occurred. However imperfect the available data, invaluable insights are still gained. The 1992 figures reflect the multiracial composition of the nation's residents: 83.3% white, 12.4% black, 9.5% Hispanic (may be black or white), and 3.3% Asian. In 1990, 8% of residents were foreign born, and almost half of them had entered the United States between 1980 and 1990.

Minority communities are found throughout the country, but their size, distinctiveness and degree of integration with surrounding communities are highly variable. Minority communities may have distinct health issues but are often medically underserved. Language and cultural differences must also be addressed to deliver quality care. It is beyond the scope of this chapter to discuss all racial and cultural variables that may affect health. Rather, the clinician must consider these variables in each patient to assess the risk of disease, available health resources, and possible outcomes to form a therapeutic partnership. The following concepts provide a framework for clinicians and will be discussed in the context of racial and cultural determinants of health.

- Does the patient *identify* with a community, culture, race, or religion?
- What are the unique *characteristics* of this physical or ideological community?
- What are the community *dynamics* that mold relationships, behavior, or health risks?
- What community *structures or resources* promote its beliefs or provide services?

Racial or cultural identity is part of the patient's self-identity discussed above. However, there may be extrinsic forces such as distinctive physical characteristics, language, discrimination, and the desire to preserve distinctive lifestyles that pressure groups to foster identity. Identity within groups is heterogeneous. Examples are first generation immigrants versus American born, older versus younger individuals, and educated versus poorly educated individuals. Identity may be regional. Blacks may be North, South, or Central American or Caribbean descendants of African slaves, or newly from Africa. Hispanics may be from North, South, or Central America, the Caribbean Islands, or Europe. Asians have origins in China, Japan, India, Southeast Asia, Korea, and the Pacific Islands. Identity may focus on language, customs, history, or diet. The potential for individual responses to identity exists, and clinicians must allow patients to express their identity and not stereotype. Open ended questions such as "What does this mean to you?" or "How does this affect your life or health?" place identity in a proper context.

Racial and cultural characteristics that influence health are those that define the concepts of health and illness and those of disease prevalence and treatment response. First, the concept of health and illness determines when and why health care is sought, frames how the problem is viewed, and defines modalities to remedy the problem. For example, the traditional Chinese view of health is that of balance between opposing hot and cold forces and that an imbalance results in illness. Treatment restores balance. Second, differences in disease prevalence and response to treatment and outcome has been noted in different racial groups. Blacks are affected by higher incidences of prostate cancer and experience poorer outcomes from hypertension and coronary artery disease compared with whites. Hispanics from Puerto Rico have higher incidences of asthma and osteoporosis. First generation Asians have high incidences of chronic hepatitis B and lower incidences of breast cancer. Pharmaceuticals' effects differ by race, e.g., angiotensin converting enzyme inhibitors are less efficacious in blacks. The relative contributions of intrinsic (genetic) and extrinsic (environmental) factors to these differences are not always clear.

Minority community dynamics that affect health include interpersonal and family relationships, views of leadership/authority, relationships to the "outside" world, and economic and social issues. It may be necessary to address a male or senior head of the family in Asian cultures. In contrast, black families often have a single woman heading the family. Extended and multigenerational families are more common among Asian, black, and Hispanic households; therefore, care or dietary instructions should be appropriate. Male dominated cultures may make discussion of reproductive choices or domestic violence difficult. Minority communities may view "mainstream" medical care as insensitive to their needs, have language and economic barriers to care, or may be insular and less likely to reach for care. Economic issues such as occupation or poverty will contribute to health concerns. For example, migrant farm workers may be exposed to pesticides or have fragmented medical records; crowded substandard living conditions encourage communicable diseases such as tuberculosis. Social issues include high incidences of alcohol or drug use in some minority communities. All these dynamics are important in assessing health risks and therapeutics.

Community structures or resources are important. Minority communities may have active alternative or traditional health care practices. Herbal or traditional patent medications, medical prayers or rituals, manipulation/massage, acupuncture, and cupping are some practices. Traditional practices most effectively address culturally based health beliefs and may be highly developed and promoted in Native American, Asian, Caribbean, or other communities. These practices and products are unregulated, and quality may be hard to ascertain. Practitioners may offer services for which they are not trained or credentialed but escape scrutiny because interactions occur in native languages. Other community institutions that may affect health are senior citizen programs, religious institutions, community self-help agencies, and "governing" bodies. These are key to outreach, home-based care and community intervention.

Patients who feel their medical provider would deem their health beliefs or practices "weird," "wrong," "old country," "old fashioned," or "stupid" are likely to keep them hidden. Clinicians working with racially and culturally diverse patients must be nonjudgmental and encourage sharing of these beliefs and practices. When the provider's instructions are in conflict with these beliefs, the patient's ability to follow through with care is impaired. Alternatives that are compatible with a patient's beliefs should be sought; e.g., vegetable soup (cool), not chicken soup (hot), should be suggested to a person with traditional Chinese beliefs who presents with a febrile viral syndrome (hot imbalance). Clinicians must avail themselves of medical information specific to their patient population.

FAMILY

The idealized family image of the 1950s—father, mother, and two or so children—is in transition. Many phenomena are contributing to this change. Divorce and separation contribute to cleavage of familial ties or to parents and children living in different households and continuing to share meaningful relationships. Children born out of wedlock and raised by a single parent, usually the mother, may never have a significant relationship with the absent parent. Children increasingly are reared by grandparents or relatives if their parents cannot because of AIDS, drug abuse, or other devastating circumstances. Families may consist of unrelated individuals as with remarriage and its consequent reshuffling of households, foster parenting, and adoptions. Extended families— multigenerational households and relatives—reflect America's diverse cultures and economic needs. "Nontraditional" gay families are increasingly visible. The clinician initiates an open discussion with, "Tell me about your family" and allows patients to define the relationships.

Traditional family relationships are also changing. Women are often working outside the home, and men are more frequently involved in child rearing. Adult children are living with parents but defining independent, interdependent, and dependent roles. As America ages, more households are involved in the care of elderly grandparents or other relatives. Household dynamics are also changing: who "brings home the bacon," manages finances, makes decisions, cooks, does laundry, or repairs is defined in each family unit. The clinician must allow patients to identify these roles.

GENDER ISSUES

The meaning of being male or female varies by family, community, ethnic group, age, and religion; therefore it is worthwhile to consider a patient's self-expectations. These factors are particularly important when a patient is faced with infertility or cancer of the breast, prostate, cervix, or testes. The expectations of a patient's family and community may coincide or conflict with his or her own and may result in health difficulties. Examples include infertility, pressure to produce an heir, and mother of a newborn returning to work. Gender issues are summarized in Table 5.2.

Table 5.2.
Essential Gender Issues

Young adult years
Women: Building calcium stores, diagnosing menstruation related iron deficiency anemia; screening for cervical cancer; using tobacco
Men: Screening for testicular cancer
Both: Reproduction and parenting choices; parenting; career development; substance use and abuse including alcohol, tobacco, and illicit and prescription drugs; sexually transmitted disease including HIV; cholesterol monitoring; exercise and physical fitness; trauma and violence

Middle years
Women: menopause; caregiving issues ("sandwich generation"); screening for breast cancer; initial cardiovascular disease surveillance
Men: cardiovascular disease; prostate symptoms
Both: reproductive and parenting choices; screening for cardiovascular disease and cancer; exercise and physical fitness; career development; sexual functioning; substance use and abuse

Older years
Women: increased incidence of coronary artery disease; breast cancer screening
Men: prostate symptoms; screening for prostate cancer
Both: maintaining independence; financial concerns; loss of significant others; retirement issues; cardiovascular disease; cancer; osteoarthritis; decreased vision and hearing

Understanding gender related cultural norms is also essential in the organization and delivery of health care for specific patient groups. Hasidic Jewish and Arabic women strongly prefer to have their medical care provided by women. Newly immigrated African women who have experienced childhood ritual surgery have special health needs that can only be effectively provided by nonjudgmental providers. Gender related cultural norms are particularly important in the provision of gynecologic and obstetrical care. Staffing flexibility is essential in these areas to encourage women to seek care. Men from many cultures may find it difficult to discuss sexual or emotional difficulties. Learning about patients' gender related cultural norms is key and requires setting aside the clinician's own assumptions about the roles of women and men. Interviewing requires reframing questions to encourage patients' views and gentle, nonjudgmental probing of guarded improbable responses.

Gender is also important to consider when critically reviewing and applying what is known in the medical literature. In general, there is a paucity of data on how women and men are different and similar in disease natural history, diagnosis, and treatment. Over the last several years, the cardio-vascular literature has begun to explore the known differences in lipid profiles in women and men and differences in the diagnosis and treatment of coro-nary artery disease. Historically, new medications have been predominantly tested in middle-aged white men. Therefore, drug side effect profiles of-ten lack information for women with respect to fertility and teratogenicity. Gender analysis is lack-ing for sexual side effects of commonly used medi-cations including antihypertensives. Recently, the Food and Drug Administration has decided that women are to be included in drug treatment trials. As new drugs being developed are tested on women as well as men, more information about pharmaco-logic gender similarities and differences will be-come available.

ECONOMICS

In 1992, the median family income in the United States was $37,000. Americans who were poorly educated, single female heads of households, or black or Hispanic had lower incomes. Income dis-parities adversely affecting minorities are further illustrated by the distribution of families below the federally determined poverty levels in 1993: 9% of whites, 12% of Asians, 26% of Hispanics, and 31% of blacks. Economic resources determine the qual-ity of housing, education and services. Health care resources, access to health care and health status are connected to economic resources. Patients' choice of therapy, dietary habits, or lifestyle priori-ties may be tied to their income. Inequities have long resulted. Examples are high rates of tuberculosis among the homeless and pockets of medically un-derserved in impoverished neighborhoods. Resolu-tion of these inequities through public health sys-tems, universal health care insurance, and subsidized care has proved elusive. Clinicians must consider a patient's economic situation in assessing health risks and proposing care plans.

EDUCATION

The level of a patient's education must be deter-mined to create an effective provider-patient rela-tionship. Education may be formal or self-attained and may not necessarily be in English. The level of education often determines how well patients can

understand their health condition(s), understand or follow medication or lifestyle instructions, and participate in creating a therapeutic plan.

It is essential to determine a patient's level of literacy. Patients who are functionally illiterate have difficulty reading labels to identify medica-tions and dosing instructions, and therefore "com-pliance" may be affected. Other sources of prob-lems are correspondence (entitlements, insurance companies, test results), medication side-effect pro-files, testing instructions, appointments, and educa-tional materials. Those who are minimally educated may misinterpret information. Technical terms are easily misunderstood, even by the educated! Medi-cation charts with sample pills and simple instruc-tions and assistance with correspondence are helpful.

Patients who lack English fluency can be found in almost any setting but are concentrated in immi-grant communities. In the 1990 census, 14% of American adults (26 million) spoke a language other than English at home. Of these people, 45% spoke English less than "very well" and 52% spoke Span-ish. Practitioners caring for patients who speak other languages must use translators to ensure com-munication of medical diagnoses and instructions, especially those that are complex or distressing. Care must be taken with confidential information, sexual issues, and many aspects of the social history if the translator is a relative, a friend, or of the opposite sex.

Educational attainment is also strongly tied to economics. Poverty has been linked with lower ed-ucational attainment and achievement. Inadequate funding and poverty's associated obstacles to learn-ing (broken families, hunger, inadequate housing, substance abuse) contribute to these poor results. Increased educational attainment improves earning potential. Educational attainment need not be static; clinicians must provide patient education as part of any therapeutic plan to improve patient participation and outcome.

DISABILITY ISSUES

In 1991, there were 49 million Americans with disabilities; half were mild and half severe. Of the 34 million with functional limitations, 8 million had limitations of activities of daily living. Disabilities affect a patient's medical needs, self-identity, self-esteem, earning potential, and lifestyle. Providers are an integral part of a patient's disability: they perform diagnostic evaluations, inform patients of diagnoses, offer treatment, and facilitate living with disabilities. Patients facing disability experience degrees of denial, depression, anger, and resolution. A patient's ability to cope with disability may be either aided or hampered by family, employers, or friends. Providers may need to speak with family members or employers to clarify the details of disability and need for modifications to the environment or responsibilities. Patients may need assistance in negotiating benefits and assistance. Clinician discussions of a disability should be honest but hopeful.

In summary, this chapter only hints at the broadness of the spectrum of patients. It is hoped that the issues and examples cited will encourage clinicians to explore each patient's individual dimensions. Open-minded, nonjudgmental encounters will enrich the provider-patient relationship and allow for an effective therapeutic partnership.

SUGGESTED READINGS

Adler NE, Boyce WT, Chesney MA, et al. Socioeconomic inequities in health: no easy solution. JAMA 1993;269: 3140–3145.

Anastos K, Charney P, Charon RA, Cohen E, Jones CY, Marte C, Swiderski DM, Wheat ME, Williams S. Hypertension in women: what is really known? Ann Intern Med 1991;115:287–293.

Woloshin S, Bicknell N, Schwarz L, et al. Language barriers in medicine in the United States. JAMA 1995; 273:724–728.

chapter 6

CARE OF THE PATIENT AT HOME
Eleanor Weinstein

Home care has been defined as the provision of services and equipment to the patient in the home for the purpose of restoring and maintaining his or her maximal level of comfort, function, and health (1). Home health care is not what it was just 5 or 10 years ago. It is one of the most rapidly growing areas of health care and has become extremely diversified in the services that can be provided. In addition to the usual physicians, dentists, nurses, and homemakers, home health care teams now include various other health care professionals (Table 6.1). This variety of professionals available to provide service in the home allows a multidisciplinary approach that is often necessary when caring for patients with complex medical and social problems. Equipment ranges from simple devices such as those for monitoring blood glucose to highly sophisticated medical devices such as ventilators, hemodialysis units, and long distance telemetry for cardiac monitoring. Diagnostic services including the use of routine x-ray, mammography, blood and urine sampling, oximetry for the measurement of oxygen saturation of the blood, and electrocardiography are commonly used in the home.

HISTORICAL PERSPECTIVE

In 1947, Montefiore Hospital in New York City established the first hospital-based home care program. This program was designed to provide care to patients in their homes with a team of physicians, nurses, and therapists. This was a novel approach to the delivery of home care services that had more traditionally used a visiting nurse model without the direct participation of physicians. Before the 1940s, physician home visits were fairly common. However, in the last 50 years there has been a sharp decline in this practice. It has been reported that in 1959 house calls represented approximately 9.2% of physician-patient contacts but that by 1979 this had decreased to 1.7%. By 1991 house calls had declined further to less than 1% of physician practice activity (2). In part, it is due to this change in physician practice activity that home care programs have generally excluded physicians from their structure. Today's physicians have cited four major explanations for their lack of involvement in home health care: (*a*) poor reimbursement, (*b*) time constraints and efficiency, (*c*) medical liability, and (*d*) fear that they cannot provide their usual quality of care in the home (3). Additionally, the general unfamiliarity with the concept of providing services for the patient outside the office or hospital setting as a result of minimal exposure to this practice is probably also involved. Although these are significant concerns, their validity and relevance must be examined closely given the recent advances in the home care industry, its increasing importance, and the need for the participation of the primary care provider.

The nation's home care industry has grown dramatically over the last 30 years. The number of home care agencies has grown from 2000 in 1967 to more than 10,000 in 1987. Gross revenues are reported to have increased from 10.3 billion in 1985 to 19 billion in 1990 (4). Funding and reimbursement for services provided in the home are complex issues that are beyond the scope of this chapter. Note, however, that there are limitations on services for which there will be reimbursement depending on the condition and stability of the patient as well as the type of health insurance. In general, most plans will only cover home care services for a defined time after the onset of a new medical/surgical problem or deterioration of a preexisting condition.

The home care industry has not only grown but has also become greatly diversified. Advances in medical technology originally led to the shift of

Table 6.1.
Professionals Involved in Care of the Patient at Home

Primary care providers: physicians, nurse practitioners, physician assistants
Field nurses: usually RNs doing most of the home visits
Allied health professionals: dentists, podiatrists
Therapists: physical, occupational, speech, and respiratory
Social workers: for assessment of psychosocial and entitlement issues
Home health aides: provide personal care and also are trained in basic skills such as monitoring vital signs, simple dressing changes, measurement of fluid input, output, etc.
Attendants, homemakers: provide personal care and homemaking services

Table 6.2.
Conditions That May Be Effectively Treated at Home

Surgical wounds requiring careful monitoring and dressing changes
Decubitus ulcers
Infectious diseases requiring long term antibiotics (e.g., septic arthritis, osteomyelitis, uncomplicated bacterial endocarditis)
Diabetes mellitus requiring improved control, e.g., daily monitoring of blood glucose and intensive patient education
Conditions requiring ongoing physical therapy or rehabilitation (e.g. patients after orthopedic surgery, neurosurgery, stroke)
Patients with respiratory compromise or failure requiring oxygen therapy and/or ventilator support

medical practice from home to office and hospital. Ironically, further advances have allowed the return of care to the home setting in many instances. This new and portable technology has supported the use of many professional services within the home that previously were not possible.

RATIONALE FOR HOME HEALTH CARE

The growth of home health care has occurred largely as an effort to contain costs. However, it has become clear that older patients and their families prefer to receive care in their homes whenever possible (4). In fact, hospitalization can be seen as a major risk for the elderly. For many patients, particularly the very old, a hospitalization is followed by a decline in functional status and independence that is often irreversible (5, 6). This result can in part be attributed to the particular disease or condition being treated in the hospital. However, many elderly patients are susceptible to the development of complications related to the hospitalization itself. Specific factors associated with usual aging when combined with certain features of hospitalization may lead to a cascade of events culminating in the functional decline of the patient at risk (Fig. 6.1) (7).

In addition to care for the elderly, home health care has become the optimal mode of health care delivery for various patients. Many acute illnesses previously felt to be treatable only in an institutionalized setting are now adequately treated at home given the advent of home intravenous therapy and

the ability to monitor patients closely (Table 6.2). For example, several studies have shown the efficacy, safety, and cost savings of intravenous antibiotic treatment at home (8). The clinician may therefore comfortably choose to treat the patient (once stabilized) at home for conditions requiring long-term antibiotic therapy including osteomyelitis, septic arthritis, and bacterial endocarditis. Advances in home care have also supported the early discharge from the hospital of many patients who previously could not have been treated at home. Patients in this group would include those requiring ongoing treatment for burns, decubiti, surgical wounds, or pulmonary or physical rehabilitation.

Many chronic conditions lend themselves to care at home (Table 6.3). Patients who are chronically disabled, physically or mentally, benefit from care at home. In addition, the quality of life of the immunocompromised, terminally ill, and essentially homebound elderly can be significantly improved by the array of multidisciplinary services that can be provided at home. Indeed, it is these patients who may find it nearly impossible to access

Table 6.3.
Patients Who May Especially Benefit from Home Care and a Multidisciplinary Approach to Health Care

Essentially homebound patients
Frail elderly
Patients with chronic physical and/or functional disabilities
Patients with psychiatric disorders
Immunocompromised patients
Patients with terminal illness

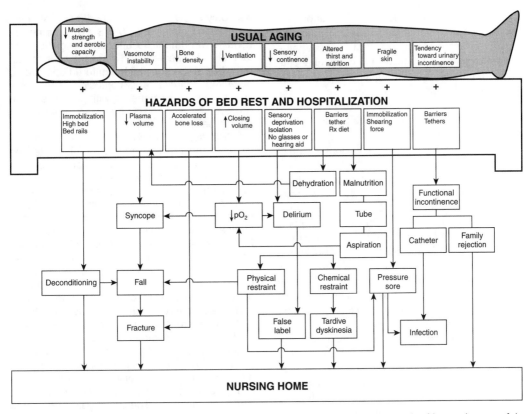

Figure 6.1. Cascade of events leading to functional decline. From Creditor MC. Hazards of hospitalization of the elderly. Ann Intern Med 1993;118:219–223.

health care in the usual manner. For these patients, providing services in the home can reduce emergency room visits and hospitalizations, decrease the need for nursing home placement, and alleviate the burden on caregivers. Additionally, in many areas hospice home care is available for care of the dying patient. These professionals are specially trained to deal with all the issues facing patients and their loved ones. There is usually a support network of volunteers and chaplains in addition to social workers who can aid during this period as well as during bereavement.

GOALS OF HOME HEALTH CARE FOR THE PRIMARY CARE PROVIDER

It is apparent that interest in home health care will grow as federal and state governments and private insurers try to contain costs by discharging patients from hospitals as quickly as possible. Also, as the elderly population expands, the need for high qual-

ity home health programs will intensify. Primary care providers, historically excluded from the structure of formal home care programs, now need to acquaint themselves with home care as a system that will increasingly supplement the service they provide in the hospital and office.

Future clinicians must be trained appropriately in this field. Curricula for medical education are undergoing major revision, and there has been a call for the formalization of exposure to home care (3, 9). Many undergraduate medical programs are including home care rotations. Home visiting is recommended as part of the curriculum of family practice and internal medicine graduate training programs. In addition, requirements for accreditation of geriatric fellowships include clinical experience in home care. The American College of Physicians published a position paper in 1986 that outlined the importance of home care and the need for physicians to become more actively involved in the provision of these services (9). Likewise, the American Medical Association Council on Scientific Affairs and Council on Medical Education have recommended that training in the principles and practice of home health care be incorporated into the undergraduate, graduate, and continuing education of physicians (3). If implemented, these revised curricula should help clinicians-in-training learn about the unique aspects of caring for patients at home through didactic teaching as well as through practical experience.

There is a broad range of benefits for the patient who receives care at home, but the benefit to the clinician may be less obvious. The home visit enables the clinician to more adequately oversee many pertinent issues than is possible in the office setting, e.g., consideration of the patient's social support system, safety and adequacy of the home environment, and patient's functional status. Also, seeing a patient at home can help the provider to become sensitive to factors that may interfere with the achievement of desired outcomes. This awareness can improve the relationship between clinician and patient and can thus be instrumental in fostering a more mutually satisfying partnership. In addition, a home visit by the clinician is a powerful statement of his or her commitment to the patient and generally wins sincere gratitude from the patient and family. This type of relationship between clinician and patient can be extremely rewarding professionally as well as personally.

Illustrative Case

This case study will illustrate the utility of home care as a component of quality, compassionate, and comprehensive health care. As has been outlined, many patients may be optimally treated at home. In this case, a patient with chronic and deteriorating illness opted to be managed in his home.

Mr. S. was an 85-year-old man with a history of progressive biventricular congestive heart failure, atrial fibrillation, and renal insufficiency who had suffered a minor stroke several years earlier. He and his wife lived in a senior housing complex in New Haven, Connecticut. Mr. S was lucky in that despite his complicated medical condition he could remain in this independent living situation because he had a supportive wife who was healthy and younger than he and two children in the area who were involved in their parents' lives.

Mr. S had experienced an episode of rectal bleeding for which he was hospitalized. Colonoscopy revealed only diverticula, and the bleeding resolved spontaneously. Although Mr. S did not suffer major complications and the hospitalization

was only a few days, this experience was trying for him and his wife. In Mr. S's own home and usual environment he appeared cognitively intact, always oriented, and pleasantly conversant but while in the hospital he suffered episodes of nighttime agitation and confusion. These episodes were easily managed with gentle sedation; however, his wife and children were greatly upset by this behavior that they had never witnessed. Additionally, Mr. S could not eat a regular diet while in the hospital because of his intestinal bleeding and preparation for colonoscopy. For many elderly patients whose daily activities have become a matter of routine, this type of disruption can be a major source of discomfort. For Mrs. S, the separation from her husband of more than 50 years was a significant strain. She had cared for her husband through bouts of congestive heart failure, pneumonia, and his stroke. Although he had been hospitalized before, this particular stay was more difficult for her. She realized he was becoming weaker generally and was concerned about his care when she was not with him.

For these reasons and probably others, Mr. S decided that he wished to avoid further hospitalizations if possible. Mrs. S and their children were aware of his feelings. Mr. S discussed this with his physician during an office visit. They had discussed advance directives previously. His physician knew that he had decided against any heroic measures and would not wish to be resuscitated. However, Mr. S had not mentioned before that he did not want to be hospitalized. She assured him that she would respect his wishes.

Mr. S's condition was stable over the next few months on a regimen of diuretics, digoxin, and afterload reduction. However, he slowly became more edematous, and his exercise tolerance diminished. Diuretics were increased to maintain fluid balance. However, with increased diuretics his renal function worsened. It became clear that it would be difficult to manage Mr. S's heart failure. His heart failure was worsening but the progressive renal insufficiency and tenuous electrolyte balance limited further adjustment of his diuretics.

Mr. S's physician met with the patient and his wife. She summarized the recent events and told them that further management was becoming problematic. She recalled their previous discussion about remaining home through deteriorating medical conditions and outlined the options for Mr. S. He could decide to go into the hospital at this time with the hope that inpatient treatment with intravenous diuretics and low-dose dopamine might temporarily improve his heart failure and renal function enough that he could return home comfortably. They understood that this stabilization would only be short term and that they would then be faced with the same dilemma sometime later. The other option would be to remain home and continue to manage him conservatively. They realized that the likelihood of achieving much improvement was low and that he would probably worsen. The physician assured Mr. and Mrs. S that whatever their decision, she would respect their wishes and do her best to improve his condition.

After a moment of thought, Mr. S decided to remain at home. A referral to a home care agency was made to help with what was likely to be a difficult period. The home care agency could provide skilled nursing visits daily if needed and a home health aide to provide some respite for Mrs. S and help with his personal care. They could also provide social services consultation to help the family deal with issues concerning the worsening illness and eventual death. The agency would also arrange for acquiring the medical equipment needed at home to make Mr. S as comfortable as possible, e.g., home oxygen therapy, a hospital bed for easy positioning, a wheelchair, and a bedside commode.

Over the next 2 weeks, Mr. S's condition continued to worsen. His response to the diuretics was diminishing, and blood samples drawn at home showed further deterioration of renal function. Mr. S and his family were pleased with the care he received at home. His physician and nurse were visiting him almost daily through this period. He was relaxed and comforted by his family, friends, and familiar surroundings. At this point, Mr. S was essentially bed bound, using his oxygen continuously. They were again given the choice to enter the hospital but declined. It was decided that no further blood samples would be taken from the patient. Mr. S's oral intake declined rapidly. He remained alert but with long periods of sleep day and night. Mrs. S asked their priest to come to the home. Also, all family members and friends who were able came to visit. Mr. S began to have worsening respiratory distress that responded to small doses of subcutaneous morphine sulfate. He slowly became less responsive. Finally , after about 3 weeks, Mr. S died during the early morning hours. His daughter, son, and wife were at his bedside.

Later, when Mr. S's physician visited the family in their home they were grieving but relieved that he had such a peaceful death. They were thankful that they carried out his wishes to the end. Mrs. S was especially appreciative of the support she was given that enabled her to have her husband remain at home. Indeed, without the involvement of the home care agency and his physician's willingness to care for the patient in his home, the family would not have felt comfortable enough to knowingly allow his deterioration and eventual death at home.

The case of Mr. S illustrates several key concepts with regard to caring for patients at home. A terminally ill patient and his family opted for conservative treatment to enable him to remain at home. The ongoing communication among clinician, patient, and family and assistance by experienced professionals were crucial. Mr. S and his family were prepared for the course that followed. They also knew that Mr. S could be transferred to the hospital or inpatient hospice if the care at home became too difficult emotionally or physically. Mr. S is an example of a patient whose quality of life at a critical time of his life was greatly enhanced by care in the home. As in the case of Mr. S, with the ability to provide comprehensive and quality care at home, clinicians of the future can help individuals live and end their lives with control and dignity.

REFERENCES

1. Council on Scientific Affairs. Home care in the 1990s. JAMA 1990;263:1241–1244.
2. Keenan JM, Hepburn KW. The role of physicians in home health care. Clin Geriatr Med 1991;7:665–675.
3. Council on Scientific Affairs. Educating physicians in home health care. JAMA 1991;265:769–771.
4. Keenan JM, Bland CJ, Webster L, Myers S. The home care practice and attitudes of Minnesota family physicians. J Am Geriatr Soc 1991;39:1101–1104.
5. Hoenig HM, Rubenstein LZ. Hospital-associated deconditioning and dysfunction (editorial). J Am Geriatr Soc 1991;39:220–222.
6. Lamont CT, Sampson S, Matthias R, Kane R. The outcome of hospitalization for acute illness in the elderly. J Am Geriatr Soc 1983;31:282–288.
7. Creditor MC. Hazards of hospitalization of the elderly. Ann Intern Med 1993;118:219–223.
8. Balinsky W, Nesbit S. Cost effectiveness of outpatient parenteral antibiotics, a review of the literature. Am J Med 1989;87:301–305.
9. Health and Public Policy Committee, American College of Physicians. Home health care. Ann Intern Med 1986;105:454–460.

SUGGESTED READINGS

Weiland D, Ferrell B, Rubenstein L. Geriatric home health care. Clin Geriatric Med 1991;7:645–664.

chapter 7

APPROACH TO THE GERIATRIC PATIENT

Eleanor Weinstein

Geriatrics is described as the discipline of medicine specifically devoted to the medical care of the elderly. The changing demographics of the American population in the last 50 years, often referred to as the "graying of America," has indeed provided the impetus for the mastery of geriatric principles and their application toward the care of the elderly by today's health care professionals. The elderly are one of the fastest growing populations in the United States. Population analysts have determined that the projected population of those age 70 and older will increase slowly from 21 million in 1990 to 25 million in 2000. After this slow growth, the elderly population will swell to 52.5 million in 2041 (Fig. 7.1) (1). It is vital that health planners and policy makers use this forecast to anticipate the needs of the future elderly population. Equally as important, in response to the growth of the elderly population health care providers must become comfortable in caring for patients who are frequently medically as well as psychosocially and ethically complex.

SPECIAL CHARACTERISTICS OF THE GERIATRIC PATIENT

The uniqueness of the growing elderly population necessitates a special and individualized approach to care. Clinicians must understand what differentiates the elderly from the young in sickness and in health to be able to provide high quality, compassionate, and comprehensive health care to the geriatric patient. They must also be alert to the special problems of the elderly that often have a significant impact on the quality of life and may be partially or totally alleviated with appropriate treatment.

When caring for an older patient the clinician must be aware of the influence of age on the presentation of illness. Three factors have been described that may influence the presentation of disease in an elderly patient: (*a*) underreporting of illness, (*b*) differences in the pattern of illness, and (*c*) altered response to illness (2).

It is a common but mistaken belief that most elderly patients are hypochondriacal and tend to focus their attention on trivial physical symptoms. The reality is, however, that many elderly may not report significant symptoms. Underreporting of illness is due to many factors including the patient's belief that usual aging is linked with the onset of certain symptoms and problems that are unavoidable (e.g., hearing impairment, incontinence, cognitive deficit, gait disturbance). Other important factors that may inhibit the elderly patient from accessing medical care or from reporting symptoms include depression as well as denial of illness. The depressed patient may incorrectly feel that there is no chance of improvement in his or her condition. The patient who denies that his or her symptoms are related to significant illness may do so for fear of economic, social, or functional consequences (2).

The differences in the distribution of illnesses in young and old must be realized when caring for a geriatric patient. There are some conditions, albeit few, that are almost exclusively found in the geriatric patient. These include conditions such as polymyalgia rheumatica and Parkinson's disease. More importantly, the clinician must be aware of the myriad conditions that have an increased prevalence in the elderly including malignancy, cardiovascular disease, and tuberculosis (Table 7.1). In addition, it is common for an elderly patient to have multiple chronic and progressive conditions.

It is clear that the presentation of disease may be atypical in the elderly patient. For instance, the elderly patient with myocardial infarction may present without chest pain; the patient with urosepsis may present without fever but with confusion and urinary incontinence. This creates a challenge

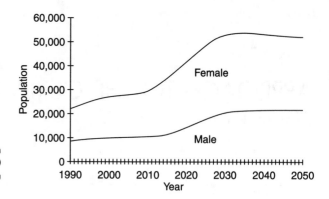

Figure 7.1. Sex-specific projected population aged 70 and over: United States, 1990–2050 (population in thousands). Source: U.S. Bureau of the Census 1989, middle series.

for the clinician who must maintain a high index of suspicion for a diagnosis that may not be obvious on first or even second glance. Another important distinction between young and old with respect to response to illness is the effect of that illness on the patient's function. An elderly patient is more commonly subject to functional decline related to a particular disease process that may affect his or her ability to live independently. For example, patients with osteoarthritis and related gait problems who suffer a hip fracture may not achieve their previous level of functioning after repair of the fracture. As another example, consider a patient with an early pneumonia that in a younger person could be easily managed as an outpatient. Due to underlying compromise of pulmonary function as a consequence of aging, this patient will be more likely to require hospitalization and supplemental oxygen.

HISTORY AND PHYSICAL EXAM OF THE OLDER PATIENT

The clinician providing care for the elderly patient must understand the importance of establishing a good relationship with the patient as well as with other family and caregivers. In addition, as opposed to the care of the younger patient where most of the data may be obtained in one encounter, the accumulation of information about an elderly patient usually occurs over several visits. Both the medical history and examination must be tailored to better address the problems and concerns of the geriatric patient.

The interview requires expansion in areas that are associated with a high prevalence of disease and disability for this group. For example, discussion

of cognitive or sensory impairments and functional status is essential in the older patient.

A detailed review of all medications, prescribed and over-the-counter, is essential. Older patients, often with multiple and complex medical problems, are subject to potential drug-drug interactions that may be harmful. Also, patients frequently will have multiple containers of the same medication with different generic and trade names, creating confusion and setting the stage for noncompliance, a common problem in the older patient. The portion of the medical interview that focuses on the patient's family history of illness may not be relevant in the very elderly patient and in some cases can be omitted entirely.

The review of systems also needs to be individualized for the older patient. In addition to the usual array of questions, some areas will require a more detailed review. Again, the primary concern should be to determine the functional impairments the

Table 7.1.
Common Conditions in the Elderly Patient

Dementia
Delirium
Incontinence
Falls and immobility
Pressure ulcers
Malnutrition
Vision and hearing impairments
Depression
Sexual dysfunction
Malignancy
Cardiovascular disease
Hypertension
Arthritis

symptoms or diseases may cause. The interviewer must remember the conditions that have a higher prevalence in the elderly (e.g., falls, urinary incontinence, visual impairment) and should ask targeted questions to detect them. If a problem is detected, a more detailed history will be taken. Cognitive function will be formally assessed during the physical examination, but questions concerning changes in the patient's memory or ability to manage personal affairs should be addressed to the patient and caregivers or family during the interview. Patients must be questioned about changes in their vision and the extent to which the impairment has affected their lives. For example, patients with significant visual loss may have difficulty reading labels on their medications or in handling money. Additionally, all patients must be asked if they drive. The clinician may decide that it is unsafe for the patient to drive if there are significant visual or cognitive impairments or if there are other medical problems that may interfere with the patient's ability to drive.

A vital component of the evaluation of a geriatric patient is a thorough assessment of the patient's ability to perform the tasks of daily living (dressing, preparing meals and eating, shopping, handling of finances, etc.). It is important to determine the patient's level of functioning to construct a comprehensive care plan. Several instruments available to standardize this evaluation will be discussed under "Comprehensive Geriatric Assessment."

The issues of advance directives and health proxy must be discussed. If the patient has not obviously made clear decisions regarding the end of life and treatment preferences, these issues may be introduced at the initial encounter and detailed on follow-up visits. Many patients may require several visits to discuss these critical issues before decisions can be made.

A few points regarding the physical examination of the elderly patient merit emphasis. Although there is little that is unique, the focus on certain aspects of the examination may be different. Much can be learned by observing the patient closely during the examination. Gait, mobility, and ability to follow instructions to cooperate with the examination can be assessed. Much information can be gained by the alert clinician in this manner.

When checking the vital signs, patients should be checked for orthostatic hypotension, which is common in the elderly and is responsible for significant morbidity. The skin should be examined for signs of cumulative sun exposure and suspicious lesions. There should be an evaluation of the patient's hearing and a check for obstructing cerumen that can cause significant hearing loss. Examination of the mouth should include an assessment of the patient's dentition. Patients should be examined with dentures in place to check the fit as well as without them to check for lesions.

Systolic murmurs, present in 30–80% of patients age 65 and older may present a diagnostic challenge (3). The differential diagnosis includes aortic stenosis, aortic sclerosis, idiopathic hypertrophic subaortic stenosis, and mitral regurgitation. These murmurs will require further evaluation depending on their characteristics as well as the overall condition of the patient.

Pelvic examination of the elderly woman may be difficult to perform if she cannot tolerate the usual position for this exam. However, the use of cushions to support the head and neck can significantly help the patient with arthritis and/or deforming kyphosis endure the exam with minimal discomfort. Interestingly, a cervix can be found in approximately one-third of all woman who give a history of having had a hysterectomy (3). This clearly has important implications regarding screening of these women for cervical cancer.

The examination of the geriatric patient must include an assessment of the patient's mental status. Abbreviated mental status tests, which will be discussed under "Comprehensive Geriatric Assessment," take only a few minutes to administer and can significantly increase the detection of dementia and delirium. A thorough neurological examination is critical in the elderly given the prevalence of cerebrovascular disease and neurological disorders.

COMPREHENSIVE GERIATRIC ASSESSMENT

Comprehensive geriatric assessment is defined as an interdisciplinary approach to the screening and diagnosis of physical and psychosocial impairments and functional disabilities in frail older patients (2). This type of assessment has been established in response to the complex medical and psychosocial problems facing many frail elderly patients. The goal of this approach is to identify problems and develop a comprehensive and interdisciplinary management plan that emphasizes patient function. The patient's cognitive ability, physical and emotional state, environment, and social support system as well as other factors interact constantly to affect the patient's functional status (Fig. 7.2). Health care professionals must be aware of the tools available to

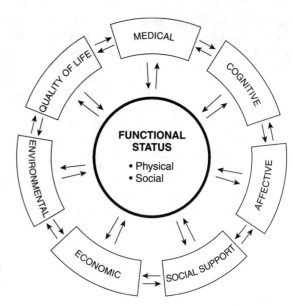

Figure 7.2. Domains of comprehensive geriatric assessment and some of their interactions. From Reference 3, p. 46.

help assess these factors and knowledgeable about the indications for their use.

Several instruments are used to assess the cognitive, emotional, and physical functional status of the geriatric patient (Table 7.2). The clinician should become familiar with those most commonly used in clinical practice. Assessment of the cognitive function of the elderly patient is a vital component of the examination. Many elderly with mild-to-moderate cognitive impairment maintain their social skills, and therefore clinically important impairment may go undetected (4). The use of a structured assessment tool often will alert the clinician to these mild impairments. Two frequently used

Table 7.2.
Assessment Tools Used to Evaluate Older Patients

Instrument	Function Assessed
Assessment of functional status	
ADL scale	basic ADL
Barthel Index	basic ADL
Instrumental ADL scale	intermediate ADL
Older Americans Resources and Services Multidimensional Function Assessment Questionnaire	intermediate ADL
Hierarchical Health Scale for the Aged	advanced ADL
Hierarchical scale of exercise-related ADLs	advanced ADL
Timed manual performance	performance of structured manual tasks
Physical performance test	physical function
Assessment of medical domain	
Braden Scale	pressure ulcer risk
Performance-Oriented Assessment of Mobility	balance and gait
Assessment of emotional state	
Structured interview guide for the Hamilton Depression Scale	depression
Geriatric Depression Scale (short form)	depression
Assessment of cognitive function	
Mini-Mental State Examination	memory, orientation, attention, constructional ability

ADL, activities of daily living; AADL, advanced activities of daily living. From Reference 3, p. 468.

Add points for each correct response.

		Score	Points

Orientation
1. What is the	Year?	_____	1
	Season?	_____	1
	Date?	_____	1
	Day?	_____	1
	Month?	_____	1
2. Where are we?	State?	_____	1
	County?	_____	1
	Town or city?	_____	1
	Hospital?	_____	1
	Floor?	_____	1

Registration
3. Name three objects, taking 1 second to say each. Then ask the patient to _____ 3
repeat all three after you have said them.
Give one point for each correct answer. Repeat the answers until patient
learns all three.

Attention and calculation
4. Serial sevens. Give one point for each correct answer. Stop after five _____ 5
answers. Alternate: Spell WORLD backward.

Recall
5. Ask for names of three objects learned in question 3. Give one point for _____ 3
each correct answer.

Language
6. Point to a pencil and a watch. Have the patient name them as you point. _____ 2
7. Have the patient repeat "No ifs, ands, or buts." _____ 1
8. Have the patient follow a three-stage command: "Take a paper in your _____ 3
right hand. Fold the paper in half. Put the paper on the floor."
9. Have the patient read and obey the following: "CLOSE YOUR EYES." _____ 1
(Write it in large letters.)
10. Have the patient write a sentence of his or her choice. (The sentence _____ 1
should contain a subject and an object and should make sense. Ignore
spelling errors when scoring.)
11. Have the patient copy the design. (Give one point if all sides and angles _____ 1
are preserved and if the intersecting sides form a quadrangle.)

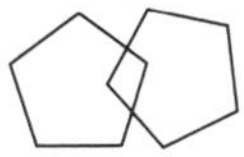

_____ 1

_____ = Total 30

Figure 7.3. Mini-Mental State Examination (MMSE). In validation studies using a cut-off score of 23 or below, MMSE has a sensitivity of 87%, a specificity of 82%, and a false positive ratio of 4.7%. These ratios refer to the capacity of the MMSE to accurately distinguish patients with clinically diagnosed dementia or delirium from patients without these syndromes. From Folstein MF, Folstein SE, McHugh PR. "Mini-mental state": a practical method for grading the cognitive state of patients for the clinician. J Psychiatric Res 1975;12:189–198.

instruments are the short portable mental status questionnaire (5) and the Folstein mini-mental status examination (6) (Fig. 7.3). Both evaluate the patient's memory, attention, and orientation. They are easy to administer and only require a few minutes of the clinician's time.

Elderly patients often have symptoms of depression. These symptoms may be significantly disabling depending on their severity and duration. Symptoms are often undetected, and use of stan-

dardized instruments may help to identify these patients and thus initiate appropriate treatment. The Beck Depression Inventory (7) and Zung Self-Rating Depression Scale (8) are two such instruments. They are both brief and simple to administer. The geriatric depression scale (9) (Fig. 7.4), another self-assessment tool, was designed particularly for the elderly.

Physical functional disability is common among the elderly. Several scales to measure the ability of

Choose the best answer for how you felt over the past week.
1. Are you basically satisfied with your life?   yes/no
2. Have you dropped many of your activities and interests?   yes/no
3. Do you feel that your life is empty?   yes/no
4. Do you often get bored?   yes/no
5. Are you in good spirits most of the time?   yes/no
6. Are you afraid that something bad is going to happen to you?   yes/no
7. Do you feel happy most of the time?   yes/no
8. Do you often feel helpless?   yes/no
9. Do you prefer to stay at home, rather than going out and doing new things?   yes/no
10. Do you feel you have more problems with memory than most?   yes/no
11. Do you think it is wonderful to be alive now?   yes/no
12. Do you feel pretty worthless the way you are now?   yes/no
13. Do you feel full of energy?   yes/no
14. Do you feel that your situation is hopeless?   yes/no
15. Do you think that most people are better off than you are?   yes/no

This is the scoring for the scale. One point for each of these answers. Cut-off: normal (0–5), above 5 suggests
depression.

1. no	6. yes	11. no
2. yes	7. no	12. yes
3. yes	8. yes	13. no
4. yes	9. yes	14. yes
5. no	10. yes	15. yes

Figure 7.4. Geriatric Depression Scale (short form). From Sheikh JI, Yesavage JA. Geriatric depression scale: recent evidence and development of a shorter version. Clin Gerontol 1986;5:165–172.

patients to care for themselves have been designed. These assessment instruments are used to describe baseline function of patients and are also useful to help determine the patient's need for regular daily assistance with basic functions such as using the toilet, dressing, eating, and walking. The Katz Activities of Daily Living Scale (ADL) (10) (Fig. 7.5) is one of the original instruments developed to measure function of basic ADLs. The Intermediate ADL Scale (11) (Fig. 7.6) and Older American Resources and Services (OARS) Multidimensional Function Assessment Questionnaire (12) are instruments most frequently used in clinical practice to supplement information on basic ADLs and focus on the more complex activities required for independent living in the community.

ISSUES IN PREVENTIVE GERIATRICS

Recommendations concerning health maintenance and prevention of illness for the general adult population have been discussed in Chapter 3. Special issues concerning recommendations and strategies for health promotion in the elderly will be discussed briefly. The United States Preventive Services Task Force was formed in 1984 to evaluate the effectiveness of clinical preventive services (13). The Canadian Task Force on the Periodic Health Examina-

tion also studied the efficacy of various preventive services (14). Their work has resulted in recommendations that can be categorized as either primary, secondary, or tertiary preventive measures.

Primary prevention refers to interventions in asymptomatic adults such as counseling about risk reduction and immunizations. Recommendations have been made to obtain a complete history of tobacco, alcohol, and drug use in the elderly, educate the patient regarding health effects of these habits, and offer counseling for cessation. Given the high prevalence of unintentional injury among the elderly, recommendations have been made to routinely discuss accident prevention strategies and the importance of the regular use of seat belts.

Recommendations have been made to counsel older persons on the importance of regular physical activity. Regular counseling regarding the patient's intake of calories, fiber, fat, and cholesterol should also be offered to the elderly patient. Patients should receive a diet and exercise prescription that have been designed to achieve and maintain ideal weight. Dietary guidelines should emphasize the reduction of total fat to less than 30% of calories and cholesterol to less than 300 mg/day.

Secondary prevention refers to strategies to improve outcomes in patients with existing but preclinical disease. Screening for disease is the major element of this form of prevention. The annual

Name _____ Day of evaluation _____

For each area of functioning listed below, check description that applies. (The word "assistance" means supervision, direction, or personal assistance.)

Bathing—either sponge bath, tub bath, or shower

☐	☐	☐
Receives no assistance (gets in and out of tub by self, if tub is usual means of bathing)	Receives assistance in bathing only one part of the body (such as back or a leg)	Receives assistance in bathing more than one part of the body (or not bathed)

Dressing—gets clothes from closets and drawers (including underclothes and outer garments) and uses fasteners (including braces, if worn)

☐	☐	☐
Gets clothes and gets completely dressed without assistance	Gets clothes and gets dressed without assistance, except for tying shoes	Receives assistance in getting clothes or in getting dressed or stays partly or completely undressed

Toilet—going to the "toilet room" for bowel and urine elimination; cleaning self after elimination and arranging cloths

☐	☐	☐
Goes to "toilet room," cleans self, and arranges clothes without assistance (may use object for support such as cane, walker, or wheelchair and may manage night bedpan or commode, emptying same in morning)	Receives assistance in going to "toilet room" or in cleansing self or in arranging clothes after elimination or in use of night bedpan or commode	Does not go to "toilet room" for the elimination process

Transfer

☐	☐	☐
Moves in and out of bed as well as in and out of chair without assistance (may be using object for support, such as cane or walker)	Moves in and out of bed or chair with assistance	Does not get out of bed

Continence

☐	☐	☐
Controls urination and bowel movement completely by self	Has occasional "accidents"	Supervision helps keep urine or bowel control, catheter is used, or person is incontinent

Feeding

☐	☐	☐
Feeds self without assistance	Feeds self except for getting assistance in cutting meat or buttering bread	Receives assistance in feeding or is fed partly or completely by using tubes or intravenous fluids

Figure 7.5. Activities of Daily Living Scale: evaluation form. From Reference 10.

screening for visual and auditory impairment as well as the measurement of thyroid function every 2–3 years has been recommended for the geriatric patient. In addition, it has been advised that a Mantoux skin test for detection of tuberculosis be performed on all elderly persons who are at increased risk, including those who live in nursing homes or other institutionalized settings and those with impaired cell-mediated immunity.

Tertiary prevention refers to strategies to pre-vent the progression of disease through identification, treatment, and rehabilitation. This form of prevention is felt to be particularly useful in the elderly, who often fail to seek medical care for common sources of disability. Thus, the clinician must remain particularly alert for conditions such as depression and sensory deprivation, functional decline, misuse of medications, and incontinence.

In many instances a seemingly modest improvement in disease may result in a significant improve-

1. Can you use the telephone _____ ?
   without help   3
   with some help   2
   completely unable to use the telephone   1
2. Can you get to places out of walking distance _____ ?
   without help   3
   with some help   2
   completely unable to travel unless special arrangements are made   1
3. Can you go shopping for groceries _____ ?
   without help   3
   with some help   2
   completely unable to do any shopping   1
4. Can you prepare your own meals _____ ?
   without help   3
   with some help   2
   completely unable to prepare any meals   1
5. Can you do your own housework _____ ?
   without help   3
   with some help   2
   completely unable to do any housework   1
6. Can you do your own "handyman" work _____ ?
   without help   3
   with some help   2
   completely unable to do any "handyman" work   1
7. Can you do your own laundry _____ ?
   without help   3
   with some help   2
   completely unable to do any laundry at all   1
8. Do you take medicines or use any medications?
   yes (answer question a)   1
   no (answer question b)   2
      a. Do you take your own medicine _____ ?
         without help (in the right doses at the right time)   3
         with some help (if someone prepares it and/or reminds you)   2
         (are you/would you be) completely unable to take your own medicine   1
      b. If you had to take medicine, can you do it _____ ?
         without help (in the right doses at the right time)   3
         with some help (take medicine if someone prepared it and/or reminds you)   2
         (are you/would you be) completely unable to take your own medicine   1
9. Can you manage your own money _____ ?
   without help   3
   with some help   2
   completely unable to handle money   1

Figure 7.6. Instrumental activities of daily living scale: self-rated version extracted from the multilevel assessment instrument. From Reference 11.

ment in the geriatric patient's functional status and quality of life. Thus, with the appropriate use of preventive care the clinician can hope to extend life and, perhaps more importantly for the patient, delay the onset of functional disability.

REFERENCES

1. Rogers RG, Rogers A, Belanger A. Active life among the elderly in the United States: multistage life-table estimates and population projections. Millbank Q 1989;67:370–379.
2. Hazzard WR, Bierman EL, Blass JP, Ettinger WH,

Halter JB. Principles of geriatric medicine and gerontology, 3rd ed. New York: McGraw-Hill, 1994.
3. Beck JC. Geriatrics review syllabus, a core curriculum in geriatric medicine, 1991–1992 edition. New York: American Geriatrics Society, 1991:50–51.
4. Applegate WB, Blass JP, Williams TF: Instruments for the functional assessments of older patients. N Engl J Med 1990;322:1207–1213.
5. Pfeiffer E. A short portable mental status questionnaire for the assessment of organic brain deficit in elderly patients. J Am Geriatr Soc 1975;26:433–441.
6. Folstein MF, Folstein SE, McHugh PR. "Mini-mental state": a practical method for grading the cognitive

state of patients for the clinician. J Psychiatr Res 1975;12:189–198.

7. Beck AT, Ward CH, Mendelson M, Mock J, Erbaugh J. An inventory for measuring depression. Arch Gen Psychiatry 1961;4:561–571.

8. Zung WWK. A self-rating depression scale. Arch Gen Psychiatry 1965;12:63–70.

9. Sheikh JI, Yesavage JA. Geriatric depression scale: recent evidence and development of a shorter version. Clin Gerontol 1986;5:165–172.

10. Katz S, Ford AB, Moskowitz RW, Jackson BA, Jaffee MW. Studies of illness in the aged the index of ADL: a standardized measure of biological and psychosocial function. JAMA 1963;185:914–919.

11. Lawton MP, Brody EM. Assessment of older people; self-maintaining and instrumental activities of daily living. Gerontologist 1969;9:179–185.

12. Multidimensional functional assessment: the OARS methodology. Durham NC: Duke University Center for the Study of Aging and Human Development, 1978.

13. United States Preventive Services Task Force. The periodic health examination of older adults: the recommendations of the U.S. preventive services task force. J Am Geriatr Sci 1990;38:817–823.

14. Canadian task force on the periodic health examination: the periodic health examination. Can Med Assoc J 1979;121:1213–1254.

chapter 8

HIV INFECTED PATIENTS
Elizabeth Jenny-Avital

Infection with the human immunodeficiency virus (HIV) results in progressive widespread immunologic dysfunction typically occurring over several years. AIDS is the clinical expression of the most severe immunosuppression that ultimately supervenes. AIDS is characterized by the occurrence of opportunistic infections, certain malignancies, marked CD4 helper lymphocyte (CD4 cell) population decline, and various other HIV related conditions.

The care of the HIV infected individual depends on the stage of infection. Early in infection, the HIV specific goals of primary care are identifying the asymptomatic patient, educating him or her about the means of HIV transmission, eradicating conditions and behaviors that favor viral transmission, and instituting measures that reduce viral replication. Later, when AIDS supervenes, prophylaxis, diagnosis, and treatment of opportunistic complications are additional goals. Supportive and compassionate care, always essential, becomes paramount in dying patients for whom palliation of symptoms is the goal.

Epidemiology

In the United States, the earliest cases of AIDS were identified among male homosexuals in 1981 and later among injecting drug users and recipients of blood products. As such, these attributes were identified as risk factors for AIDS and suggested that AIDS was caused by a transmissible agent. Ultimately, the causative agent, HIV, and the means of transmission were identified. HIV is transmitted sexually by HIV infected semen and cervicovaginal secretions, parenterally by HIV infected blood, blood products, or other infected body fluids, and from mother to child during pregnancy, childbirth, and breastfeeding. Globally, heterosexual transmission is numerically most im-

portant and is the fastest growing component of the epidemic in the United States and Europe where male homosexuals and injecting drug users still constitute the first and second largest groups of HIV infected persons. Screening of blood products and organs for HIV since 1985 has virtually eliminated transfusion associated HIV in the United States.

A person's risk for HIV infection depends not only on his or her own risk behavior but also on the risk behavior of his or her sexual contacts. Although sexual promiscuity increases the opportunity for encountering HIV, the presence of genital ulcer disease, such as herpes, chancroid, and syphilis, appears to facilitate transmission. A particularly high prevalence of HIV infection is present in certain geographic regions, e.g., sub-Saharan Africa, parts of Southeast Asia (Thailand), and parts of South America and the Caribbean, and especially among prostitutes and their clients in these areas.

Pathophysiologic Correlation

Primary HIV infection results in an intense viremia that may be associated with a febrile illness occurring several weeks after infection. An intense immunologic response results in the clearance of viremia and coincides with the appearance of HIV antibodies and the disappearance of HIV p24 core antigen. The patient enters a clinically latent phase of the infection during which HIV virus is sequestered in lymphoid tissue where there is ongoing viral replication and during which progressive subclinical immunologic dysfunction ensues. Reverse transcribed viral RNA results in proviral DNA that integrates into the host genome in infected cells. Individuals may be entirely asymptomatic or may have minor clinical or laboratory abnormalities referable to HIV at this stage. Patients may transmit their infection with variable efficiency during all phases of infection, even during clinical latency.

Table 8.1.
AIDS Defining Conditions

Candidiasis: esophageal, tracheal, bronchial
Cervical cancer, invasive
Coccidiomycosis, extrapulmonary
Cryptococcus, extrapulmonary
Cryptosporidiosis, chronic intestinal (>1 month)
Cytomegalovirus retinitis or in a structure other than
    liver, spleen, and/or lymph nodes
Herpes simplex mucocutaneous ulceration of >1
    month
Histoplasmosis, disseminated, extrapulmonary
HIV encephalopathy
Isosporiasis, chronic, >1 month
Kaposi's sarcoma
Lymphoma: Burkitt's, immunoblastic, CNS
Mycobacterium avium complex or *M. kansasii*,
    extrapulmonary
Pneumocystis carinii pneumonia
Pneumonia, recurrent (two or more episodes in 1 year)
Progressive multifocal leukoencephalopathy
Salmonella bacteremia, recurrent
Toxoplasmosis, cerebral
Wasting syndrome caused by HIV

The onset of AIDS is defined by the occurrence of a CD4 cell count of <200/mm^3 (normal is around 1000/mm^3) or by the occurrence of certain indicator conditions in HIV seropositive persons (Table 8.1). Immunologically, advanced HIV infection results in impaired cell mediated immunity, impaired specific serologic antibody responses (B lymphocyte dysregulation), and abnormalities in monocytes and macrophages. Most opportunistic infections result from the markedly impaired cell mediated immunity.

The occurrence of many opportunistic infections appears to result from reactivation of quiescent infections acquired in the remote past. For example, toxoplasmosis and cytomegalovirus (CMV) infections almost invariably occur in patients who had preexisting antibody. Histoplasmosis and coccidiomycosis can occur in patients who have previously resided in areas endemic for these fungi. Diarrheal diseases are more common in homosexual men and in persons having resided in areas where diarrheal diseases are common. Cervical cancer and progressive multifocal leukoencephalopathy appear to be linked to preexisting human papilloma virus and papova (JC) virus infection, respectively. By contrast, *Pneumocystis carinii* pneumonia (PCP), and *Mycobacterium avium* complex (MAC) infections may result from envi-

ronmental acquisition of these fairly ubiquitous organisms or may represent reactivation disease. Tuberculosis may result from reactivation or recent acquisition.

Clinical and Laboratory Evaluation

The physical examination and laboratory evaluation of the patient with HIV infection are by necessity comprehensive. History focuses on past infections, current symptoms, and behaviors.

HISTORY

Any history of male homosexual sex, injection drug use, receipt of blood products before 1985, sexual promiscuity, sexually transmitted diseases or cervical dysplasia, sex with prostitutes, or sex with persons from geographic areas with a high prevalence of HIV should prompt consideration of HIV infection. Certainly any history of an opportunistic infection should suggest HIV infection as should certain conditions that occur especially in HIV infected persons, e.g., tuberculosis, dermatomal herpes zoster in a young person, immune thrombocytopenia, demyelinating neuropathies including Guillain-Barre syndrome, nephrotic syndrome, cardiomyopathy, recurrent bacterial infections (sinusitis, pneumonia, soft tissue), new onset or exacerbation of skin disease and, in patients with advanced HIV infection, persistent fever, weight loss, prolonged diarrhea, or dementia.

Other important elements are those suggesting prior exposure to pathogens that might reactivate. Patients should be questioned about travel history (to areas endemic for opportunistic fungi, diarrheal diseases, and/or tuberculosis); history of tuberculosis, exposure to tuberculosis, prior tuberculin testing or residence in a congregate facility, prison, or shelter; history of sexually transmitted disease and any treatment (particularly for syphilis); and history of jaundice or hepatitis (prior hepatitis B or C infection).

PHYSICAL EXAMINATION

Characteristic findings on physical examination that might suggest HIV infection depend on the stage of infection. "Healthy" asymptomatic patients with a high CD4 count (>500/mm^3) would likely have generalized symmetric, painless, firm, rubbery lymphadenopathy and an otherwise normal exam. The physical examination remains fairly normal in asymptomatic patients with CD4 cell counts in the 200–500/mm^3 range, and in this group the generalized lymphadenopathy regresses as lymphoid depletion ensues. When patients have significant immunodeficiency (AIDS, CD4 <200/mm³) physical findings will be related to the various opportunistic conditions described under "Laboratory Evaluation." Nonspecific physical findings such as wasting, diffuse hyperpigmentation, hair loss, dry skin, long eyelashes, pallor, hepatosplenomegaly, linear hyperpigmentation along the axis of the fingernails, psychomotor slowing, lower extremity sensory peripheral neuropathy, and various skin disorders including seborrheic dermatitis, atypical and nonhealing herpes lesions, and pustular folliculitis can be seen in patients with advanced HIV disease. All patients should be carefully examined for sexually transmitted diseases because many can be easily treated.

LABORATORY EVALUATION

Serologic confirmation of suspected HIV infection is accomplished with an enzyme immunoassay (99% sensitive, 95–99% specific). A reactive enzyme immunoassay is confirmed with a more specific Western blot test. Other tests, e.g., those for core p24 antigen or for HIV nucleic acid by polymerase chain reaction, can be done in special circumstances such as in primary infection, before the antibody response, or in neonates in whom passively acquired HIV antibody does not prove congenital infection. Once HIV infection is ascertained, the CD4 count should be measured. The decrement in CD4 count roughly correlates with the patient's level of immune suppression and is the clinician's best "surrogate marker" for use in decision making.

Patients should further have a complete blood count and automated chemistry panel. Hematologic abnormalities such as anemia, leukopenia, and neutropenia are common, increasing in prevalence and severity with more advanced HIV infection. Immune thrombocytopenia may be seen in all stages of HIV infection and typically has a benign course. Pancytopenia suggests a disseminated opportunistic infection (fungal, mycobacterial) or lymphoma. An elevated globulin-to-albumin ratio can be seen at all stages of disease, reflecting B lymphocyte dysfunction. Cholesterol levels decline in tandem with immunosuppression. Triglycerides may be elevated. Renal function is typically normal except with HIV nephropathy. Electrolyte and liver chemistry abnormalities are referable to opportunistic infections, medications, malnutrition, and chronic liver disease.

Other elements in the initial laboratory evaluation include chest x-ray (looking for evidence of old tuberculosis), serology for diseases that may reactivate (toxoplasmosis, CMV, syphilis, hepatitis B and C), urine analysis for asymptomatic proteinuria, cervical cytology, and a tuberculin test placed concurrently with a panel of common recall antigens (anergy panel).

Differential Diagnosis

Differential diagnoses for HIV positive patients presenting with various symptom complexes are discussed in this section. Pulmonary, central nervous system (CNS), gastrointestinal, and skin disease are reviewed. A short section about fever is also included.

PULMONARY COMPLAINTS

Possible diagnoses include bacterial pneumonia, PCP, pulmonary tuberculosis, fungal pneumonia, and pulmonary involvement by lymphoma or Kaposi's sarcoma.

Bacterial pneumonias in HIV positive patients present similarly as in other patients and are more often accompanied by bacteremia. Common pathogens are pneumococcus and *Haemophilus influenzae*. *Pseudomonas aeruginosa* is seen in patients with advanced disease, possibly reflecting bacterial selection from chronic antibiotic use. Patients present with pleuritic chest pain, purulent sputum, fever, segmental consolidation on chest x-ray, pleural effusion (variable), and a relative leukocytosis. These may occur at all stages of HIV disease and may occur repeatedly in patients with advanced HIV disease—especially those with underlying chronic lung disease.

PCP typically occurs in patients with CD4 counts of <200/mm³ who are not on effective PCP prophylaxis. PCP is a common AIDS defining diagnosis in patients not previously known to be HIV positive. The dominant symptom of PCP is dyspnea occurring over weeks that is associated with fever, anorexia, dry cough, and fatigue. Purulent sputum and pleuritic chest pain are so unusual that they suggest another diagnosis. The chest x-ray shows interstitial infiltrates, usually diffuse and typically without hilar lymphadenopathy or pleural effusion. Hypoxemia, elevated lactic acid dehydrogenase, and a normal white blood cell count are usual. Diagnosis is made by identifying the organisms in bronchoalveolar lavage fluid on lung biopsy or in saline induced sputa.

Tuberculosis may present as a pulmonary disease with cough, sputum, and chest pain or as a nonspecific febrile illness with anemia and weight loss. It is thought that typical cavitary upper lobe reactivation disease occurs in patients with higher CD4 counts and that patients with lower CD4 counts present with nonspecific pulmonary infiltrates and/or mediastinal/hilar lymphadenopathy or with normal chest x-rays. In these latter patients, sputum AFB smears are typically negative, but cultures are positive.

Fungal infections caused by *Histoplasma capsulatum* and *Cryptococcus neoformans* may present as a febrile illness with a markedly abnormal chest x-ray, with diffuse reticulonodular infiltrates, possibly with lymphadenopathy, but with less prominent pulmonary complaints than with PCP. High lactic acid dehydrogenase is common, causing confusion with PCP. Serum cryptococcal antigen and urinary Histoplasma antigen are useful, sensitive, and specific tests. Histology with culture are diagnostic. Disseminated histoplasmosis, which may present as a nonspecific febrile illness with pancytopenia and positive blood cultures, occurs in HIV positive patients with CD4 counts of <100/mm^3 who reside in or have resided in endemic areas. Isolator tubes may facilitate blood culture isolation of fungi, and Wright stained buffy coat of peripheral blood may reveal intraleukocytic fungi. In patients with advanced HIV disease, Aspergillus may cause cavitary lesions that resemble those seen in reactivation tuberculosis.

Kaposi's sarcoma may involve the lungs, resulting in endobronchial lesions, parenchymal lesions visible as nodular infiltrates on chest x-ray, and/or pleural effusion, usually hemorrhagic. Dyspnea may be pronounced. Diagnosis is by gross visualization of lesions on bronchoscopy, biopsy, or presumptive in the setting of widespread mucocutaneous Kaposi's sarcoma.

Dyspnea associated with a normal chest x-ray and without fever should suggest an acute drop in hematocrit. This is somewhat frequent because commonly used drugs in AIDS may cause anemia.

CENTRAL NERVOUS SYSTEM DISEASE AND NEUROLOGIC COMPLAINTS

Relevant diagnoses are toxoplasmosis, cryptococcosis, CNS lymphoma, progressive multifocal leukoencephalopathy, AIDS dementia complex, AIDS encephalopathy, and other fungal, tuberculous, or bacterial meningitides or abscesses. Patients who present with focal neurologic signs, symptoms of elevated intracranial pressure (nausea, vomiting, and/or papilledema), or a change in mental state

should be evaluated with a neuroimaging study such as computed tomography or with magnetic resonance imaging. CNS toxoplasmosis is the most common CNS mass lesion in AIDS patients, typically occurring in toxoplasma seropositive (IgG) persons with CD4 cell counts of <100/mm^3. Computed tomography typically shows multiple lesions with peripheral enhancement with iodine contrast that involve the basal ganglia. Magnetic resonance imaging may demonstrate lesions not visible on computed tomography.

Cryptococcal meningitis typically presents with fever and dull headache. Altered sensorium, photophobia, and meningismus are less common. Elevated intracranial pressure is fairly common and requires aggressive cerebrospinal fluid (CSF) drainage. CSF cell counts and chemistry are often unremarkable. Cryptococcal disease occurs in AIDS patients with CD4 counts of <100/mm^3. Cryptococcal disease may present as fungemia, pneumonitis, skin disease, or prostatitis but presents most commonly (80%) as meningitis. Diagnosis is by identification of the organism in culture in the relevant body fluid. A rapid presumptive diagnosis can be made based on a positive india ink preparation of CSF (one drop each of CSF and india ink demonstrating budding yeast on microscopy) and/or a positive test for cryptococcal polysaccharide antigen in blood or CSF.

Progressive multifocal leukoencephalopathy is a demyelinating disease of cerebral white matter characterized by multiple discrete foci of disease visible on computed tomography scan as noncontrast enhancing low density lesions of periventricular white matter that are not associated with mass effect or edema. Patients typically present subacutely with symptoms of headache, ataxia, hemiparesis, or confusion. Most patients with progressive multifocal leukoencephalopathy are diagnosed late in their HIV disease.

CNS non-Hodgkin's lymphoma is typically a manifestation of late HIV disease (CD4 <50/mm^3). Imaging studies typically reveal a single lesion, although multiple lesions are possible. There is no distinct pattern of contrast enhancement on computed tomography. Diagnosis is by biopsy.

Other infections (e.g., tuberculosis, cryptococcus, nocardia, or histoplasma) can occasionally cause inflammatory CNS lesions that require biopsy for diagnosis except perhaps in the setting of widely disseminated documented disease where specific therapy results in a rapid clinical response of the CNS lesions.

HIV encephalopathy or AIDS dementia complex can occur when HIV infects the brain. It is seen in 15–20% of AIDS patients, typically with advanced immunodeficiency. Early symptoms are memory loss, impaired concentration, and mental slowness. Late HIV encephalopathy is characterized by marked cognitive abnormalities, profound psychomotor retardation, memory loss, and behavioral change. Imaging studies generally reveal cerebral atrophy. Spinal fluid shows normal glucose, slightly elevated protein, and perhaps a mild pleocytosis.

Symptomatic ocular disease is most commonly caused by CMV that results in a hemorrhagic exudative retinitis in patients with CD4 counts of <50/mm^3. Symptoms include floaters and blurring that progress to painless visual loss. Diagnosis is based on the characteristic appearance of the retina when examined by an ophthalmologist. Treatment is effective in halting disease progression.

The peripheral nervous system is affected in 20–40% of AIDS patients. The most common peripheral neuropathy is a distal, axonal, predominantly sensory neuropathy and typically occurs in late HIV infection. Patients complain of chronic, painful, symmetric dysesthesia in a stocking distribution especially on the soles. Absent ankle jerks are common. An identical peripheral neuropathy can result from didanosine, zalcitabine, isoniazid, and dapsone.

GASTROINTESTINAL COMPLAINTS

Common problems in the oral cavity include oral thrush (pseudomembranous candidiasis), which is characterized by an uncomfortable cheese-like exudate on the buccal mucosa or soft palate; oral hairy leukoplakia, characterized by painless raised white lesions on the tongue; and painful oral ulcers caused by herpes simplex, medications, or idiopathic aphthous ulcers. Esophageal disease is caused by the same pathogens as oral disease. Esophageal *Candida* infection causes dysphagia, often described as "sticking in the chest." Esophageal ulcer disease requires biopsy for diagnosis.

Important gut pathogens can be associated with small bowel symptoms (bloating, nausea, cramping, malabsorption, profuse diarrhea) or large bowel symptoms (lower quadrant pain and cramping, urgency, tenesmus, and/or bloody or purulent stools), and they can be categorized as invasive or superficial. Fecal leukocytes suggest an invasive pathogen. Noninvasive evaluation should include bacterial culture of stool for enteric pathogens (Salmonella, Shigella, or Campylobacter, which are associated

with acute diarrhea and fever), multiple specimens for analysis for ova and parasites (Cryptosporidium, *Isospora belli*, and microsporidia, which are small bowel noninvasive pathogens associated with voluminous diarrhea without fever; *Entamoeba histolytica*, which is associated with bloody diarrhea and fever; Giardia, which is noninvasive upper tract pathogen associated with abdominal pain and diarrhea), and an assay for *Clostridium difficile* toxin in stool (antibiotic associated pseudomembranous colitis). Giardia and amoebae cause illness at any stage of HIV infection and are associated with usual risk factors such as sexual practices and travel. Cryptosporidium, Isospora, and microsporidia are causes of refractory diarrhea in patients with advanced HIV disease. Other pathogens may require invasive evaluation with upper and lower endoscopy for their demonstration. CMV and MAC can affect the gastrointestinal tract in patients with low CD4 cell counts (<50/mm^3), typically resulting in colitis (CMV) and either small or large bowel infiltration (MAC). Proctocolitis may be associated with agents of sexually transmitted diseases, especially in homosexual men.

SKIN COMPLAINTS

Skin disorders are extremely common in HIV infected patients. Psoriasis and seborrheic dermatitis are more common in and can be exacerbated by HIV infection. Symptoms of xerosis and pruritus are also common. Other skin disorders include Kaposi's sarcoma, a multifocal neoplastic vascular lesion that can involve skin, mucous membranes, and visceral organs and is characterized by purple skin lesions often associated with edema; molluscum contagiosum, characterized by fleshy 2- to 5-mm umbilicated papules; eosinophilic pustular folliculitis consisting of urticarial follicular papules with characteristic histology; herpes simplex or zoster ulcerations that may be chronic and atypical in appearance; staphylococcal folliculitis; cutaneous lesions of disseminated fungal disease; fungal nail infections; and dermatomal herpes zoster. Cutaneous drug reactions are common in HIV infected patients, especially in association with sulfa drugs, penicillins, and other antibiotics and rarely in association with antiretrovirals or acyclovir.

FEBRILE SYNDROME WITHOUT LOCALIZING COMPLAINTS

Fever and constitutional symptoms without localizing symptoms should suggest a disseminated infection. Disseminated MAC may present in this manner in association with anemia, elevated alkaline phosphatase (reflecting liver infiltration), anorexia, and wasting. Disseminated MAC can be diagnosed on blood culture using special media or by culture of tissue biopsy (liver, bone marrow). MAC colonization in sputum or stool does not necessarily correlate with disseminated infection. Disseminated MAC is so common in HIV infected patients with a CD4 cell count of $<50/mm^3$ that prophylaxis is recommended although somewhat controversial. Disseminated fungal disease, Salmonella bacteremia, and disseminated tuberculosis are some infections that may present as a nonspecific febrile illness with wasting and anemia. Appropriate evaluation includes routine blood cultures, blood isolator tubes for fungus, blood culture for mycobacteria, serum cryptococcal antigen, urine histoplasma antigen, Wright stain of buffy coat looking for intraleukocytic organisms and induced sputum for tuberculosis.

Management

Routine management of HIV infected patients entails the use of antiretroviral agents to forestall the onset of HIV related immunodeficiency, the use of prophylactic antimicrobial agents to primarily prevent predictable opportunistic infections and to secondarily prevent relapses of opportunistic infections that have already occurred, and the use of agents to palliate various symptoms. Specific management is dictated by the stage of HIV infection.

All patients should be counselled regarding the mechanisms of HIV transmission. Patients should be instructed that the consistent and correct use of condoms dramatically reduces sexual transmission of HIV. Patients should be referred to services, e.g., drug treatment programs, that may assist in reducing high risk behavior. All patients should be screened for tuberculosis yearly, with tuberculin testing and with chest x-ray if they are anergic. Cervical cytology should be obtained in women every 6–12 months with further evaluation if there is dysplasia. Patients should have periodic determinations of blood count, chemistry, and CD4 cells: less frequently when they are well (CD4 $>500/mm^3$, every 6–12 months), more frequently when they are receiving antiretroviral therapy or are approaching a landmark CD4 count ($200/mm^3$) (CD4 $200–500/mm^3$, every 3 months), and most frequently (monthly) for symptomatic AIDS patients who are likely to be receiving multiple medications. Some authorities recommend immunization against pneumococcus, *Hemophilus influenza* B,

and hepatitis B based on the high frequency of these infections in HIV infected persons, although there is little evidence of benefit and there is a theoretical risk of HIV activation with immune stimulation. Seasonal influenza vaccine is also recommended.

ANTIRETROVIRAL TREATMENT

Despite the fact that HIV replication is a dynamic process throughout all stages of infection, beneficial effects of available therapy have so far only been conclusively demonstrated for patients with CD4 counts of $<500/mm^3$. Zidovudine (ZDV, Retrovir, AZT) was the first drug to show a survival advantage over placebo in a clinical 24-week trial in AIDS patients, thus leading to its initial approval for patients with CD4 counts of $<200/mm^3$. The use of ZDV at earlier stages of HIV disease (CD4 $200–500/mm^3$) has been shown to delay the onset of AIDS and to reduce various minor HIV related events. On this basis, the use of ZDV was later approved for use in patients with CD4 counts of $<500/mm^3$.

However, several studies have been interpreted as failing to show a survival advantage attributable to ZDV in patients with CD4 counts of $>200/mm^3$. There is controversy over that interpretation. ZDV, initiated after the first trimester of pregnancy, has been shown to reduce maternal-fetal transmission of HIV in women with CD4 counts of $>250/mm^3$. Other antiretroviral drugs developed later [ddI (didanosine, Videx), ddC (zalcitabine, Hivid), and d4T (stavudine, Zerit)] have been evaluated in comparison with ZDV. As initial therapy, ZDV remains the initial choice. However, changing to or adding a second agent may be appropriate in patients who have been on one agent for a period, especially when there is clinical deterioration or a drop in CD4 counts. Combination antiretroviral therapy shows more impressive improvements in surrogate markers of immune function; whether this translates into clinical and survival benefit remains to be proven.

General recommendations for therapy are as follows. For patients with CD4 counts of $>500/mm^3$, there is no compelling evidence favoring therapy other than intuitive belief that therapy makes sense; hence therapy should not routinely be prescribed. For patients with CD4 counts of $200–500/mm^3$, it should be explained to patients that monotherapy may forestall HIV related complications but will not necessarily change overall life expectancy. Patients may reasonably elect ther-

Table 8.2.
Antiretroviral Agents

Agent	Dosage/Formulation	Indication	Toxicity
Zidovudine (ZDV, Retrovir, AZT)	100-mg capsules 100 mg five times a day 200 mg TID 100 TID (dose reduction for toxicity)	CD4 <500/mm^3 delays onset of AIDS CD4 <200/mm^3 survival advantage HIV associated thrombocytopenia—may improve platelet counts; neurologic dysfunction—may improve HIV related cognitive dysfunction; reduces maternal-fetal transmission	(a) Transient, at initiation, gastrointestinal complaints, lassitude, fatigue, headache (b) Macrocytosis (predictable) (c) Hematologic toxicity (dose related) (more common in advanced HIV disease), anemia, leukopenia, neutropenia (d) Myopathy—characteristic histology—discontinue ZDV
Didanosine (ddl, Videx)	25-, 50-, 100-, 150-mg buffered tablets 167-, 250-mg sachets (powder) Tablets: 125 mg BID (<60 kg) 200 mg BID (>60 kg) 300 mg BID (>75 kg) Sachet: 167 mg BID (<60 kg) 250 mg BID (>60 kg) 375 mg BID (>75 kg) ddl must be administered 1 hr before meals or 2 hr after meals on an empty stomach because acid interferes with its absorption; regardless of dose, patients must always take two tablets to ingest proper amount of buffer; tablets must be thoroughly crushed or chewed; powder must be dissolved in water	Intolerant of ZDV initial treatment; delays disease progression after prior ZDV	(a) Unpleasant taste (b) Gastrointestinal symptoms (c) Peripheral neuropathy—can rechallenge with reduced dose (d) Hyperamylasemia (e) Pancreatitis—requires permanent drug discontinuation
Dideoxycytidine (ddC, Hivid)	0.75 mg TID 0.375 mg TID (dose reduction for toxicity)	Intolerance of ZDV and ddl; improved survival after prolonged ZDV therapy (>18 months)	(a) Transient, during initiation (1–4 weeks), fever, rash, aphthous ulcers (b) Peripheral neuropathy, reversible with drug withdrawal
Stavudine (d4T, Zerit)	30 mg BID (<60 kg) 40 mg BID (>60 kg) Tablets must be thoroughly crushed or chewed; powder must be dissolved in water	Intolerant of ZDV, ddl, ddC; progression of disease while on ZDV, ddl, ddC	(a) Peripheral neuropathy (b) Elevated hepatic transaminases (c) Pancreatitis (<1%)

TID, three times a day; BID, twice a day.

Table 8.3.
Primary and Secondary Prophylaxis of Selected Opportunistic Infections

Candidiasis

Secondary or as needed prophylaxis of oral *Candida* may be accomplished with topical nystatin suspension, swish and swallow 5–10 ml four times daily, or with clotrimazole troches five times a day. For esophageal *Candida* a systemic drug must be used: oral ketoconazole (200 mg/day) or fluconazole (50–200 mg/day). Achlorhydria impedes absorption of ketoconazole. Ketoconazole is more often associated with hepatitis. Intermittent intravenous amphotericin is used in azole refractory cases.

Coccidiomycosis

Primary prophylaxis is under investigation for patients with history of exposure. Secondary prophylaxis is with itraconazole 200 mg BID or weekly intravenous amphotericin 1 mg/kg. Fluconazole 400 mg/day is an alternative. Itraconazole can be associated with hypokalemia.

Cryptococcosis

Primary prophylaxis is not recommended. Secondary prophylaxis is with fluconazole 200–400 mg/day and is well tolerated. Itraconazole 200 mg/day or weekly intravenous amphotericin B (1 mg/kg) are alternatives. Infusion related side effects of amphotericin include fever, rigors, and phlebitis, and renal insufficiency associated with potassium and magnesium wasting occurs regularly.

Cryptosporidiosis

There is no standard treatment. Paromomycin 500–750 mg three to four times daily may work and could be used for prophylaxis.

Cytomegalovirus

Primary prophylaxis makes sense but is not recommended. Secondary prophylaxis for retinitis is standard and is also frequently necessary for gastrointestinal disease. Intravenous ganciclovir (5 mg/kg/day) or foscarnet (90–120 mg/kg/day, adjusted to renal function) is used. Their toxicities are hematologic (leukopenia and anemia) and renal (including potassium and magnesium wasting and infusion related hypocalcemia), respectively. Oral ganciclovir became available recently and appears to be a reasonable alternative to intravenous ganciclovir.

Herpes simplex

Acyclovir 200 mg three to four times daily can prevent recurrent herpes outbreaks and is well tolerated.

Histoplasmosis

Secondary prophylaxis is with itraconazole 200 mg twice daily or with intravenous amphotericin 50 mg weekly or biweekly; fluconazole 400 mg/day may be an alternative.

Isosporiasis

Secondary prophylaxis is with TMP/SXT double strength three times a week or with pyrimethamine 25 mg/day with folinic acid 5 mg/day.

Mycobacterium avium Complex

Primary prophylaxis with rifabutin 300 mg/day is recommended for patients with CD4 counts of <100/mm. Higher doses (450 mg/day) are associated with uveitis. Side effects may include thrombocytopenia, hepatitis, and leukopenia. Discolored urine (reddish-orange) occurs frequently. Clarithromycin 500 mg twice daily is a promising, possibly superior alternative. Its main side effect is gastrointestinal intolerance.

PCP

Primary prophylaxis is indicated for patients with CD4 cell counts of <200/mm^3. Secondary prophylaxis is recommended after an episode of PCP. TMP/SXT is the most effective agent. Dosage is one double strength tablet every day or every other day. Its toxicity is rash (frequent), possibly with fever, leukopenia, and hepatitis. Alternative agents are dapsone 100 mg/day (toxicity is anemia, methemoglobinemia, and hemolytic anemia in association with glucose-6-phosphate dehydrogenase deficiency) and aerosolized pentamidine 300 mg via nebulizer monthly (toxicity is wheezing and possibly dysglycemia and pancreatitis secondary to systemic absorption). The main problem with pentamidine is inadequate distribution of drug resulting in upper lobe breakthrough PCP. Other agents including atovaquone, periodic intravenous trimetrexate, and oral clindamycin-primaquine might be useful in some situations.

Salmonella Bacteremia

Secondary prophylaxis is recommended for patients with recurrence. Double strength TMP/SXT every day for sensitive strains accomplishes PCP prophylaxis at the same time. Ciprofloxacin 500 mg twice daily can also be used (according to the sensitivity of the isolate).

Table 8.3.—*continued*

Toxoplasmosis

Primary prophylaxis makes sense in *Toxoplasma* IgG seropositive persons but is not standard practice. TMP/SXT 1 double strength every day is effective. Secondary prophylaxis is mandatory, usually with whatever regimen induced remission of active disease. (Sulfadiazine 1 g four times daily or clindamycin 300 mg four times daily plus pyrimethamine 50 mg every day with folinic acid 10 mg/day). Both sulfadiazine and clindamycin are both associated with rashes. Sulfadiazine may also be associated with leukopenia and hepatitis. Clindamycin may be associated with pseudomembranous colitis. Pyrimethamine predictably results in neutropenia that can be prevented with adjunctive folinic acid.

apy or a wait-and-see approach of following their disease and instituting therapy based on clinical or laboratory parameters. For patients with CD4 counts of <200/mm³, it is reasonable to strongly encourage the use of ZDV as an initial agent followed by combination therapy or a change to an alternative agent when there is disease progression. Many authorities recommend the use of maintenance acyclovir (600–800 mg/day) in patients with a history of herpes because some data, both in vitro and observational, suggest that concurrent acyclovir with ZDV confers an additional survival advantage. For dosages, side effects, and indications for the various approved antiretroviral agents, see Table 8.2.

PROPHYLAXIS OF OPPORTUNISTIC INFECTIONS

An essential part of the management of HIV infected persons is the primary prophylaxis of predictable opportunistic infections and the chronic suppression or secondary prophylaxis of opportunistic infections that have already occurred. Some opportunistic infections are less opportunistic than others and occur at lower CD4 counts so that the institution of opportunistic infection prophylaxis may be stepwise as CD4 counts drop.

PCP prophylaxis is instituted at CD4 counts of <200/mm³. All patients are considered at risk. Prophylaxis has been shown to increase survival. Patients who take trimethoprim/sulfamethoxazole (TMP/SXT) daily virtually never get PCP. Other agents are not as reliable. MAC prophylaxis with rifabutin is recommended for CD4 counts of <100/mm³. This agent reduces the incidence of MAC bacteremia. Clarithromycin may prove to be a superior alternative. *Toxoplasma* antibody positive persons could conceivably benefit from primary prophylaxis at CD4 counts of <100/mm³, but this is not currently recommended. Interestingly, TMP/SXT used for PCP prophylaxis prevented CNS toxoplasmosis in some studies, making it an even better choice for PCP prophylaxis. CMV prophy-

laxis at CD4 cell counts of <50/mm³ likewise is a reasonable goal. Oral ganciclovir only became available in early 1995 and has not yet been studied for primary prophylaxis. Studies of other drugs for CMV prophylaxis have not resulted in a recommendation for prophylaxis. Patients with positive tuberculin reactions should receive at least 1 year of INH prophylaxis or another agent if their PPD reactivity can be ascribed to exposure to INH resistant tuberculosis.

Prophylaxis against systemic fungal infections is not routinely recommended. Chronic suppression of oral or esophageal *Candida* infections is optional because these infections are not life threatening. It is unresolved whether chronic therapy or intermittent therapy will be more likely associated with the selection of species resistant to antifungal agents. Prophylaxis against recurrent herpes with acyclovir may be appropriate because it may be associated with a survival advantage. Except for tuberculosis, there is uniform agreement that lifelong secondary prophylaxis or chronic suppression be maintained after an episode of opportunistic infection. See Table 8.3 for indications, dosages, and side effects of prophylactic agents.

TREATMENT OF OPPORTUNISTIC INFECTIONS

Specific treatment of opportunistic infections is reviewed in this section. As under "Differential Diagnoses," the organization of systems is pulmonary, nervous, and gastrointestinal followed by a short section about fever.

Pneumocystis Pneumonia. The most effective treatment for PCP, TMP/SXT (5 mg/kg every 8 hours, oral or intravenous), is complicated by an appreciable occurrence of side effects (rash, fever, leukopenia, and/or hepatitis). Alternative treatments include pentamidine (intravenous), trimetrexate (intravenous) with folinic acid, trimethoprim-dapsone (oral), atovaquone (oral), and clindamycin-primaquine (oral). Glucose-6-phosphate dehydrogenase deficiency should be excluded if primaquine or dapsone is used. Treatment is given for 14–21 days followed by lifelong prophylaxis. Adjunctive steroids are recommended for severe hypoxemia with the caveat that a definitive diagnosis be pursued because other pulmonary infections concurrent with or mistaken for PCP might be worsened.

Tuberculosis. Treatment of tuberculosis depends on the drug susceptibility of the isolate and regimens that do not contain rifampin and must be given for longer periods (at least 18 months) because of a higher risk of relapse. The issue of lifelong prophylaxis after treatment is unsettled; it is probably warranted when it is practical and when the patient developed tuberculosis in the setting of a low CD4 count ($<200/mm^3$).

Fungal Pneumonia. Treatment of fungal pneumonia with amphotericin B (intravenous) is followed by lifelong therapy with an oral azole: fluconazole for cryptococcus and itraconazole for Histoplasma. Oral azoles may be used as first line therapy in patients who are not gravely ill.

Central Nervous System Toxoplasmosis. In patients with typical neuroradiologic findings, positive *Toxoplasma* serology, and no other infection (e.g., tuberculosis, fungal, or Nocardia) or malignancy known to disseminate to the brain, a trial of empiric therapy for toxoplasmosis is warranted. A marked improvement, clinically and neuroradiologically, with therapy can be expected within 2 weeks and will be diagnostic for toxoplasmosis provided that neither steroids nor other therapies were used concurrently. Recommended treatment regimens are pyrimethamine with folinic acid plus either sulfadiazine or clindamycin (both are associated with a high rate of side effects). Alternative regimens include pyrimethamine with folinic acid plus either clarithromycin, atovaquone, azithromycin, or dapsone.

Cryptococcal Meningitis. Treatment is with amphotericin, possibly with 5-fluorocytosine. This treatment is followed by lifelong maintenance with oral fluconazole or periodic (usually weekly) intravenous amphotericin.

Other CNS Disease. Although there is no proven therapy for progressive multifocal leukoencephalopathy, there are reports of remission with high dose antiretrovirals and with intravenous cytarabine. Treatment of non-Hodgkin's lymphoma with radiation and/or steroids may significantly palliate symptoms.

Several studies have indicated that AIDS dementia complex responds favorably to ZDV and that a lower prevalence of AIDS dementia complex appears to be attributable to use of ZDV. Treatment of CMV retinitis is with ganciclovir (intravenous), foscarnet (intravenous), and possibly with scleral implants of ganciclovir. Maintenance therapy must be continued for life. Newly available oral ganciclovir may be a promising new alternative to intravenous therapy.

Gastrointestinal Infection. In general, dysphagia, especially if associated with oral thrush, merits an empiric trial with antifungal therapy with an oral azole (fluconazole, ketoconazole). If there is no resolution, a biopsy diagnosis should be pursued. Idiopathic aphthous ulcers may respond to steroid therapy or thalidomide (experimental in the United States). Ulcers caused by herpes can be treated with acyclovir. Oral Candida, without esophageal involvement, can be treated with topical antifungal agents such as nystatin liquid or clotrimazole troches.

Febrile Syndrome without Localizing Complaint. Rifabutin reduces the incidence of MAC bacteremia but does not necessarily improve survival. Clarithromycin may prove to be a better alternative.

ILLUSTRATIVE CASES WITH SELF-ASSESSMENT QUESTIONS AND ANSWERS

Case 1

C.H. is a 20-year-old Senegalese woman who comes to the emergency room during her 24th week of pregnancy complaining of 3 weeks of fever without localizing symptoms. She was previously admitted to another hospital for 2 weeks but left "because they did not do anything" for her. Her physical exam is unremarkable; her chest x-ray is difficult to interpret because of high diaphragms and crowding of vessels, but bilateral infiltrates are suggested. Her labs are remarkable for mild anemia (hemoglobin = 9.3).

QUESTION: *Why should you consider HIV infection?*

ANSWER: *ZDV in pregnancy reduces the risk of congenital HIV infection, so all pregnant women should be offered HIV testing and counseling, especially if they come from an area highly endemic for HIV (west Africa in this case) and if they present with a subacute febrile illness.*

QUESTION: *What is in your differential diagnosis?*

ANSWER: *Although the differential diagnosis is extremely broad, HIV testing might narrow it. The chronicity of her symptoms and the fact that her prior 2-week hospitalization did not result in definitive treatment suggests that she has an unusual pathogen or a complication of a usual pathogen (e.g., a renal abscess as a consequence of pregnancy associated pyelonephritis). Important considerations in an HIV positive African woman would be Salmonella bacteremia and tuberculosis, both of which could present as a fever without source. The suggestion of pulmonary involvement makes tuberculosis, PCP, and fungal diseases more of a consideration. As it turned out, a call to the previous hospital revealed that an AFB smear negative sputum specimen had grown M tuberculosis.*

Case 2

D.B. is a 34-year-old former injection drug user currently receiving methadone in a drug treatment program. He feels entirely well and even lifts weights. Routine labs at the program are normal except for a platelet count of 38,000 and an elevated protein-to-albumin ratio (8.9:3.9).

QUESTION: *What does this suggest?*

ANSWER: *Despite the patient's subjective well-being, the lab abnormalities and clear HIV risk factor are compatible with early HIV infection. Certainly other conditions, e.g., chronic liver disease, could also give these findings.*

QUESTION: *What do you do next?*

ANSWER: *Explain to the patient that part of the*

evaluation of his thrombocytopenia is an HIV test. You can further explain that if his decreased platelets are HIV related, he may not have bleeding problems and that ZDV can be involved in increasing his platelet count. Also, question the patient about medication and alcohol use.

Case 3

R.V. is a 42-year-old man presenting with a 3-week history of progressive exercise intolerance, fever, mild cough, and anorexia. His past medical history is remarkable for episodes of *Giardia* and amoebic dysentery that he ascribes to frequent vacations to Mexico and the Caribbean. His only medication is acyclovir as required for recurrent perirectal herpes. When questioned further about sexually transmitted diseases he indicates that he had gonorrhea many years ago. His physical exam reveals a well developed man in no distress with a respiratory rate of 30. His chest x-ray reveals a fine diffuse reticular interstitial infiltrate. His labs are remarkable for a normal white blood cell count and a lactic acid dehydrogenase of 432.

QUESTION: *Why should you consider HIV infection?*

ANSWER: *The patient has a history of sexually transmitted diseases (herpes and gonorrhea) and also gives a history of diarrheal diseases that can also be transmitted sexually by genital-rectal contact even though an explicit statement of homosexual sex as a risk factor was not elicited.*

QUESTION: *What is in your differential diagnosis?*

ANSWER: *For a patient without prior knowledge of HIV infection or a patient not on PCP prophylaxis, PCP is a common first AIDS defining occurrence, especially if the patient presents with dyspnea as the dominant complaint. Viral pneumonia, fungal pneumonia, tuberculosis, and bacterial pneumonia (less likely without an elevated white blood cell count and with diffuse infiltrate on x-ray) are also in the differential diagnosis. The next step would be an induced sputum or bronchoalveolar lavage.*

SUGGESTED READINGS

Chaisson RE, Volberding PA. Clinical manifestations of HIV infection. In: Mandell GL, Bennett JE, Dolin R, eds. Principles and practice of infectious diseases. New York: Churchill Livingstone, 1995;1:1217–1253.

Chamberland ME, Ward JW, Curran JW. Epidemiology and prevention of AIDS and HIV infection. In: Mandell GL, Bennett JE, Dolin R, eds. Principles and practice of infectious diseases. New York: Churchill Livingstone, 1995;1:1174–1202.

Sande MA, Volberding PA. The medical management of AIDS. Philadelphia: Saunders, 1995.

chapter 9

OCCUPATIONAL HEALTH ISSUES

David M. Ackman

Occupational exposures cause as many as 400,000 new cases of disabling illness each year in the United States and as many as 100,000 deaths, including more than 6000 deaths from injuries. Despite the importance of occupational disease, and the potential for preventing or limiting it by prompt medical diagnosis and intervention, most United States medical students have little or no instruction in occupational health (1). Because many occupational illnesses are clinically indistinguishable from other diseases and because many have a long latency between exposure and illness, they are often misdiagnosed. The terminology, epidemiology, and criteria for diagnosis of occupational disorders differs from diseases covered in preclinical courses. These factors make the relationship between diseases and the work place easy to overlook.

Nevertheless, there are important reasons for students to learn to take an occupational history, recognize common occupational disorders seen by primary care physicians, and understand the basic steps in managing occupational illnesses, including public health measures. First, because many physicians never ask about occupation or job duties, many occupational diseases are never recognized. Unlike most diseases, which are diagnosed on the basis of symptoms, physical findings, and tests, the diagnosis of an occupational disorder starts with a history of an appropriate exposure. For example, the early stages of byssinosis, a restrictive lung disease caused by inhalation of cotton dust, may be indistinguishable from intrinsic asthma on the basis of symptoms, physical findings, or pulmonary function tests. However, obtaining a history of employment in a cotton mill and finding a relation of symptoms to work schedule would suggest this occupational disorder. Second, only through an appreciation of occupational disorders can the primary care physician take advantage of interventions to prevent further exposure and illness. In the above

example, the primary intervention would be to eliminate exposure to plant fibers, either by changing jobs, modifying the manufacturing process, or using a personal respirator, not prescribing inhaled beta-agonists or steroids. Third, the diagnosis of one patient may be the first indication of a more widespread public health problem. The identification of a single case of byssinosis could prevent many additional cases by changing a manufacturing process, improving ventilation in the mill, or improving industrial hygiene.

This section reviews the basic elements of an occupational history, gives examples of common occupational disorders encountered by primary care providers, and introduces some important public health concepts for practicing clinicians. Students should be able to identify potential occupational and environmental exposures, understand the variable relationship between exposure and symptoms, and appreciate the importance of primary care physicians in identifying sentinel health events. Although environmental medicine (the relationship between toxins in the home or environment and disease) will not be addressed here, the general concepts of hazard identification and assessment apply equally to those exposures as well.

ELEMENTS OF AN OCCUPATIONAL HISTORY

The diagnosis of most occupational diseases depends on uncovering a pertinent exposure. While obtaining a complete occupational history, detailing all potential exposures to toxins, may take over an hour, the student should allow several minutes to cover the most important elements (Table 9.1). At a minimum, a student should obtain a history of current or most recent employment, past occupations, and the duties performed at those jobs. In the review of systems, students should ask about

Table 9.1.
Essentials of an Occupational History

Current occupation
  a. What do you do?
  b. How long have you been doing this job?
  c. Describe your work, including materials or
     agents you work with or are exposed to.
  d. Under what circumstances do you use protective
     equipment?

Other employment
  a. List your previous jobs, in reverse chronological
     order.
  b. List any part-time jobs, second jobs, or summer
     jobs.
  c. On any of these jobs did you work with or were
     you exposed to chemicals, fumes, or hazardous
     materials?

Military or wartime exposure (if applicable)

Symptoms or illnesses related to work
  a. Describe your symptoms in relation to work
     hours or schedule. Do your symptoms improve
     when you are away from work, or worsen when
     you return?
  b. Has anyone at work suffered the same or similar
     problems?
  c. Have you seen a physician at your job, and if
     so, have you learned what he or she thought
     was causing your problems?

Nonoccupational exposures that could be related to
illness or could be expected to produce problems
  a. Smoking. Do you smoke now or have you in the
     past? What do you smoke? About how many
     cigarettes do you smoke per day and for how
     long have you been smoking?
  b. Alcohol. Do you drink alcohol? (See also
     Chapter 10.)
  c. Geographic history. Did you ever live near a
     facility that could have contaminated the
     surrounding area (smelter, mine, plant)?
  d. Family exposure. Does anyone in your
     household work with hazardous materials?
  e. Hobbies. What are your hobbies? Are you
     exposed to any hazardous materials?

Modified and reproduced with permission from Rom WN, ed.
Environmental and occupational medicine. Boston: Little,
Brown, 1992.

any other history of exposure to dust, fumes, chemicals or other potential toxins, whether on the job or at home. Most importantly, the student should explore the relationship between the work place and the chief complaint. This relationship may not

be obvious to the patient. For example, a typist who just started a new job might not relate hand and finger pain to his or her work. Questions like, "Describe your symptoms in relation to your job," or, "Has anyone else at your job had similar problems?" may help focus a patient's attention on the relationship of work place activities or exposures to their illness. If the initial questions suggest an occupational exposure, more detailed questions should be asked about the use of protective devices (respirators, gloves), contact with specific chemicals, and activities that produce or worsen symptoms.

The student should not expect the occupational history to immediately lead to a diagnosis. The criteria for diagnosing an occupational disorder include demonstrating that the exposure or activity can cause the disease; the time, duration, and extent of exposure are consistent with the diagnosis; and no other condition more readily explains the patient's complaints and findings. Rather, the information collected should be used to generate hypotheses. Testing the hypothesis of the relatedness of work and disease requires information on the specific effects of chemicals or work place practices, latencies between exposure and disease, and additional tests, including biopsies. Information on toxic effects of chemicals is readily available from poison control centers or textbooks, and details on particular industrial practices are available from local or regional occupational medicine clinics, the Occupational Safety and Health Administration, or local health departments. Internists and general practitioners often need to consult with specialists in occupational medicine, and students should be comfortable doing so as well.

COMMON OCCUPATIONAL DISEASES

The National Center for Occupational Safety and Health has published a list of the 10 leading work-related diseases and injuries (Table 9.2). Others have published the leading problems that have been referred to occupational medicine clinics. There are no good data on the frequency of presentation of persons with occupational disorders to primary care clinicians. The disorders presented below were chosen either because of their prevalence (asbestosis, dermatoses), because of the potential for limiting exposure (occupational asthma), or because they are often sentinel health events (asthma, infections).

Table 9.2.
Ten Leading Work-Related Illnesses or Injuries

1. Occupational lung diseases: asbestosis, byssinosis, silicosis, coal worker's pneumoconiosis, lung cancer, occupational asthma
2. Musculoskeletal injuries
3. Occupational cancers (other than lung): leukemia, mesothelioma, cancers of the bladder, nose, and liver
4. Severe occupational traumatic injuries: amputations, fractures, eye loss, lacerations, and traumatic deaths
5. Cardiovascular diseases: hypertension, coronary artery disease, acute myocardial infarction
6. Disorders of reproduction: infertility, spontaneous abortion, teratogenesis
7. Neurotoxic disorders: peripheral neuropathy, toxic encephalitis, psychoses, extreme personality changes (exposure related)
8. Noise-induced loss of hearing
9. Dermatologic conditions: dermatosis, burns and scaldings, chemical burns, contusions and abrasions
10. Psychologic disorders: neuroses, personality disorders, alcoholism, drug dependency

Based on frequency of occurrence, severity, and preventability. Developed by the National Institute for Occupational Safety and Health.

Asbestos-Related Diseases

Asbestos is a ubiquitous material in American industry. It is used in the manufacture of asbestos-cement pipes in water systems, brake linings, textiles, insulating tiles, and paints and fillers. Millions of workers living today were exposed to asbestos, especially between 1940 and 1970. These people comprise a cohort at risk for the development of asbestosis (a restrictive lung disease characterized by dyspnea, reduced forced vital capacity and diffusing capacity, and hypoxemia), bronchogenic carcinoma, and malignant mesothelioma. Still, only 5% of all exposed workers will develop disease, usually after as much as 40 years. Asbestos-related disease is the most common cause of referral to occupational medicine clinics.

ASBESTOSIS

Patients presenting with chronic or exertional dyspnea should be questioned about a history of exposure to asbestos. Cough, sputum production, pleuritic chest pain, and inspiratory rales on physical exam are characteristic. Chest x-rays show sym-

metrical basilar opacities, often with pleural thickening, but in some patients the chest film is normal. Some asymptomatic patients are diagnosed by chest x-rays taken for another reason. Because asbestos was widely used, and because of the long latency between exposure and disease, the patient may not be aware of an exposure. Some occupations where exposure was common are insulators, pipe fitters, automobile workers, and demolition workers. Although there may be little to do for patients when they present with advanced disease, patients with early disease can be reassured that asbestosis is usually mild and slowly progressive.

BRONCHOGENIC CARCINOMA AND MALIGNANT MESOTHELIOMA

Asbestos exposure is related to pulmonary neoplasms. The effect of smoking and asbestos on the development of bronchogenic carcinoma is synergistic. Conversely the risk for malignant mesothelioma is almost totally related to asbestos exposure. The period between exposure and disease is up to 40 years.

Occupational Asthma

Patients with asthma make up a significant portion of a general medical practice. A conservative estimate is that 2% of these patients, and perhaps 15% of persons with adult onset asthma, have occupational asthma, defined as "variable air flow limitation caused by a specific agent in the work place" (3). The pathology of occupational asthma may be allergic (sensitization to a specific antigen with specific and nonspecific airway hyperresponsiveness) or nonallergic (caused by airway inflammatory or irritant effects). Because symptoms and pulmonary function tests cannot distinguish occupational from other types of asthma and because many occupations and hundreds of substances have been linked to asthma, eliciting a pattern of symptoms related to work or specific exposures is critical to the diagnosis. Some patients may improve after a few hours away from the work place, and others may not notice a change in symptoms until after a prolonged vacation. It is often helpful to ask whether coworkers have similar symptoms.

A recent Centers for Disease Control and Prevention (CDC) study found that a follow-up of individual case reports of occupational asthma identified many other unreported workers suffering from asthma and that many of the work places inspected had inadequate environmental controls or respiratory inspection programs (4). Most of the initial case reports came from physicians, demonstrating the importance and effect of correctly diagnosing and reporting one case of occupational asthma. Some states require the reporting of occupational asthma.

Occupational Dermatoses

Work-related dermatoses are the most common type of occupational disease. Most are due to direct contact with an irritant or allergen that can cause acute or chronic skin inflammation. The lesions usually resemble eczema and may be pruritic. Vesicles or bullae may occur, and photoallergic responses or postinflammatory depigmentation may occur at sites of injury. Some workers, particularly farmers, florists, fishermen, and other outdoor workers, are at risk for cutaneous infections.

In acute cases, the patient may identify the exposure, although many common chemicals, including soaps or detergents, are not considered irritants. Lesions may occur on exposed skin surfaces, under elastic clothing bands, or on surfaces touched by a gloved hand (face, neck). The student should look for these patterns and ask about the use of even common chemicals, particularly while doing housework or hobbies.

Infectious Diseases

Infections, once among the most common of occupational disorders, are now relatively rare because of effective vaccination and infection control measures in the animal and meat processing industries. Still, an occupational history may lead to the diagnosis of rare or unusual diseases, particularly zoonoses. For example, poultry workers, veterinarians, and bird handlers are at risk for psittacosis, which usually presents as an interstitial pneumonia. Brucellosis, an insidious infection characterized by fever, malaise, myalgias, and anorexia, still occurs in outbreaks among slaughterhouse workers. Most work-related infections are reportable to state health departments.

One industry where infections are still of major concern is health care. Clinicians are at increased risk for several potentially fatal infections, all of which are preventable by vaccination or proper infection control practices. In the late 1980s and early 1990s, several outbreaks of nosocomially transmitted tuberculosis demonstrated that transmission can readily occur in hospitals, particularly when patients with undiagnosed pulmonary disease are not isolated. The Centers for Disease Control and Prevention recommend that all patients with

Table 9.3.
Methods for Prevention of Nosocomial Infection

Wash hands
Employ universal precautions
Wear gloves, gowns, and masks as indicated
Isolate patients when necessary (e.g., early tuberculosis)
Vaccinate (e.g., Recombivax HB) high risk personnel
Treat presumptively (e.g., exposure to meningococcemia or needle stick exposure to viral hepatitis)

suspected tuberculosis be placed in a negative pressure, single bed respiratory isolation room pending diagnostic sputum examinations for tuberculosis. Health care workers are also at increased risk for blood-borne infections, including hepatitis B and C and human immunodeficiency virus (HIV). Vaccination (for hepatitis B) and practicing universal precautions, including washing hands and wearing gloves, can greatly reduce the risk to workers. In addition, proper infection control practices, particularly hand washing, also reduces the spread of pathogens between patients, a problem of growing concern given the emergence of antibiotic-resistant bacteria, especially vancomycin-resistant enterococcus. Table 9.3 lists recommended measures for health care workers to prevent nosocomial infection.

Sentinel Health Events

A sentinel health event is a preventable disease or death whose occurrence serves as a warning that the quality of therapeutic or preventive medical care may need improvement. In the field of occupational disease, a sentinel health disease is "an unnecessary disease, disability, or untimely death which is occupationally related and whose occurrence may (1) provide the impetus for epidemiologic or industrial hygiene studies; or (2) serve as a warning signal that materials substitution, engineering control, personal protection, or medical care may be required" (5). For example, health departments investigate all cases of elevated lead levels in workers to identify potentially dangerous work practices and prevent additional cases of lead poisoning. As important as it is for the physician to recognize an occupational disorder, the beneficial effect may be magnified by the opportunity to prevent additional disease among coworkers. Students should realize that any case of occupational illness may be only the tip of an iceberg but that prompt reporting and investigation can prevent additional cases. Although reporting requirements vary by state, most local or state health departments will accept and pursue reports of occupational disease.

ILLUSTRATIVE CASES

Case 1

R.S., a 26-year-old medical student, was completing her clinical clerkship when she developed fever, cough, and sputum production. After 1 month of ineffective treatment for bronchitis, she had a chest x-ray that showed an upper lobe cavity suggestive of pulmonary tuberculosis. After a positive sputum culture for *Mycobacterium tuberculosis*, she was treated and improved. The student health office required all third and fourth year students to undergo yearly tuberculin skin testing and found that six students, including four others from R's medicine rotation, were also recent convertors.

The student health office and infection control staff conducted an investigation to determine the cause of transmission. They found that all six students were working on ward 6B while patients with tuberculosis were admitted. An environmental assessment of the ventilation system showed that air vented from newly constructed isolation rooms was entering the house staff lounge where morning conferences were held.

This case shows that health care workers are at risk for occupational diseases, including tuberculosis, HIV infection, and hepatitis. Although vaccines, universal precautions for body fluid exposures, and environmental safeguards can greatly reduce the risk of nosocomial infections, lapses occur. The maintenance of an infection control program and regular tuberculin testing of all health care workers prevented additional cases of tuberculosis in this hospital. This case also demonstrates the importance of sentinel health events. Tuberculosis in one health care worker should prompt an investigation or review of regular surveillance records for evidence of possible work place exposures.

Case 2

G.D., a 41 year-old actor, presents complaining of 2 weeks of bilateral hand paresthesias and occasional pain. The symptoms occur over the distribution of the median nerve. He has a positive Phalen's sign (reproduction of symptoms with wrists maximally flexed). You diagnose carpal tunnel syndrome and prescribe nonsteroidal antiinflammatory drugs.

He returns 2 weeks later with no improvement in symptoms. On further history, you find that in the past month he has worked as a word processor. Adjustment of his work station, including a pad to extend his wrists while typing, leads to an improvement in symptoms.

This case illustrates that occupational disorders occur outside factories and heavy industries. The important exposure and relationship to the patient's symptoms were initially missed because of an incomplete occupational history. The clinician should ask about all current jobs, including part-time work.

REFERENCES

1. Burstein JM, Levy BS. The teaching of occupational health in US medical schools: little improvement in 9 years. Am J Public Health 1994;84:846–849.
2. National Institute for Occupational Safety and Health. Proposed national strategies for the prevention of leading work-related diseases and injuries. Association of Schools of Public Health, 1986.
3. Chan-Yeung M. Occupational asthma. Chest 1990; 98:148s–161s.
4. Reilly MJ, Rosenman KD, Watt FC, et al. Surveillance for occupational asthma—Michigan and New Jersey, 1988–1992. In: CDC Surveillance Summaries (June 10). MMWR 1994;43(SS-l):9–17.
5. Rutstein DD, Mullan RJ, Frazier TM, et al. Sentinel health events (occupational): a basis for physician recognition and public health surveillance. Am J Public Health 1983;73:1054–1062.

SUGGESTED READINGS

Cullen MR, Cherniack MG, Rosenstock L. Occupational medicine (parts I and II). N Engl J Med 1990;322:594–601, 675–683.

Division of Health Promotion and Disease Prevention, Institute of Medicine. Role of the primary care physician in occupational and environmental medicine. Washington DC: National Academy Press, 1988.

Goldman RH, Peters JM. The occupational and environmental health history. JAMA 1981;246:2831–2836.

LaDou J, ed. Occupational medicine. Norwalk: Appleton & Lange, 1990.

Landrigan PJ, Baker DB. Using occupational history to pinpoint the diagnosis. Geriatrics 1991;46:61–67.

McCunney RJ, ed. Handbook of occupational medicine. Boston: Little, Brown, 1988.

Rom WN, ed. Environmental and occupational medicine, 2nd ed. Boston: Little, Brown, 1992.

Rubenstein E. Occupational safety and health. In: Rubenstein E, Federman DD, eds. Scientific American medicine. New York: Scientific American, 1994.

chapter 10

AN APPROACH TO SUBSTANCE ABUSE
Joseph Conigliaro

Health professionals have reported a reluctance and an inability to properly diagnose and treat patients with substance abuse. This feeling of ineffectiveness has been well described for alcohol abuse but can be generalized to abuse of all substances and stems from four distinct impediments. First, clinicians feel they lack knowledge of the many varied manifestations and presentations of substance abuse and lack a general approach to detect such patients. Second, clinicians may possess certain attitudes and values about substance abuse that may interfere with the patient-clinician relationship. Third, substance abusing patients can be some of the most difficult patients encountered, at times exhibiting hostile, dependent, and anxious behaviors. They may be untruthful and misleading. Finally, substance abuse especially in its early presentations may not fit the traditional biomedical or psychosocial model of illness. These reasons may explain why the diagnosis and treatment of substance abusing patients have often been considered the domain of psychiatrists or specialists. The goal of this chapter is to heighten the awareness of the problem in general medicine as well as to present a clear and effective diagnostic and early treatment strategy.

The problem of substance abuse is staggering: 90% of United States adults drink or have drunk alcohol, and nearly 14% report a history of abuse or dependence. Up to 3 million Americans are regular users of cocaine, and more than 2 million use heroin. The health and social consequences of substance abuse are a major factor in hospital and emergency visits, sick days, and accidents. Trauma is increasingly associated with alcohol and cocaine use, usually of a greater severity and with a higher mortality. The economic burden of substance abuse is enormous in terms of health care costs and lost productivity.

Primary care clinicians are in a unique position

Table 10.1.
Commonly Abused Substances

alcohol
amphetamines (diet pills, stimulants)
caffeine
cocaine (crack)
hallucinogens (ergot, LSD)
benzodiazepines (Valium, Ativan)
barbiturates (secobarbital)
opioids (heroin, methadone, morphine, codeine)
cannabis (hashish)

to control this problem in its early stages. Patients suffering from substance abuse first present with minor medical problems. Because early treatment is simple, cheap, and more likely to be effective clinicians must be knowledgeable and comfortable with early diagnosis and intervention. Screening should be routinely performed at the initial evaluation and as an ongoing part of health care maintenance for all patients. Furthermore, recognize that the list of substances that can be abused should not be limited to alcohol and "street drugs" but should include over-the-counter and prescription medications as well (Table 10.1).

Pathophysiologic Correlation

Disorders involving substance abuse and dependence consist of a constellation of cognitive, behavioral, and physiologic symptoms that share certain features. Early diagnosis relies less on recognizing physical or chemical derangement and more on cognitive and behavioral symptoms. Therefore it is useful to approach the diagnosis of dependence and abuse from a psychosocial perspective.

Abuse and Dependence

The casual use of an illicit (or licit) substance becomes abuse when evidence of loss of control oc-

73

curs. Drug use becomes frequent and begins to interfere with other aspects of a person's life. The drug begins to be used in situations that are physically hazardous. Legal problems occur, and social and interpersonal relationships are adversely affected. When evidence of psychological and physical tolerance develops, the patient then becomes dependent. Physical tolerance develops as the patient requires more of the substance to achieve the same mood altering effect. If the substance is not consumed, physical withdrawal will occur. Loss of control in the use of the drug begins when the patient takes the drug in larger amounts or for longer periods. The patient makes frequent attempts to cut down. Life begins to revolve around the drug. The time and effort to obtain the drug and recover from its effect leave less time for work and leisure activities. This pattern of use escalates despite the patient's knowledge of these ill effects.

Clinical Evaluation

Upon presentation to the primary care clinician, substance abusers often complain of nonspecific problems, many of which do not follow logical pathophysiologic patterns. Many manifestations of abuse are behavioral rather than physical, so screening should be heavily based on the history and not on the physical exam or laboratory data. The physical exam and laboratory work-up should be reserved for confirmation of the diagnosis and a search for secondary manifestations.

HISTORY

During the routine history there are many clues that should be associated with a substance abuse problem. Complaints are vague and varied and include fatigue, insomnia, headaches, sexual problems, anorexia, and weight loss. There is frequently a history of multiple episodes of minor trauma. Physical symptoms include abdominal pain, nausea and vomiting, diarrhea, and palpitations. Psychologically, patients exhibit symptoms of anxiety, paranoia, depression, and changes in personality (Table 10.2). The social history may reveal current and/or past history of substance abuse.

PHYSICAL EXAMINATION

The physical exam can uncover much evidence about substance abuse, but the findings are generally nonspecific although many occur as later manifestations. In general the patient may be hypertensive with tachycardia or bradycardia. The skin may

Table 10.2.
Symptoms Associated with Substance Abuse

General
minor trauma
insomnia
fatigue
anorexia and weight loss

Skin
flushing
sweating
palmar erythema
ecchymoses

Cardiovascular
palpitations
chest pain

Gastrointestinal
dyspepsia
abdominal pain
nausea
vomiting
diarrhea

Genitourinary
impotence
spontaneous abortion
birth defects (fetal alcohol syndrome)

Neurologic
tingling of extremities
memory loss
headaches
confusion
hallucinations

reveal erythema of the palms, areas of previous injections, or old abscesses. The pupils can be pinpoint (heroin) or dilated (cocaine). Recent drinkers may have alcohol noticeable on their breath. A runny nose or engorged nasal mucosa may be evidence of recent use of intranasal cocaine. The musculoskeletal exam can reveal evidence of old trauma, e.g., prior fractures. The most common neurologic finding is tremulousness.

Differential Diagnosis

Because of the varied presentations and the need to screen for the early abuser, clinicians require a strategy for detection that does not simply rely on the patient's symptoms and physical findings. This strategy can be used for different substances of abuse. Screening is based on the history with confirmation from the physical exam and laboratory data.

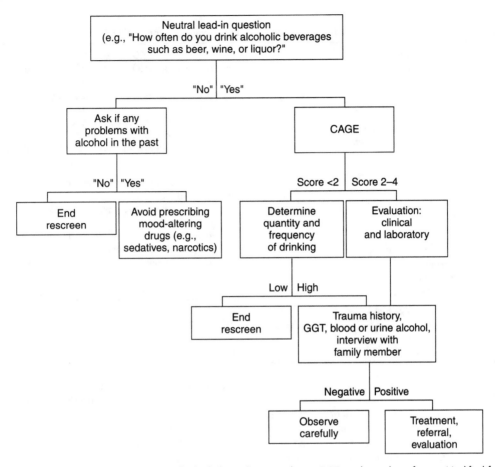

Figure 10.1. Approach to the patient with alcohol or substance abuse. GGT, γ-glutamyltransferase. Modified from National Institute of Alcohol Abuse and Alcoholism: 7th Special Report to the U.S. Congress on Alcohol and Health. Washington DC: Department of Health and Human Services, 1990:196 (DHHS publication no. ADM90-1656).

The clinician must possess a high index of suspicion when screening any patient for substance abuse. Difficult diagnoses, frequent vague complaints, and numerous episodes of minor medical or surgical problems are key signals of a problem and should prompt further inquiry. Providers must break the constraints that all historical information is obtained from the patient. Collateral data from family and friends are important sources of information. Evidence of the social morbidity (driving under the influence, divorce or separation, isolation, drug use among peers, etc.) associated with substance abuse aids in the diagnosis.

A general approach to addressing the problem of drugs and alcohol abuse is offered in Figure 10.1. The example is outlined for alcohol, but it can be modified for other substances including caffeine and cigarettes. The initial question should be open-ended, e.g., "How often do you drink alcoholic beverages such as beer, wine, or liquor?" Questions such as "Do you drink?" allow the patient to end the discussion with a simple "no." Remember to define the terms "alcoholic beverage" or "drug." Some patients do not consider beer and wine to be alcoholic beverages.

ALCOHOL

Patients who abuse alcohol present with several medical problems including dyspepsia, hypertension, minor trauma, anxiety, and insomnia (Table 10.3). Many of these complaints are a direct manifestation of the use of alcohol, whereas some may be secondary manifestations from intoxication or dependence. Alcohol screening should occur at the initial visit because many of these medical and social comorbidities occur later in a patient's addiction.

Table 10.3.
Common Disorders Associated with Substance Abuse

Cardiovascular
hypertension
tachycardia
cardiac ischemia
atrial and ventricular arrhythmia

Neurologic
paresthesia and anesthesia
seizures

Gastrointestinal
gastritis
peptic ulcer disease
pancreatitis
hepatitis

Hematologic
anemia
macrocytosis
thrombocytopenia

Psychiatric
anxiety
depression
insomnia

Table 10.4.
Initial Evaluation for Alcohol Abuse

CAGE questions[a]
Have you ever felt you ought to cut down on your drinking?
Have people annoyed you by criticizing your drinking?
Have you ever felt bad or guilty about your drinking?
Have you ever had a drink first thing in the morning to steady your nerves or get rid of a hangover ("eye-opener")?

Skinner trauma questions[b]
Since your 18th birthday
  Have you ever had any fractures or dislocations of your bones or joints?
  Have you ever been injured in a traffic accident?
  Have you ever injured your head?
  Have you ever been in an assault or fight (excluding sports)?
  Have you ever been injured while drinking?

[a]From Reference 1.
[b]From Reference 2.

Determining the amount of alcohol consumed as a measure of abuse is an inadequate and insensitive measure. The clinician must determine in an efficient manner not only quantity and frequency of alcohol consumed but its impact on life. Two simple and effective screens that clinicians should be comfortable using are the CAGE and Skinner trauma questions (Table 10.4) (1, 2).

The CAGE enables the clinician to explore the impact of alcohol on a person's life (annoyed, guilty) as well as ascertain if an element of dependence exists (cut down, eye opener). CAGE questions are used systematically in a nonthreatening manner for all health related habits. For instance, a caffeine CAGE may be followed by one for alcohol and then cigarettes. Although intended to be used sequentially, CAGE questions may also be incorporated into the screening history piecemeal or in a different order. A "yes" to any of these questions should be followed with further questions of how or why. The Skinner trauma scale asks five questions dealing with accidents, assaults, head injuries, motor vehicle accidents, and any injury associated with alcohol (Table 10.4). It can be used alone or in conjunction with the CAGE. It is especially useful in approaching the patient who presents to the emergency or medical walk-in area for care. Affirmative responses to two or more of the questions suggests excessive drinking or alcohol abuse.

The amount of alcohol consumed is determined only after the CAGE or Skinner questions have been asked. Remember that consumption is measured not only in amount consumed but also its frequency. Specific questions should be asked separately for wine, beer, and liquor. Men who consume four drinks at a time and women who consume three drinks at a time three times per week are considered hazardous users and are at risk to develop problems (3).

The laboratory evaluation of alcohol abuse is confirmatory and can help in maintaining abstinence. The blood alcohol level can confirm that the patient is tolerant to alcohol when the level exceeds 150 mg/dl and the patient appears sober. If the level is 300 mg/dl or above, regardless of the patient's state of inebriation, the patient is tolerant. Elevated levels of γ-glutamyltransferase correlate with chronic alcohol consumption. γ-Glutamyltransferase usually rises within 2 weeks of heavy drinking and subsequently takes 2 weeks to return to normal with abstinence. It may be elevated with other disorders of the liver as well as with use of prescription drugs such as phenytoin or phenobarbital. Other laboratory abnormalities that can occur later in addiction are anemia secondary to vitamin deficiency or as a direct toxic effect of the alcohol and thrombocytopenia.

STREET DRUGS

The key to diagnosing abuse of drugs such as cocaine and opiates is the realization that abuse is common and occurs in those patients where it is least expected. Screening instruments specifically designed for drug use have not been as well studied as the CAGE and are certainly not as brief. The CAGE and trauma screens can be modified to accommodate abuse of cocaine and other drugs. A general screen for substances of abuse including alcohol, drugs, and tobacco should be employed. As with alcohol, patients who abuse these substances have frequent medical problems that are vague and frustrating to interpret.

Like early alcohol abuse the physical stigmas of early drug abuse may not be evident. Hypertension, tachycardia, and tremulousness are common with the use of cocaine. Patients may present with cardiac arrhythmia or evidence of ischemia. Weight loss, fatigue, and depression can be seen with the use of narcotics (Table 10.2). Social manifestations are equally common, e.g., problems and absenteeism at work or school, marital discord, and social isolation.

Urine toxicology is widely used for the detection of street drugs and usually employs an immunoassay technique. Confirmatory tests are necessary to reduce false positive results that may occur with certain foods (e.g., poppy seeds) or medications (e.g., decongestants). Furthermore certain drugs may not be detectable in urine screens, either because of short half-lives (e.g., cocaine, LSD) or a different route of elimination (inhalants).

PRESCRIPTION DRUGS

Patients maintained on drugs such as barbiturates, benzodiazepines, and narcotics for prolonged periods or for questionable indications are abusing those drugs. The best way to deal with this form of abuse is to prescribe these medications with extreme caution for short periods and only for specified indications, with the goal of therapy clearly stated. This should be clarified for the patient at the outset and should be well documented in the medical record. Suspect patients who present for a first visit already on such medication from other practitioners. Making it clear from the beginning that other modes of therapy (e.g., physical therapy or bed rest for low back pain, biofeedback for chronic pain, and counseling for anxiety) are the preferred treatments will make discontinuation of an abused drug easier. Also, especially in the case of chronic pain, emphasize that the goal of therapy is not total absence of pain but control of pain.

Management

Management of substance abuse has many components. The primary care practitioner is pivotal not only in bringing the problem to attention but also in providing early counseling and advice that has proven to be beneficial in the case of alcohol abuse.

If the patient is actively using the substance during the 3 days before the visit, an admission to a medical or detoxification unit may be appropriate. If the patient has a supportive social environment, has no history of delirium tremens (DTs) or seizures, and does not possess signs of hallucinosis, mental status changes, or signs of withdrawal (e.g., tachycardia, hypertension, and seizures), detoxification can be accomplished as an outpatient. Withdrawal and evidence of DTs are medical emergencies and should be treated as such with admission to a medical unit before rehabilitation.

Early and brief intervention should be the therapy for alcohol and substance abusers who do not fit the definition of dependence. Brief intervention includes continued assessment of the patient's problem as well as direct feedback of the results of that assessment to the patient, contracting and goal setting of a specific drinking (or drug use) level, review of health consequences and how they relate to the patient, and self help materials. Meeting lists for self-help groups such as Alcoholics Anonymous, Narcotics Anonymous, Al-Anon, and Alateen should be readily available. These techniques have been studied extensively for alcohol abuse but can be used as an initial strategy for all substance abusers.

Primary care clinicians must be knowledgeable about treatment and counseling resources available at their institution. If there is evidence of loss of control, negative consequences, or physical dependence, then the patient is considered dependent and should be referred to a specialized treatment program. The clinic social worker should get involved and can help with referral to an outpatient or inpatient program.

Regardless of whether the patient will be counseled or referred the primary care provider must be involved in the maintenance of recovery. Frequently when the clinician encourages the relationship this provides a constant resource and a place to turn should relapse occur.

ILLUSTRATIVE CASES WITH SELF-ASSESSMENT QUESTIONS AND

ANSWERS

Case 1

A 45-year-old white male postal worker is referred by an orthopedic surgeon because of elevated blood pressure. He was well until 3 weeks ago when he presented to the local emergency department with a fractured wrist sustained when slipping on the ice outside his home. The patient states that he feels fine and has no complaints.

QUESTIONS:

What more in the history would you like?
a. Does he have prior history of trauma?
b. Does he have a history of a motor vehicle accident?
c. Has he ever been assaulted or involved in a fight?
d. How often does he drink?
e. Has he cut down on his drinking?

ANSWER: *All these questions are useful in this evaluation. The first three are part of the Skinner trauma scale and the last is part of the CAGE. Further questions will be important including the following. Has he felt guilty about his drinking? Does he feel annoyed when approached about his drinking? Does he need an "eye opener" in the morning?*

Case 2

A 31-year-old colleague presents to the emergency department with crushing substernal chest pain, diaphoresis, and severe nausea with vomiting. Her symptoms were not relieved by antacids. She had no prodromal symptoms. She is the chief resident of the ENT service at a neighboring hospital and the mother of two children. She was relaxing with her husband and some friends when the pain began. Physical examination reveals a thin pale diaphoretic female in moderate distress with alcohol fumes on her breath. Her heart rate is 104; her blood pressure is 195/90; her respirations are 24. She is afebrile. Her nasal mucosa is hyperemic. Her ECG reveals sinus tachycardia with Q waves and ST segment elevations inferiorly.

QUESTIONS:

a. What is the diagnosis?
b. What should be done next?

ANSWERS: *A young person presenting with an acute myocardial infarction may be the initial presentation for cocaine intoxication. Given this patient's profession and physical findings, urine toxicology for cocaine metabolites as well as blood levels for alcohol should be obtained. She should be hospitalized.*

REFERENCES

1. Ewing JA. Detecting alcoholism. The CAGE questionnaire. JAMA 1984;252:1905–1907.
2. Skinner HA, Holt S, Schuller R, Roy J, Israel Y. Identification of alcohol abuse using laboratory tests and a history of trauma. Ann Intern Med 194;101:847–851.
3. Sanchez-Craig M, Israel Y. Pattern of alcohol consumption associated with self-identified problem drinking. Am J Public Health 1985;75:178–180.

SUGGESTED READINGS

Bradley KA. The primary care practitioner's role in the prevention and management of alcohol problems. Alcohol Health Res World 1994;18:97–104.

Maly RC. Early recognition of chemical dependence. Primary Care 1993;20:33–50.

National Institute on Alcohol Abuse and Alcoholism. The physician's guide to helping patients with alcohol problems. Bethesda MD: National Institutes of Health, 1995 (NIH publication no. 95-6769).

Section III

EVALUATION AND MANAGEMENT OF COMMON PROBLEMS IN ADULT AMBULATORY CARE

chapter 11

HEAD, EARS, EYES, NOSE, AND THROAT

Charlotte Deutsch, Christine Oman, and Lisa M. Rucker

EARACHE AND HEARING LOSS

Ear pain and hearing problems are commonly encountered by the primary care provider. Acute problems of ear pain usually can be managed by the primary care provider. Chronicity may imply complex or serious entities and will probably need referral to the otolaryngologist or audiologist.

Pathophysiologic Correlation

The external ear is composed of the pinna or auricle (on the side of the head) and the external auditory canal (leading into the temporal bone to the tympanic membrane). The external opening to the canal is termed the meatus. The outer portion of the external ear is composed of cartilage covered by perichondrium, then epithelium that contains hair follicles, wax-forming cerumen and sebaceous glands. The inner portion is composed of bone covered by epithelium that is continuous with the tympanic membrane. Anatomical and physiological mechanics keep the canal clean; hairs and wax trap foreign matter; mastication pushes wax outward; the inner epithelium migrates outward. These natural barriers to infection and conductive hearing loss are commonly overcome by excess moisture (otitis externa or "swimmer's ear") and opposing forces such as cotton swabs (impacted wax). Blood vessels and nerves of the external ear are very near the surface and are easily traumatized. Sound waves are collected and mechanically funneled to the tympanic membrane and middle ear.

The middle ear is a cavity situated in the temporal bone adjacent to the sinus and cerebellum. It contains air, the tympanic membrane, three ossicles held together by muscle and ligament, and the eustachian tube. The three ossicles are the malleus, whose end is attached to the tympanic membrane, the incus, and the stapes, which lies in contact with the thin membrane separating middle and inner ears.

The middle ear and external ear conduct sound waves mechanically. Sound waves emanating from the external canal produce vibrations of the tympanic membrane that are transmitted to the ossicular chain and then to the thin membrane covering the fluid filled inner ear that sets the fluid in motion. The middle ear also amplifies sound owing to the relatively larger surface area of the tympanic membrane (compared with the round window where the waves are dissipated) and to the mechanical motions of the ossicles. If this were not the case, sound energy would be reflected away from the tympanic membrane surface. The tympanic membrane can be a site of infection (otitis media) and its spread to the central nervous system.

The facial nerve runs through the middle ear and can be damaged by inflammation. The eustachian tube runs from the middle ear to the nasopharynx and shares the mucosa of the middle ear. It equalizes pressure in the middle ear by replenishing air that is absorbed by the middle ear mucosa. Although it is usually closed, it opens with yawning, sneezing, nose blowing, and swallowing. Middle ear inflammation, upper respiratory infections, sinus infections, and pharyngitis inflame the eustachian tube mucosa and prevent the tube from opening and closing properly. The mucosa secretes fluid that fills the middle ear, and hearing declines (serous otitis media). Fluid may burst through the tympanic membrane (perforation). Profuse discharge from the external ear implies middle ear infection or cholesteatoma.

The inner ear is comprised of fluid, cochlea (the hearing portion containing hair cells and the eighth cranial nerve), and vestibular labyrinth. Sound wave transmission in the inner ear is converted from mechanical energy of the external and middle ears to a neurological impulse (action potential). Fluid waves, produced by movement of the stapes footplate, act on the organ of Corti to generate action potentials in the nerve cells (hair cells and first order neurons). These electrical impulses are transmitted along the eighth cranial nerve to the brainstem, thalamus, and temporal lobes of the cortex.

Hearing loss can be localized in these systems. First, the number of neurons increases from few in the cochlea to many in the central nervous system. Second, tonotopic organization allows specific frequencies to correlate with specific areas in the neurological system. Most sensorineural hearing loss is due to lesions in the inner ear (whereas conductive loss usually occurs in the external or middle ear).

Clinical and Laboratory Evaluation

The diagnosis of ear pain can nearly always be made without the aid of laboratory tests. Hearing loss may require special testing. The key to diagnosis is knowing what to ask and how to look. Symptoms of ear disease are few and specific.

HISTORY

The history is focused on the main symptom of pain, hearing loss, drainage, tinnitus, and vertigo. Onset and duration, bilateral versus unilateral, course (progressive worsening or improvement or fluctuating), and significance of the disability are important descriptive characteristics of pain or hearing loss. Presence of associated symptoms such as upper respiratory infection, pharyngitis, stridor, or hoarseness aid in diagnosis because pain in the ear is often referred from other head and neck structures. Predisposing factors to investigate are a positive family history for hearing loss, ear surgery, ear trauma (flying, diving, head injury), noise exposure (employment or recreational), and medications (including previous hospitalizations and use of intravenous antibiotics). Intercurrent disease is always important to ascertain.

PHYSICAL EXAMINATION

Except for palpation of the pinna, tragus, mastoid, and pertinent lymph nodes, most of the examination of the ear is done by observation. In addition, the head, neck, and chest are completely examined. A basic neurological examination with attention to the cranial nerves is also done in particular if a unilateral or asymmetrical hearing loss is the case.

Ear Examination. The pinna, external canal, meatus, and the mastoid are inspected for any ab-

normalities (Fig. 11.1A). The pinna, tragus, and mastoid are palpated for tenderness. The remainder of the examination of the ear itself utilizes the pneumatic otoscope, an insufflator bulb attachment for the otoscope, and a 512-Hz tuning fork. The otoscope is used to visualize the tympanic membrane and with the insufflator to evaluate its mobility. The tuning fork detects substantial hearing impairment and can determine conductive hearing loss (external and middle ear damage or air conduction) versus sensorineural hearing loss (inner ear and nerve damage or bone conduction).

If cerumen and debris obscure the view of the tympanic membrane, they should be removed. Wax can be removed with a curette and debris with a thin cotton tipped applicator. Irrigation should be reserved for those cases where wax is impacted and difficult to remove with a curette. Irrigation can confuse the examination when residual fluid remains in the ear. Irrigation is discussed in further detail in the context of conductive hearing loss and impacted cerumen.

A speculum is chosen that fits into the external ear canal with the least discomfort and affords the best view of the tympanic membrane. The right hand with the speculum examines the right ear and vice versa. The hand without the speculum maintains upward, outward, and backward traction on the pinna. It is necessary to decrease the distance to the viewing lens and adjust the line of sight and speculum position to obtain a complete view of the membrane.

There are four main features of the tympanic membrane (Fig. 11.1B): color, cone of light, malleus (handle and short process), and membrane mobility (Fig. 11.1C). The normal tympanic membrane is pearly gray and slightly concave (caused by the malleus adhering to the membrane). The handle of the malleus appears as a white line extending from the center of the tympanic membrane. At the top, the short process can be seen. With inflammation, the membrane becomes thickened and less concave (Fig. 11.1D). This obliterates the bony landmarks. At the bottom of the handle is the cone of light, which is a reflection of the otoscope light. It may be splayed or absent. This may be due to an abnormality, e.g., inflammation, or due to senile changes, the angle of the external canal, or the shape of the membrane. Whether it is abnormal or normal depends on the appearance of the remainder of the tympanic membrane. The annulus is a fibrous layer forming the periphery of the membrane and is a common spot for perforations. It appears whiter and denser than the rest.

Examining tympanic membrane mobility is an aid to diagnosis of middle ear disease. Squeezing and releasing the insufflator bulb attached to the otoscope produce positive and negative air pressure changes in the external canal. A tight air seal will allow the examiner to see pressure changes reflected in the mobility of the eardrum. A normal eardrum will move with positive and negative pressure. If the eardrum moves with negative pressure only, middle ear serous fluid, an upper respiratory infection, or eustachian tube dysfunction may be indicated. If the eardrum is immobile, fluid in the middle ear space or a perforation may be indicated. Dizziness or eye movement with this test suggests a perforation or inner ear anomalies. Pneumatic otoscopy is insensitive if the air seal is inadequate.

Hearing Examination. Before using the tuning fork, make a rough assessment of hearing threshold (but not discrimination) by performing the watch tick test (or whispered voice or finger rub). Both sides are tested. By using the words baseball or hot dog, one can test first for speech threshold, then speech discrimination (the patient understands what was said).

A 512-Hz tuning fork can best detect hearing impairment. Air conduction (sound wave transmission via the external and middle ears) can be tested by holding the vibrating tuning fork near the external auditory canal with the broad side of one of the prongs facing the ear. Impairment of air conduction is termed a conductive hearing loss. Bone conduction (sound wave transmission in the inner ear and nerve) can be tested by placing the base of the vibrating fork on the skull, upper teeth or dentures, mastoid, or mandible (thus bypassing the external and middle ear areas). Impairment in bone conduction indicates a sensorineural hearing loss.

The Rinne test aids in determining conductive versus sensorineural loss. The fork is struck hard and alternately placed beside the ear (as in testing air conduction) and on the base on the mastoid. It is moved back and forth rapidly until the patient can determine if there is a difference in the sound level between the two. Hearing the sound louder on the mastoid indicates bone transmission is stronger than air, suggesting a conductive hearing loss and a problem in the external or middle ear.

The Weber test confirms the Rinne. A vibrating fork is placed midline on the skull. The patient is asked to which ear the sound is transmitted. If the sound lateralizes to the affected ear, a conductive loss is suggested. Sound lateralizing to the unaffected ear indicates a sensorineural loss. In all of these tests the untested ear should be masked, if possible, with a piece of paper being crumpled, as sounds transmit around the head or through the skull. Tuning forks cannot determine minimal high frequency loss nor quantify hearing loss. For this, further audiometric testing is needed and is discussed briefly under "Laboratory Evaluation."

LABORATORY EVALUATION

Cultures of the external auditory canal are generally not required unless the patient is a diabetic, or otherwise immunosuppressed, or there is no response to treatment. If fungal growth is suspected, a potassium hydroxide preparation can be examined. The individual with probable sensorineural deafness will need audiometric testing that can determine the degree of loss. Many tests are required, and computed axial tomography and magnetic resonance imaging may be necessary. Serologic and chemical screening is determined by the history and physical examination.

Differential Diagnosis

Patients may present with ear pain, hearing loss, or both. In this section, the problems will be addressed separately. Remember, there is considerable overlap of these symptoms, particularly with infections or inflammatory disease.

EAR PAIN

Common problems involving ear pain or discomfort as the primary symptom are acute otitis externa, bacterial otitis media, and serous otitis media. These will be discussed. Other less common entities are listed in Table 11.1.

Acute Otitis Externa. The most common site of an otitis externa is the ear canal (not the pinna). The usual cause is traumatic abrasion or maceration from excessive moisture. These destroy the cerumen barrier or change the acid pH to alkaline, allowing bacteria to invade. Gram-negative and anaerobic bacteria, especially *Pseudomonas aeruginosa*, are common invaders. Predisposing factors include swimming or cleaning the canal with cotton swabs or bobby pins. The history should inquire into these factors. The patient will present with complaints of itching and pain. Pain on movement of the tragus is a significant diagnostic sign. It does not occur in otitis media. However, this does not exclude otitis media, which may be concomitant, unless the eardrum can be seen.

A foul odor to the discharge indicates a choles-

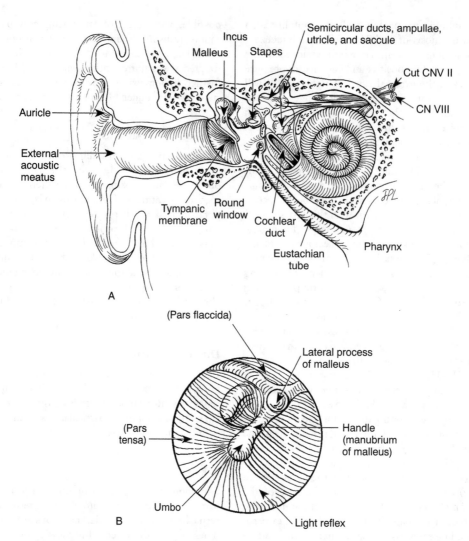

Figure 11.1. Examination of the ear. **A.** Coronal section through the ear. **B.** Normal right tympanic membrane. **C.** Otoscopic appearance of normal right tympanic membrane. **D.** Otoscopic appearance of abnormal right tympanic membrane (in otitis media). From Willms JL, Schneiderman H, Algranati PS. Physical diagnosis: bedside evaluation of diagnosis and function. Baltimore: Williams & Wilkins, 1994:35 (**A** and **B**) and Fleisher GR, Ludwig S, eds. Textbook of pediatric emergency medicine, 3rd ed. Baltimore: Williams & Wilkins, 1993:610 (**C** and **D**).

teatoma (an eroding cyst within a perforation). The external auditory canal in otitis externa is edematous, erythematous, and weepy. Hearing may be decreased because of edema. Included in the differential of otitis externa should be otomycosis (fungal infections) because they are often indistinguishable from bacterial infections unless there is a distinctive fluffy or black appearance caused by hyphae or black material. Otomycosis is associated with extended use of antimicrobial drops. Diabetics are

particularly at risk for malignant otitis, which appears benign, without systemic signs, but actually involves the cartilaginous-bony junction of the external canal and extends into the skull. A characteristic finding is visible granulation tissue at the aforementioned junction of the canal. Other more serious forms of otitis externa are usually distinguished by fever or other systemic symptoms.

Bacterial Otitis Media. Bacterial otitis media is commonly a secondary infection, the cause being

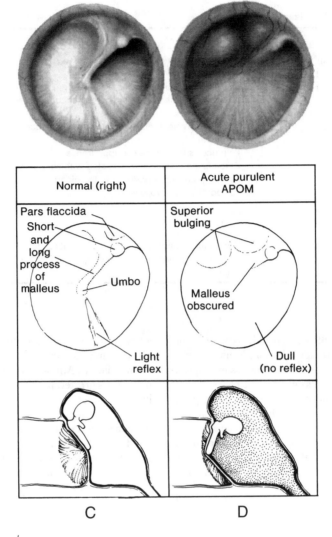

Normal (right)	Acute purulent APOM
Pars flaccida / Short and long process of malleus / Umbo / Light reflex	Superior bulging / Malleus obscured / Dull (no reflex)

C   D

Figure 11.1.—*continued*

external to the ear. Usually it is an ascending infection from the nasopharynx through the eustachian tube. Predisposing conditions include viral upper respiratory infections, chronic middle ear effusions, and sinus anomalies and allergy. Common bacteria are *Streptococcus pneumoniae, Haemophilus influenzae,* group A streptococcus, and *Branhamella catarrhalis. Mycoplasma pneumoniae* can cause a bullous myringitis. One-third of otitis media infections are viral. A common complication is an eardrum perforation that occurs when the purulent material in the middle ear is allowed to accumulate.

Complaints are primarily of pain. This is generally accompanied by hearing loss. There may be an associated fever, rhinitis, cough, or pharyngitis. Otorrhea will be the major complaint, with a notable absence of pain subsequent to the onset of the discharge if the membrane has perforated.

Physical examination quickly determines the cause of the patient's pain. The tympanic membrane is red. Bony landmarks are obliterated because of inflammation of the membrane and buildup of purulent fluid behind the membrane. The cone of light is absent or is splayed. The mem-

Table 11.1.
Uncommon Causes of Ear Pain

Etiology	Symptoms
Malignant (necrotizing) otitis externa	Immunosuppression, indolent course
Cellulitis	Pinna involvement, fever
Perichondritis	Infectious extension into the ear cartilage, fever
Furuncle/folliculitis	Involvement of the outer third of the canal (lined with hair follicles), localized swelling
Dermatitis	Pinna involvement, eczema, seborrhea, contact dermatitis localized to the source
Herpes zoster	Pain occurs before vesicle appearance
Cholesteatoma	Keratinizing epithelium associated with chronic suppurative otitis media
Mastoiditis	Swelling, erythema posterior to the pinna
Petrositis	Temporal bone involvement
Trauma	
Foreign body	
Tumor	
Referred	Pharyngitis, sinusitis, dental infection, parotiditis, tumor, temporomandibular joint dysfunction, other head, neck, cervical spine, or chest anomalies

brane is immobile. Blisters, possibly dark brown or purple from hemorrhagic effusion, located on the tympanic membrane indicate a bullous myringitis. Other symptoms such as pharyngitis or cough and fever usually accompany this entity. Fever, pain, and a reddened tympanic membrane make a clinical diagnosis of otitis media. Purulent material in the canal indicates the membrane has perforated, in which case direct visualization of the membrane is usually impossible. Uncommon complications, which usually occur in developing nations, include cholesteatoma and mastoiditis (patient is toxic and swelling and erythema posterior to the pinna are present). Chronic otitis media, another complication, is seen more commonly in children (as is acute bacterial otitis media). In an adult, chronic otitis media indicates a cholesteatoma or a perforation in the pars tensa.

Serous Otitis Media. Serous otitis media in adults is caused by an acute effusion resulting from pathology external to the middle ear. Most commonly a viral upper respiratory infection is the cause. Other less common causes include barotrauma, allergic rhinosinusitis, and, in an older adult, a primary head or neck carcinoma. When the mucosal lining of the middle ear is inflamed, the eustachian tube becomes blocked. This prevents the middle ear from gaining access to air needed to balance middle ear pressure with that in the external auditory canal. The air already present in the middle ear is absorbed by the mucosa, which

allows a negative pressure to build in the middle ear, drawing fluid from the middle ear lining into the middle ear. Atmospheric pressure in the external canal is greater, pushing in the tympanic membrane ("retraction").

The patient presents with a feeling of blockage or fullness in the ear that is associated with diminished hearing. There is no severe pain. There may be some vertigo or tinnitus. There may also be a complaint of bubbling or crackling sounds with head movement.

The tympanic membrane is dull and/or retracted. An amber or dark gray membrane indicates prolonged fluid stasis. There may be an air-fluid level or air bubbles in fluid visualized though the eardrum (if the eustachian tube is only partially occluded). Pneumatic otoscopy demonstrates decreased mobility with negative pressure only or with both positive and negative pressure. A perforation may be associated. A conductive hearing loss is present. If recurrent and unilateral, a serous otitis media in an adult is considered to be a head or neck carcinoma unless otherwise demonstrated.

HEARING LOSS

The most common cause of conductive hearing loss is impacted cerumen. Other notable causes are tympanosclerosis and otosclerosis. The most common cause of sensorineural loss is presbycusis. Ménière's disease, acoustic neuroma, and viral-induced and noise-induced hearing loss will be discussed. Other causes of hearing loss are listed in Table 11.2.

Conductive Hearing Loss. The most essential characteristic of conductive loss is that bone conduction is better than air conduction, with bone conduction being normal. This is known as an air:bone gap. Other characteristics include pain or fullness in the ear or discharge. The patients will say they hear better in noisy areas or they hear well as long as people speak loud enough (discrimination is not affected, only threshold). The patient will speak with a soft voice. The physical examination will usually detect some abnormality in the external auditory canal or the tympanic membrane. The exception is a problem emanating from the ossicles in which case otoscopic findings will be normal. Even though a conductive loss is suspected, the examiner must always eliminate sensorineural loss

Table 11.2.
Uncommon Causes of Hearing Loss

Etiology	Symptoms
Conductive	
Chronic suppurative otitis media	Copious discharge associated with cholesteatoma or perforation
Tuberculosis	Similar presentation to chronic supporative
Trauma	Concussions, fractures, barotrauma
Tumor	Primary or metastases
Immune mediated	
Sensorineural	
Ototoxicity	Loop diuretics, salicylates, erythromycin, aminoglycosides, antineoplastics
Infection	Tuberclosis, syphilis
Trauma	
Tumor	Primary or metastases
Immune medicated	Lupus, multiple sclerosis, with or without systemic symptoms
Congenital	Majority are nonsyndromal, a minority are conductive
Circulatory	Emboli, hemorrhage, migraine
Idiopathic	

Adapted with permission from Nadol JB. Hearing loss. N Engl J Med 1993;329:1090.

by determining the air:bone gap (Rinne test). The Weber test demonstrates lateralization to the affected ear and helps confirm the diagnosis.

Impacted Cerumen. Impacted cerumen occurs for several reasons. Either it was pushed there or it accumulated because of abnormal external auditory canal structure, quantity of hairs, or consistency of the cerumen. It is a common occurrence in the elderly and industrial workers.

The patient will complain of an acute onset of hearing loss, usually after chewing or probing. There is commonly a history of using cotton swabs, toothpicks, or bobby pins to clear the canal. Other symptoms include pain or mild discomfort, itching, tinnitus, or hearing the heartbeat.

The otoscopic findings will immediately determine the cause of discomfort. Cerumen may partially or completely obstruct the meatus. Cerumen varies from yellow to deep brown and can be soft or hard, forming a plug. An otitis externa may be present if an over-the-counter preparation was used debride the cerumen. These medications are caustic to the canal and can cause the cerumen to swell.

Tympanosclerosis. Tympanoscerotic plaques are postinflammatory thickened hyalinized collagen fibers. They can deposit in the fibrous layer of the tympanic membrane or within the joints of the ossicles. The patient will present with a symptom of a unilateral conductive hearing loss. There will be a history of a past ear infection. Visualization of the tympanic membrane will demonstrate thick yellow or white deposit unless the deposits are within the ossicles, in which case visualization of the eardrum will produce normal findings.

Otosclerosis. The cause of otosclerosis is unknown. Excessive formation of spongy bone actually begins with changes in the cochlear bone that involve the stapedial footplate, which becomes fixated in the oval window. This fixation of the stapes produces a conductive hearing loss and the classic picture of otosclerosis. Notable historical factors are that the individual is a white female with a positive family history for hearing loss. Pregnancy may precipitate the event. The otoscopic examination findings are normal. Otosclerosis often leads to sensorineural damage, but even if there is such hearing loss, bone conduction is still better than air conduction.

Sensorineural Hearing Loss. The essential characteristic of sensorineural hearing loss is reduced bone conduction. The important complaint is hearing loss manifested by an inability to understand speech. These individuals have impaired speech discrimination because of an inability to distinguish consonants. Consonants occur at higher frequencies than vowels. Loudness does not clarify the sounds, it worsens the understanding of speech owing to the cochlea's loss of ability to accommodate its intensity range. Background noise makes it more difficult for the patient to discriminate, and men's voices are easier to discriminate; both for the identical reason that they are at lower thresholds. Usually the individual does not respond during conversation. This lack of response is often interpreted as inattentiveness. If tinnitus is present, it is a high-pitched hiss or ring (however, tinnitus in Ménière's is seashell or roaring).

On physical examination the patient's voice may be loud and strained. There is no air:bone gap. Air conduction and bone conduction are reduced to the same level. The tuning fork will lateralize to the unaffected ear if there is a notable difference between the ears. Otoscopic findings are normal. Audiometric testing is indicated.

The most common cause of sensorineural hearing loss is presbycusis. Less common but notable causes are viral-induced, Ménière's, noise-induced, and acoustic neuroma.

Presbycusis. Presbycusis is the most common cause of sensorineural hearing loss. There is a gradual onset of bilateral and symmetrical loss; higher frequencies are lost first and then lower. The process actually begins in childhood. As hair cell loss progresses from outer to inner, the individual gradually becomes more aware of the hearing loss. This awareness usually begins at about age 50 years. Risk factors to be determined in the history include age, male sex, illness, a positive family history, Ménière's disease, and noise exposure.

Ménière's Disease. The pathology of Ménière's disease entails an excess of endolymph fluid in the vestibular portion that increases pressure in the hair cells in the cochlea. The cause for this pathology is unknown. The presentation is clear-cut. There is a history of acute recurrent attacks of rotary vertigo, ocean-roaring or seashell tinnitus, and hearing loss (reduction in discrimination). Tinnitus and hearing loss are almost always unilateral. Before the attacks there is a sensation of pressure or fullness in the ears. Risk factors include female sex and ages 35–55. The patient is most concerned with the tinnitus and the vertigo and is very apprehensive. Symptom frequency declines with stress reduction. Weber lateralization in Ménière's disease is an unreliable test. Computed axial tomography or magnetic resonance imaging will exclude acoustic neuroma.

Noise-Induced Hearing Loss. History must indicate noise exposure, either prolonged or acute. An individual with acute acoustic trauma will complain of hearing loss with fullness in the ear and tinnitus. Some of these individuals retain a degree of permanent hearing loss. There is no progression. Those with prolonged occupational exposure usually present with loss advanced to the degree that it interferes with communication. The loss is irreversible because of hair cell loss. This permanent loss occurs after a period of reversibility.

Management

Problems involving ear pain can usually be managed by the primary care provider. Those cases needing referral are generally the rare cases involving lack of response to treatment, severe disease, or the potential for life-threatening systemic illness. Hearing loss can often be managed by the primary care provider and the audiologist.

EAR PAIN

Ear pain that can be managed by the primary care provider usually has an infectious etiology. Management with antibiotics and analgesics is required. Referral may be necessary in refractory cases.

Otitis Externa. In otitis externa, the canal must first be cleansed by curettage or irrigation. Local antibacterial medication is prescribed. Neomycin, polymyxin B, and hydrocortisone (Cortisporin) solution is instilled three to four drops into the ear three times a day for 5–7 days. If allergic, chloramphenicol drops, two to three drops into the ear three times a day, can be used. If a fungal infection is suspected, a topical antifungal agent such as hydrocortisone 1% with acetic acid 2% (VoSol HC) four drops three times a day, are instilled into the ear. In the patient whose canal is swollen shut, a wick can be inserted. Medication is added to the wick. When it dries, it is replaced by another. Patients in whom a wick has been inserted must return to the clinic within 2 days. The medications should be applied three to four drops four to six times a day for 10 days. If the clinician is in doubt or if extensive canal swelling makes it impossible to visualize the tympanic membrane, an oral antibiotic should be prescribed. Ciprofloxacin is used because it is active against Gram-negative bacilli including *Pseudomonas*. The dosage is usually 500 mg every 12 hours for 7 days. Analgesics may be needed for 3 days. The ear should be kept dry. Prophylaxis with 2% acetic acid dries the canal and restores the natural acidity. It can be utilized once the infection has resolved.

If the patient is diabetic or is otherwise immuno-compromised, a malignant otitis externa is possible owing to *Pseudomonas*. A consult is advised, and aggressive management is indicated. Fungal and bacterial cultures should be taken. Another complication may be cellulitis of the pinna for which hospitalization may be required. A consult is advised.

Bacterial Otitis Media. Treatment of acute bacterial otitis media entails use of antibiotics and analgesics. Ampicillin 500 mg four times a day for 10 days will cover *S. pneumoniae* and *Haemophilus influenzae.* Erythromycin 250 mg four times a day can be substituted if the patient is allergic to penicillin. There should be a response to treatment within 48 hours of starting antibiotics. Persistence of symptoms usually is due to a remaining serous effusion or resistant bacteria. The antibiotics should be changed to either cefaclor or amoxicillin-clavulanic acid.

Bullous myringitis has the potential to cause pneumonia. It should be treated with erythromycin 250 mg four times a day for 10 days. The patient should return to the clinic for follow-up in 1 month. If hearing loss persists, a consult with the otolaryngologist is advised. A persistent middle ear effusion, progressive infection, or neoplasm may be the cause. A consult is advised in the case of perforations also.

Serous Otitis Media. Serous otitis media generally resolves spontaneously when the eustachian tube opens again. Treatment is directed to the cause in the nasopharynx and to the relief of ear symptoms. Pseudoephedrine, 30–60 mg four times a day for 3 days, can reduce inflammation of the mucosa and the fluid transudation. If the effusion is chronic, then a referral to the otolaryngologist is advised.

HEARING LOSS

Conductive hearing loss is amenable to surgical or medical treatment. Prognosis for sensorineural loss is generally poor. Those with sudden onset have the best prognosis. The United States Preventive Services Task Force recommends no screening for asymptomatic individuals younger than 65 years except for those regularly exposed to excess noise. For those older than 65 years and for those exposed to noise, the periodic screen would consist of history and otoscopic examination and patient education regarding availability of hearing aid devices.

Conductive Hearing Loss—Cerumen Impaction. The common causes of conductive hearing loss that are amenable to medical treatment rendered by the primary care provider have been discussed under "Ear Pain" except for cerumen impaction. Other causes of conductive loss would be referred to the specialist for further evaluation and for possible surgical correction. The risk of surgery is subsequent sensorineural hearing loss. A hearing aid may be useful in conductive hearing loss because the inner ear is normal and all that is needed is amplification.

If the curette cannot debride the cerumen and the patient does not wish to soften the wax at home for a few days with a few drops of warm olive oil, irrigation should be attempted. Hydrogen peroxide drops should be instilled first, and the patient should be instructed to lie on his or her side opposite to the affected ear for about 10 minutes. Warm or room temperature water is instilled with a 50-ml syringe and a butterfly with the tip removed. Cold water risks labyrinthine stimulation that induces nausea, vomiting, and vertigo. The water is directed at the superior/posterior wall. This protects the eardrum from the force of the water and allows the stream to be directed around and behind the impaction. The patient's head should be tilted toward the affected side during the irrigation process. Irrigation is contraindicated in cases of a suspected perforation, recent ear injury, or presence of myringotomy tubes. The canal should be dried afterward. The patient may continue to use hydrogen peroxide ear drops, two drops in each ear, two or three times a week. Use of cotton buds, sharp objects, or over-the-counter cerumenlytics should be discouraged.

Sensorineural Hearing Loss. Presence of sensorineural hearing loss indicates the need for referral to an audiologist by the primary care provider. The mainstay of management is the hearing aid unless a cause amenable to treatment is discerned, e.g., syphilis or acoustic neuroma. Hearing aids offer no reduction in sound distortion. They amplify background noise, which interferes with speech intelligibility. Many cannot adjust to hearing aid use. Hearing therapists offer services that may be useful to these patients. Cochlear implants have proven useful to those who are totally deaf.

ILLUSTRATIVE CASES WITH SELF-ASSESSMENT QUESTIONS AND ANSWERS

Case 1

E.L. is a 55-year-old female who has been hearing a swishing sound in her right ear for 2 weeks. She is also experiencing some fullness and pain in the same ear after she tried to cleanse the canal with hydrogen peroxide 1 week ago. She denies discharge, vertigo, fever, dysphagia, weakness, or change in vision. She had this problem before, and after receiving antibiotics the problem resolved. Past medical history also includes a right deep vein thrombosis and hypertension. Medications include Coumadin and Lopressor.

On physical examination, the right tympanic membrane is obscured by cerumen and cotton. The left tympanic membrane displays good landmarks and a cone of light. Tuning forks show bone better than air conduction on the right. Weber testing lateralizes to the right. Irrigation removes wax and cotton from the right ear. The right tympanic membrane appears intact and slightly injected. After irrigation, air and bone are equal on the right, and the tuning fork lateralizes to the left. Air is better than bone conduction on the left. The neurological exam is normal, and there are no bruits. Fullness and noise sensations have gone.

QUESTION: *What is the most likely diagnosis?*

a. Conductive hearing loss
b. Sensorineural hearing loss
c. Mixed hearing loss
d. Cerumen impaction

ANSWER: d. *The final diagnosis would be cerumen impaction with unilateral (right) sensorineural hearing loss. Before irrigation, this was a mixed hearing loss (conductive and sensorineural). The patient was unaware of the sensorineural loss. The "swishing" sound is a common complaint when wax is pushed against the tympanic membrane. The patient could hear a rushing tinnitus or her own heartbeat. It is best to do hearing tests before and after wax removal and before a diagnosis is made.*

QUESTION: *What is the appropriate management?*

ANSWER: *The patient should be educated regarding the correct cleansing of the external canals. A referral to the audiologist or otolaryngologist is necessary to determine the cause of the unilateral sensorineural hearing loss. If acoustic neuroma is present, early removal may be accomplished.*

Case 2

A 48-year-old male comes to the clinic with pain in his left ear for 3 days. He also is experiencing a decline in hearing in the same ear. He denies discharge, vertigo, or tinnitus. There is a history of an upper respiratory infection 2 weeks ago. There is no history of swimming. On physical examination there is pain palpable over the tragus. There are no nodes or swellings. There are good landmarks visible in the right tympanic membrane. The left ear has some exudate, and the left bony external auditory canal (beyond the cartilaginous pinna and meatus) is inflamed. The tympanic membrane can be partially seen. It appears to be red, without visible bony landmarks or cone of light. There is no perforation visible. Tuning forks indicate a conductive hearing loss in the left ear.

QUESTION: *What are the most likely diagnoses?*

a. Otitis externa
b. Bacterial otitis media
c. Chronic otitis externa
d. Furuncle

Answer: a *and* **b.** *The diagnoses are otitis externa and bacterial otitis media. Otitis externa is most likely bacterial. Fungal infections may show a black exudate or white patches. Pain, discharge, and a feeling of blockage are typical complaints of otitis externa. A chronic otitis externa is characterized by dryness and pruritus in the ear canal. The usual cause is fungal. Although the left tympanic membrane can only partially be seen, the redness and the absence of landmarks or cone of light indicate a bacterial otitis media. A furuncle is a highly localized swelling that is extremely tender. It is found in the external canal* *where hair follicles are located. The exudate may also indicate an otitis media and associated perforation.*

QUESTION: *What is the appropriate management?*

ANSWER: *Cultures may be done to determine if any fungal infection is present. Either an antibacterial (e.g., neomycin, polymyxin B, and hydrocortisone (Cortisporin)) or an antibacterial, antifungal, yeast, and mold (Cortic) may be prescribed. These treat the otitis externa. Otitis media is treated with oral antibiotics. Ampicillin is effective against S. pneumoniae, the most common cause of otitis media in adults. Erythromycin or Bactrim may be given if the patient is allergic to penicillin. If the patient does not improve within 48–72 hours after antibiotics are started, the patient should return for reevaluation. The antibiotic may be changed to either Augmentin or Ceclor, which are effective against beta-lactamase producing organisms. If a perforation is suspected, a referral to an otolaryngologist is necessary. Otherwise, the patient should return in 2 weeks. An effusion may persist, in which case a second referral is necessary.*

RED EYE AND VISION PROBLEMS

The inflamed eye and disorders in visual acuity are commonly encountered in primary care settings. Causes range from the innocuous and self-limited to the complex and vision threatening. The presentation may belie the seriousness of the cause. For example, the patient with common bacterial conjunctivitis presents with a dramatically swollen, red, draining eye, whereas the individual with 40% optic nerve destruction caused by open-angle glaucoma is completely asymptomatic.

Pathophysiologic Correlation

The anatomy of the eye is illustrated in Figure 11.2. The conjunctiva contains glands that contribute to the tear film (a mixture of water, lipids, and proteins), which protects cornea and conjunctiva. Conjunctival arteries anastomose at the limbus with ciliary arteries that also produce the deeper scleral vessels. If there is an inflammation, these vessels dilate, making the tissue red. In conjunctival inflammation the conjunctival vessels can be moved with the conjunctiva, as opposed to inflammation associated with deeper ocular structures where involved and dilated scleral and perilimbal vessels

("ciliary flush") cannot be moved and are also less distinct.

The outer coat of the eye consists of the sclera and its anterior continuation, the cornea. Both are made of the same collagen fibers, but a different arrangement allows the cornea to be transparent. The cornea begins the process of bending (refracting) and transmitting the light to the optic nerve. Problems with the cornea entail refractive errors (excessive or inadequate curvature), astigmatism (uneven curvature), abrasions or ulcers (producing lack of light transmission and/or pain). There are five layers to the cornea. The epithelium, most anterior, can regenerate itself in 8 days. Minor abrasions can heal in a few hours. Damage to deeper layers (Bowman's membrane, stroma, Descemet's membrane, and endothelium) leads to scarring opacities. The cornea merges with the sclera at the limbus. Sensory innervation from the ophthalmic nerve allows for highest corneal sensitivity at the apex away from the limbus. Sensitivity decreases with contact lens use, aging, and herpetic infection. Traversing the opening in the sclera for the optic disc is a thin supporting network (lamina cribrosa) that is the site of pathological excavation of the disc in glaucoma. The area surrounding the opening is the thinnest part of the sclera.

The uvea is made up of the iris, ciliary body, and choroid. The ciliary body produces aqueous humor that nourishes all transparent ocular structures. The aqueous humor flows through anterior and posterior chambers and maintains shape and pressure. It exits mainly through the trabecular meshwork in the anterior chamber. Aqueous humor is produced fairly constantly. There is no feedback system so that blockage of the exit does not result in stoppage of production. If the exit is obstructed as it is in angle-closure glaucoma, the pressure increases, the eyeball hardens, and blood has difficulty getting into the eye at the back through the optic disc where the central retinal artery enters the eye. Aqueous humor carries sodium, chloride, glucose, oxygen, and proteins to ophthalmic tissues and carries away carbon dioxide and lactate.

The lens is made of a central hard nucleus surrounded by a soft cortex and outer capsule. With aging, the nucleus enlarges, comprising almost the entire lens. This contributes to hardening of the lens and presbyopia.

Behind the iris and lens is vitreous gel, which is high in water content. With aging it deteriorates, becoming increasingly liquid, causing an increase in floaters, and loosening its natural adhesion to the retina. With trauma, this loosening leaves the

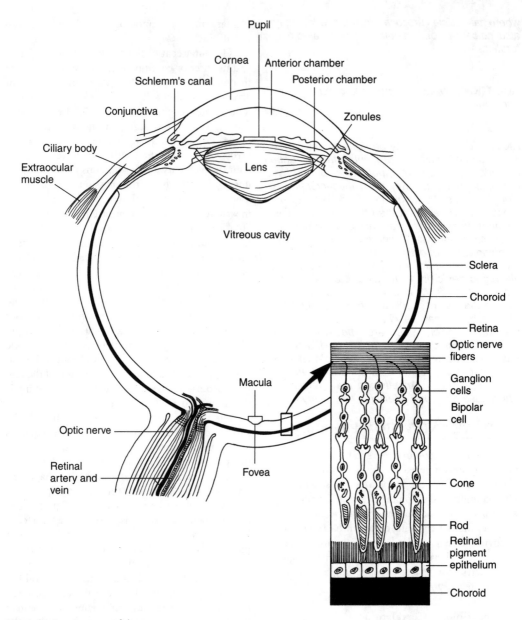

Figure 11.2. Anatomy of the eye.

vitreous gel inclined to prolapse, which can produce retinal tears. A shower of floaters is a symptom of a retinal tear.

The retina is the neural layer and is a continuation of the optic nerve. The eye possesses two distinct types of visual acuity: central and peripheral. Central vision does not merge gradually into field vision. Central vision is dominated by the macular retina. The macular retina is responsible for dis-

tinct, precise visual acuity. Cones dominate. The extramacular retina contains much less detailed visual information of the periphery. Rods predominate. This, combined with the fact that the surviving field in one eye can mask a missing field in the other and that peripheral vision loss begins as islands of reduced sensitivity, account for the tremendous damage to the optic nerve before an individual is aware of such a loss. The nerve fibers of the retina leave the eye through the optic disc. The number of axons that pass through the disc varies among individuals. The cup is not required for axon transmission. The cup may be absent in an individual with hyperopia or large in an individual with myopia.

Clinical and Laboratory Evaluation

Diagnosis is most often accomplished by a careful history alone. Physical examination will help to confirm the diagnosis. Laboratory evaluation is usually not required in an inflamed eye. Visual acuity problems in the absence of an inflamed eye indicate the need for an extended physical examination and funduscopy through a widely dilated pupil done by an ophthalmologist rather than a laboratory evaluation.

HISTORY

An ophthalmic history places emphasis on certain particulars. Questions regarding similar episodes, previous symptoms, treatments given, preexisting trauma, surgery, infections, and prior treatments and their effectiveness should be asked. Any ophthalmic disorder and medications used should be noted. The color of the bottle top of topical ophthalmic medications correlates with a certain class of medication. Yellow or blue tops indicate a beta-blocker. White indicates steroids, antibiotics, or artificial tears. Red indicates anticholinergic or sympathomimetic medications that dilate the pupil or treat glaucoma. Green indicates a cholinergic medication used to constrict the pupil or treat glaucoma. A family history specific for incidences of poor vision of unknown cause or of ophthalmic disorders that may be inherited is useful to elicit. The general past medical history concentrates on the presence of cardiac, cerebrovascular, respiratory, immune, and/or collagen vascular disorders or tumors. A review of medications and allergies is necessary.

PHYSICAL EXAMINATION

The same physical examination should be performed to evaluate any optical complaint. Both eyes should always be examined. The examination should be performed systematically from the outward structures inward.

Acuity. Visual acuity, central and peripheral, is always determined first unless the patient needs topical anesthetics or irrigation. Central vision is determined with the Snellen distance chart or, as a practical alternative, the Rosenbaum chart or newsprint examination for near vision (read at a distance of 14 inches, newsprint signifies 20/40 vision). Failure at any of these requires that the examination be repeated with use of a pinhole card or disc that contains a small hole and aids the patient in focusing. Improvement with the pinhole indicates probable refractive error. If unsuccessful with the pinhole, the patient attempts counting fingers, hand motions, and light perception. No light perception designates failure of all. Peripheral acuity is determined by confrontation examination—a gross screen. The patient covers one eye while the examiner covers his or her own contralateral eye. The patient fixes on the examiner's exposed eye. The examiner's fingers are moved equidistant between both parties from 5 cm outward into each quadrant. Defects are quantified as identifying the correct number of fingers versus gross motion.

External Structures and Tissues. Periorbital and lid structures and, if implicated, associated structures such as temporal arteries, lymphatic system, head, and neck are examined. The lower lid is everted by traction on the skin below. Eversion of the upper lid, done when there are complaints of a red or uncomfortable eye, is accomplished by pulling downward and away on the lashes while a cotton tip pushes downward on the outer surface. The patient should be told that this will feel uncomfortable but will not be painful. Conjunctival tissue is inspected with the ophthalmoscope.

Cornea. Implications of insult to the cornea are such that the cornea is considered separately from other external structures. The cornea surface light reflex is normally smooth and even. Corneal sensitivity is tested with the light stroke of a sterile wisp of cotton. Next a fluorescein strip is moistened and stroked on the conjunctival surface of the lower lid. The cobalt blue filter on the ophthalmoscope can then illuminate corneal disease such as abrasion or ulcer (which is not obviously white or hazy) as green patches or lines that do not move after the patient blinks.

Pupil. The pupil (and iris) should be inspected for irregularities and the pupils for equality of size, round shape, light reaction, and accommodation (PERRLA). Equality of pupil size is checked in the dimmest light possible. Inequality of pupil size (anisocoria) signifies serious eye disease in a unilateral red eye. Light directed at one eye will constrict that eye (direct reflex) and the opposite eye (consensual response). The swinging light test (swinging a light in a wide arc) can demonstrate consensual constriction before the normal direct light takes over. A relative afferent pupillary defect occurs when a pupil reopens to light continuously directed toward that eye. Painful accommodation indicates serious eye disease.

Anterior Chamber. The anterior chamber is inspected with the ophthalmoscope light. The eclipse test of anterior chamber depth can detect potential for acute angle-closure and help determine whether it is safe to dilate the eye. The light is aimed from the temporal side of the corneal margin. Normally the entire iris will be illuminated because iris and lens lay almost on a flat plane. In those individuals with potential for angle-closure glaucoma, the anterior chamber is shallow, caused by an iris or lens that lays more convex. This leaves the nasal side of the iris in shadow (positive eclipse test). The digital examination (palpation of the globe for elevated pressure) can aid in the evaluation. With the lid closed, the eye looks downward, and the palpating index fingers are placed under the outer angle of the orbit. Leaning on the patient's forehead with the sides of the ring and little finger, the two index fingers meet and one index finger palpates with tiny movements while the other feels for fluctuations. The softer the eye, the greater the fluctuations. Digital comparison with the unaffected eye increases the sensitivity of this examination.

Funduscopy. The examiner's (and patient's) eyeglasses or lenses can be worn, or the strength can be rotated into the ophthalmoscope (clockwise for hyperopia and counterclockwise for myopia). If the pupil is not dilated, the optic nerve may not be seen. The red reflex is visualized; a vessel is focused on; and the arrows made by vessel branches are followed to the disc. The disc outline should be well defined, and the cup, a pale central area, is usually less than half the radius of the disc. The cup should be about the same size in both eyes. The retina is red-orange and the macula a dark smudge temporal to the disc. Without pupil dilation these will be hard to visualize. Retinal arteries are brighter and thinner than the veins.

Medications Used in the Exam. Phenylephrine 2.5%, a sympathomimetic, induces mydriasis in 30 minutes, and risk of angle-closure is negligible. However, dilating drops should not be used if angle-closure is possible, if the patient has a neurological disease or a severe neurologic injury, or if there is a lens implant. Because of systemic absorption, caution is advised if the patient has heart disease or hypertension.

Proparacaine 5%, a topical anesthetic can be used. There are no systemic side effects. Topical anesthetics should never be prescribed because they prevent healing and lead to corneal perforation with loss of vision.

Referral to Ophthalmology for a Comprehensive Eye Examination. It is recommended by the American Academy of Ophthalmology that the physical examination be performed every 2–4 years in individuals aged 40–64 years and every 1–2 years beginning at age 65. Because of the risk of glaucoma, African Americans aged 20–39 years should be examined every 3–5 years. Diabetics need a comprehensive eye exam every year. Individual risk factors for ocular disease must be evaluated, and appropriate patients should be referred for comprehensive examination as indicated.

LABORATORY EVALUATION

Conjunctivitis is usually a clinical diagnosis. Laboratory evaluation is recommended when conjunctivitis is resistant to treatment. In viral conjunctivitis, Gram's stain of conjunctival scrapings will show a dominance of polymorphonuclear leukocytes in the first few days followed by a lymphocytic dominance. Rapid detection of adenovirus is available (antigen detection immunoassay and enzyme immunofluorescent assay). Viral cultures will confirm diagnosis. For a bacterial conjunctivitis, Gram's stain and cultures of the exudate can be helpful. Gram's stain can demonstrate fungi. Many polymorphonuclear leukocytes and intracellular Gram-negative diplococci found on Gram's stain indicate a neisseria conjunctivitis. Patients with neisseria conjunctivitis should be suspected of having a concomitant chlamydia infection. A conjunctival scraping of epithelial cells stained with Giemsa will demonstrate cytoplasmic paranuclear inclusion bodies of a chlamydia infection. Rapid detection of chlamydia conjunctivitis is available via fluorescent monoclonal antibody or enzyme immunoassay testing of discharge. The presence of eosinophils can be helpful in identifying an allergic conjunctivitis; however, they are not reliably present and are often present in those individuals without allergic conjunctivitis. An ophthalmic consult is mandatory if neisseria is suspected.

Differential Diagnosis

The differential diagnoses for an inflamed eye form a wide range from simple, self-limiting etiologies such as conjunctivitis to manifestations of systemic disease. Major etiologies to consider are conjunctivitis, blepharitis, iritis, keratitis, and angle-closure glaucoma, which are described in greater detail in the following sections. Other less commonly occurring entities are outlined (Table 11.3).

Disorders of visual acuity may be divided into two categories: sudden and gradual onset. Those of gradual onset are frequently encountered in primary care settings. Major diagnoses to be considered are cataract, refractive error, and open-angle glaucoma. These are discussed in greater detail. Other etiologies less commonly encountered and not discussed here are macular degeneration caused by aging (central vision loss, drusen identified in the macular area), diabetic retinopathy, and other optic disc atrophies or neuropathies such as tumor, retinitis pigmentosa (peripheral vision loss and night blindness), or Alzheimer's disease. Sudden onset of deterioration in visual acuity is less commonly encountered and is generally vascular in origin or occasionally neuropathic. Entities include retinal artery or vein occlusion, giant cell arteritis, vitreous hemorrhage, amaurosis fugax, ocular migraine, and hyperglycemia or hypoglycemia.

RED EYE

The most common cause of an inflamed eye is a simple viral, allergic, or bacterial conjunctivitis.

Blepharitis, an inflammation of the lids frequently associated with conjunctivitis, is also commonly encountered. The primary task for the practitioner is to differentiate these simple entities that are innocuous and self-limiting from keratitis, iritis, and angle-closure glaucoma, which are less common but threaten vision.

Blepharitis. Blepharitis, caused by staphylococcus or by hypersecretory or inflamed sebaceous glands, is often associated with a conjunctivitis. Prominent in the presentation are complaints of bilateral lid margins that are flaking, crusting, and possibly red and sore. There is usually a history of sties (staphylococcus abscess of a sebaceous gland) and chalazions (an aseptic granulomatous derivative of a sty). Scales at the bases of the lashes and reddened lid margins are found on physical examination. Rosacea, seborrhea, or a complaint of dry eyes may be associated with blepharitis.

Conjunctivitis. Conjunctivitis is commonly caused by viruses (adenovirus), bacteria (ataphylococcus), and allergies. Onset for viral and bacterial causes occurs sequentially, the second eye becoming involved within 2–3 days. Allergic conjunctivitis is always bilateral. A thick, purulent discharge that causes the lids to stick together in the morning is

Table 11.3.
Uncommon Causes of Red Eye

Etiology/Problem	Symptoms and Indications for Treatment
Neisseria gonorrhea	Indication for hospitalization
	Hyperacute onset (<12 hours)
	Copius purulence, genitourinary symptoms
Chlamydia	Chronic, refractory to treatment
Herpes simplex*	Corneal involvement, unilateral
Herpes zoster*	Nasal tip vesicles
Scleritis*	Severe pain, bluish hue to sclera
Episcleritis*	Mild pain, recurrent, young adult
Subconjunctival hemorrhage	Sectorial redness, no pain or discharge, history of abuse
Dry eye syndrome	Most common cause of red eye for those older than 65; irritation, burning; induced by sedatives or beta-blockers
Preseptal or orbital cellulitis	Indication for hospitalization; lid swelling, lymphadenopathy, fever
Canaliculitis or dacrocystitis	Swelling over the nasal section of the lower lid, discharge
Pediculitis	Inflamed lids and conjunctiva, nits
Contact dermatitis	Inflammation of surrounding tissue
Injected pingueculum	Minimal pain
Pterygium	Excision if encroaching the visual axis
Corneal abrasions	History of poke in the eye; foreign body sensation; fluorescein diagnosis; antibiotics, patch, and return to clinic in 24 hours; ophthalmic referral
Foreign bodies	Foreign body sensation, pain, blepharospasm
Conjunctival	Remove with moistened cotton swab and treat as abrasion
Corneal*	History of tools, metal fragments
Intraocular*	Assume diagnosis based on history

* = urgent ophthalmology referral.

a prominent complaint in bacterial conjunctivitis. Itching is the major complaint of allergic conjunctivitis along with a chronic history of fluctuating symptoms dependent on weather or seasonal changes. A history of recent viral illness or exposure to an individual with red eye indicates a viral etiology. There are no complaints of pain, photophobia, loss of visual acuity, or trauma in cases of simple conjunctivitis.

The major finding on physical examination is inflammatory edema and hyperemia of the conjunctiva caused by vessel engorgement. The redness is diffuse and intense, indicating a bacterial etiology or mild and diffuse or patchy suggestive of an allergic or viral etiology. A heavy thick discharge indicates bacterial infection; a mucoid discharge indicates a viral etiology, and a thin watery discharge indicates an allergic etiology. Follicular hypertrophy of the inner lids and preauricular adenopathy suggest a viral cause. Visual acuity is normal, as are the cornea, pupil, anterior chamber, and funduscopy findings. Routine bacterial and viral cultures and Gram stain are generally not required.

Corneal Abrasion/Foreign Body. Patients with corneal abrasion or foreign body in the eye complain of sudden onset of pain and tearing immediately after the injury. Fluorescein testing localizes the injury. Small superficial foreign bodies can be removed by an experienced primary care provider or ophthalmologist. Ophthalmology referral is indicated for large foreign bodies and deep abrasions.

Keratitis. Keratitis (inflammation of the cornea) is a nonspecific diagnosis associated with viral infections (particularly herpes), trauma, other infections, or an immunological process triggered by conjunctivitis. Anatomical or physiological factors such as an inward turned eyelash or dry eye syndrome may also cause a keratitis. Presentation usually involves complaints of pain. However, when a subepithelial viral infection or herpetic infection is the cause, there will be little to no pain. Accompanying the pain may be a foreign body sensation, photophobia, and tearing. Physical exam demonstrates an uneven corneal light reflex that stains with fluorescein. Keratitis can be ulcerative or non-ulcerative. Nonulcerative keratitis (caused by some irritation) is illustrated by small pinpoint corneal epithelial erosions (superficial punctuate keratitis) that can lead to scarring. Ulcers indicate necrosis and destruction of corneal tissue. A dendritic ulcer pattern indicates a herpes infection. Rarely, fluorescein stain can be normal when an infection has begun in the deeper layers of the cornea.

Iritis. Iritis (inflammation of the iris or anterior chamber) is usually caused by trauma but can be idiopathic or associated with immune diseases or infections. Inflammatory exudates (protein and red or white cells) in the anterior chamber produce the signs and symptoms. The prominent symptom is deep, dull, aching eye pain accompanied by photophobia. On physical examination the affected pupil is small with a poor and irregular response to light. Visual acuity and pattern of redness vary. Ciliary flush (involvement of deeper scleral vessels) may not be apparent. Cells collecting at the bottom of the chamber will produce a hypopyon (white cells) or hyphema (red cells) if present. Diagnosis is made with a slit lamp that will visualize "cells and flare" (inflammatory exudates) in the anterior chamber.

Angle-Closure Glaucoma. Angle-closure glaucoma rarely presents in individuals younger than 50 years unless there are secondary causes (injury; eye surgery, particularly retinal; or inflammation, e.g., iritis). Other historical factors of importance are a positive family history, Asian or Eskimo ancestry, hyperopia, and use of medications (e.g., topical mydriatics, miotics, or systemic anticholinergics). Dim lighting also may precipitate a glaucoma attack. Multiple factors combine to occlude enough of the trabecular meshwork to cause an elevation of intraocular pressure. These factors include a small eye, a disproportionately large lens (usually caused by aging), and pupillary block (pupil attaches to the lens). Presentation consists of complaints of poorly localized pain, blurry vision, rainbow halos around lights, headache, abdominal pain, nausea, and vomiting. Systemic complaints may dominate the picture and lead the examiner away from the red eye. On physical examination acuity is reduced. There is a unilateral red eye. The cornea is hazy, whereas the iris is gray due to edema. The pupil is dilated and fixed. The anterior chamber is shallow (positive eclipse) in the affected eye and also in the unaffected eye, if primary angle-closure is the case. If secondary to other pathology, the anterior chamber will be of normal depth in the unaffected eye.

DISORDERS OF VISUAL ACUITY

Commonly encountered disorders of visual acuity include cataracts, refractive errors, and open-angle glaucoma. Cataracts are opacities in the lens. They have multiple causes, the most common being senility or age, which is discussed under "Cataracts." Refractive errors signify problems with bending or focusing of light. Optic nerve destruction, the exact mechanism of which is unknown, accounts for the loss of visual acuity in open-angle glaucoma.

Cataract. Normal aging changes include alterations in the largely anaerobic metabolism, protein and fluid concentration within the lens that leads to hardening of fibers and reduced transmission of light. When opacity and decline in acuity are significant, a cataract has formed. The most significant effect of a cataract is to scatter light toward the retina, producing a weaker image received by the retina and accounting for symptoms of glare and reduced contrast and acuity. Other symptoms include diplopia or halos of one or two colors. A history of risk factors should be obtained. These include tobacco and alcohol use, ultraviolet radiation, diabetes, poor antioxidant vitamin status, dehydration, and steroid, antipsychotic, or diuretic use. Findings on physical examination may include diminished acuity with worsening of vision upon pinhole occlusion, a diminished red reflex, or a blurry retinal view despite changes in the focusing lens.

Refractive Error. Common refractive errors include myopia, hyperopia, and presbyopia. Myopia can be either simple (stable in the third decade) or degenerative (progressively destructive of central vision). Commonly there is a long axial length or an exaggerated curve to the cornea and lens or a combination of both. Parallel light rays are focused anterior to the retina. Refractive power is excessive, producing a complaint that distance vision is out of focus. Myopia is associated with an increased vulnerability to trauma and risk of retinal tears or detachment caused by the elongated axis that stretches and thins the retina.

Hyperopia is universal at birth and lessens with increasing years. A short axial length and/or shallow curve to the cornea and lens allow parallel light rays to focus beyond the retina. The individual actively uses accommodation to achieve normal acuity for near or distance vision. Accommodation, via the ciliary muscles, is the additional refractive power normally needed for near vision besides the other refractive abilities of lens and cornea. Constant use of accommodation causes eye strain.

Presbyopia, or hyperopia of aging, occurs when aging causes proteins in the lens to degenerate and the lens to resist changing its shape. Accommodative powers cannot overcome this sclerotic resistance. Persons with hyperopia or presbyopia offer similar complaints of headaches and fatigue caused by constant use of the ciliary muscles to accommodate. Both conditions will cause difficulty with near vision.

During the physical examination, the examiner must ensure that acuity is checked without allowing the patient to squint, or myopia may be missed.

If the Snellen examination is improved with the pinhole occluder, the problem is one of refractive error. The remainder of the ophthalmic examination should be completed.

Open-Angle Glaucoma. History includes an inquiry into risk factors and associated pathologies. Risk factors include age, African ancestry, and a positive family history. Associated pathologies include myopia, hypertension, diabetes, migraine, and vasospasm. The patient is asymptomatic, making the history and a recommendation for complete ophthalmological examination crucial. Recommendations of the American Academy of Ophthalmology are reviewed under "Physical Examination." Ophthalmological examination consists of Goldmann's applanation tonometry and inspection of the optic nerve head. Unique characteristics of glaucoma include a deeply excavated appearance of the optic disc, a twice normal cup-to-disc ratio, and an hourglass pattern of atrophy (Fig. 11.3). The entire pathological mechanism of optic nerve destruction in open-angle glaucoma is unknown. Vascular hyperaggregability, reduced blood flow velocity, and accelerated loss of cells from the trabecular meshwork have been implicated. Although high intraocular pressure is the most consistent risk factor, it is no longer included in the definition because some who have glaucoma have normal pressures. Automated field testing gives the definitive diagnosis. All other methods lack adequate sensitivity.

Open-angle glaucoma is defined as a uniquely abnormal appearance of the optic nerve head and a progressive, slow, asymptomatic loss of peripheral vision followed by central vision loss.

Management

Early recognition and prompt management of serious causes of red eye can prevent vision loss and possibly systemic illness. This is the primary task for the practitioner. Visual acuity problems, in the absence of an inflamed eye, are primarily managed by the ophthalmologist or optometrist, and the situation is not commonly acute.

RED EYE

Indicators of a serious red eye demonstrate the need for an immediate ophthalmologic referral. These indicators include extreme pain, significant photophobia, trauma, pupillary abnormalities, corneal abnormalities, or elevated pressures. If a simple conjunctivitis is determined to be the case, the question becomes one of the infectiousness of the conjunctivitis. Although simple conjunctivitis is generally self-limited and innocuous, topical medi-

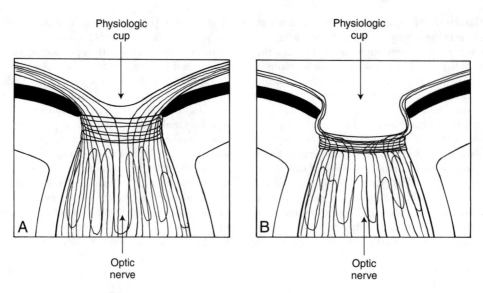

Figure 11.3. Glaucoma. **A.** Cross-sectional view of optic disc showing enlarged physiologic cup. **B.** Cross-sectional view of optic disc showing enlarged cup and hourglass pattern of atrophy.

cations may shorten the course, reduce risk of spread to others, prevent secondary bacterial infection if the etiology is viral, and lesson the potential for corneal disease or systemic infection.

Blepharitis. The key to management of blepharitis is controlling the source of the conjunctivitis and lid irritation. This means treating the scalp with selenium sulfide shampoo, dry eyes with artificial tears, and rosacea with systemic tetracycline. Eyelid hygiene (warm compresses followed by baby shampoos, diluted with water 50%, applied to the lids twice a day, then daily) is practiced in addition to controlling the source. If moderately severe, erythromycin ophthalmic ointment 0.5% or Bacitracin ophthalmic ointment 500 units/g applied topically once or twice daily can be used to treat staphylococcus infection. Resistance has been found with sulfonamide use. The patient should be informed that medical treatment is not a cure but a measure used to control symptoms and prevent complications. Eyelid hygiene may be needed indefinitely. Sties and chalazions are initially treated with warm compresses and topicals.

Conjunctivitis. Topical sulfacetamide sodium ophthalmic solution 10%, one or two drops instilled into the lower conjunctival sac four times a day for 7 days, is the most frequently prescribed medication for first time coverage and is the least expensive. Adverse effects include local irritation, hypersensitivity, and, rarely, Stevens-Johnson syn-

drome in patients previously allergic to systemic sulfur administration. Erythromycin ophthalmic ointment 0.5% twice a day or gentamicin sulfate ophthalmic solution 0.3% every 4 hours may be used alternatively for those who are allergic to sulfur medications. Patients should be educated in hygiene measures such as washing hands, not sharing towels, and avoiding touching of eyes. Medications to be avoided are neomycin (frequently causes contact dermatitis) and steroids (cannot be used without an ophthalmological consult because they mask a viral and fungal infection, leading to loss of vision).

Either topical or systemic medication or a combination of the two may be used for an allergic conjunctivitis. The standard topical prescribed is naphazoline ophthalmic solution 0.3%, one to two drops four times a day. It is sympathomimetic and has no systemic effects. Prolonged use is to be avoided because it may lead to rebound congestion and conjunctivitis medicamentosa. Medications similar to cromolyn sodium (lodoxamide trometha- mine ophthalmic solution) are preventive medications and must be used four times a day daily. Patients generally tire of the regimen. Chlorpheniramine maleate, 4 mg orally four to six times a day, is a commonly used antihistamine that is well tolerated but causes sedation. Other antihistamines such as terfenadine, 60 mg every 12 hours, or astemizole, 10 mg once daily, do not cause sedation but are expensive and can rarely cause lethal cardiac arrhythmias, either as overdoses or in combination with other medications, e.g., erythromycin, that inhibit hepatic metabolism.

Patients should return to the clinic within 3 days. If there is no response, antibiotics should be changed (erythromycin or gentamicin); the patient should be reexamined; and cultures obtained. An ophthalmologic consult is necessary.

Corneal Abrasion/Foreign Body. Treatment of corneal abrasion after removal of foreign body is to instill sulfacetamide sodium ophthalmic solution 10% to the affected eye two drops four times a day for 2–3 days. If pain is severe, the eye is patched for 24 hours, after which most corneal abrasions have effectively healed. If there is no improvement or a worsening of symptoms after 2–3 days, the patient should be referred to an ophthalmologist.

Keratitis. Clinical features suggestive of keratitis also demand urgent referral to an ophthalmologist because there is risk of active infection and permanent damage caused by corneal scarring. In the interim, contact lenses should be removed and artificial tears and erythromycin ointment instilled. Patching is contraindicated if an infection or an ulcer is suspected—which is especially the case when a contact lens is involved.

Iritis. If clinical features are suggestive of iritis, an urgent referral to an ophthalmologist is required. Definitive diagnosis depends on slit lamp visualization of cells and flare. Treatment requires steroids.

Angle-Closure Glaucoma. A presumptive diagnosis and emergent referral are required. Emergent treatment begins first with the unaffected eye at risk. Pilocarpine 0.5 or 1% is instilled every 6 hours. Pilocarpine 2% is instilled in the affected eye, one drop every 15 minutes for 2 hours, then every 4 hours as necessary. Pilocarpine constricts the pupil to pull the iris from the trabecular meshwork. Topical timolol can reduce pressure and help with corneal penetration of pilocarpine. In severe cases, a topical miotic may not work until the intraocular pressure is lowered with hyperostotic agents (glycerol, mannitol, or isosorbide in the case of diabetics) or with acetazolamide, a carbonic anhydrase inhibitor. Morphine sulfate is used for pain and to encourage miosis. Vision loss cannot be restored.

DISORDERS OF VISUAL ACUITY

The only completely successful management of cataracts today is surgery. Management of refractive errors consists of use of corrective lenses and, in the case of myopia, a surgical option. Treatment of glaucoma, whether surgical, medical, open-angle, or angle-closure, aims at lowering intraocular pressure.

Cataract. If cataract is suspected, a referral to an ophthalmologist is made. The best way to visualize a cataract is through a dilated pupil with a slit lamp. Once abnormalities in acuity are found to attribute to cataract, the question becomes one of the indication for surgery. Many cataracts are nonprogressive or increase slowly; only a small proportion need surgery. Nonsurgical management consists of correcting refractive errors, performing a pupil dilation trial, and ensuring adequate lighting, although glare may obviate any benefits. Lifestyle risk factors should be addressed. Follow-up examinations are at least once a year.

Indications for surgery include visual disability based on the Snellen, cataract effect on function, presence of lens-induced disease (glaucoma), and cataract interference with the ability to visualize the fundus to manage other vision-threatening ocular diseases. The risk-to-benefit ratio of surgery is weighed. Risks of surgery include retinal detachment, macular edema, glaucoma, and keratopathy. Left unattended, mature cataracts produce glaucoma and iritis. Surgery restores visual acuity in most. Surgical techniques include extracapsular cataract extraction (anterior lens capsule, nucleus, and cortex of the lens are removed) or phacoemulsification (nucleus is broken up by ultrasound). Half of postoperative patients develop posterior lens capsule cataracts that are repaired by laser and have favorable outcomes. After extraction, the patient suffers from hyperopia. To resolve the severe hyperopia, an intraocular lens is implanted at the time of surgery, or thick glasses or contact lenses are used.

Refractive Error. Myopia can be corrected with concave lenses or surgery. Surgical interventions (incision and laser) are effective for mild to moderate myopia but not for severe. Adverse effects include overcorrection and retinal detachment. Hyperopia is corrected with a convex lens that adds refractive power to bring light rays inward onto the retina. Reading glasses or bifocals correct presbyopia. Myopic shift occurs when a person with presbyopia can see close work clearer without glasses.

Open-Angle Glaucoma. All patients suspected of having glaucoma should be referred to an ophthalmologist for definitive diagnosis and individualized treatment. Current treatment modalities (medication or surgery) aim at lowering intraocular pressures. A step-down additive format is used to prescribe medication. Topicals are first line. Beta-blockers followed by the addition of epinephrine and then pilocarpine are used to reduce formation (beta-blockers) or increase outflow (epinephrine and pilocarpine) of aqueous humor. Systemic absorption of topical medications can be allayed by instructing the patient to apply pressure over the lacrimal sac for 30 seconds after administration. When topicals have not decreased pressures sufficiently, oral acetohexamide is added. It suppresses aqueous humor formation. Common side effects of these medications include ocular irritation with epinephrine; blurry vision with pilocarpine; and lethargy, gastritis, and paresthesias with acetohex-

amide. Bone marrow suppression is a rare adverse effect of acetohexamide.

Surgical intervention consists of laser treatment and then drainage channels, shunts, or ciliary body destruction to improve outflow. Adjuncts to medical and surgical therapies include control of hypertension and diabetes and treatment of vascular disease. Lifestyle issues including cessation of smoking and use of aerobic exercise should be addressed.

Few studies have focused on clinically relevant points. None have involved long-term follow-up. The National Eye Institute is conducting a long-term multicenter clinical trial to answer questions regarding the clinical efficacy of open-angle glaucoma therapeutics.

ILLUSTRATIVE CASES WITH SELF-ASSESSMENT QUESTIONS AND ANSWERS

Case 1

A young woman complains of awakening for a few days with a discharge and redness in her right eye and her lids sticking together. The left eye is beginning to appear similar to the right. There is some mild irritation but no pain or vision problem. There is no history of past eye problems or trauma, allergies, or recent upper respiratory infection. She is sexually active with her husband, who had a similar problem last week. He went to a clinic near his job where they gave him some drops, but she does not remember the name. He is better now. She feels well and has no systemic complaints.

On exam, there is diffuse injection of the conjunctiva of the right eye with minimal involvement of the left. A mucopurulent discharge is apparent at the nasal canthus. Acuity, lids, cornea, and pupil are normal.

QUESTION: *What is the most likely diagnosis?*

a. Blepharitis
b. Iritis
c. Bacterial conjunctivitis
d. Viral conjunctivitis
e. Episcleritis

Answer: c. *This is most likely common bacterial conjunctivitis. Blepharitis is characterized by scaly lids and episcleritis by local injection. Iritis would have been indicated by pain or photophobia or pain on accommodation. Because her husband responded quickly to antibiotics and because lymphadenopathy is absent, this is probably not a viral or chlamydial conjunctivitis. A profuse discharge and hyperacute onset (<12 hours) would have indicated a gonococcal infection.*

QUESTION: *What treatment is indicated?*

ANSWER: *One drop of sodium sulfacetamide ophthalmic solution should be instilled into the conjunctival sac of each eye four times daily. Cool compresses may help the irritation. The patient should be instructed in hygiene measures such as washing hands, not sharing towels, and avoiding touching of eyes. The patient should return to clinic in 3 days, and by that time the infection should have cleared. If the infection is still present, a chlamydia infection or a reaction to the medication may be considered. The medication should be stopped, cultures taken, and an ophthalmology consult obtained.*

Case 2

A 62-year-old man complains that his left eye has been swollen and painful for a few days. There has been no change in his acuity and no photophobia. There is no previous history of eye problems or skin disorders. He is otherwise feeling well.

On physical examination, the left eyelid has a tender, red, swollen area at the lower lid margin. Otherwise the lids are normal, as is the remainder of the exam.

QUESTION: *What is the most likely diagnosis?*

a. Chalazion
b. Hordeolum (sty)
c. Septal cellulitis
d. Blepharitis
e. Dacryocystitis

ANSWER: b. *The diagnosis is hordeolum (sty). A chalazion is a nonpainful nodule that points inside and can produce a foreign body sensation. This patient is 62, so the possibility of a sebaceous or basal cell carcinoma increases, especially if the chalazion is recurrent or resistant to treatment. Septal cellulitis is indicated by swollen, reddened eyelids with lymphadenopathy and fever. An urgent ophthalmologic consult is needed. Treatment entails intravenous antibiotics. Dacryocystitis presents with pain over the lacrimal sac. Blepharitis often accompanies a hordeolum but with involvement of the entire lid. An asymmetric involvement of the lid is another indicator of a possible carcinoma.*

SORE THROAT

Clinicians frequently evaluate patients with sore throats. Despite the high prevalence of the complaint, the most important questions regarding diagnosis and management of pharyngitis remain unanswered. This section will explore some common causes of pharyngitis; the clinically most challenging pathogen, *S. pyogenes* (strep) will be discussed in detail because recognition and treatment of streptococcal pharyngitis can prevent serious complications.

Pathophysiologic Correlation

Inflammation of the tissues of the nasopharynx causes the patient to experience a sore throat. Surrounding lymphatic tissues, including the tonsils, adenoids, and cervical nodes, react to contain infec-tion. Viral infections are especially noted for causing extensive inflammation of sinus and nasopharyngeal tissues. As drainage from the sinuses and middle ears is blocked, sinusitis or otitis can complicate pharyngitis.

Although the most common cause of sore throat is a viral upper respiratory infection, there are important nonviral infectious causes (1). Streptococcal pharyngitis is caused by *S. pyogenes* (strep), a Gram-positive beta-hemolytic group A streptococcus. The organism produces numerous molecules facilitating virulence and inducing antibody formation in the host (2) (Table 11.4). Bacterial products attach bacteria to epithelial membranes and assist penetration into deeper tissues. They foil host defenses by blocking phagocytosis of the bacteria. The atypical pathogens such as *M. pneumoniae* and *Chlamydia pneumoniae* (TWAR strain) frequently cause sore throat in adults. Unlike viruses, which invade the cells lining the upper respiratory tract, the mycoplasma remain attached to the epithelial surface, damaging the cells and impairing ciliary motion (3). *C. pneumoniae*, a recently described pathogen, enters the respiratory mucosal cells and multiplies within them (4). Although *C. pneumoniae* usually causes pneumonia, many patients have pharyngitis as an initial symptom (5).

Clinical and Laboratory Evaluation

When evaluating a patient with a sore throat, the clinician must determine whether the cause is beta-hemolytic group A streptococcus, whether the illness is potentially life-threatening, and whether the sore throat is a symptom of disease whose true anatomic locus lies elsewhere. Remember that sore throat is a subjective symptom. Pharyngitis, or inflammation of the pharynx, is an objective finding of reddened, injected, edematous mucosa. Tonsillitis exists when the tonsils are reddened and enlarged; exudative tonsillitis means that a patchy exudate adheres to the tonsils.

HISTORY

Knowledge of the setting in which the sore throat appeared will prove helpful. The time of year is useful in determining infectious and allergic causes. The contacts of the patient and any illnesses in those contacts or in the family aids in identifying an infectious cause. If an epidemic of influenza or streptococcus is ongoing, the patient probably has the same illness. Recent confinement in a closed, crowded space such as an airplane or bus is another clue to an infectious cause.

Table 11.4.
Streptococcal Products and Pathogenic Effects

Product	Effect
M proteins	More than 80 distinct serotypes
	Filaments projecting beyond cell surface
	Resistance to phagocytosis
	Antibodies to M proteins confer protective immunity to that serotype
Lipotechoic acid	Adhesin: binds to oral epithelium
Hyaluronate capsule	Antiphagocytic
	Heavily encapsulated strains are more virulent
	Causes mucoid appearance of colonies
Streptolysin A&O	Causes hemolysis in culture on sheep's blood agar
	Antistreptolysin O can be assayed to confirm recent infection
Streptokinase	Clot lysis
	Commercially produced as a treatment for acute myocardial infarction
Deoxyribonucleases (DNase A, B, C, and D)	Anti-DNase A can be assayed to confirm recent infection
Hyaluronidase	Spreading factor
	Destroys collagen, allowing bacteria to invade host tissues
Streptococcal pyrogenic exotoxins (erythrogenic toxins A, B, and C)	Cause rash of scarlet fever
	Induce shock
	Impair immune function
	Disrupt blood brain barrier
	Multiorgan damage
	Strains producing erythogenic toxin A are most virulent

Adapted from material presented in Bisno AL. Group A streptococcal infections and rheumatic fever. Engl J Med 1991;325:783–792.

Exposures to new pets, plants, foods, medications, or geographic location may bring out a previously unrecognized allergy. Sore throat after a meal of fish raises the possibilities both of allergy and of a fish bone lodged in the throat. Symptoms after meals, while lying flat, and associated with sour taste in the mouth suggest gastroesophageal reflux with inflammation of the pharyngeal tissues. Intimate contact with a new partner can transmit Epstein-Barr virus and gonorrhea.

The course and associated symptoms often provide the most valuable clues. Acute presentations are more likely to be infectious, and prolonged symptoms often are associated with other disease processes such as chronic allergies, reflux, or tumor, although symptoms from unrecognized sinusitis will persist. Fever, chills, sweats, myalgias, and arthralgias all indicate an infectious cause. Cough is usually not associated with streptococcal infection but instead is induced by many other causes of pharyngitis, especially viruses and the atypical respiratory pathogens such as mycoplasma and chlamydia. In addition, patients with allergies or with sinusitis often have cough accompanying their sore throats because secretions pass from the nose and sinuses into the posterior pharynx. Conjunctivitis and runny or stuffy nose also signal viral or allergic causes and virtually exclude strep.

As always, the underlying health of the patient must be ascertained. Patients with human immunodeficiency virus (HIV) infection complaining of sore throat are likely to have thrush or herpes simplex. Smokers with sore throat present special challenges: they may have simple irritation from smoke, viral infections to which they are especially vulnerable, or cancer of the pharynx or larynx. Rarely, a patient with angina could have pain radiating to the neck and perceive this as an intermittent sore throat.

PHYSICAL EXAMINATION

When examining a patient with sore throat, carefully compare the severity of physical findings with the reported intensity of symptoms. A patient complaining of extreme sore throat with intense pain on swallowing but whose pharynx looks quite normal on exam could have epiglottitis, which is fatal if untreated. Patients who are drooling should undergo immediate ear, nose, and throat evaluation, because this can be a sign of impending airway obstruction. Patients with high fevers may have influenza or systemic streptococcal infection. Hypotension and tachycardia raise the specter of toxic shock syndrome. A pink, sandpaper-like rash is pathognomonic for scarlet fever.

Examine the patient for evidence of conjunctival inflammation, the unilateral periorbital swelling that accompanies sinusitis, and reddened nose from rhinorrhea. Listen for hoarseness or nasal voice. Examine the oral mucosa carefully for lesions such as canker sores, viral enanthems, thrush, vesicles (herpangina), or petechiae on the palate. Inspect the pharynx for inflammation and the tonsils for exudates; without exudates, strep is less likely. A cobblestone appearance to the posterior pharynx is correlated with allergy. Occasionally drainage from the nose and sinuses visibly coats the pharyngeal wall. A peritonsillar abscess displaces the tonsil medially and deflects the uvula away; this patient may also have trismus.

Examine the lymph nodes. Adenopathy is associated with various infectious causes of sore throat, although an isolated enlarged node can be from lymphadenitis (tender) or cancer (nontender). More prominent later in the disease, adenopathy of the anterior cervical nodes is a clue to streptococcal pharyngitis. Posterior cervical adenopathy is associated with viral infections, especially Epstein-Barr infection (mononucleosis) or HIV.

LABORATORY EVALUATION

Laboratory tests for strep, the traditional throat culture and the newer rapid antigen detection kits, suffer from variable sensitivity (6). Although the sensitivity for a throat culture can be as high as 90% through a commercial laboratory, in-office incubation and interpretation of cultures can miss up to 70% of cases. Studies of trained technicians performing the newer rapid office tests for strep reveal sensitivities of 80–95%; however, a sensitivity of only 67% was reported from a study evaluating a rapid test in a system of urgent care centers (7).

To collect an adequate specimen for throat culture, swab the tonsils and posterior pharynx briskly. The rapid antigen tests often specify a particular swab; this swab and the culture swab can be held together when sampling the throat. Send the culture swab to the laboratory in the appropriate transport container. When the bacteria are cultured on agar containing red blood cells, streptolysins secreted by *S. pyogenes* lyse the red blood cells, clearing a halo around the colony. Group A strep are identified by confirming the presence of group specific antigen in the cultured bacteria.

The throat culture incubates for 48 hours before results are available; this is a major disadvantage. The rapid test gives results quickly, but the low sensitivity dictates simultaneous culturing to pick up any missed cases, obviating some of the time advantage. Cost of the rapid test can be a factor, but one analysis revealed that this can easily be offset by savings in unneeded antibiotics (8).

Gonococcal pharyngitis can be cultured as for genital infection. Epstein-Barr virus infection can be identified by the serum Monospot test; if initially negative, this test should be repeated several days later, allowing the patient time to mount the antibodies measured by the test. *Hemophilus influenzae* causing epiglottitis is usually confirmed by blood cultures. Cultures for particular respiratory viruses are not of clinical use, although in certain circumstances when confirmation of influenza infection would be useful in containing an epidemic, serological tests for influenza A and B can be obtained.

Differential Diagnosis

Seemingly endless lists of causes of sore throat can be generated, but Table 11.5 lists the most frequently encountered etiologies and summarizes key findings on history and physical exam. The most pertinent diagnoses will be discussed in more detail below.

STREPTOCOCCAL PHARYNGITIS

Pharyngeal infection from streptococcus spreads by droplet from person to person, with highest prevalence in the late winter and early spring. The disease most commonly afflicts school-age children, but adults in contact with children or living in crowded situations (e.g., military barracks) are also at risk. Streptococcal pharyngitis can infect many members of a family, especially when multiple generations or large numbers of children constitute the household. Asymptomatic carriers of strep may act as a reservoir for infection of others. The prevalence of streptococcal pharyngitis ranges from a baseline of 5% of patients with sore throats (1) to 44% of patients who had throat cultures performed during an epidemic (9).

Streptococcal pharyngitis can initiate several suppurative and nonsuppurative complications (Table 11.6). Tissue proteases expressed by the bac-

Table 11.5.
Important Differential Diagnoses of Sore Throat

Causes of Sore Throat	Identifying Signs and Symptoms
Infectious	
Viral	
Common cold	Rhinorrhea and conjunctival inflammation
Adenovirus	Herpangina, gastrointestinal complaints possible
Influenza A and B	High fever, arthralgias and myalgias, cough
Epstein-Barr virus (mononucleosis)	Posterior cervical adenopathy, fatigue
Herpes simplex virus	Characteristic ulcerated lesions
Viral enanthems	Rash
Bacterial	
Streptococcus pyogenes	Fever, anterior cervical adenopathy, tonsillar exudates, absence of cough
Hemophilus influenzae (epiglottitis)	Pharynx normal in contrast to severe symptoms, airway obstruction
Neisseria gonorrhea	History of sexual contact
Atypical pathogens	
Mycoplasma pneumoniae	Cough, vesicles in ear canals
Chlamydia pneumoniae (TWAR)	Cough
Fungal	
Thrush	Scattered white patches on erythematous bases
Deep tissue infection	
Peritonsillar abscess	Deflection of tonsil and uvula, trismus
Retropharyngeal abscess	Dysphagia, respiratory compromise
Ludwig's angina	Cellulitis of tissues of neck, respiratory compromise
Lymphadenitis	Tender enlarged node
Allergic	
Hayfever or other environmental allergies	History of prior seasonal or exposure-related symptoms
Angioedema	Perioral or periorbital edema, hives
Mechanical	
Postintubation	History of intubation
Trauma	Ecchymoses, abrasions
Foreign body	History of ingestion
Pharyngeal or laryngeal cancer	History of smoking
Lymphoma or leukemia with infiltration of tonsils and adenoids	Fatigue, anemia, thrombocytopenia, fever, night sweats, weight loss
Irritative	
Smoking or other inhalations	History
Overuse	History
Persistent cough	History
Postnasal drip	Evidence of allergy or sinusitis
Gastroesophageal reflux	History suggestive of reflux

teria, allowing extension of the original infection into deeper tissues, facilitate complications such as abscesses, cellulitis, and bacteremia. Streptococcal pyrogenic toxin, especially exotoxin A, causes life-threatening scarlet fever and shock, which are becoming increasingly prevalent (2, 10).

Acute rheumatic fever (ARF), which occurs in approximately 1.6–3% of patients with streptococcal pharyngitis (11), follows the acute infection by 1–3 weeks. Patients present with any of the mani-

festations listed in Table 11.7 (12). The illness is confirmed by demonstration of recent streptococcal infection by culture or by high antistreptolysin O titers. The disease has traditionally affected patient groups without ready access to medical care, but recent outbreaks have occurred in middle-class suburbs and military bases (2, 11). Patients who have had ARF are at increased risk of repeat episodes during new episodes of streptococcal pharyngitis, so they require long-term antibiotic prophylaxis. It is a leading cause of valvular heart disease worldwide and in older patients who contracted streptococcal pharyngitis before the use of antibiotics.

Why only some patients develop ARF after streptococcal pharyngitis remains mysterious. Characteristics of both host and pathogen seem to be involved: serotyping of streptococcus during outbreaks of ARF reveals that only a few strains are associated with outbreaks of the disease (13), and patients with certain human lymphocyte antigen types appear to be more susceptible (2). ARF was even thought to have disappeared in the 1970s in industrialized countries (14), but it has reappeared in several outbreaks since 1986 (11, 15). These observations support the longstanding theory that some aspect of the immune response to streptococci, possibly antibodies against M protein of certain strains, cross-reacts with human tissues such as cardiac muscle. Vaccines, exploiting type-specific and durable immunity to M proteins, are being designed to prevent strep infection and ARF.

Diagnosing streptococcal pharyngitis is important because cases recognized and treated within 9 days of onset will not progress to ARF. The most commonly used decision rules concentrate on the features of fever, exudates, cervical adenopathy, and absence of cough (16). The predictive value of clinical criteria increases when the prevalence of strep pharyngitis is higher, as in an epidemic, but at other times physicians will overestimate the diagnosis of strep by 69–93% (15, 16). Providers more accurately identify who does not have strep (17). The 1% of adult patients who are asymptomatic carriers of the bacterium (6) complicate the determination of which patients have strep pharyngitis. A carrier presenting with viral pharyngitis would nonetheless have a positive culture and receive unnecessary treatment.

VIRAL UPPER RESPIRATORY INFECTION

The most common viral upper respiratory tract infection causing pharyngitis is the common cold, which is characterized by widespread inflammation in the nose and paranasal sinuses, the pharynx, and the middle ear. It readily spreads from person to person via droplets and hand-to-hand contact. The illness is self-limiting but can be complicated by otitis media, sinusitis, and bronchitis. Because there are a plethora of strains of cold viruses, an individual remains susceptible to the syndrome throughout life.

GONOCOCCAL PHARYNGITIS

Oral sexual contact with infected individuals can transmit *Neisseria gonorrhoeae*, which will cause

Table 11.6.
Complications of Streptococcal Pharyngitis

Suppurative
  Local
    Peritonsillar abscess
    Retropharyngeal abscess
    Ludwig's angina (cellulitis of the neck)
    Lymphadenitis
  Systemic
    Septicemia
    Toxic shock syndrome
    Scarlet fever
Nonsuppurative
  Acute rheumatic fever
  Poststreptococcal glomerulonephritis

Table 11.7.
Jones Criteria (Revised) for Guidance in Diagnosis of Rheumatic Fever

Major Manifestations	Minor Manifestations	Evidence of Streptococcal Infection
Carditis	Previous rheumatic fever or rheumatic heart disease	Increased titer of antistreptococcal antibodies such as antistreptolysin O
Polyarthritis	Arthralgia	Positive throat culture for Group A streptococcus
Chorea	Fever	Recent scarlet fever
Erythemia marginatum	Prolonged P-R interval	
Subcutaneous nodules	Acute phase reactants: erythrocyte sedimentation rate, leukocytosis	

The presence of two major criteria, or of one major and two minor criteria, indicates a high probability of acute rheumatic fever, if supported by evidence of preceding Group A streptococcal infection. Adapted from the American Heart Association. Jones Criteria (revised) for guidance in the diagnosis of rheumatic fever. Circulation 1984;69:204A–208A.

pharyngitis. Evidence of genital or rectal infection support the diagnosis, but the patient may present solely with sore throat. This infection is probably widely underdiagnosed.

MYCOPLASMA

An atypical bacterial pathogen, mycoplasma causes a range of upper and lower respiratory infections, including pharyngitis. Cough is usually present, and there may be bullous myringitis as well. Infection may progress to bronchitis or even pneumonia in patients with mycoplasma pharyngitis.

CHLAMYDIA

The strain of chlamydia called TWAR has been renamed *C. pneumoniae*. It is distinct from *C. trachomatis*, which causes genital and ocular infection, and from *C. psittaci*, which is transmitted by birds. Although early reports of the disease included a patient who had pharyngitis alone (5), in most patients the pharyngitis is an early manifestation of chlamydia infection, which progresses to bronchitis or pneumonia.

MONONUCLEOSIS

The "kissing disease," caused by infection via droplet with Epstein-Barr virus, is common among teenagers and young adults. Characterized by exudative pharyngitis, posterior cervical adenopathy, and splenomegaly, the illness may also involve the liver, causing tender hepatomegaly and abnormal liver function tests. A rash can accompany episodes of viremia, and hemolytic anemia can complicate the course. Although suffering from profound fatigue, most patients remain stable. Mononucleosis

is named for the atypical lymphocytes that dominate the differential white blood cell count in infected patients.

EPIGLOTTITIS

Although *H. influenzae* is widely known to cause life-threatening epiglottitis in children, it can also infect the epiglottis of adults. The disease can be fatal from respiratory compromise if unrecognized and untreated. Patients complain of extremely painful, rapidly progressive sore throats and may drool because of severe odynophagia. Because the epiglottis is not normally visible during exam of the pharynx and because of the danger of precipitating acute airway obstruction during indirect laryngoscopy, refer patients suspected of epiglottitis to an otolaryngologist for emergent evaluation.

Management

A reasonable approach to the patient with pharyngitis is outlined in Figure 11.4. The principles underlying this algorithm are prevention of suppurative complications and ARF by presumptive treatment of patients who are the most ill-appearing or at greatest risk for ARF and allowing the patients with lower clinical probability to await results of rapid test and culture. For patients with none of the four clinical features of strep pharyngitis and who are not at increased risk for ARF, the clinician could elect not to culture, but only if the presentation fits convincingly with another etiology.

Streptococcal pharyngitis is treated with penicillin, which is inexpensive, effective, and available everywhere. Treat adults with oral penicillin V 250

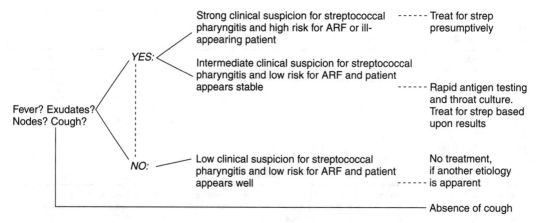

Figure 11.4. Approach to patient with pharyngitis.

mg every 6 hours for 10 days. The full course is needed for maximum effectiveness in prevention of ARF. A single intramuscular dose of benzathine penicillin, 1.2 million units for adults, is an excellent choice in patients at high risk for ARF, patients who may not comply with the full regimen, and patients who appear more ill. Whether penicillin treatment shortens the course of streptococcal pharyngitis or improves symptoms rapidly has not been convincingly demonstrated; in one placebo-controlled study of acetaminophen vs. penicillin with acetaminophen, there was little symptomatic improvement with the addition of penicillin (18).

Erythromycin 250 mg orally every 6 hours for 10 days is the choice for patients who are allergic to penicillin. It would seem to be a good first-line agent for pharyngitis given its usefulness in treating mycoplasma, but there are some strains of strep that are resistant. Tetracycline cannot be used to treat strep infections because of widespread resistance.

Mycoplasma is treated by erythromycin 250–500 mg orally every 6 hours for 7–10 days, and chlamydia is treated by a tetracycline such as doxycycline 100 mg orally every 12 hours for 10 days. Pharyngeal gonorrhea is treated as for genital infection. Epiglottitis from *H. influenza* requires admission with intravenous antibiotics active against beta-lactamase producing organisms and prophylactic intubation.

Antibiotics are ineffective against viral pharyngitis; however, as with all the infectious causes of sore throat, advising the patient to use analgesic agents such as acetaminophen will give symptomatic relief.

ILLUSTRATIVE CASES WITH SELF-ASSESSMENT QUESTIONS AND ANSWERS

Case 1

A 26-year-old elementary school teacher presents in March with 2 days of sore throat.

QUESTION: *Identify features of her presentation that place her at risk for strep.*

ANSWER: *Her occupational exposure to children and the time of year are both risks for strep throat but also are consistent with viral infection.*

QUESTION: *The patient tells you on further history that the sore throat is mild, she has had no fever, and she has noted a nonproductive cough at night. She has had a runny nose and feels like her ears are clogged. Her temperature is 99.3°F; you find mild conjunctival injection, clear tympanic membranes, no sinus tenderness, and mild pharyngeal inflammation without exudative tonsillitis. There is no adenopathy. What is your leading diagnosis at this point?*

ANSWER: *This presentation is most consistent with viral infection. Because there are none of the clinical features of strep infection, you could elect not to culture.*

QUESTION: *As you begin to tell her to rest and take acetaminophen, she interrupts you, stating she came in because several students in her class had been diagnosed with strep, so she really wants a culture. In addition, she says that she lives with her mother, who was born in the Caribbean and who has a heart murmur; the cardiologist thinks the patient's mother has had rheumatic fever. How does this new data change your management?*

ANSWER: *Her proximity to documented strep infections should prompt a culture. Her mother likely had ARF as a child and thus may be at some increased risk of recurrence should she contract strep, although with increasing time the risk of recurrence diminishes. If the patient had a history of ARF, she should be treated presumptively for strep.*

Case 2

A 46-year-old man presents to the emergency room late one evening with 3 days of malaise, arthralgias, fever to 102°F, and sore throat without cough. On exam he has no exudates, but he does have impressive pharyngitis with beefy red swollen tonsils.

QUESTION: *What is your assessment, and how will you diagnose his illness?*

ANSWER: *He has some but not all clinical features of strep; in particular there are no tonsillar exudates. He may have a viral infection, perhaps influenza, although he is without cough. You should do a rapid test for strep if this is available and send a confirmatory culture as well.*

QUESTION: *The rapid test comes back negative, and you send him home with acetaminophen and instructions to return immediately if his condition worsens; 2 days later the follow-up nurse calls to tell you that his throat culture was positive. You call the patient to tell him, and he says he is much improved. Should you treat him at this point for strep?*

ANSWER: *Yes. Although his acute infection appears to be self-limiting, you still can protect him from ARF by treating now, because it is within 9 days from the start of symptoms. You may consider intramuscular penicillin, because he is unlikely to comply to a course of oral antibiotics if he is feeling well.*

SINUSITIS

Sinusitis is a highly prevalent disease condition. The incidence of sinusitis is particularly increased during "allergy season" (spring and fall) and "cold season" (winter). To understand the multiple causative factors of sinusitis, including anatomical defects, allergies, and infections, it is imperative to have a firm knowledge of the structure and physiology of the sinuses.

Pathophysiologic Correlation

The paranasal sinuses are hollow air-filled spaces lined with ciliated epithelium. The cilia function to clear the sinuses of contaminants, either biological or chemical. The sinuses—maxillary, frontal, ethmoid, and sphenoid—are sterile under normal conditions. Each individual sinus drains into the nose, through an ostium, an opening averaging 2 mm in diameter. Blockage of the ostia and/or malfunction of the ciliated epithelial cells are common findings in sinusitis.

A sagittal view of the paranasal sinuses and lat-

eral wall of the nose is depicted in Figure 11.5. Structural abnormalities, particularly those in proximity to the ostia, can predispose to sinus infection. Defects, such as septal deviation and nasal polyps, can impair drainage of the sinuses and lead to the accumulation of mucus and subsequent infection. Patients who are immunocompromised, such as diabetics, are at increased risk for infection. Asthmatics also are at increased risk.

Any condition causing local edema and blockage of the ostia can result in sinus infection. Allergy and extremely dry air both cause local edema and blockage of the ostia. Even without infection, inflammation of the sinuses can cause pain. The pain of sinusitis is positional and probably related to the inflammatory process and small changes in the structure of and pressure within the sinuses.

Viral and bacterial infections are very common. Pneumococcus and *H. influenzae* are the most frequently cultured bacterial pathogens in adults, accounting for about three-fourths of cases of acute bacterial sinusitis. In chronic sinusitis, these pathogens, staphylococcus, other streptococci, and Gram-negative bacilli are the bacteria most frequently cultured. The bacteria infect the epithelia, ultimately causing local inflammation, edema, and mucus production and leading to blockage of the ostia.

Clinical and Laboratory Evaluation

The importance of a focused history and physical examination cannot be overemphasized. Laboratory tests are helpful in some cases and essential in fewer. In general, the diagnosis of acute sinusitis is made on the basis of clinical evaluation only, without the aid of the laboratory.

HISTORY

The clinician must learn if the patient has a past history of allergy or hayfever, recurrent symptoms and time of these symptoms, structural abnormality of the sinuses or the septum, asthma, or a condition causing immunocompromise, such as diabetes or HIV disease. Although a creative clinician could think of several other questions, there are three related to current symptoms that are worth asking every patient with sinusitis (Table 11.8). Ask about

- Maxillary toothache;
- Improvement with decongestants;
- Colored nasal discharge.

Certain facts are relevant in the history of a patient with chronic sinusitis. Be sure to inquire what ther-

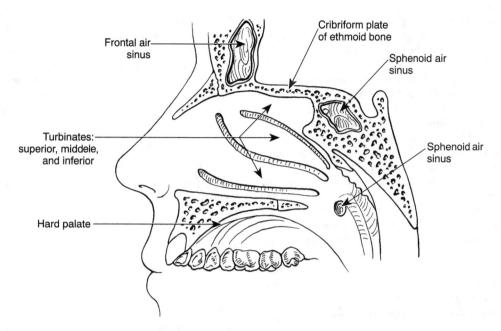

Figure 11.5. Lateral wall of the nose. From Willms JL, Schneiderman H, Algranati PS. Physical diagnosis: bedside evaluation of diagnosis and function. Baltimore: Williams & Wilkins, 1994:137.

apies have been used and which have been successful. Find out which antibiotics were helpful and how long they were used. If there was a culture-proven diagnosis from the most recent infection, try to obtain the name of the pathogen and the results of the antibiotic sensitivities.

PHYSICAL EXAMINATION

Abnormal transillumination of the maxillary sinuses and visualization of purulent secretions on examination of the nares are the two physical findings that best predict the presence of sinusitis. In fact, these two findings and the three key questions

Table 11.8.
Performance Characteristics of and Signs and Symptoms for Sinusitis in 247 Patients

Symptoms	Sensitivity (%)	Specificity
Maxillary toothache	18	93
No improvement with decongestants	41	80
Hyposmia	56	64
Colored discharge	72	52
Preceding upper respiratory infection	50	61
Malaise	56	47
Headache	68	30
Facial pain	52	48
Fever, chills, or sweats	45	51
Purulent secretion	51	76
Nasal speech	45	73
Abnormal transillumination (mini-MagLite)	73	54
Sinus tenderness	48	65
Temperature >38°C[a]	16	83

Adapted with permission from Williams JW, Simel DL, Roberts LR, Samsa GP. Clinical evaluation for sinusitis: making the diagnosis by history and physical examination. Ann Intern Med 1992;117;705–710.
[a] $n = 187$ (data not recorded for 60 patients).

listed under "History" combine to form a five factor checklist for diagnosing sinusitis. If all five factors are present, the probability of sinusitis is 92% (Table 11.9).

The classic finding of tenderness to palpation over the maxillary and/or frontal sinuses is neither sensitive nor specific for sinusitis. Fever or nasal speech is an insensitive finding but has some specificity. The nose must be examined for structural defects and foreign bodies and the mouth examined for dental caries and abscesses.

Transillumination of the maxillary sinuses is accomplished by shining a transilluminator from the infraorbital area and observing any light transmitted through the palate. This technique must be performed in a dark room, and the clinician's eyes must be accustomed to the dark. The frontal sinus is examined by transilluminating superiorly through the supraorbital ridge and observing light transmitted through the palate. Pus and mucus buildup in the sinus will block light transmission.

LABORATORY EVALUATION

X-rays of the paranasal sinuses are often ordered but are usually not necessary. Films showing opacification or air-fluid levels are relatively specific for sinusitis but are not very sensitive. Films showing mucosal thickening are fairly sensitive but not specific. The maxillary and frontal sinuses are easily visualized on x-ray (Fig. 11.6); the ethmoids and sphenoids are difficult to visualize. In general, x-rays of the paranasal sinuses should be ordered if the diagnosis is not certain or if the symptoms have

not responded to therapy. Computed tomography is reserved for diagnosis of ethmoid or sphenoid sinusitis, for preoperative evaluation, or for diagnosis of suspected structural abnormality.

Culture and sensitivity are useful in chronic or recalcitrant sinusitis. When culture is indicated, a nasal swab is inadequate. Sinus aspirates are the only reliable culture source.

Differential Diagnosis

The differential diagnosis of sinusitis can be overwhelmingly broad, but the most common diagnoses can be categorized as follows:

- Allergies/inflammations
- Infections
- Anatomic/structural defect
- Dental processes
- Upper respiratory tract infection without sinusitis

Allergies and infections account for the vast majority of cases of sinusitis. Although the symptoms can be identical for the diagnoses listed above, the history and physical examination will usually lead the clinician to the correct diagnosis. Patients with a history of allergies, hayfever, or postnasal drip are likely to have allergic sinusitis. Those with visible structural defects in the nasal passages are more likely to have symptoms related to the defects. Patients with abscesses or inflammation of maxillary teeth are at risk for maxillary sinusitis (by direct extension). Most other patients who do not have these specific findings on history or physical examination will have infectious sinusitis. Stuffy nose does not equal sinusitis; however, some patients equate the two conditions.

Infection can spread from the sinuses to other local sites. Patients who present with abnormal mental status, or signs of uncontained infection (e.g., significant facial swelling, proptosis, severe pain, or a toxic appearance) could have spread of infection to the cranial bones, orbit, brain, or meninges. They should be hospitalized for evaluation and parenteral antibiotic therapy.

Management

Allergic sinusitis can be controlled by using several different modalities. Initial treatment in the noninfected patient includes oral antihistamines and decongestants, either inhaled or oral. An inexpensive initial prescription would include an antihistamine such as diphenhydramine 25 mg or chlorphenira-

Table 11.9.
Predicted Probability of Sinusitis

Number of Predictors Present[a]	Predicted Probability of Sinusitis (95% confidence interval)
0	9 (5–17)
1	21 (15–28)
2	40 (33–47)
3	63 (53–72)
4	81 (69–89)
5	92 (81–96)

From Williams JW, Simel DL, Roberts LR, Samsa GP. Clinical evaluation for sinusitis: making the diagnosis by history and physical examination. Ann Intern Med 1992;117:705–710.
[a]Predictors of sinusitis from the logistic regression model are maxillary toothache, history of colored nasal discharge, poor response to nasal decongestants, abnormal transillumination, and purulent secretion on examination.

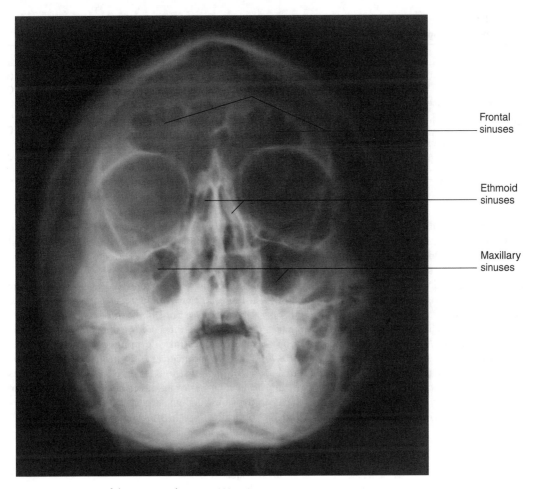

Frontal
sinuses

Ethmoid
sinuses

Maxillary
sinuses

Figure 11.6. X-ray of the paranasal sinuses: Water's view.

mine 4 mg orally every 8 hours and a decongestant such as pseudoephedrine 30 mg orally every 8 hours or oxymetazoline nasal spray topically every 12 hours. Patients who get too drowsy from standard antihistamines may benefit from a more expensive, newer formulation such as terfenadine 60 mg orally twice daily. Inhaled corticosteroids such as flunisolide or beclomethasone twice daily should be added if symptoms persist. Mucolytics such as guaifenesin may be helpful, as well. Desensitization therapy is reserved for those whose symptoms persist despite multiple drug trials. Desensitization works by cumulatively overwhelming the immune system with a specific allergen to the point that more of that allergen produces little to no response. After skin testing to determine which antigen(s) is the allergen, small then increasingly larger doses

of it are injected serially over months. Usually by 6–12 months the patient is effectively desensitized.

The goals of treatment of infectious sinusitis are to promote drainage and eradicate infection. Unless drainage is reestablished, infection will be difficult to treat. Decongestants such as pseudoephedrine or oxymetazoline should be prescribed. Humidification of the patient's bedroom and the inhalation of water vapor are effective and safe treatments. The choice of antibiotic should reflect the most likely pathogen. For acute sinusitis a 10- to 14-day course of ampicillin, amoxicillin, trimethoprim/ sulfamethoxazole, or erythromycin is an effective and inexpensive treatment. Please refer to Table 11.10 for recommended dosages. If there is no resolution of symptoms, x-rays of the paranasal sinuses should be ordered. If x-rays are

Table 11.10.
Recommended Dosages of Antibotics Used to Treat Acute Bacterial Sinusitis

Antibiotic	Dosage	Cost
Ampicillin	250–500 mg every 6 hours for 10 days	$10
Amoxicillin	250–500 mg every 6 hours for 10 days	$10
Trimethoprim/sulfamethozizole	Two tablets every 12 hours for 10 days	$10
Erythromycin	500 mg every 6 hours for 10 days	$10
Cefaclor	500 mg every 12 hours for 10 days	$50
Amoxicillin-clavulanate	500/125 mg every 8 hours for 10 days	$50
Azithromycin	Two tablets first day, one tablet daily for the next 4 days; note 5-day treatment because of long half-life	$50

consistent with sinusitis, a 14-day course of a second line antibiotic along with continuation of decongestants should be prescribed. If symptoms persist, the patient should be referred to an otorhinolaryngologist (ENT) for evaluation. Please refer to Figure 11.7 for the treatment algorithm of acute sinusitis.

Treatment of chronic sinusitis is similar to that of acute sinusitis. Antibiotic treatment should be prescribed for 21 days, however, and local corticosteroids should be prescribed as part of the initial therapy. If a patient has had success previously with a certain antibiotic, it is reasonable to initiate therapy with that same drug. Because of the wider variety of potential pathogens in chronic sinusitis and the possibility of resistance, consideration of initial therapy with second line antibiotics is not inappropriate.

If the patient's symptoms do not resolve, the astute clinician should reconsider the diagnosis. Previously overlooked diagnoses such as HIV disease, nasal cocaine use, or undiagnosed anatomic abnormalities may be present. If the patient remains symptomatic, ENT referral is indicated. The ENT specialist uses powerful local decongestants and then performs direct fiberoptic endoscopy of the sinuses. Even surgery can be conducted fiberoptically.

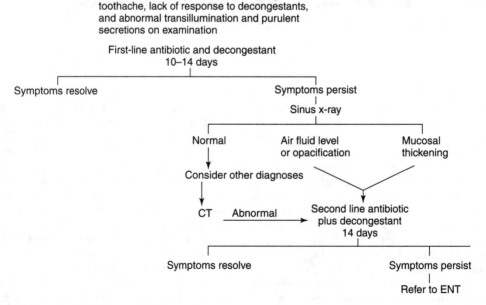

Figure 11.7. Algorithm for treatment of acute sinusitis. CT, computed tomography.

ILLUSTRATIVE CASES WITH SELF-ASSESSMENT QUESTIONS AND ANSWERS

Case 1

H.F. is a 43-year-old woman with a 1-week history of right facial pain and toothache, yellow nasal discharge, and stuffy nose. She has taken diphenhydramine and pseudoephedrine for 3 days without relief of her symptoms. She is allergic to penicillin. She has purulent nasal discharge and no dental abnormalities on examination.

QUESTION: *What is your diagnosis?*

a. Viral upper respiratory infection
b. Acute bacterial sinusitis
c. Allergic sinusitis

ANSWER: b. *The answer is acute bacterial sinusitis. She has typical symptoms and findings.*

QUESTION: *What antibacterial treatment do you recommend?*

a. Trimethoprim/sulfamethoxazole for 10–14 days
b. Ampicillin for 10–14 days
c. Amoxicillin for 10–14 days
d. Azithromycin for 5 days

ANSWER: a. *Trimethoprim/sulfamethoxazole is the least expensive drug that may be effective. She is allergic to penicillin, so ampicillin and amoxicillin should be avoided.*

Case 2

M.R. is a 35-year-old man with a 6-year history of worsening hayfever. He is having a particularly bad week symptomatically, with complete nasal stuffiness and sore throat from postnasal drip. Diphenhydramine and pseudoephedrine are making him sleepy and shaky.

QUESTION: *What is the most likely diagnosis?*

a. Viral upper respiratory infection
b. Acute bacterial sinusitis
c. Allergic sinusitis

ANSWER: c. *The answer is allergic sinusitis. Less likely is a viral upper respiratory infection. He lacks maxillary toothache, colored nasal discharge and purulent secretions that would suggest acute bacterial infection.*

QUESTION: *What treatment do you recommend?*

a. Inhaled corticosteroids
b. Inhaled decongestants
c. Both a and b

ANSWER: *Any answer is reasonable.*

Case 3

J.F. is a 53-year-old man who is HIV positive. He has had symptoms of acute sinusitis for 1 week and now has left frontal tenderness and redness, fever of 103°, and questionable confusion.

QUESTION: *What treatment do you recommend?*

a. Hospitalization and parenteral antibiotics
b. Ampicillin for 10–14 days
c. Cefaclor for 10–14 days, with a decongestant

ANSWER: a. *The answer is hospitalization. This immunocompromised patient is at risk for severe infection by unusual organisms. His examination and symptoms are compatible with complicated infection, such as frontal osteomyelitis or meningoencephalitis.*

REFERENCES

Sore Throat

1. Huovinen, P, Lahtonen, R, Ziegler, T, et al. Pharyngitis in adults: the presence and coexistence of viruses and bacterial organisms. Ann Intern Med 1989;110:612–616.
2. Bisno AL. Group A streptococcal infections and rheumatic fever. N Engl J Med 1991;325:783–793.
3. Relman DA, Schoolnick GK, Swartz MN. Infections due to mycoplasmas. Sci Am Med 1987;7:1–7.

4. Relman DA, Swartz MN. Diseases due to chlamydia. Sci Am Med 1994;7:1, 8–9.
5. Grayston JT, Kuo C, Wang S, Altman J. A new *Chlamydia psittaci* strain, TWAR, isolated in acute respiratory tract infections. N Engl J Med 1986; 315:161–168.
6. Centor RM, Meier FA, Dalton HP. Throat cultures and rapid tests for diagnosis of group A streptococcal pharyngitis. Ann Intern Med 1986;105:892–899.
7. Reed BD, Huck W, French T. Diagnosis of group A β-hemolytic streptococcus using clinical scoring criteria, Directigen 1-2-3 group A streptococcal test, and culture. Arch Intern Med 1990;150:1727–1732.
8. Meier FA, Howland J, Johnson J, Poisson R. Effects of a rapid antigen test for group A streptococcal pharyngitis on physician prescribing and antibiotic costs. Arch Intern Med 1990;150:1696–1700.
9. Centers for Disease Control. Acute rheumatic fever at a Navy training center—San Diego, California. MMWR 1988;37:101–104.
10. Ferrieri P, Kaplan, EL. Invasive group A streptococcal infections. Infect Dis Clin North Am 1992;6: 149–161.
11. Wallace MR, Garst PD, Papadimos TJ, Oldfield EC. The return of acute rheumatic fever in young adults. JAMA 1989;262:2557–2561.
12. American Heart Association. Jones criteria (revised) for guidance in the diagnosis of rheumatic fever. Circulation 1984;69:204A–208A.
13. Kaplan EL, Johnson VD, Cleary PP. Group A streptococcal serotypes isolated from patients and sibling contacts during the resurgence of rheumatic fever in the United States in the mid-1980's. J Infect Dis 1989;159:101–103.
14. Land MA, Bisno AL. Acute rheumatic fever: a vanishing disease in suburbia. JAMA 1983;249:895–898
15. Bisno AL, Shulman ST, Dajani AS. The rise and fall (and rise?) of rheumatic fever. JAMA 1988;259: 728–729.
16. Poses RM, Cebul RD, Collins M, Fager SS. The importance of disease prevalence in transporting clinical prediction rules: the case of streptococcal pharyngitis. Ann Intern Med 1986;105:586–591.
17. Shank JC, Powell TA. A five-year experience with throat cultures. J Fam Pract 1984;18:857–863.
18. Middleton DB, D'Amico F, Merenstein JH. Standardized symptomatic treatment versus penicillin as initial therapy for streptococcal pharyngitis. J Pediatr 1988;113:1089–1094.

SUGGESTED READINGS

Earache and Hearing Loss

Albert DM, Jakobic FA. Clinical practice—principles and practice of ophthalmology. Philadelphia: Saunders, 1994.

Reilly B. Practical strategies in outpatient medicine, 2nd ed. Philadelphia: Saunders, 1991.

Rosen P, Barkin RM. Emergency medicine—concepts and clinical practice, 3rd ed. St. Louis: Mosby-Yearbook, 1992.

Sataloff RM, Sataloff J. Hear loss, 3rd ed. New York: Marcel Dekker, 1995.

Trobe JB. The physician's guide to eye care. Am Acad Ophthamol 1993.

Eye and Vision Problems

Albert DM, Jakobiec FA. Clinical practice: principles and practice of ophthalmology. Philadelphia: Saunders, 1994.

Cullom RD, Chang B. The Wills eye manual. Philadelphia: Lippincott, 1994.

Reilly BM. Practical strategies in outpatient medicine, 2nd ed. Philadelphia: Saunders, 1991.

Rosen P, Barkin RM, eds. Emergency medicine, concepts and clinical practice, 3rd ed. St. Louis: Mosby-Year Book, 1992.

Trobe JD. The physician's guide to eye care. San Francisco: American Academy of Ophthalmology, 1993.

Sore Throat

Bisno AL. Group A streptococcal infections and rheumatic fever. N Engl J Med 1991;325:783–793.

MayoSmith MF, Hirsch PJ, Wodzinski SF, Schiffman FJ. Acute epiglottitis in adults: an eight year experience in the state of Rhode Island. N Engl J Med 1986; 314:1133–1139.

Sinusitis

Willett LR, Carson JL, Williams JW. Current diagnosis and management of sinusitis. J Gen Intern Med 1994;9:38–45.

Williams JW, Simel DL, Roberts LR, Samsa GP. Clinical evaluation for sinusitis: making the diagnosis by history and physical examination. Ann Intern Med 1992; 117:705–710.

chapter 12

NEUROLOGY

Susan Dresdner, Rafael Pelayo, Lisa M. Rucker, Kathleen Ward, Eleanor Weinstein, and Kin M. Yuen

HEADACHE

Headache is the fourth most common ailment that brings patients to outpatient medical attention (1). It affects 50 million Americans per year (2). The time lost from work costs between $5.6 and $17.2 billion annually from migraine headache alone (3). However, most headache sufferers are not treated by health professionals because only 5% of the population seek medical help for headaches.

The International Headache Society has published extensive new guidelines on the diagnosis of headaches (Table 12.1). This section will discuss headache from the type most common to the least common.

Pathophysiologic Correlation

Headache can be the symptomatic manifestation of various pathological or physiological processes. Imbalances in neurotransmitters, episodic alterations in hypothalamic function, and undefined postcoital changes are among the etiologies in the more benign types of headache. Bleeding or mass lesions that impair blood flow and apply traction onto the meninges and infection on inflammation of cranial structures can cause more serious types of headache, as can infection or inflammation of cranial structures.

Clinical and Laboratory Evaluation

The patient's history is often diagnostic of the particular type of headache. The physical examination is key to clinically confirm the diagnosis. Laboratory tests are ordered if structural headache is suspected.

HISTORY

The clinician should focus on the history of headache, including when the symptoms began. The duration of each headache, the description and location of the pain, and exacerbating and remitting factors should be sought. History of trauma, drugs/alcohol/medication use, past medical history, and family history are important to elicit. Headaches can be classified by time of onset (Table 12.2).

PHYSICAL EXAMINATION

Performance of the neurologic examination is essential when evaluating a patient with headache. Specifically, cranial structures and the neck; speech, gait, and mental status must be examined, and cranial nerves, motor, sensory, cerebellar function, and reflexes must be tested. Vital signs should be assessed in each patient. The presence of papilledema or a focal finding alerts the examiner to a serious type of headache.

LABORATORY EVALUATION

Neuroimaging studies are indicated if the clinician suspects a serious or dangerous etiology of headache. The merits of computed tomography (CT) and magnetic resonance imaging (MRI) are discussed under "Abnormal Mental Status: Dementia and Delirium," but in general either test is acceptable. Lumbar puncture (assuming that papilledema is absent) and cultures of cerebrospinal fluid (CSF) and blood are indicated if the clinician suspects meningitis. Lumbar puncture is necessary to diagnose subarachnoid bleeding if the clinical suspicion is high but neuroimaging is nondiagnostic.

Differential Diagnosis

The accurate diagnosis of headache is essential for therapeutic and economic reasons. The diagnoses of common and dangerous headache will be reviewed in this section.

Table 12.1.
International Headache Society Classification
of Headache

1	Migraine
1.1	Migraine without aura
1.2	Migraine with aura
1.3	Ophthalmoplegic migraine
1.4	Retinal migraine
2	Tension-type headache
2.1	Episodic tension-type headache
2.2	Chronic tension-type headache
3	Cluster headache and chronic paroxysmal hemicrania
4	Miscellaneous headaches not associated with structural lesion
4.1	Idiopathic stabbing headache
4.2	External compression headache
4.3	Cold stimulus headache
4.4	Benign cough headache
4.5	Benign exertional headache
4.6	Headache associated with sexual activity
5	Headache associated with head trauma
5.1	Acute posttraumatic headache
5.2	Chronic posttraumatic headache
6	Headache associated with vascular disorders
7	Headache associated with nonvascular intracranial disorder
8	Headache associated with substances or their withdrawal
9	Headache associated with noncephalic infection
10	Headache associated with metabolic disorder
11	Headache or facial pain associated with disorder of cranium, neck, eyes, ears, nose, sinuses, teeth, mouth, or other facial or cranial structures
12	Cranial neuralgias, nerve trunk pain, and deafferentation pain
13	Headache not classifiable

Reprinted with permission from Olesen J. Headache classification committee of the International Headache Society. Classification and diagnostic criteria for headache disorders, cranial neuralgia, and facial pain. Cephalagia 1988;8 (suppl 7):1–96.

TENSION HEADACHE

Formerly termed "muscle contraction headache," tension headaches affect 19–32% of the outpatient population (4, 5). It is uncertain what induces tension headaches; there is no underlying neurologic abnormality. Muscle spasm often occurs with the acute variety but is not reproduced with the chronic type. Electromyographic recordings of muscle contractions do not correlate with pain perception consistently. It has been postulated that tension headaches and migraines are part of a continuum.

Tension-type headaches are separated into epi-

sodic or chronic types. If the headache frequency is less than 15 per month, it is termed episodic; if the frequency of headache is more than 15 per month, it is termed chronic (4). Table 12.3 lists the features of tension headaches. The astute clinician realizes that about one of every four patients complaining of headache has tension headache. However, if symptoms are not typical or the vital signs and neurological examination are abnormal, other more serious causes must be considered.

MIGRAINE HEADACHE

The etiology of migraines remains unclear. It is thought that cranial vasoconstriction followed by dilation induces headaches; the resulting sterile inflammation and muscle contraction further potentiate the pain. The most recent theory hypothesizes that neurotransmitters such as serotonin are purported to be responsible. It has been observed that serotonin levels tend to decline before the onset of migraine. Other vasoactive peptides such as acidic lipid, catecholamine, peptic kinin, and slow-reacting substance of anaphylaxis may also be involved in inducing vascular dilation or permeability. The subsequent edema correlates with pain.

About 50% of individuals who seek help for vascular headaches have migraines. Most migraine headaches can be classified with or without aura. Less common are the ophthalmoplegic and retinal migraines. There is a 55–70% family history correlation. It is unknown whether migraine headaches result from familial clustering or are hereditary. Alcohol and caffeine are known precipitants of migraine headaches; caffeine intake during an attack may alleviate the intensity. Diets rich in tyramine containing substances such as canned or processed meat, avocados, or cheeses can precipitate migraine attacks. Pregnancy tends to inhibit headaches. Migraine sufferers are often described as ambitious, persistent, fearful, tense, and easily frustrated. A higher frequency of migraine headache is reported in patients with panic attacks.

The examination may be completely normal except in familial hemiplegic migraine that produces neurologic deficits during an attack. Also corresponding neurologic findings are prominent features of other rare migraine syndromes (retinal, ophthalmoplegic). Most deficits resolve once the headache subsides. Table 12.4 reviews the features of migraine headache.

Migraine headaches may be associated with focal neurologic findings. Ophthalmoplegic migraine headaches usually present in childhood; nausea,

Table 12.2.
Headache Classification by Time of Onset

Acute Single Same Day	Acute Recurrent Days	Subacute Days-to-Weeks	Chronic Daily Months-Years	Chronic Relapsing Years
Trauma	**Structural**	**Trauma**	**Structural**	Chronic fatigue
Concussion	Intracranial	Subdural bleed	Intracranial	Sleep apnea
Postlumbar puncture	Cerebral tumors	**Structural**	Pseudotumor	Facial neu-
Infectious	Cerebral vascular	Tumors	cerebri	ralgia
Intracranial	disease	Pseudotumor cerebri	Tumors/metastases	
Encephalitis	Extracranial	**Infectious**	Extracranial	
Meningitis	Pheochromocytoma	Brain abscesses	Cervical spon-	
Extracranial	Idiopathic intracran-	**Inflammatory**	dylosis	
Sinusitis	ial hypertension	Temporal arteritis	Temporal mandibu-	
Otitis	Intermittent hydro-	**Vascular**	lar joint arthritis	
Orbital cellulitis	cephalus	Intracranial sinus	**Vascular**	
Inflammatory	**Vascular**	thrombosis	Chronic tension	
Optic neuritis	Cluster	**Systemic**	headache	
Vascular	Migraine	Hypo/	**Medication related**	
First migraine	Subarachnoid bleed	hyperthyroidism	Rebound headache	
Subarachnoid hem-			off NSAIDs	
orrhage			**Psychiatric**	
			Malingering	

Table 12.3.
Features of Tension-Type Headache

Age of Onset
Usually around middle age; female-to-male ratio is about 5 : 4
Location
Bilateral temples, occiput, and neck are the most common sites
Character of Pain
Vice- or band-like pressure sensation is typically described; it is also *non*pulsatile; pain is often mild to moderate but does not limit daily activities
Duration
From 30 minutes to 7 days
Frequency
Daily is the norm
Precipitants
Stressful life situations appear to increase the occurrence; physical exertion does not correlate with intensity

Anxiety and depression have been reported in patients with tension-type headaches. There is no physical abnormality except for muscle tenseness or trigger points at the upper shoulder or neck muscles.

vomiting, and photophobia are commonly associated. Ipsilateral oculomotor nerve involvement, inducing ocular muscle palsy and ptosis, can last for hours to days. Retinal migraine is rare in this type of headache and may be preceded by amaurosis aura or monocular blind spots. The aura typically lasts for 1 hour.

In familial hemiplegic migraine, hemiplegia or aphasia with disorientation usually present 1–2 hours before the onset of headache. Familial history (autosomal dominant transmission) and duration of hemiplegia often indicate the diagnosis. Rarely the hemiplegia may be persistent; other organic causes should be excluded before this diagnosis is made.

CLUSTER HEADACHE

The cluster headache is also called histamine cephalalgia. The intensity of pain in cluster headaches is one of the most important distinguishing features. The attack is usually associated with signs of autonomic dysfunction. Therefore it is postulated that the trigeminal vascular system is affected secondary to a disordered central hypothalamic pacemaker. Table 12.5 reviews the diagnosis of cluster headache.

Unlike patients with chronic daily headache, patients with cluster headache usually work despite the severe attacks. Cigarette smoking and heavy alcohol use have also been reported in the profiles of cluster headache patients. Depression and thoughts of suicide are common.

On physical exam, parasympathetic hyperactivity-like signs may be noted. Miosis may be subtle

Table 12.4.
Features of Migraine Headaches

Age of Onset

Usually begins during childhood or early adolescence. There is a slight predominance of migraine headache in females after puberty: female-to-male ratio is 2.5 : 1 (8); highest prevalence rate is among women between the ages of 25 and 44. Prevalence rate is 15–17% among women and about 6% among men. Menopause is associated with cessation.

Location

More likely to be unilateral and affect the temporal area; however the pain can be bilateral and affect any part of the face and head.

Character of Pain

Dull or pulsating are typical descriptions. Severity usually is quite variable depending on the chronicity and precipitating factors.

Duration

Typically less than 24 hours. Sleep aborts the headache; however, the headache may recur during the subsequent days to weeks.

Frequency

Highly variable, ranging from once to twice a year in its mild form to 15 to 16 a month. The most common reported frequency is one to four attacks monthly.

Precipitants

Environmental factors such as bright lights, loud noises, and change in barometric pressure may trigger as well as exacerbate. Physiologic changes such as menstruation, fatigue, hypoglycemia, and sleep loss can also trigger migraines. Exertion or lying down tends to exacerbate the headache, whereas standing up relieves it. Ingestion of alcohol and new medications, especially oral contraceptives, are other precipitants.

Associated Symptoms/Signs

"Aura" may manifest as the following forms
  Fortification spectra: zigzag patterns
  Metamorphosia: visual distortion of objects (in size and shape)
  Photopsia: flashing lights or colors
  Scotomata: blind spots
  Teichopsia: bright shimmering lines/waves (see fortification spectra)
Symptoms
  Anorexia, nausea, vomiting, diarrhea, constipation, flatulence, dizziness, lightheadedness, blurred vision, diplopia, decreased concentration or memory, mood change, decreased libido, pessimism, fatigue
Signs
  Ataxia, dysarthria

When symptoms or signs persist after the resolution of the headache, especially neurological signs, one must be suspicious of other etiologies.

---

to the examiner, but the patient can certainly discern the difference.

INDOMETHACIN RESPONSIVE HEADACHE

The following heterogeneous types of headache, although having varying features, all respond to low doses of indomethacin (initial dosage of 25–75 mg two to three times a day).

Chronic paroxysmal hemicrania syndrome resembles cluster headache but occurs more often in women. The characteristic response to low dose indomethacin sets it apart from migraine and cluster headaches. The duration of attack is usually 2–45 minutes, an average of 16 times a day. Recurrence rates range from 1–5 days monthly to daily

for years. The ipsilateral temporoorbital region is affected; Horner's syndrome, conjunctival hyperemia, and rhinorrhea are present.

Postcoital headache usually presents during sexual excitement, orgasm, or after coitus. Typically the headache is described as severe, throbbing, or explosive. Onset is abrupt and lasts for minutes to hours. There is no associated neurologic sequela. If the headache persists, other diagnoses, such as ruptured aneurysm, must be considered.

Ice pick headache is reported to be intense lightening jabs or sharp intermittent stabs. These headaches often affect migraine patients but can also occur independently in otherwise asymptomatic individuals.

Table 12.5.
Features of Cluster Headaches

Age of Onset
Usually at the third or fourth decade of life; pattern is more consistent in middle age. Male-to-female ratio is 4.5–6.7 : 1 (10).

Location
Typically the retroorbital, frontal, and facial regions; may rapidly spread to the parietal, occipital, or cervical areas.

Character of Pain
Initially a dull discomfort is followed by a severe, burning, boring pain within 30 minutes. Peak intensity occurs about 10–15 minutes after onset; then within 1–2 hours, the pain subsides. Patients are often awakened by cluster headaches during the first period of sleep with rapid eye movements (90 minutes from onset of sleep). There may be tenderness along the anterior neck and carotid artery areas.

Duration
Headaches usually last 10–120 minutes.

Frequency
1–3 headaches daily for 1–2 months then none for a year or more

STRUCTURAL HEADACHE

Structural headaches are serious and may be life threatening. The common structural etiologies are reviewed in this section.

Intracranial Lesions. Any space occupying lesion that applies traction onto the pain-sensitive meninges or displaces or impinges upon the vasculature can induce headache. Tumor (primary or metastatic), hematomas, and abscesses are apt to cause pain if they encroach onto pain-sensitive cranial nerve fibers. This type of headache increases in intensity, usually affecting one localized area. It is associated with nausea and stereotypical "projectile" vomiting. Abscesses are linked to fever and rigors.

A thorough neurologic examination and funduscopy are essential. For those with suspected early lesions and no papilledema, diagnostic neuroimaging of the head is warranted. If no significant abnormality is found, then expectant periodic neurologic evaluation is prudent.

Of cerebrovascular diseases, subarachnoid bleeds invoke the most dramatic clinical picture. "The worst headache in my life" is typically a pathognomonic phrase used to help make the diagnosis. Saccular aneurysm or arteriovenous malformation ruptures are the most common causes of subarachnoid bleed. Other structural abnormalities

inducing subarachnoid bleed include amyloid angiopathy, arteritis, brain tumor, and hemorrhagic diathesis. The mechanism for pain is likely linked to increased intracranial pressure, abrupt expansion of vessels, and blood's irritation of pain sensory fibers on the meninges. Table 12.6 reviews the headaches from vascular bleeds.

Signs of meningeal irritation such as Kernig's and Brudzinski's signs are commonly found. Papilledema should be suspected in all patients. Patients having a transient loss of consciousness linked with the onset of a severe headache should raise the suspicion of a subarachnoid bleed. Emergent neuroimaging is essential in locating the site of the bleed and any sign of parenchymal shift. If no bleeding is seen, a lumbar puncture may be diagnostic. Typically, xanthochromic CSF is revealed by the spinal puncture. If the above methods are nondiagnostic, a cerebral angiogram may be needed.

Table 12.6.
Features of Headaches from Vascular Bleeds

Age of Onset
Patients with a subarachnoid bleed from a ruptured atrioventricular malformation tend to be younger than those with ruptured berry aneurysms; onset is usually in the thirties compared with the fifties or sixties. Patients with atrioventricular malformation ruptures may also have a history of recurrent seizures.

Location
Often generalized throughout the head. If the middle cerebral or internal carotid/posterior communicating vessels are involved, it can be unilateral; if the anterior communicating artery ruptures, it is more likely to be bilateral.

Character of Pain
Usually severe with the actual rupture and reaches peak intensity within 1–2 minutes of onset. The premonitory headache that may precede the event is often milder in intensity.

Duration/Frequency
Constant and may last for several days to 1–2 weeks. Rebleeding is heralded by recurrence of a headache within 2–14 days of the first episode. Time from onset of warning signs to actual rupture may be 20 days.

Precipitant
Physical exertion is almost always linked with the onset of the headache.

Associated Signs and Symptoms
Nausea and vomiting are typically associated with the acute rupture. A stiff neck and an altered level of consciousness may result.

The frequency of headache varies from 23–57% for cerebral hemorrhage to 65–80% for cerebellar hemorrhage (7). Acute onset of nausea, vomiting, and sudden headache are the usual presentations. The pathophysiology is similar to intracranial lesions. The diagnosis is made by a thorough neurological exam, and confirmation is made by neuroimaging of the head.

Patients with infection and inflammation of the meninges often complain of a throbbing, generalized, severe headache. The mechanism of pain is felt to be similar to that of subarachnoid bleed. Movement usually increases pain, and lying on one's side with the knees and hips flexed but head extended decreases pain. Cervical rigidity elicited by Kernig's and Brudzinski's maneuvers are diagnostic aids. Lumbar puncture serves as a diagnostic and therapeutic test; it often relieves the headache temporarily.

After a lumbar puncture, CSF may continue to leak through the dura, resulting in lower CSF pressure. Traction on the pain-sensitive intracranial venous vessels may produce headache. Pain increases with elevation of the head and decreases with lying supine. The headache usually starts a few hours after the procedure and lasts 24–72 hours. Nausea and vomiting may follow the throbbing headache if the patient maintains an erect body position.

Epidural and subdural hematomas may occur after direct trauma to the head. Epidural bleeds are less common but can be present during severe trauma with injury to the ipsilateral middle cerebral artery. Loss of consciousness occurs with the initial phase; thereafter the patient may appear lucid for minutes to days. Subsequent onset of headache with nausea and vomiting usually signals a relapse. Coma and rapid neurological deterioration may ensue. Diagnosis is usually facilitated by neuroimaging; treatment is surgical evacuation. Subdural hematomas may have a slower onset. Family members may report a change in the patient's personality if the frontal region is affected. In general, if there is any sign of head injury such as Battle's sign, otorrhea, rhinorrhea, or cranial bone depression, rapid intervention is warranted. Postconcussive headache usually has its onset within hours to days of minor head injury. It may slowly intensify over days to weeks and then subside over weeks. The headache is typically diffuse and nonpulsatile and worsens with Valsalva or changes in head position. Resting and sleep reduce the headache. There may be associated fatigue, vertigo, impaired concentration, or insomnia. Event amnesia is not uncommon. Con-

Table 12.7.
Features of Headaches Related to Giant Cell Arteritis

Age of Onset
Usually individuals between the ages of 50 and 70, and women (female-to-male ratio of 2 : 1) are most commonly affected.

Location
Invariably the temporal area.

Character of Pain
Boring, lancinating severe pain along with scalp tenderness.

Duration/Frequency
Onset and duration are variable. Sometimes headache is abrupt and severe; sometimes it is more insidious.

Associated Signs and Symptoms
Fatigue, jaw claudication, scalp tenderness, anorexia, and weight loss are the early presenting complaints. Polymyalgia rheumatica, visual changes (blurring, diplopia), tongue and jaw claudication, sore throat, and stiffness of the hand, wrist, neck, and shoulders are commonly reported.

servative observation and avoidance of exertion are the most effective therapies.

Pseudotumor cerebri affects 1 per 100,000 of the population per year. However, 90% of the cases are comprised of obese women between the ages of 20 and 40. The headache originates from an increased intracranial pressure, although no displacement of the ventricles occurs. Reports of linkage with medical diseases (e.g., hypo- or hyperthyroidism) and medications (e.g., birth control pills, nitrofurantoin) have not been proven and are mostly anecdotal. Corticosteroids, however, may be associated with pseudotumor cerebri. Headaches are often described as constant. Associated symptoms may be stiff neck, paresthesia of the limbs, and arthralgias. Signs may include visual changes or loss. Relief of intracranial pressure ought to be performed with periodic lumbar puncture before the development of severe or permanent visual loss (5–15% of patients).

Extracranial Lesions. Giant cell arteritis more commonly affects the elderly. The prevalence increases with age to about 850 per 100,000 people age 80 or older. Pathologically, focal granulomatous inflammations of the small and medium-size arteries are seen. The inner portion of the media is usually most affected. Fibrinoid necrosis and thromboses of vessels may also cause pain. Table 12.7 reviews headaches related to giant cell arteritis.

Tenderness, nodularity, or decreased pulsation

may be found along the temporal arteries. In more severe cases, optic nerve pallor, optic disc edema, scattered cotton wool spots, and small hemorrhages may be seen before impending permanent visual loss. Neurologic findings may be present in 30% of the patients whose cranial vessels may be involved. Transient ischemic strokes and neuropathies are the most common manifestations. Mild anemia and elevation of the erythrocyte sedimentation rate to 90 mm/hour are typical findings. A minimum of a 1-inch segment biopsy of one or both temporal arteries is needed for definitive diagnosis.

Acute sinusitis frequently presents as a dull, throbbing headache. Pain is usually felt over the involved paranasal sinus. Movement of the head, especially over a dependent position, would increase the pain. Headache is often worse in the morning. Associated nasal discharge, fever, and localized tenderness frequently yield good clues to the diagnosis. Previous history of allergic rhinitis or sinusitis further supports the diagnosis. Physical examination using transillumination of the sinuses is sometimes helpful; x-rays are usually not useful unless they demonstrate air-fluid levels. In cases of recurrent sinusitis, CT scan of the sinuses would be more appropriate.

The cause of trigeminal neuralgia or tic douloureux is mostly unknown. This syndrome may occur in association with systemic diseases—multiple sclerosis, basilar artery aneurysm, or tumor involving cranial nerve V distribution. Pressure over the trigger areas reproduces the characteristic pain. The neurologic exam is otherwise normal. Table 12.8 lists the features of trigeminal neuralgia.

SYSTEMIC DISEASES

Patients with hypertension often notice a mild to moderate throbbing headache on awakening. The occipital area is most commonly reported although the location can also be at the top of the head. This type of headache may represent a kind of tension headache from vascular dilatation. Malignant hypertension can cause cerebral swelling and therefore a more severe headache. Nausea and vomiting may also be observed in malignant hypertension. Pheochromocytomas typically generate paroxysms of hypertension and headache. Associated features include flushing of the face, diaphoresis, and possibly diarrhea. Hyperthyroidism may cause hypertension and a similar headache as well.

Recrudescence of herpes zoster can cause an acute headache at the ophthalmic branch of the trigeminal cranial nerve. The pain may precede

Table 12.8.
Features of Trigeminal Neuralgia

Age of Onset
After age 30.

Location
Unilateral pain affecting the second (maxillary) or third (mandibular) branch of the fifth cranial nerve commonly; extension to the other branches is not rare.

Character of Pain
Short, sharp, stabbing pain that is often intense has been described.

Duration
Paroxysms of pain last 20–30 seconds to minutes at a time. Pain-free intervals also last for a few seconds to a minute.

Frequency
Pain may recur daily for weeks at a time; remission may last for longer periods. Attacks may occur during day or night.

Precipitants
"Trigger zones" of face, lips, or gums when stimulated by touch or cold would often induce pain within seconds. For example, brushing one's teeth, yawning, and chewing would cause paroxysms rapidly. Patients often have involuntary winces resembling "tics."

the vesicular eruptions by 4–5 days. Tearing and rhinorrhea may be accompanying features. When the geniculate ganglion is involved, pain at the pinna, external auditory meatus, and palate may become evident. This second variety is known as Ramsay Hunt's syndrome. Deafness, tinnitus, vertigo, and concomitant occipital headaches are common.

Management

After diagnosing the headache, the treatment must be addressed. Therapies, both abortive and prophylactic, will be discussed in this section. Discussion of outpatient treatments only will be presented. Table 12.9 reviews key features of diagnosis and management of headache.

TENSION HEADACHE

Episodic tension headache usually responds well to rest, over-the-counter analgesics, and avoidance of stress. Occasionally, nonsteroidal anti-inflammatory drugs (NSAID) may be needed. Behavioral modifications such as biofeedback, relaxation training, and psychotherapy are helpful for motivated patients with tension headache.

NSAIDs (e.g., naproxen and ibuprofen) are ef-

Table 12.9.
OIH Management Outline for Headaches

Severity	Location	Symptoms	Signs	Labs	Procedure	Differential Diagnosis	Treatment
Acute Onset							
Severe	Generalized	Projectile vomiting	Meningeal	CT of head	Lumbar puncture if no shift midline on CT of head	Subarachnoid bleed, intracranial mass	Neuro/neurosurgery evaluation
Moderate-severe	Focal	Periorbital pain	Diminished vision			Acute glaucoma Temporal arteritis	Ophthalmology evaluation
Moderate	Generalized	Change in mental status	Papilledema/seizures	CT of head		Malignant hypertension, metastases	Control high blood pressure and seizures
Mild-moderate	Focal	Change in personality	Trauma: Battle's sign/rhinorrhea	CT of head		Subdural hematoma, epidural hematoma	Evacuation of hematoma
Mild-moderate	Site typical	Stress induced	Maybe none	Normal		Vascular headache	Medications
Chronic							
Moderate	Generalized		Papilledema	CT of head	Lumbar puncture/neurosurgery consult	Pseudotumor cerebri/neurosurgery consult	
Moderate	Generalized	NSAIDs use	Normal neurological exam			NSAIDs rebound headache	Withdraw NSAIDs
Moderate	Focal	Paranasal sinus pain/snoring	Temporomandibular joint tenderness			Sleep apnea Sinusitis, temporomandibular joint arthritis	Treat underlying disease

fective analgesics. However, the potential for developing rebound headaches with chronic use of NSAIDs is great. Naproxen or fenoprofen are popularly used due to their longer half-lives. Dosages of all medications in this class should be modified for the elderly. Rarely, muscle relaxants are needed for acute exacerbations. Benzodiazepines are not usually recommended because of their abuse potential.

Tricyclic antidepressants have been known to be efficacious in the treatment of tension headaches and especially in patients with depressive features; 20 mg amitriptyline at bedtime increasing to 100 mg as needed is often prescribed. Doxepin, desipramine, imipramine, and trazodone are other alternatives. Both amitriptyline and doxepin tend to cause more sedation than the others. Monoamine oxidase inhibitors such as phenelzine have been effective. Their use has been limited because of the extensive dietary restrictions, sedation, and weight gain.

MIGRAINE HEADACHE

Typically, treatment of migraine is divided into abortive and prophylactic interventions. Therapy to abort migraines must be given at the first sign of the headache for it to be effective. Environmental interventions such as the attenuation of sound and light often are sufficient in aborting or decreasing the severity of attacks. Sleep helps terminate the headache.

Abortive Interventions. Abortive interventions are summarized in Table 12.10. Ergotamines remain the mainstay of therapy. The induction of vascular constriction is presumed to be the mechanism of action. Nausea may limit the use of oral doses. Aerosolized spray, suppositories, and intramuscular forms are recommended in cases of severe nausea and vomiting. Contraindications include signs and symptoms of peripheral vascular disease or vasoocclusive disease (e.g., claudication, Raynaud's phenomenon, angina, signs of basilar insufficiency), and pregnancy.

Dihydroergotamine is a derivative of ergotamines. It is more effective than ergotamines in blocking the development of neurogenic inflammation at the trigeminal nerve and central sites; thus it reduces the intensity of migraines. With chronic use, it causes less rebound headache than other ergotamines. Although the intranasal formulation is not yet approved, the intravenous, subcutaneous, and intramuscular forms are available.

Caffeine is utilized in combination with ergotamines in medicinal preparations. Its role in migraine was described under "Differential Diagnosis." NSAIDs (e.g., ibuprofen) and acetaminophen, if used early, are effective abortive agents. Mostly, these agents are effective in stopping pain.

Opioid preparations with and without NSAIDs are widely available. These may be required in headache not responding to ergotamines or common NSAIDs. The risk of habituation, especially in chronic headache, should be considered. Nonetheless these are effective in terminating nausea and inducing sedation and sleep, which is essential in stopping migraines. Butorphanol is a synthetic opioid analgesic. In intranasal form, its rapid onset of action (15 minutes after administration) and moderate half-life (4–5 hours after a 1-mg dose) have made it an important adjuvant agent.

Sumatriptan is a serotonin agonist. It is one of the newest medications on the market that is effective. Its mechanism of action presumably is in elevation of serotonin levels in cerebral vessels; 72% of patients experience relief at the prescribed dosages. It reaches peak concentration in 20 minutes, and pain relief is usually within 1–2 hours. Patients with hypertension and cardiac disease should not be given sumatriptan because it can cause chest tightness and hypertension. Patients that found the subcutaneous injections intolerable may use the oral formulation. Although widely available in Europe, oral sumatriptan is still being investigated in the United States.

Antiemetics such as metoclopramide and promethazine function by promoting gastric emptying of abortive agents and suppressing vomiting, respectively. Ondansetron is a serotonin antagonist that has been used in treatment of nausea related to chemotherapy. It is also an effective but expensive antiemetic now used in the treatment of migraines. An oral dose of either 8 mg or an intravenous dose of 0.15 mg/kg in 50 ml dextrose (or normal saline) can be administered.

Valproic acid has been reported to be effective in aborting migraine. It increases the level of gamma-aminobutyric acid either by interfering with its degradation or by enhancing the postsynaptic response to gamma-aminobutyric acid. Doses of 800–1000 mg have been used in randomized trials. Migraine headaches are prevented by ensuring a plasma level of 70–90 units valproate (8).

In headaches unresponsive to the above agents, corticosteroids can be effective when given in short courses of 1–3 days per month.

Prophylactic Interventions. Prophylactic interventions are recommended for patients having frequent attacks or headaches resistant to abortive

Table 12.10.
Abortive therapy

Medication	Dosage	Route
Ergotamines		
Ergotamine and caffeine	2 tablets with onset; repeat in 1 hour; maximum 4/attack	po
Ergotamine	1 tablet, repeat in 30 min; 2/attack	Sublingual
Ergotamine and caffeine	½ to 1 tablet; repeat in 1 hour; maximum 2	Suppository
Ergotamine		Aerosolized
DHE	0.5–1.0 ml	sc, im, iv
Serotonin agonists		
Sumatriptan	6 mg, repeat in 1 hour; maximum 4/attack	sc
NSAID		
Naproxen	550–750 mg, repeat in 1–2 hours; maximum three times/week	po
Meclofenamate	100–200 mg, repeat in 1–2 hours; maximum 3 times/week	po
Ketorolac	10 mg every 4–6 hours	po
Ketorolac	30–60 mg loading, repeat half dose every 6 hours; maximum 150 mg/first day, 120 mg/second day	im
Mixed barbiturate analgesic		
Bultabital/caffeine and ASA or acetaminophen; bultabital and acetaminophen	1–2 tablets every 4–6 hours; maximum 4/day, two times/week	po
Corticosteroids (Dexamethasone)	2–6 mg, repeat in 3 hours	po
Dexamethasone	4 mg	im
Prednisone	80 mg every day/7 days; taper over 7 days	po

Adapted from Baumel B. Migraine: a pharmacologic review with newer options and delivery modalities. Neurology 1994;44(suppl 3):S13–S17.

therapy. Menstruation related migraines (catamenial) may not respond to prophylaxis. Drugs used to prevent migraine are reviewed in Table 12.11.

Among beta-adrenergic blockers, propranolol is the drug of choice. Its mechanism of action is not entirely clear. Its anxiolytic effect may contribute to its effectiveness. It also can stabilize pericapillary membranes and reduce cerebral arterial spasm experimentally. Atenolol and metoprolol, beta$_1$ selective agents, are successful in prevention therapy. Nonetheless, at the doses required for prophylaxis, most agents tend to lose their selectivity. Therefore, for patients with asthma, congestive heart failure and depression, one may consider other agents. Likewise, in patients with bradycardia and postural hypotension, beta-blockers should not be used.

Calcium channel blockers such as verapamil, diltiazem, and nifedipine are all effective prophylactic medications. Their ability to prevent arterial vasospasm and inhibit platelet serotonin release and aggregation may be the mechanism of action. Constipation and fluid retention may limit the utilization of this class of medications. Nimodipine has

Table 12.11.
Prophylactic Therapy for Migraine

Medication	Daily Dosage (mg)
Beta-blockers	
Propanolol	20–240
Atenolol	50–150
Metoprolol	50–300
Calcium channel blockers	
Verapamil	120–240
Diltiazem	90–180
Nifedipine	30–180
Methysergide	4–8
Antidepressants	
Amitriptyline	10–200
Nortriptyline	10–125
Fluoxetin	20–80
NSAIDs	
Naproxen	550–1100
Ibuprofen	300–1200
Sulindac	150–200

Adapted from Baumel B. Migraine: a pharmacologic review with newer options and delivery modalities. Neurology 1994;44 (suppl 3):S13–S17.

a greater effect on cerebral vessels than others in this class; its utilization thus far is restricted to reduction of vasospasm from subarachnoid hemorrhage. Its efficacy for migraines is still being assessed. Flunarizine is also being investigated; it has promising results from European studies.

Tricyclics have long been thought to increase serotonin levels by inhibiting serotonin and norepinephrine reuptake. Similarly the new serotonin reuptake inhibitors, fluoxetine and sertraline, have been employed in prophylactic therapy. Serotonin reuptake inhibitors have fewer systemic side effects than the tricyclics and tend to be well tolerated. Caution should be exercised when using monoamine oxidase inhibitors with tricyclics because uncontrollable hypertension may result.

Methysergide maleate is a lysergic acid derivative. It potentiates the action of ergotamines and catecholamines. It induces serotonin inhibition and mild vasoconstriction. Although effective, it is not recommended for long term use because of the production of retroperitoneal and cardiopulmonary fibrosis. After 4–6 months of use, a hiatus free of methysergide should be observed for 4–6 weeks. Regular patient evaluation ought to be performed, and an intravenous pyelogram obtained to evaluate for retroperitoneal fibrosis. Monoamine oxidase inhibitors and cyproheptadine have also been reported to be effective, but their uses are limited by the many dietary restrictions with monoamine oxidase inhibitors and sedation with cyproheptadine.

NSAIDs have been used in prophylactic therapy; they reduce the severity and duration of attacks. Naproxen sodium, 550 mg twice a day, is commonly prescribed for this purpose. Corticosteroids are effective in recalcitrant chronic migraines but are not ideal for long term use because of the resulting immunosuppression. Psychotherapy may assist in stress reduction and behavioral response to pain; however, its role may be limited in pain abolishment.

CLUSTER HEADACHE

Abortive interventions can have profound results on cluster headache duration and can often lessen the severity of pain. Dihydroergotamine is an effective abortive agent. Patients administer 1 mg i.m. at bedtime, then 0.5 mg twice daily as needed. Sublingual and inhaled ergotamines are also helpful, although oral ergotamines are ineffective. Aside from oxygen, ergotamine is the most effective medication for treating acute headache. Sumatriptan has also been successful in reducing attacks within 15 minutes (9). Intranasal lidocaine has also been found to offer some relief.

All medications used in the prophylaxis of migraine headaches are generally effective in cluster. The notable exception are antihistamines, which are of little value. Lithium carbonate in dosages of 300 mg twice daily alone or in combination with ergonovine or verapamil may be more helpful in treating chronic cases. For those with pain refractory to medical therapy, radiofrequency trigeminal rhizotomy has been providing optimistic long term results (10).

OTHER CAUSES OF HEADACHE

Treatment of pseudotumor cerebri consists of surgical shunt placement or medications such as acetazolamide 500 mg or 1000 mg in divided doses per day; 40 mg furosemide twice a day can also be used. In refractory cases, 40–60 mg prednisone may also be effective.

Corticosteroid in doses of 60 mg or more a day for 1–2 years is recommended especially when there is ophthalmic involvement with giant cell arteritis. Headache, erythrocyte sedimentation rate elevation, and visual symptoms should subside within days of therapy.

Treatment of sinusitis is comprised of antibiotics (if fever is present) and decongestants. Referral to an ear, nose, throat specialist may be required in more resistant cases. Please refer to Chapter 11 for more details.

Anticonvulsants have been found to depress synaptic transmission in trigeminal neuralgia. They do not possess any anesthetic effect. Carbamazepine at 200–600 mg a day in divided doses may be effective in suppressing or shortening the symptoms. If effective, a maintenance dose of 200 mg per day may be needed to prevent relapses. Nausea, vomiting, sedation, and blood dyscrasias may limit the use of this drug. Continual monitoring of blood therapeutic levels is necessary.

Muscle relaxants such as baclofen can be used with carbamazepine as a second agent. Because of the short half-life, baclofen 5 mg should be given twice daily; this dosage may be increased to 20 mg twice daily. Phenytoin 200–400 mg a day may provide relief to some patients that do not respond to carbamazepine alone or in combination with baclofen. Similarly, blood levels should be monitored. Side effects include drowsiness, dizziness, and diplopia. Ataxia, slurred speech, nystagmus, gum hypertrophy, and megaloblastic anemia, although sometimes seen with routine use, may signify toxicity.

ILLUSTRATIVE CASES WITH SELF-ASSESSMENT QUESTIONS AND ANSWERS

Case 1

A 28-year-old stockbroker reports to the emergency room with a severe headache that he has had for 3 hours. He noticed a sensitivity to light. He felt nauseous about 30 minutes ago but has not vomited. His lunch was 4 hours earlier and consisted of a turkey sandwich and a bottle of soda. His neck has become increasingly stiff, and he had felt a loud "popping" sound with the onset of his headache. Physical exam reveals a febrile man in some distress who is vomiting in the emergency room; he has meningeal signs.

QUESTION: *What is the type of headache he most likely has?*

a. Food poisoning with dehydration
b. Tension
c. Migraine
d. Subarachnoid bleed
e. None of the above

ANSWER: *d. Subarachnoid bleed. The acuteness in onset, severity, and associated mechanical sound strongly suggest a subarachnoid bleed. Because of his age, it probably is from an aneurysmal rupture.*

Food poisoning from staphylococcal enterotoxin has an onset within 1–6 hours of ingestion of dairy products, cream-filled pastries, or improperly refrigerated meats. However, the amount of nausea, vomiting, diarrhea, and abdominal pain that are typically associated with food poisoning is not seen here. Although this patient has photophobia, the cause is from meningeal irritation and is not a migraine component. The severity at onset of the headache and its generalized nature are uncharacteristic of migraine. Tension headaches, although frequently associated with stressful work environment, are not seen with neurological signs.

Case 2

A 35-year-old executive presents to you with a recurrent headache that she has had for the last 3 hours. She has been experiencing this type of headache since she was 12. Normally, if she rests in a quiet room, the headache will subside. She has extensive board meetings scheduled and could not rest. She normally takes naproxen 1 tablet every 8 hours, but it provided no relief. Her headache is usually at the right side of her face; however, today it is bilateral.

Her last attack before today's episode was 1 month ago. She is expecting her menses in the next 2 days but is unwilling to stop the usage of her birth control pills.

QUESTION: *What is the best treatment for her migraine headache now?*

a. Corticosteroids
b. Methysergide
c. Subcutaneous sumatriptan
d. Tegretol
e. None of the above

ANSWER: *c. Migraine headache associated with menstrual cycles is quite difficult to treat. Because of the acute recurrence, abortive methods should be used first. This patient is a likely candidate for prophylaxis therapy as well if she experiences about two to five episodes per month. Pain control with narcotics and antiemetics may be used in more indolent cases. Ergotamines would be a good alternative. Corticosteroids ought to be used in resistant cases secondary to the side effects. Because of the numerous options, steroids should be reserved. Methysergide is inappropriate as an abortive agent. In reproductive age women, the concern of retroperitoneal fibrosis is great. Tegretol is effective in controlling trigeminal neuralgia and chronic pain but is not indicated in stopping migraine headache.*

Case 3

A 63-year-old hypertensive woman returns for a follow-up appointment with you in the office. She reports a new earache at her temples that she has had for about 1 month. There have been no changes in her vision. However, she feels more "tired" lately, especially in the jaw area after chewing tough meats. She has been having a low-grade temperature but has no sinus pain.

She states that she takes all her medications. Her blood pressure is 150/92 and pulse is 80. She has tenderness along her temporal arteries and has a decreased pulse on the right. Her fundi revealed grade 1–2 hypertensive changes. The remainder of her examination is unremarkable.

QUESTION: *Which of the following diagnostic laboratory tests would you select next?*

a. Sedimentation rate
b. Sinus CT scan
c. CT scan of the head
d. Serum renal function panel
e. None of the above

ANSWER: *a. Sedimentation rate. In patients suspected of having temporal arteritis, the erythrocyte sedimentation rate is often elevated. Temporal biopsies and early treatment would be prudent to prevent progression. Although this patient does not seem to have ophthalmic involvement, blindness from involvement of the ciliary, ophthalmic vessels or central retinal artery can present precipitously. Low grade fevers, malaise, and jaw claudication are some common features of temporal arteritis.*

There is no physical finding to support an acute sinusitis or an intracranial head lesion; therefore the sinus and head CTs are not warranted. The renal function panel, although useful for medication adjustment for her hypertension, is not likely to contribute to the diagnosis.

DIZZINESS

"There are few physicians so dedicated to their art that they do not experience a slight decline in spirits on learning their patient's complaint is of dizziness" (1). The most feared of all symptoms—dizziness. Crushing substernal chest pain or melena do not engender such a response. Why is dizziness so intimidating? The complexities of the human balance system and the diverse possibilities for malfunction make diagnosis difficult.

Pathophysiologic Correlation

The interaction of the visual, proprioceptive, and vestibular systems maintains equilibrium and sense relation to surroundings. The eyes, muscles, joints, and otic labyrinths continuously supply information about body position at the unconscious level.

The body then makes adaptive movements to maintain equilibrium.

VERTIGO

All vertigo represents dysfunction of the vestibular system at some level. The vestibular system is extremely complex, as depicted by Figure 12.1. It is divided into peripheral and central components. The peripheral vestibular apparatus (see Fig. 11.1) includes the labyrinth and the vestibular portion of cranial nerve eight (CN VIII). The labyrinth consists of the semicircular canals that sense head rotation and the utricle and saccule that provide information about the body orientation with respect to gravity. It is embedded in the petrous portion of each temporal bone, which makes it vulnerable to trauma, blood-borne toxins, and infections of the inner ear and meninges.

The labyrinths supply balanced impulses of head position and movement to the central nervous system (CNS). Vertigo occurs when the input from one labyrinth is disrupted. The CNS accommodates to unilateral input, and the vertigo disappears. The vestibular portion of CN VIII connects the labyrinth to the brainstem, entering the brainstem just below the pons and anterior to the cerebellum and proceeding to the four vestibular nuclei of the brainstem and the cerebellum (Fig. 12.2). Impulses travel from the nuclei to two pathways, the medial longitudinal fasciculus and the vestibulospinal tract that contribute to the clinical manifestations of vertigo.

The central vestibular apparatus consists of vestibular nuclei at the pontomedullary junction in the brainstem. The latter receives impulses from CN VIII and has elaborate connections with the nuclei controlling eye movements and the cerebellum. The medial longitudinal fasciculus coordinates contraction of the ipsilateral medial rectus muscle (CN III) and the contralateral lateral rectus muscle (CN VI) as illustrated in Figure 12.3. Nystagmus occurs when the synchronized vestibular information is unbalanced and causes asymmetric stimulation of the medial and lateral rectus muscles. This unopposed activity will cause a slow movement of the eyes toward the affected side. The cerebral cortex corrects for these eye movements and rapidly brings the eyes back to midline only to have the process begin again. The vestibulospinal tract connects with motor neurons of the extremities and accounts for the abnormal gait or other movements seen in a person with a defective vestibular apparatus. Connections between the vestibular nuclei and

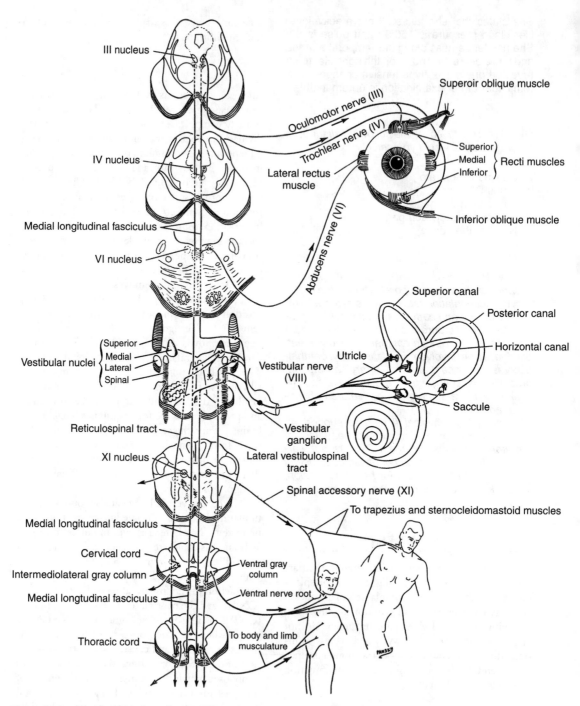

Figure 12.1. Simple vestibular reflex pathways. From House EL, Pansky B, Siegel A. A systematic approach to neuroscience, 3rd ed. New York: McGraw-Hill, 1979:240.

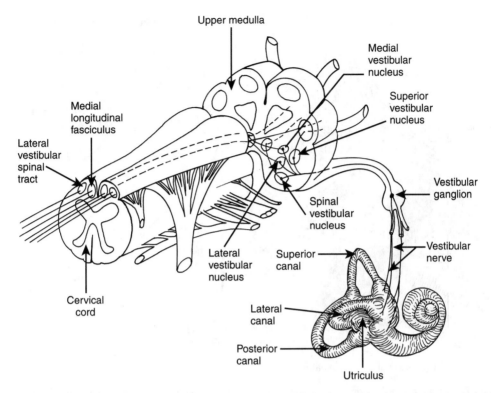

Figure 12.2. Central connections of vestibular apparatus. Adapted from Elia JC. The dizzy patient. Springfield IL: Charles C. Thomas, 1968:6.

the autonomic system explain the sweating, nausea, and vomiting that accompany vertigo.

DISEQUILIBRIUM

As mentioned before, equilibrium is maintained by the visual, proprioceptive, and vestibular systems. Three elements are needed to maintain upright posture and smooth ambulation: accurate sensory input to the CNS regarding body position, proper processing of this sensory input by the CNS, and appropriate motor response from the CNS. Disequilibrium results when any pathways are disturbed. The four sensory inputs needed are vision, hearing, vestibular system, and position and touch in the lower extremities.

PRESYNCOPE

Lightheadedness or feelings of faintness can be described by patients as dizziness. These are more often symptoms of a cardiovascular problem rather than a neurologic one. These symptoms are due to globally diminished cerebral blood flow, as distin-

guished from a transient ischemic attack (TIA) that is due to a focal area of cerebral ischemia.

Clinical and Laboratory Evaluation

Three diagnoses encompass three-fourths of patients with dizziness. The initial task is to categorize the patient's symptoms into one of three classes of dizziness: vertigo, disequilibrium, or presyncope. The physical examination determines the need for more specialized otoneurologic testing.

HISTORY

Dizziness means different sensations to each individual. The most critical aspect of obtaining a history about dizziness is to determine exactly what the patient means by "feeling dizzy." This may not be easy, but a careful history can frequently make the diagnosis before the physical examination. The best approach is to ask open-ended questions that require the patient to describe what he or she experienced without using the word dizzy. Restrain the urge to ask leading questions about spinning, light-

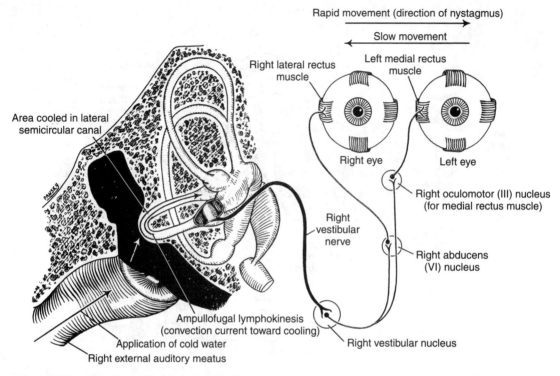

Figure 12.3. From House EL, Pansky B, Siegel A. A systematic approach to neuroscience, 3rd ed. New York: McGraw-Hill, 1979:248.

headedness, or unsteadiness. The best information is in the patient's own words.

The history allows the symptoms to be put into one of three categories: vertigo, disequilibrium, or presyncope. Vertigo is the hallucination of movement. It most frequently is described as rotational, but sometimes it is a sense of movement forward, backward, or to the side. The sensation that follows getting off a merry-go-round is an example to which most patients can relate. Disequilibrium is a sense of being unbalanced and insecure when walking. Patients report a fear of falling and the absence of symptoms when sitting or supine. A distinguishing feature is that this symptom is usually associated with the "legs" rather than the head. Presyncope is the sensation that loss of consciousness is about to happen. The patient can describe lightheadedness, wooziness, or fuzziness but usually ascribes the symptom to the head rather than the legs.

After the category is determined, other aspects of the history should be obtained. These include associated symptoms (tinnitus, hearing loss), temporally related events (position, urination), pattern, and medications. For a listing of key parts of the history see Table 12.12.

PHYSICAL EXAMINATION

The examination begins by observing the patient walking into the room—gait, use of upper extremities or appliances for support. Blood pressure is measured in both arms, and orthostatic blood pressure and pulse are determined to identify subclavian-steal syndrome, orthostatic hypotension, or arrhythmia as a cause of presyncope. Respirations, especially frequent sighing, may suggest anxiety and hyperventilation. Auscultation of the carotids for bruits could reveal atherosclerosis.

The ears are examined for cerumen or foreign body, fluid behind the tympanic membrane, retraction of the tympanic membrane suggesting occlusion of the eustachian tube, perforated or scarred tympanic membrane that may suggest a perilymphatic fistula, and a whitish plaque on the tympanic membrane suggesting cholesteatoma. Hearing should be evaluated by the Weber and Rinne tests using a 512-Hz tuning fork.

Table 12.12.
Specific Symptoms of Vertigo and Presyncope

	Vertigo		Presyncope
Associated symptoms	Hearing loss	Ataxia	Paresthesias
	Tinnitus	Diplopia	
	Nausea/vomiting	Dysarthria	
	Sweating	Sensory symptoms	
Temporal events			Urination
			Coughing
			Head movement
			Valsalva
			Painful viscera
			Prostate exam venipuncture
Pattern	Positional		Standing
	Intermittent or constant		Reproduced by hyperventilation
	Once or recurrent		
Medications	Alcohol		Diuretics
	Antibiotics		thiazides
	aminoglycosides		furosemide
	chloramphenicol		Vasodilators
	vancomycin		nitrates
	minocycline		nifedipine
	erythromycin		hydralazine
	Barbiturates		prazosin
	Phenytoin		minoxidil
	Diuretics		Antihypertensives
	ethacrynic acid		methyldopa
	flurosemide		reserpine
	Phencyclidine		guanethidine
	Quinine		Antipsychotics
	Quinidine		chlorpromazine
	Salicylates		thioridazine
			Antidepressants
			tricyclics
			monoamine oxidase inhibitors
			L-Dopa
			Barbiturates

Examination of the eyes includes visual acuity with correction, pupils, extraocular muscles, fundi, and observation for nystagmus. Pupillary abnormalities may suggest CN II or CN III problems. A cerebellar hemorrhage compressing the brainstem may cause CN VI palsy. Papilledema or absent spontaneous venous pulsations suggest increased intracranial pressure. Hollenhorst plaque (cholesterol embolus) may suggest atherosclerosis.

Nystagmus is irregular jerking movements of the eyes. As mentioned before, nystagmus occurs when there is an asymmetry of vestibular information, causing a slow movement of the eyes toward the affected side and a cortical (fast) component that brings the eye to midline. "Normal" nystagmus can be elicited when the eyes are maximally horizontally deviated (end-point nystagmus) or when the examiner does not move his or her finger slowly and smoothly. The eyes should not be deviated more than 30 degrees when looking for nystagmus. With symptoms suggesting vertigo, the type of nystagmus can determine if the source of the vestibular problem is peripheral or central.

Peripheral nystagmus is bilateral, unidirectional (fast component of the nystagmus always beats in the same direction regardless of which direction the patient is looking), horizontal or rotatory, and is suppressed by fixation of eyes and repetition of movements. Eye movements may be observed with the patient's eyes closed. If jerking movements of the eye are more pronounced with the eyes closed, it is peripheral nystagmus. Central nystagmus can be unilateral or bilateral, unidirectional or bidirectional, and may be vertical.

A focused neurological examination completes the physical. Other cranial nerve abnormalities would suggest a central origin of the vertigo. Corneal reflex will give information about the sensory component of CN V and motor component of CN VII. A diminished corneal reflex may be an early sign of an acoustic neuroma.

Cerebellar function should be tested by checking for abnormalities in finger-to-nose pointing (dysmetria) and alternating fast movements (dysdiadokokinesia). If not done already, gait and turning should be evaluated. Vertiginous ataxia has coordinated limb movements compared with cerebellar ataxia and is present only during the episode of vertigo. Observation of turning is important and may often be slow, short-stepped, and wavering.

Testing proprioception is necessary to help determine deficits that may cause disequilibrium. The patient is asked to touch the nose with the index finger with both eyes closed, to determine position of the great toe with both eyes closed, and to touch thumb to fingers with eyes open and closed. A Romberg test assesses the ability to maintain posture without visual input, which requires proprioception. It tests posterior column function, not cerebellar function. Unless the patient can stand steadily, even with wide base with eyes open, Romberg testing is not possible.

Stimulation tests to reproduce the symptoms of dizziness are frequently recommended to help confirm a diagnosis. Although they may be valid, the tests may produce significant distress without yielding any new information not already gleaned from the history and focused physical examination. Stimulation tests for vertigo include the Nylen-Bárány maneuver, fistula test (putting air into the ear with a pneumatic otoscope), and caloric testing. The latter should be reserved for patients who are not conscious. Presyncope can be demonstrated by voluntary Valsalva maneuvers and voluntary hyperventilation. Carotid sinus massage should be done only in a monitored setting. Disequilibrium can be reproduced during certain parts of the physical examination, such as gait, turning, and Romberg testing.

LABORATORY EVALUATION

Laboratory studies are generally not useful in the evaluation of dizziness. An electrocardiogram (ECG) may be indicated if an abnormal heart rate or rhythm is noted during the examination. Hearing loss, tinnitus, and/or nystagmus of central origin would warrant a radioimaging study focusing on the posterior fossa and cerebellopontine angle.

Differential Diagnosis

The diagnoses of the three most common dizziness syndromes (vertigo, disequilibrium, and presyncope) are discussed in this section. Vertigo is the most common diagnosis in a young, healthy patient. Disequilibrium and presyncope are seen in older individuals.

The causes of peripheral and central vertigo are summarized in Tables 12.13 and 12.14. Peripheral vertigo is usually not a symptom of underlying serious disease. Central vertigo may be. It is extremely important to differentiate the two (Table 12.15).

As mentioned under "Disequilibrium," disequilibrium results from processes that disturb equilibrium at any of its three points: sensory input, integration, or motor response. Frequently, patients with disequilibrium will have problems in more than one area, making diagnosis more difficult. Diminished vision, hearing, and tactile sense in the lower extremities can limit sensory input. Distortion of vision will cause more problems with equilibrium than visual loss alone. The elderly will often have multiple sensory deficits that produce disequilibrium.

Central integration of sensory input is affected by any global impairment in CNS function. Dementia, metabolic encephalopathy, and medication with sedative side effects are the most common etiologies.

Motor function has three major components: pyramidal system, extrapyramidal system, and cerebellum. Problems in any of these can produce disequilibrium. Frontal lobe dysfunction (degenerative disease, hydrocephalus, neoplasm), Parkinson's disease, and cerebellar disease (alcohol-related, degenerative, neoplasm) are examples of the most common etiologies, respectively.

Globally diminished cerebral blood flow is the underlying pathology of presyncope with transient impairment in venous return as the most common etiology. Symptoms of the autonomic nervous system such as nausea, diaphoresis, and palpitations accompany decreased cerebral blood flow. The differential diagnosis includes vasovagal (vasodepressor) presyncope, hyperventilation, orthostatic hypotension, vagotonia/Valsalva mechanisms, carotid sinus sensitivity, and cardiac presyncope. Table 12.16 presents additional information on each of these diagnoses.

Management

The initial management for patients is found in Tables 12.13, 12.14, and 12.16, which summarize

Table 12.13.
Causes of Peripheral Vertigo

Cause	Symptoms/History	Physical Exam	Definitive Diagnosis	Treatment
Otitis media	Ear pain	Inflamed tympanic membrane; unusual in adults (conductive hearing loss)	Physical exam	Antibiotics
Serious otitis	Ear pain, ear fullness	Fluid behind tympanic membrane, (conductive hearing loss)	Physical exam	Decongestants
Cerum/wax	Ear fullness, decreased hearing	Impaction (conductive hearing loss)	Physical exam	Wax removal
Cholesteatoma	Tinnitus, hearing loss, history of chronic otitis or tympanic membrane rupture	Opaque density on tympanic membrane (conductive hearing loss)	Fistula test	ENT referral for surgery
Menier's disease	Tinnitus, hearing loss, episodic	Sensorineural hearing loss during attack	Audiogram	ENT referral
Vestibular neuronitis	+Tinnitus, acute onset, maybe positional after upper respiratory infection	Nystagmus	History, physical exam, normal audiogram	Antiemetics and/or anxiolytics
Labyrinthitis	Similar to vestibular neuronitis, trauma (whiplash, ear), toxic (alcohol, aspirin, loop diuretics, aminoglycosides), viral infection, severe otitis media	Nystagmus	History, physical exam, normal audiogram	Eliminate toxin, antiemetics, anxiolytics
Benign positional vertigo	Only positional	Positional nystagmus	History, physical exam	Antiemetics, anxiolytics, adaptation exercises
Acoustic neuroma	Unilateral tinnitus, unilateral gradual hearing loss	Progressive sensorineural hearing loss	Audiogram, CT/MRI of posterior fossa and cerebellopontine angle	ENT referral for surgery
Internal auditory artery infarction	Sudden hearing loss, tinnitus	Permanent hearing loss, vertigo resolves	Audiogram	Aspirin, consider angiography

the differential diagnoses. With an appropriate history and physical examination, most patients with dizziness can be reassured as to the cause of their problem and the likelihood of correction and/or impairment. A distressing or annoying problem is sometimes better tolerated by patients when they know its cause, possible treatments, and prognosis.

Management of outer and middle ear pathology and stroke are discussed elsewhere in this book. Treatment of benign positional vertigo or vertigo caused by labyrinthitis is similar. Any suspicious toxins should be eliminated. Ear infections should be treated, if possible. Of course avoidance of head motion should be recommended. For severe nausea and vertigo the patient should take an antiemetic such as prochlorperazine 10 mg po four times daily or promethazine 25 mg po four times daily and temporarily withhold solid food. Pregnant women may take trimethobenzamide 250 mg po four times daily. Patients who are vomiting should take prochlorperazine or promethazine 25 mg per rectum every 6 hours. Because labyrinthitis is self-limited,

Table 12.14.
Causes of Central Vertigo

Cause	Symptoms/History	Physical Exam	Definitive Diagnosis	Treatment
Drugs (alcohol, anticonvulsants, sedatives, opiates)	Alcohol or drug use	Fruity breath, tremor, mental status change, constricted pupils	History, serum levels	Remove or adjust offending agent
Vertebrobasilar vascular insufficiency	Vertigo less severe than peripheral, associated symptoms (CN VII—sensory; CN III/IV—motor, diplopia; dysarthria; dysphagia)	Ataxia present only with vertigo	History, CT, MRI	Antiplatelet treatment, evaluation of carotids indicated
Multiple sclerosis	Vertigo mild recurrent attacks seen in the young (<40)	Hearing loss is rare; intranuclear ophthalmoplegia is pathognomonic	MRI, evoked potentials, cerebrospinal fluid exam	Steroids for acute demyelination, phenothiazine/antihistamines for vertigo
Basilar artery migraine	Vertigo, associated symptoms (scintillating scotomata, homonymous hemianopsia, diplopia, dystharia, ataxia)	No hearing loss or tinnitus, can be migraine equivalent if not followed by headache	History	Same as for other migraines
Head trauma	History of trauma	Basilar skull fracture, laceration of vestibular portion of CN VIII, postconcussive syndrome may persist for months	CT, history, (CT will be negative in postconcussive syndrome)	Refer to neurosurgery, reassurance follow-up
Seizure	Aura prior to seizure		EEG with vertigo	Treatment of seizures

Table 12.15.
Differentiation of Peripheral from Central Vertigo

Symptoms	Peripheral	Central
Hallucination of movement/intensity	Definite, severe	Less definite/never severe
Onset	Abrupt, paroxysmal	Gradual, constant
Duration	Usually short	Longer
Influence of head position	Frequent	Seldom
Autonomic symptoms	Definite	Less intense or absent
Hearing loss	Can be present	Not present
Tinnitus	Can be present	Not present
Altered sensorium	Absent	Can be present
Nystagmus	Present, bilateral, unidirectional, horizontal/rotating, fatigues	Present or absent, unilateral or bilateral, unidirectional or bidirectional, horizontal, rotatory, or vertical, does not fatigue, persists

Table 12.16.
Causes of Presyncope

Cause	Symptoms/History	Physical Exam	Definitive Diagnosis	Treatment
Vasovagal (common faint)	Patient upright when symptoms begin; associated with hot/crowded room, acute injury/pain, or emotional stress; prodromal symptoms (nausea, sweating, weakness); pallor frequent	May find bradycardia	History Normal examination	Avoid precipitating conditions, lie down
Vagotonia/Valsalva-micturition syncope	Seen only in men during urination, usually nocturnal, bladder full to distended	Sudden peripheral vasodilation at the end of urination	History	Empty bladder at bedtime
Carotid sinus hypersensitivity	Seen in elderly	Carotid massage (done in monitored setting) reproduces symptoms	History	Permanent pacemaker
Orthostatic hypotension	Symptoms when patient is standing, maximal symptoms when patient rises from sitting or supine position, Associated history (antihypertensives, rapid blood loss, autonomic neuropathy)	Orthostatic change in blood pressure	Reproduction of symptoms with fall in blood pressure Documentation of blood loss	Adjust or change medications Determine cause and treat blood loss
Hyperventilation Acute	Seen in young women, associated symptoms (lightheadedness, visual blurring, perioral/digital paresthesas), patient describes anxiety and sensation of shortness of breath	Important to eliminate panic attacks	Reproduction of symptoms with 3 minutes of observed hyperventilation	Reassurance, rebreathing into paper bag
Chronic	Seen in men, usually no associated symptoms, patient unaware of hyperventilation, occurs in stressful situations	Diagnosis frequently not accepted, more difficult to manage, usually underlying anxiety or depression	Reproduction of symptoms with 3 minutes of observed hyperventilation	Same as acute

these treatments are required for a few days only. Diazepam 5 mg po three times daily decreases dizziness, nausea, and the anxiety they cause.

Benign positional vertigo may recur, so a long term strategy for its treatment is essential. Adaptation exercises are effective for controlling symptoms. The patient identifies the specific motion that initiates symptoms and then repeats that motion

several times. The brain ultimately is "trained" to ignore the stimulus.

Treatment of disequilibrium focuses on its causes (abnormalities, sensory inputs, integration in the CNS, and motor response). Hearing, touch, and vision should be assessed and deficits corrected. Processing of sensory input can be altered by drugs that affect the CNS. Review of the patient's medications and discontinuation of any potentially offending agent is indicated. Abnormal motor response is difficult to treat; however, avoidance of alcohol and treatment of Parkinson's disease can improve symptoms in selected patients.

Patients with simple vasovagal or orthostatic dizziness are best treated by educating them to avoid precipitating conditions. If shock or strong emotions lead to symptoms, patients should leave or at least sit down in such situations. Patients should dangle their legs on the side of the bed for 2 minutes before standing. If medical conditions allow, patients may note fewer symptoms if they liberally salt their food. Patients with other cardiovascular causes of presyncope require specific treatment (e.g. pacemaker) as indicated by the specific diagnoses.

ILLUSTRATIVE CASES WITH SELF-ASSESSMENT QUESTIONS AND ANSWERS

Case 1

A 42-year-old man comes to the walk-in clinic because of dizziness, which began 1 week ago but has progressively gotten worse. On further questioning he describes an unsteady gait and walking "like a drunk." His past medical history is remarkable only for cerebral aneurysm that was surgically clipped 2 years ago. He takes phenytoin for seizure prophylaxis. Your examination is negative except for an ataxia and unsteady gait and vertical nystagmus.

QUESTION: *What is the most appropriate next step in the management of this patient?*

a. Cerebral angiogram
b. Blood alcohol level
c. Head CT with contrast
d. Blood phenytoin level
e. MRI of the head

ANSWER: *d. Blood phenytoin level is the correct answer. As Willy Sutton, the infamous bank robber said, "Go where the money is." The examination showed vertical nystagmus, which indicates a central etiology. The lack of other focal findings and a potential toxic cause would suggest drug induced symptoms and signs.*

Once the elevated phenytoin level is documented, it is extremely important to determine what triggered the toxicity—inadvertent overdosage, drug-drug interaction, impaired metabolism, or excretion.

Case 2

A 69-year-old woman tells you about "dizziness" at her regular follow-up visit. On further descrip-tion, the dizziness is really a sense of unsteadiness when walking. She has never fallen but is afraid she will do so. She has restricted activities outside of her home to those during which family can accompany her.

Her medical problems include hypertension and diabetes for which she takes a diuretic and an oral hypoglycemic agent. The only complication of diabetes she has experienced was an ulcer at the base of the first metatarsal joint that developed from an irregularity in the insole of her shoe. On walking into the exam room, her gait seemed steady, but she was holding onto her daughter's arm. The findings on your examination are new eyeglasses and no response when you talk to her through the curtain.

QUESTION: *Which of the following would not help in making a diagnosis?*

a. Visual acuity with correction
b. Audiogram
c. Noninvasive arterial studies of the lower extremities
d. Electromyogram with testing of nerve conduction
e. Mini-mental status exam

ANSWER: *c. Noninvasive arterial studies would contribute little, if anything, to the diagnosis. New eyeglasses may account for the sudden onset of symptoms in this patient. Distortion of vision, as happens with bifocals or lens implants, causes more problems with equilibrium than just diminished visual acuity. (Remember the hall of mirrors?) The history suggests a peripheral neuropathy, probably from diabetes and some degree of hearing loss. The patient may have accommodated to these changes over time only to have a* *sudden decompensation with another sensory deficit.*

Case 3

A 58-year-old woman is brought to the office by her husband. He says he found her in the bedroom lying on the floor. She said suddenly "everything was moving around so fast and I felt sick to my stomach." The patient has no known medical problems and takes no medications. She denies hearing deficits and tinnitus. As she reclines on the exam table, she has another episode of dizziness and nausea.

QUESTION: *What would you expect to find on physical examination?*

a. Hemiparesis
b. Orthostatic changes in blood pressure and pulse
c. Resting tremor
d. Spontaneous nystagmus
e. Stool positive for occult blood

ANSWER: *d. You would expect to find either rotary or horizontal nystagmus. The profound vertigo in this patient suggests a peripheral cause. The lack of tinnitus and hearing problems directs attention to the labyrinth. The medical history is noncontributory, so an acute, self-limited process is the most likely etiology.*

STROKE AND TRANSIENT ISCHEMIC ATTACK

Stroke is the most common cause of major neurologic disability and third most common cause of death in the United States after heart disease and cancer. Stroke is diagnosed approximately 400,000 times yearly in the United States and contributes to about 150,000 deaths annually (11). Although new methods to treat patients with stroke have been proposed, the most effective strategies for reducing the incidence of stroke-related disabilities continue to concern the primary prevention of stroke and prevention of recurrent stroke.

Cerebrovascular diseases consist of disorders of the blood or blood vessels that cause infarction of brain tissue or hemorrhage into or around the brain. These diseases are classified based on their duration. A TIA is defined as a transient episode of focal cerebral dysfunction that usually lasts from 2 to 15 minutes but always resolves completely within 24 hours. A reversible ischemic neurological

Table 12.17.
Distribution of Diagnosis Subtype (Stroke Data Bank)

Stroke Subtype Diagnosis	%
Cerebral infarctions	
Infarct, unknown cause	32
Embolic	14
Atherosclerotic	6
Lacune	19
Hemorrhages	
Intracerebral	13
Subarachnoid	13

From Foulkes MA, Wolf PA, Price TR, et al. The stroke data bank: design, methods and baseline characteristics. Stroke 1988;19: 547–554. Reproduced with permission.

deficit or resolving ischemic neurologic deficit is defined as an episode of focal cerebral dysfunction that lasts longer than 24 hours but resolves completely within 3 weeks. A completed stroke is defined as an episode of focal cerebral ischemia that has not resolved completely after 3 weeks.

These disorders are further classified as either ischemic or hemorrhagic disorders. Ischemic disorders are subtyped as those caused by disease of large vessels, small deep vessels known as lacunar infarcts, or cardiogenic emboli. Hemorrhagic disorders are further described as either intraparenchymal hemorrhage or subarachnoid hemorrhage (Table 12.17). This classification will be used to further discuss cerebrovascular disorders with respect to their etiology, presentation, diagnostic evaluation, and management.

Cerebrovascular disorders may occur at any age but are most common in the elderly, especially those with risk factors for vascular disease such as hypertension, atherosclerosis, smoking, or hyperlipidemia; 85% of the patients suffering from stroke are older than 65 years (12). In fact, when stroke is diagnosed in a patient who is younger than 45 years special diagnostic considerations are warranted. A major challenge for the primary care clinician with respect to cerebrovascular disease is the detection and management of those patients who are at risk for stroke. Another challenge is the provision of optimal care for the many stroke survivors that are found in one's practice.

Pathophysiologic Correlation

Atherosclerosis is the underlying process leading to ischemic cerebrovascular disease in most stroke patients. Atherosclerosis most commonly affects the larger vessels at the base of the brain and in the neck at bifurcations. Therefore the internal

Table 12.18.
Etiologies of Intracerebral or Subarachnoid
Hemorrhage

Chronic hypertension
Hypertensive crisis
Ruptured aneurysm
Ruptured arteriovenous malformation
Blood dyscrasias
  Hemophilia
  Thrombocytopenia
  Use of anticoagulants
Tumors
Trauma
Drugs related to sudden hypertension
  Cocaine
  PCP
  Amphetamines
  Monoamine oxidase inhibitors in the presence of
    foods containing tyramine
Vasculitis

carotid artery, carotid siphon, proximal middle cerebral artery, and vertebral and basilar arteries are all common sites of atherosclerotic narrowing. These narrowed sites collect atherosclerotic plaque (and eventually hemorrhage within the plaque), cholesterol debris, platelet-fibrin material, and thrombus. This is the process that eventually leads to clinically significant stenosis and cerebral ischemia.

Lacunar infarcts are small infarcts that occur most commonly in deep white and gray matter of the cerebral hemispheres and in the brainstem. They are believed to be due to thrombotic occlusion of small deep perforators off of primarily the middle cerebral artery and basilar artery.

Just as in ischemic strokes, hypertension is the primary risk factor for intracerebral hemorrhage. The pathogenesis is likely related to the formation and rupture of microaneurysms of small penetrating arterioles. In younger patients without chronic hypertension, ruptured aneurysms, arteriovenous malformations, and angiomas are often implicated. Other less common etiologies include hemorrhage caused by blood dyscrasias, tumors, drugs etc (Table 12.18). Subarachnoid hemorrhage is most commonly due to rupture of a berry aneurysm. Other etiologies of subarachnoid hemorrhage include rupture of arteriovenous malformations and coagulopathy.

Risk Factors for Cerebrovascular Disease

A special discussion of the risk factors for cerebrovascular disease is warranted given the data that supports the relationship between therapeutic interventions and management of some of these factors and the decreased incidence of stroke. Risk factors for ischemic cerebrovascular disease include, among others, advanced age, male sex, hypertension, hyperlipidemia, smoking, and diabetes mellitus. Although these factors are clearly associated with an increased risk of stroke, their modification or improvement has not been shown to reduce the risk in all instances.

Hypertension remains the paramount risk factor for stroke. Both systolic and diastolic blood pressure levels have been found to be strongly and independently related to the incidence of stroke. In addition, many treatment trials have demonstrated that antihypertensive therapy reduces the risk of stroke significantly. A meta-analysis of several studies with a combined population of 37,000 revealed that therapy which reduced diastolic blood pressure an average of 5–6 mmHg produced a 42% reduction in stroke during the study (13). Likewise there is evidence that smoking cessation reduces the risk of stroke (14). There is no convincing body of data that links the improvement in hyperlipidemia or diabetic control with a reduction in the risk for cerebrovascular disease.

Another group of patients who are at high risk for stroke are those with cardiac conditions that predispose them to cardioembolic events (Table 12.19). Certainly, the early detection of these conditions and their appropriate management may lower the risk for stroke in this group. The proper management of these patients as well as the aggressive treatment of hypertension is felt to be responsible for the recent decline in the incidence of stroke. The management of these patients will be discussed under "Management."

Other less common conditions that have been

Table 12.19.
Cardiac Conditions Associated with Cerebral Emboli

Nonvalvular atrial fibrillation
Ischemic heart disease
  Acute myocardial infarction (usually anterior)
  Ventricular aneurysm
Prosthetic cardiac valves
Rheumatic heart disease
Mitral valve prolapse
Cardiac myxoma
Nonbacterial thrombotic endocarditis
Cardiomyopathy
Infective endocarditis

Table 12.20.
Common Clinical Features of Cerebral Ischemia
Involving Major Vascular Territories

Anterior circulatory system
Hemiparesis
Hemisensory deficit
Aphasia—expressive or receptive
Loss of vision in one eye or part of one eye (amaurosis fugax)
Posterior circulatory system
Vertigo
Diplopia
Dysphagia
Paresis in any combination of all four extremities
Sensory loss in any combination of all four extremities
Ataxia
Dysarthria
Facial parasthesia
Hemianopia or bilateral visual loss

associated with ischemic stroke include hematologic conditions such as polycythemia, sickle cell anemia, thrombocytosis, and hypercoagulable states. Specific interventions such as transfusion therapy in patients with sickle cell disease or the use of agents to decrease platelet count in patients with thrombocytosis may be effective in reducing the risk for stroke.

Clinical and Laboratory Evaluation

HISTORY

As in many neurological diseases, a thorough history is vital in diagnosing and further classifying stroke. Details concerning the onset of symptoms are important. Additionally, associated symptoms such as headache, palpitations, chest pain, or fever should be elicited. Information about previous events such as TIAs or stroke should be obtained from the patient or family. Relevant medical history such as knowledge of hypertension, arrhythmia, or heart disease should also be obtained.

In ischemic stroke or TIA, the presenting symptoms will depend chiefly on the site of the occlusion to blood flow, more specifically whether it is in the anterior circulation (common carotid, internal carotid, middle cerebral, or anterior cerebral arteries) or posterior circulation (vertebral, basilar, or posterior cerebral arteries). Table 12.20 lists the clinical features of anterior and posterior circulation ischemia. In intracerebral hemorrhage, the symptoms are produced by direct tissue damage, compression of surrounding tissue, elevation of in-

tracranial pressure, and herniation. In subarachnoid hemorrhage, severe headache, often described as the worst headache the patient has ever experienced, is the most prominent symptom.

PHYSICAL EXAMINATION

A thorough general physical exam as well as detailed neurological evaluation are essential to the evaluation of a patient with presumed stroke. The patient's blood pressure must be followed closely, given the association between hypertension and stroke. In stroke thought to be due to large vessel occlusive disease, there may be physical findings in the general exam that support this diagnosis. The clinician should look for signs of atherosclerosis elsewhere, such as abdominal or femoral bruits or diminished pedal pulses. The clinician must also check for stenosis of the cervical vessels by auscultating for bruits in the neck. Bruits are felt to first become audible with a stenosis of about 40% of the cross-luminal diameter. This degree of stenosis, however, is not usually clinically significant. It is important for clinicians to realize that bruits will disappear at about 90% stenosis. There must be careful auscultation of the heart to detect cardiac conditions (e.g., mitral stenosis, atrial fibrillation, etc.) that may predispose the patient to a cardioembolic stroke.

A detailed review of the variety of neurological findings in stroke is beyond the scope of this chapter, but specific key features deserve mention. Hemiparesis is usually the most prominent finding in a contralateral cerebral lesion. An ischemic stroke involving the anterior cerebral artery is more likely to cause maximal weakness of the leg, whereas a stroke involving the middle cerebral artery will lead to maximal weakness of the arm. Deep tendon reflexes are usually increased on the side opposite the cerebral lesion. Also, a positive Babinski reflex may be present. The presence or absence of aphasia also helps the clinician determine the site of the lesion. Most aphasias are associated with left hemispheric lesions. Cranial nerve abnormalities as well as patterns of sensory loss also are helpful in clinically localizing a lesion. Lesions of the right cerebral hemisphere classically produce a depressed mental status and, often, the hemineglect syndrome where the patient may not recognize the hemiplegia or any external object to the left of his or her own midline.

LABORATORY EVALUATION

Routine laboratory as well as radiological studies must be done to define the etiology of stroke as

Table 12.21.
Diagnostic Evaluation in a Patient with
Presumed Stroke

Basic studies
Complete blood counts
Electrolytes, blood urea nitrogen, creatinine, glucose
Prothrombin time, partial thromboplastin time
Erythrocyte sedimentation rate
Lipid profile
Chest x-ray
Electrocardiogram
CT scan or MRI
Other studies as clinically indicated
Echocardiography—two-dimensional or transesophageal
Holter monitor
Toxicology screen
Blood cultures
Cerebral angiogram
Doppler ultrasound studies of the carotid arteries
Lumbar puncture

well as to detect other possible etiologies of the presenting neurological symptoms (Table 12.21). For example, hypoglycemia that usually causes global encephalopathy may present with focal neurological signs and symptoms. Additionally, anemia, thrombocytosis, and polycythemia can also cause focal cerebral ischemia. A CT scan without contrast should be done early in all patients with presumed stroke to help differentiate bland infarct (Fig. 12.4) from hemorrhage (Fig. 12.5). The CT scan will also detect other lesions that may not be expected such as intracranial tumors or subdural hematomas that can cause neurologic presentations similar to stroke. MRI scanning, now available at most major diagnostic centers, may detect lesions that current CT scans cannot, such as those smaller than 5 mm or small lesions in the brainstem. Also, MRI may detect infarcts as early as 2 hours after the onset of symptoms. CT scans are unlikely to detect infarcts before 12 hours after the onset of symptoms.

Additional studies that may be used to search for the etiology of stroke will be individualized based on the clinical scenario. For example, the patient who presents with what appears to be an embolic stroke but whose neck vessels are without apparent stenosis requires a thorough evaluation for a cardiac source of emboli. This would include echocardiography, either two-dimensional or, ideally, transesophageal. Holter monitoring to find unsuspected arrhythmias is also warranted in this

clinical situation. This evaluation is not appropriate for most patients presenting with infarction.

As mentioned earlier, the patient who presents with ischemic stroke who is younger than 45 years requires a more exhaustive search for the etiology of stroke. In some cases, a hypercoagulable state may be responsible for the cerebral ischemia. This condition may be due to proteins C or S or antithrombin III deficiency, presence of antiphospholipid antibodies, or lupus anticoagulant. In addition, cerebral vasculitis related to systemic conditions such as lupus erythematosus or polyarteritis nodosa may present with cerebral ischemia. There are myriad other less common etiologies for ischemic stroke in the younger patient, the discussion of which is beyond the domain of this chapter.

Differential Diagnosis

Certain metabolic abnormalities such as hypo- or hyperglycemia may present with focal neurological deficits. Other conditions that may lead to stroke-like syndromes include complicated migraine, subdural hematoma, or intracranial tumor. In addition, patients with seizure disorders may be left with a hemiparesis after a seizure that is known as a Todd's paralysis. This form of paralysis may last up to 24 hours or more.

Management

Admission to the hospital is indicated for any patient with a newly diagnosed stroke with a neurologic deficit. It has been demonstrated that it is not possible to accurately predict which patients with a recent stroke will deteriorate further. Therefore early hospitalization allows for close monitoring and observation as well as prompt therapy and multidisciplinary rehabilitation.

The patient who has suffered a probable TIA does not usually require emergent hospitalization. These patients require a prompt and efficient evaluation, but this may often be done in the ambulatory setting. Although the period immediately after TIA carries a higher risk for stroke, there is little evidence that immediate hospitalization is of benefit (15). However, if symptoms recur during the evaluation, then prompt hospitalization is recommended.

The basic care of the patient hospitalized for stroke will include monitoring of vital signs and close observation for deterioration of neurologic function. The patient's blood pressure should be maintained within reasonable limits. However, hypertensive patients should not have their blood

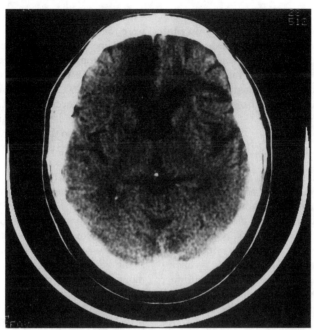

Figure 12.4.   Cerebral infarction anterior cerebral artery distribution. Infarct is a low density area in the frontal lobe.

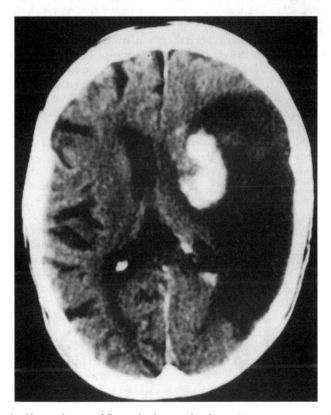

Figure 12.5.   Intracerebral hemorrhage middle cerebral artery distribution. Intravenous contrast leaks from the hemorrhage site into the lateral ventricle.

pressure treated aggressively because this may result in cerebral hypoperfusion. Depending on the clinical scenario, patients may require cardiac monitoring and treatment of cardiac arrhythmias, supplemental oxygen, endotracheal intubation, or treatment of seizures. Specific therapy will depend on the underlying neurologic process and will be outlined in the next section.

TRANSIENT ISCHEMIC ATTACKS AND RESOLVING ISCHEMIC NEUROLOGICAL DEFICITS

Studies of the natural history of TIAs have shown that approximately one-third of patients with TIA continue to experience attacks without permanent sequela; one-third experience remission, and one-third go on to brain infarction. Most patients that will develop infarction usually do so within 3–6 months after the onset of TIA (16). Management of these patients thus focuses on reduction of the risk for future stroke. This may involve improvement of blood pressure control, smoking cessation, and appropriate treatment of cardiac conditions that may predispose the patient to stroke (e.g., arrhythmias and valvular heart disease).

Antiplatelet Agents. The most widely used medical therapy for TIAs is aspirin. At low doses aspirin will diminish platelet aggregability. Several studies have attempted to address the efficacy of aspirin in the treatment of TIA. It has been concluded from analysis of these trials that aspirin is effective in reducing the risk of stroke and myocardial infarction in high-risk patients, including those with TIA (17). There is still some debate about the optimal dose of aspirin; however, most clinicians will prescribe enteric coated aspirin in a dose of 80–325 mg/day for their patients with symptoms of TIA.

Ticlopidine hydrochloride is a new antiplatelet agent recently approved for prevention of stroke in patients with TIA or minor stroke. Two large, multicenter, randomized trials have evaluated the efficacy of ticlopidine. The Canadian American Ticlopidine Study (CATS) enrolled 1053 patients who had had a recent moderate to severe atherothrombotic or lacunar stroke. Patients were randomly assigned to receive ticlopidine at 500 mg/day or placebo. The relative risk reduction for important vascular events in patients randomized to receive ticlopidine was 23.3% with a benefit being seen in both men and women (18).

The Ticlopidine-Aspirin Stroke Study (TASS) compared the efficacy of ticlopidine and aspirin in reducing the risk of stroke and death in patients with a recent stroke or TIA. A total of 3069 patients were randomized to receive either 500 mg/day of ticlopidine or 650 mg aspirin twice a day. This study demonstrated an overall risk reduction for stroke of 21% by the use of ticlopidine compared with aspirin (19). Side effects of ticlopidine include diarrhea that occurred in 12.5% of patients in TASS, rash, and neutropenia. The neutropenia may be severe, so therefore it is recommended that patients receiving ticlopidine be monitored with a complete blood count every 2 weeks during the first 3 months of therapy.

Ticlopidine certainly can be seen as an alternative and perhaps even more effective antiplatelet medication for the prevention of cerebrovascular ischemia. However, consideration of the increased cost of the medication as opposed to aspirin as well as the side effect profile and need for hematologic monitoring has led the American Heart Association Ad Hoc Committee on Guidelines for the Management of TIA to recommend aspirin as the appropriate initial antiplatelet agent in most cases (20). Ticlopidine may be useful in patients who are intolerant to aspirin or who have continued ischemic symptoms despite aspirin therapy.

Anticoagulants. Oral anticoagulation with warfarin has been commonly used to prevent stroke in patients who have had TIAs. Actually, to date, there are no conclusive data to support this practice. There is, however, general agreement that patients with stroke or TIA due to cardiac embolism should be treated with anticoagulants. In addition, long term anticoagulation is also recommended for the prevention of cerebral embolism in the setting of mitral valve disease and recent myocardial infarction. Until recently there had been no trial specifically examining cardioembolic TIAs. The European Atrial Fibrillation Trial compared warfarin, aspirin, and placebo in 1007 patients with nonvalvular atrial fibrillation and TIA or minor stroke (21). This trial demonstrated a 66% reduction in subsequent stroke with warfarin as opposed to placebo. Aspirin therapy was responsible for a 14% reduction in stroke compared with placebo. This study strongly supports the use of anticoagulation in patients with atrial fibrillation and TIA or stroke provided there are no major contraindications.

Surgical Therapy. Carotid endarterectomy was first performed in 1954. Its use as a means of preventing stroke grew steadily until 1984 when several studies appeared questioning its efficacy and appropriateness. In the last decade the issue of whether and when to perform carotid endarterectomy has been controversial. Recently, results from two large prospective trials have begun to answer some of the questions about the use of carotid endarterectomy in the management of cerebrovascular disease.

The North American Symptomatic Carotid Endarterectomy Trial (NASCET) included 659 patients with high grade carotid stenosis, defined as 70–90% stenosis, who had had TIA or minor stroke within 120 days. Patients were randomly assigned to surgical or medical therapy. After 2 years ipsilateral stroke had occurred in 26% of the medically treated group and in 9% of the surgically treated group (23). Due to these dramatic findings the trial was discontinued for those with high grade stenosis. The trial is continuing to look at those patients with 30–69% carotid artery stenosis.

The European Carotid Surgery Trial (ECST) included 2518 patients over 10 years. As in the NASCET trial there was a significant benefit in the surgically treated patients with high grade stenosis (24). Once these results were obtained, this part of the trial was discontinued. This trial also continues to enroll patients with 30–69% carotid artery stenosis.

Clinicians must realize that the anticipated benefit of carotid endarterectomy for a particular patient is clearly dependent on the perioperative complication rate of the procedure. This rate may vary considerably among institutions. When attempting to make a decision about whether to refer a patient for carotid endarterectomy, the primary care provider may enlist the advice of a consulting neurologist to help determine the patient's risk for recurrent stroke if treated medically. This will be dependent on the degree of stenosis of the carotid artery as well as on the particular characteristics that put the patient at risk for cerebrovascular disease. However, the clinician must also factor in the patient's risk for surgery as performed by a particular surgeon at a specific hospital. Obviously, this may be a complicated decision.

CARDIOGENIC EMBOLISM

Approximately 20% of cerebral infarcts are thought to be caused by emboli from a cardiac source. The use of long term anticoagulation in patients at risk for cardiogenic embolism has been discussed. The management of the patient with acute infarct caused by cardiac embolus is somewhat controversial owing to the risk of bland infarct becoming hemorrhagic with the use of heparin. The usual recommendation is a 2- to 3-day delay in heparinization for those with large infarcts due to cardiogenic embolus.

INTRACEREBRAL AND SUBARACHNOID HEMORRHAGE

The acute management of those with intracerebral and subarachnoid hemorrhage is similar to that outlined in the preceding section. These patients must be observed closely, often in an intensive care unit. Careful monitoring of their vital signs, neurologic function, and fluid and electrolyte balance is essential. In addition, these patients may require special measures to control intracranial pressure such as hyperventilation and mannitol. Other management issues such as the surgical treatment of arteriovenous malformations and berry aneurysms are complex and beyond the scope of this chapter.

Rehabilitation

Although the incidence of stroke in the United States is declining, because of the increasing elderly population, stroke will continue to be a prevalent problem and will thus continue to have a significant impact on health care costs and the quality of life for many individuals. Stroke rehabilitation has been defined as the process of minimizing or resolving a handicap or disability that results from the permanent impairment caused by the stroke (22). Rehabilitation can play a major role in the improvement of quality of life for those survivors of stroke.

Stroke rehabilitation can take many different forms. At one end of the spectrum, rehabilitation may merely involve the management of the patient after stroke to minimize complications while spontaneous recovery occurs. At the other end of the spectrum, rehabilitation may involve admission to an inpatient unit where the patient is cared for by a multidisciplinary team of professionals including speech, occupational, and physical therapists. Alternatively, stroke rehabilitation may occur at home with delivery of services coordinated by a home health care agency. Certainly the form of rehabilitation program that is prescribed for the patient will depend on many factors including the patient's overall medical condition and functional status, availability of family support, as well as the bias of the primary care provider.

There have been many studies that attempt to quantify the effectiveness of comprehensive rehabilitation programs. Indeed there has been some controversy about the contribution of rehabilitation to the functional improvement of the stroke patient. However, in general these studies suggest that rehabilitation adds to the functional improvement of the patient beyond what can be expected from spontaneous recovery (18). It must be noted that even a small improvement in functional capacity could represent the difference between institutionalization and remaining at home. It is the responsibility of the primary care provider, with the advice of a consulting neurologist in some instances, to decide if a patient is appropriate for referral to an intensive rehabilitation program. Not all patients are appropriate for such a program, but there are several factors that may help select the most appropriate patients. Primarily, the patient must be motivated to participate in rehabilitation. Successful rehabilitation is not likely in the unwilling patient. Additionally, the patient must possess the cognitive ability to follow simple commands. He or she must also have the short term memory capacity to remember the lessons learned in therapy sessions.

Rehabilitation for the stroke patient is usually accomplished via a multidisciplinary team of physical, occupational, and speech pathology therapists as well as nurses, physicians, and social workers. The goal of the rehabilitation program is to limit the functional impairment caused by the stroke. The basic functional activities that are considered include safe mobility, activities of daily living, and communication skills. Successful rehabilitation after a stroke that allows the patient to return home in an independent fashion can be extremely gratifying for the patient as well as for those professionals on the rehabilitation team who have worked with the patient to achieve his or her goals.

ILLUSTRATIVE CASES WITH SELF-ASSESSMENT QUESTIONS AND ANSWERS

Case 1

A 75-year-old woman with a history of hypertension and diabetes mellitus presents to her primary care provider with left-sided weakness that began about 2 hours before. On examination the patient is alert and oriented; blood pressure is 170/100; and there is mild weakness of the left upper and lower extremities.

QUESTION: *Immediate management of this patient would include _____. (Choose all that apply.)*

a. Referral to the hospital for admission
b. Reduction of the patient's blood pressure to normal
c. Evaluation of the patient's blood glucose and electrolytes
d. CT scan of the brain
e. transesophageal echocardiogram

ANSWER: *a, c, d. Any patient with a new neurologic deficit should be managed as an inpatient. Evaluation of blood chemistries and glucose is necessary to search for possible other causes of the neurologic symptoms. A CT scan of the head is necessary to distinguish among hemorrhage, bland infarct, and other less common causes of* the neurologic deficit. Acute reduction of the patient's blood pressure may cause cerebral hypoperfusion. A transesophageal echocardiogram is only indicated if there is a reason to suspect cardiogenic embolus, and this would probably not be part of the initial management even if indicated.

Case 2

A 68-year-old man with a history of poorly controlled hypertension, hypercholesterolemia, and a long smoking history presents to his clinician's office reporting an episode of transient visual loss of the right eye about 1 week earlier. Neurological examination at the time of his office visit is normal.

QUESTION: *Management of this patient would include _____.*

a. Referral to the hospital for admission
b. Doppler ultrasound studies of the carotid arteries
c. CT scan of the brain
d. Close follow-up and immediate communication if neurologic symptoms occur
e. Carotid angiography

ANSWER: *b, c, d. A patient with recent TIA probably does not need hospital admission as long as the evaluation can proceed quickly. If symptoms recur one would consider hospitalization. Noninvasive testing of the carotid arteries is indicated to evaluate the patient for the presence of high-grade stenosis. CT scan of the brain is indicated in the patient with TIA to look for signs of undetected cerebrovascular disease as well as for unusual causes of TIA.*

QUESTION: *The patient's carotid study reveals 60% stenosis on the right side. CT scan of the brain was negative. He has had no further symptoms. What recommendations can the clinician make regarding the management at this point?*

a. Immediate referral to a vascular surgeon for evaluation for carotid endarterectomy
b. Initiation of aspirin at 325 mg daily
c. Immediate smoking cessation
d. Improved control of the patient's hypertension
e. Improved compliance with a low fat, low cholesterol diet and pharmacologic therapy if necessary

ANSWER: *b, c, d, e. Current data do not support surgical treatment for moderate carotid stenosis. However, this is continuing to be studied. Management of TIA should focus on risk reduction such as cessation of cigarette smoking and better control of his hypertension. Although improvement in blood lipid levels has not been proven to be associated with a reduced risk of cerebrovascular disease, treatment of hyperlipidemia is recommended for reduction in coronary artery disease. Antiplatelet therapy with aspirin is indicated unless there is a contraindication.*

SEIZURES

Seizures affect about 1% of the population. A seizure may be classified by electroencephalogram (EEG) as partial (involving only a portion of the brain) or generalized (involving the entire brain) or by observation as simple (not affecting consciousness) or complex (affecting consciousness). For example, a clonic seizure of the arm of a conscious person would be classified as a partial simple seizure. Lip smacking (a focal neurologic finding) by a person with impaired consciousness would be classified as a partial complex seizure. An absence seizure is a generalized complex seizure that does not cause abnormal motor activity. The grand mal seizure is a generalized complex seizure that causes clonic movements of the limbs. This chapter will focus mainly on the common tonic-clonic, generalized, grand mal seizure and its evaluation and treatment.

Pathophysiologic Correlation

Seizures are initiated by electrochemical abnormalities in the brain, such as alterations in the concentration of excitatory or inhibitory neurotransmitters. Abnormal electrical discharge from one site quickly spreads to involve the entire brain, causing changes in perception, motor control, attention, and consciousness. The generalized tonic-clonic seizure may uncommonly be preceded by an aura, a vague warning heralding the onset of the seizure. Next there is sudden unconsciousness and tonic muscle contraction that lasts a few seconds. This is followed by a clonic flexion and extension of the muscles causing uncontrollable jerking of the limbs (lasting about 1 minute), biting of the tongue, and incontinence of urine and feces. After seconds or minutes, the muscles relax. The postictal period is characterized by amnesia of the seizure, confusion, headache, and drowsiness that may last for several hours.

Normal electrical discharge in the brain of an awake person is disorganized and irregular. During a generalized tonic-clonic seizure the electrical activity is characterized by regular rhythmic electrical discharges (spikes) followed by slow waves. Many processes can alter the electrochemical functioning of the brain. Ischemia, drugs, metabolic disorders, infection, and structural abnormalities may cause seizures. However, particularly in adolescents, idiopathic causes are also common. There may be genetic reasons for certain types of seizures.

Clinical and Laboratory Evaluation

The history, physical examination, and laboratory evaluation are equally important in diagnosing a seizure. The diagnostic workup should be guided by the patient's age and specific risks. In this fashion, the workup is cost-effective.

HISTORY

The history begins with the description of the seizure. Often the patient cannot recall the seizure, in which case a witness should be questioned. The patient and witness are asked about warning symptoms, movements (focality, tonic-clonic), and the postictal period. The recent and past history should

Table 12.22.
Causes of Seizure by Age Group

Adolescent—Young Adult
Idiopathic
Alcohol or drug related
Traumatic
Infection

Older Adult—Elderly
Alcohol or drug related
Brain tumor
Circulatory causes
Metabolic causes
Infection

include questions pertaining to fever, headache, neurologic symptoms, head injury, drug use, concomitant disease (especially cardiovascular, hepatic, pulmonary, and renal), and diabetes.

The most likely etiologies vary by age. Adolescents may have idiopathic seizures or seizures secondary to infection or drug use. In adults seizures are more likely to be secondary to a preexisting known illness, a mass lesion, or drug or alcohol use. For a listing of common etiologies of seizure by age group see Table 12.22.

PHYSICAL EXAMINATION

A complete physical examination is performed, noting in particular the vital signs, cardiovascular system, and neurologic system. The heart is carefully examined for signs of valvular disease and arrhythmia. The neurologic examination, including assessment of the head, eye grounds, cranial nerves, neck, speech, gait, mental status, and motor (including cerebellar), sensory, and deep tendon reflexes must be performed. Signs of a focal neurologic defect and history of focal seizure correlate with a structural brain abnormality. A normal neurologic examination is often found in those with idiopathic seizures.

LABORATORY EVALUATION

The laboratory evaluation of seizure is guided by the findings on history and physical examination. In general, the laboratory evaluation of a first seizure includes a chemical profile, noting the glucose, sodium, and calcium concentrations in the serum. EEG is performed in search of characteristic spike and wave discharges. Imaging studies, CT scans, or MRI are useful in diagnosing bleeds, mass lesions, and scars and necrotic areas in the brain.

If an infection is suspected, lumbar puncture is

performed, and CSF is sent for cell count, immediate staining, and culture. Peripheral blood cultures should also be sent. Lumbar puncture can be used to confirm the diagnosis of subarachnoid hemorrhage if imaging studies are not diagnostic.

When a seizure disorder has been previously diagnosed but a breakthrough seizure occurs, the serum concentration of the patient's prescribed anticonvulsant should be checked. Missing even one day's dose can cause anticonvulsant levels to fall, allowing a seizure. Concentrations of alcohol, cocaine, or other drugs may be measured if indicated.

Differential Diagnosis

Although the causes of seizure are multiple, there are a handful of causes likely to be seen in the office of the practitioner who cares for adolescents and adults. With the aid of modern imaging studies, these diagnoses are relatively easy. One entity, syncope, does not cause seizures, but it is so often confused with seizure that it is included in this section.

IDIOPATHIC SEIZURE

Known as epilepsy, the idiopathic seizure often begins in childhood or adolescence. As suggested by its name, the cause is unknown. There may be a hereditary predisposition to idiopathic seizures. Neurologic examination is normal as are all laboratory tests. The EEG is often abnormal.

TRAUMATIC CAUSES

Birth and perinatal injuries can cause early seizures, but usually these are diagnosed before adulthood. Head trauma from vehicular accidents, sports, or falls can cause seizures. Seizures that occur more than 1 day after an injury may recur. The more severe the head injury, the greater the likelihood of developing posttraumatic seizures. Penetrating head wounds and trauma resulting in amnesia for more than 1 day are likely to lead to posttraumatic seizures. Brief loss of consciousness is not considered a high risk for subsequent seizures.

INFECTIOUS CAUSES

Infection of the brain, encephalitis, is associated with seizures during and after the infection. Septic emboli and abscesses seen in endocarditis also cause seizures. Clues to the diagnosis of infection include recent history of a febrile illness, change in mental status, and presence of an epidemic of encephalitis. In the case of infected emboli or abscesses, a history of parenteral drug use, AIDS, recent dental work, and murmur or valvular heart disease should be sought. The causative microbiologic agent must be identified. This usually is accomplished by staining and culture of CSF and blood. Serologic identification of viral infection may not be helpful in the short term diagnostic search.

ALCOHOL AND DRUG CAUSES

Alcohol can cause seizures because of associated malnutrition and increased risks of head trauma. One or two alcohol withdrawal seizures may be seen in the first 24–48 hours after an alcoholic abstains from drink. These early withdrawal seizures do not suggest underlying structural disease.

Cocaine and similar stimulants are associated with increased incidence of seizure. Diagnosis is based on history, physical examination supporting stimulant use (hypertension, tachycardia, diaphoresis, dilated pupils), and demonstration of drugs in the blood or urine. Withdrawal from barbituates can also cause seizure.

MASS LESIONS

Primary tumors, either benign or malignant, and metastatic tumors are responsible for a significant number of seizures in older adults. Melanoma, lymphoma, and tumors of the breast, kidney, and lung may metastasize to the brain. Patients often have a history of malignancy, although many years may elapse between initial diagnosis and the appearance of metastatic disease. Focal findings on neurologic examination and documentation of a mass or masses by neuroimaging help secure the diagnosis. If there is doubt about the diagnosis, a biopsy must be performed.

Nontumor mass lesions include abscesses and arteriovenous malformations. An arteriovenous malformation may be diagnosed in a young healthy patient. Some patients have symptoms of headache or focal motor or sensory deficits. Sometimes the diagnosis is made after rupture of the arteriovenous malformations. Neuroimaging (CT with contrast or MRI) will make the diagnosis. Angiography is often required if surgical correction is planned.

CIRCULATORY CAUSES

In older adults, circulatory abnormalities account for many seizures. Hypertension and hypercholesterolemia, leading to atherosclerosis or cardiomyopathy, predispose to stroke, either ischemic or embolic. Valvular heart disease and arrhythmia can also cause ischemic or embolic stroke. Seizure may occur at the time of a stroke or after the affected area develops a scar.

METABOLIC CAUSES

Severe pulmonary, hepatic, cardiac, or renal disease can cause seizure. Hypoxemia in pulmonary disease and many metabolic disturbances in uremia and liver failure can cause seizure. Hypoglycemia most often seen in treated diabetics can cause seizures. Hypocalcemia and hyponatremia can also be causative. History, physical examination, and evaluation of serum chemistries will aid in diagnosis.

PSYCHOLOGICAL CAUSES

Hysterical seizures are usually enacted in front of a witness. The seizure lasts longer (>1 minute) and does not follow the phases of a typical tonic clonic seizure. A history of psychiatric disorder is common. The EEG is normal.

SYNCOPE

Witnesses may use the term seizure to describe syncope. Some useful historical and physical examination clues that favor the diagnosis of syncope over seizure are listed in Table 12.23. If the diagnosis remains unclear, it is reasonable to evaluate with an ECG and a complete neurologic examination. Further diagnostic testing with EEG, 24-hour continuous cardiac monitor, or echocardiogram is ordered selectively based on the history, physical examination, and ECG findings.

Management

The basic premises in management of generalized tonic-clonic seizures are to minimize their occurrence and to educate the patient about the risks. If there is an underlying cause that is highly treatable or curable, then no further long-term treatment of seizure is needed. However, if the risk of seizure remains or the defect cannot be corrected, institution of anticonvulsants is indicated.

ANTICONVULSANTS USED IN GENERALIZED TONIC-CLONIC SEIZURE

Anticonvulsants are the mainstay of therapy for seizures (Table 12.24). The anticonvulsants used for generalized tonic-clonic seizures all work by blocking sodium channels and inhibiting high frequency repetitive electrical discharges. The drug dosages can be titrated to a therapeutic level, the concentration most likely to prevent seizures but

Table 12.23.
Comparison of Syncope and Seizure

	Syncope	Seizure
Movement	None	Tonic clonic jerking
Incontinence	None	Often
Initiation of event	Fright, hot surroundings	Staring, focal movement of one body part
Tongue biting	No	Often

not cause undue adverse reactions. Drug levels can be misleading. Hypoalbuminemic patients (those with renal or hepatic disease) may have low levels of anticonvulsants because most assays measure free and protein-bound drugs. Only the free (un-bound) drug is active. In general, dosing of anticonvulsants is based on the patient's current seizure symptoms and adverse reactions, in addition to drug levels.

As a group the anticonvulsants are moderately to highly protein bound. Administration of an anticonvulsant with another highly bound drug may cause an increase in the concentration of the free anticonvulsant and a decrease in the other drug or vice versa depending on which bonds tighter. These drugs are metabolized by the liver and can induce hepatic drug metabolizing enzymes, thereby reducing the half-life of other drugs metabolized by these enzymes. The exception is valproic acid, which inhibits the same enzymes. Knowledge of the special attributes of the anticonvulsants and strict minimization of prescribed medications will help prevent dangerous drug interactions. Single drug therapy is recommended.

Phenytoin. Phenytoin is often the drug of choice for treatment of seizure. It is nonsedating

and does not dull the intellect. Its oral bioavailability is variable depending on the manufacturer. Be certain that the same brand is prescribed each time. The clearance of phenytoin is different from that of most drugs; it is nonlinear. Therefore very small adjustments in dosage can result in large changes in serum concentration. Although the usual adult dosage is 300 mg once daily or in divided doses, dosage adjustments should be small (e.g., 50 mg), and levels should be rechecked in 4–7 days. Patients taking therapeutic doses of phenytoin have lateral nystagmus. More problematic is gingival hyperplasia (especially in the young), hirsutism, nausea, and lymphadenopathy.

Carbamazepine. Carbamazepine in doses of 200–400 mg twice daily does not affect cognitive function. It is sedating at high doses and may cause liver toxicity and bone marrow suppression. For this latter reason blood counts and liver function tests should be checked early in the treatment. Also, the drug induces its own metabolic enzymes, so dosages often must be increased a few weeks after initiating therapy.

Barbiturates. Phenobarbital has a long half-life (3–5 days) and is only 50% protein bound, making it a good choice for poorly compliant pa-

Table 12.24.
Comparison of Four Common Anticonvulsants

Anticonvulsant	Dosage	Half-Life	Advantage	Adverse Effects	Therapeutic Level (μg/ml)
Phenytoin (Dilantin)	300 mg every day	1 day	Nonsedating, does not dull intellect	Gingival hyperplasia, hirsutism, nausea, lymphadenopathy	10–20
Carbamazepine (Tegretol)	200–400 mg twice daily	Half day	Nonsedating (at low doses), does not dull intellect	Sedating at high doses, liver toxic, bone marrow toxic	4–12
Phenobarbital	90–120 mg every day	3–4 days	Long half-life for drug interactions	Sedating, dulls intellect	10–20
Valproic acid (Depakene)	250–500 mg twice daily	Half day	Nonsedating, does not dull intellect	Liver toxic, bone marrow toxic, gastrointestinal irritation, alopecia	50–100

tients or those who must take multiple medications. It depresses cognitive function and is sedating, causing it to be less frequently prescribed than phenytoin, although it is probably the safest drug used for the treatment of generalized tonic-clonic seizures. Usual doses are 90–120 mg daily.

Valproic Acid. Valproic acid does not sedate or impair cognition, but it has been associated with hepatic dysfunction, bone marrow suppression, stomach irritation, and hair loss. It is usually prescribed in doses of 250–500 mg twice daily. Because of possible hematologic and hepatic toxicities, a complete blood count and liver function should be checked periodically.

EDUCATION AND FOLLOW-UP

The challenge of education is that the practitioner must be aware of the odds of recurrence of seizures and the risks involved. After a first seizure, if the workup is normal, there is about a 50% chance of recurrence. The decision regarding whether to begin drug therapy is based on the patient's wishes, provider's preferences, and risks of recurrence and adverse reactions to treatment. It is intuitively likely that a patient employed as a bus driver would have a higher risk of harm to self and others than would someone who neither drives nor works. Regardless of the decision, the patient must be seen for follow-up evaluation (and testing of drug levels as doses are titrated to the therapeutic range). Small lesions that may have been missed on initial evaluation may be more obvious on reexamination. The patient and family should be taught what a seizure is, what to expect if another one occurs, and how to intervene. In general, families are told not to try to stop the tonic-clonic movements or to insert anything into

Table 12.25.
Discontinuation of Anticonvulsant Therapy—Assessment of Risk Factors for Recurrent Seizure

High Risk	Low Risk
Frequent seizures	No seizures for 2–4 years
Repeated status epilepticus	Control with one anticonvulsant
	No structural brain lesion
	Normal neurologic examination
	Normal EEG

the patient's mouth to prevent tongue biting. The exception is the seizure occurring when the patient is in a dangerous position or situation, such as on the edge of a bed or in the water. Patients and families should be reassured that most seizures do not kill patients even though they are frightening. However, if tonic-clonic activity lasts more than 20–30 minutes, the patient should receive emergency medical treatment.

There is a long religious and folk history of seizures being a form of punishment. It is reasonable to explain to some patients that a seizure, like a heart attack or a toothache, is a physical malady with no spiritual connotation.

DISCONTINUATION OF ANTICONVULSANT THERAPY

Many patients require lifelong anticonvulsant therapy. However, patients with the characteristics outlined in Table 12.25 are low risk for recurrent seizures. The decision to discontinue treatment is based on the preferences of the patient and the doctor, the patient's environmental risks, and the occurrence of adverse drug reactions.

ILLUSTRATIVE CASES WITH SELF-ASSESSMENT QUESTIONS AND ANSWERS

Case 1

M. G. is a 58-year-old woman with a history of mitral valve stenosis, hypertension, and type 2 insulin-requiring diabetes. She had a seizure today. She has no past history of seizure. A witness described the seizure by saying, "She became sweaty, then fell down and her eyes rolled back in her head." Other than amnesia for the event, Mary's neurologic examination is normal.

QUESTION: *What is the diagnosis?*

a. Epilepsy
b. Syncope
c. Partial complex seizure

ANSWER: *b. Mary has risks for seizure, but more risks for syncope.*

QUESTION: *What diagnostic studies are indicated first?*

a. Serum chemistry
b. ECG
c. Lumbar puncture
d. MRI of the brain

ANSWER: *a, b. After finishing the history and physical examination, serum chemistries (including sodium, glucose, and calcium) and an ECG should be done. If the diagnosis is unclear, an EEG and 24-hour ambulatory cardiac monitor and possibly an echocardiogram should be ordered.*

Case 2

J. A. is a 68-year-old mechanic who has been healthy until his first seizure this morning. He now feels well but confides that he is losing weight. Neurologic examination reveals that he has decreased light touch sensation in his right upper extremity. He is a moderate drinker and a heavy smoker.

QUESTION: *What is his diagnosis?*

a. Seizure secondary to intracranial mass
b. Alcohol withdrawal
c. Syncope

ANSWER: *a. He has a focal neurologic abnormality and risks for malignancy. About 30% of first seizures in adults are related to intracranial masses.*

QUESTION: *Should he take anticonvulsants?*

ANSWER: *Yes, phenytoin would be a good choice in the case of a brain tumor because it does not impair cognition and is nonsedating. Steroids would be useful to decrease edema around the tumor.*

ABNORMAL MENTAL STATUS: DEMENTIA AND DELIRIUM

Assessment of the patient with altered mental status can be challenging. A patient who is suddenly confused is shockingly easy to identify, but a busy practitioner may overlook a patient who develops confusion over months. Memory worsens with age. As more people survive until the eighth, ninth, or tenth decade of life, the issue of a normal decline in mentation versus abnormal mental status will loom

larger in clinical practice. This section will review dementia and delirium.

Pathophysiologic Correlation

To maintain normal mental status, the parts of the brain that control awareness (brainstem and reticular activating system) and cognition (several cortical areas) must function properly. Any process that interferes with the function of these key areas can cause changes in mental status. For the purpose of this chapter mental status changes refer to dementia or delirium. Dementia is defined as a loss of intellectual capacity with attendant change in personality. Delirium is defined as an acute disorder of mentation characterized by agitation, extreme excitement, and hallucination. Systemic processes (e.g., septicemia, hypoxemia, hypotension, or hypoglycemia) or intoxication with alcohol, drugs, or heavy metals can impair the function of the neurons. Local processes, such as infection, bleeding, tumor, high blood pressure, hydrocephalus, or degeneration of the neurons, can likewise cause changes in mental status. Psychiatric disorders with imbalances of neurotransmitters have the same effect. Alzheimer's disease accounts for over 50% of newly diagnosed dementias, with multiinfarct dementia a distant second. Of reversible dementias, drugs, depression, normal pressure hydrocephalus, and metabolic disorders are the most common causes.

Clinical and Laboratory Evaluation

History and physical examination can determine the etiology of altered mental status. Different from other adult disease processes, the history should be verified by a family member or other close contact of the patient. Because of the seriousness of the symptoms and the possibility of a cause, laboratory testing and expensive diagnostic imaging are ordered in most cases.

HISTORY

Although a routine, complete history is sufficient, special emphasis should be placed on certain questions when interviewing the patient and family. The timing of the onset of the change is essential to elicit. Intracranial bleeds, drugs, and meningitis cause changes in mental status over minutes to hours. Tumors, primary neuronal diseases, and some toxins cause symptoms over weeks to months. Be certain to inquire about family history of similar symptoms, drug, alcohol, or medication use, and recent trauma. Elicit medical history including history of cancers. Specifically inquire about recent fevers or weight loss.

PHYSICAL EXAMINATION

The mental status examination begins when the patient enters the room and continues through the history and physical examination. The examiner notes the general appearance of the patient. The patient's alertness (can he or she concentrate enough to subtract sevens serially starting at 100?) and orientation (name, date, place) are then noted. His or her mood is elicited directly ("Can you describe your mood?") or indirectly (observed). Note the patient's language: diction, appropriateness of chosen words, speed of response. A simple assessment of visual-spatial relations is done by having the patient draw a clock (complete with numbers). To assess memory, ask the patient to remember three words; then ask him or her to repeat the three words immediately and 5 minutes later. Distant memory is checked by asking about date of birth, schooling, and employment. Cognition is assessed by asking about parables, such as "What does 'Don't cry over spilled milk' mean?" Ask about hallucinations or delusions.

A screening neurologic examination should be done, noting the integrity of the face and skull, gait, neck, funduscopy, oral/nasal area, and function of cranial nerves. Peripheral motor examination should test at least a large muscle and a small muscle group in both of the upper and lower extremities. Sensory examination should include at minimum tests of light touch and pinprick sensation in both upper and lower extremities, proximally and distally. Cerebellar testing (Romberg test, finger-to-nose and heel-to-shin test) follows. The screening examination ends with assessment of deep tendon reflexes. If abnormalities are discovered, more complete assessment, including motor testing of all muscle groups and testing for temperature, vibratory sensation, and proprioception, is indicated.

LABORATORY EVALUATION

There is considerable debate about the cost effectiveness of laboratory or radiological tests for dementia. Most dementia is of the Alzheimer's variety, for which there is no readily accessible confirmatory test. Findings on the history and physical examination should guide laboratory workup. A complete blood count, thyroid-stimulating hormone, and serum chemistry profile with glucose, creatine, liver functions, and electrolytes including calcium should be checked. Testing for syphilis should be done if the patient has risks for or findings consistent with infection. Checking levels of vitamin B_{12} can be helpful if the mean cor-

puscular volume is elevated. Selected patients should have cultures, drug levels, HIV tests, erythrocyte sedimentation rate, and urinalysis sent. Chest x-ray and ECG are recommended by some groups

Radiographic imaging of the brain is indicated for patients with new onset mental status change unless the diagnosis is certain and imaging would not aid management. Examples of when imaging is not necessary include routine meningitis, drug use, change in mental status secondary to another disease, and primary psychiatric disorders. CT scans and MRI are the most widely used imaging studies. CT is preferred for evaluation of bony abnormalities and acute intracranial bleeding. MRI gives better definition of gray and white matter and is preferred for diagnosis of diseases such as multiple sclerosis. Also, the MRI more reliably views the cerebellum. Currently, MRI is more expensive than CT scan.

Lumbar puncture and analysis of CSF are indicated when CNS infection or subarachnoid hemorrhage is suspected. Lumbar puncture should not be performed if there is evidence of increased intracranial pressure, such as papilledema. Often an imaging study is quickly performed before lumbar puncture, reassuring the clinician that the procedure can be conducted safely. However, if bacterial meningitis or meningoencephalitis is suspected and there is no papilledema, diagnostic lumbar puncture should not be delayed.

Differential Diagnosis

The incidence of disorders causing altered mental status varies according to diagnosis, age, social class, profession, and underlying disease. It is useful to try to determine the patient's risks for a disease before ordering diagnostic tests. Clearly an octogenarian is more at risk for dementia than a teenager. An exterminator is more at risk for organophosphate poisoning than is a homemaker. A patient with AIDS is at risk for opportunistic CNS infection and if an elicit drug user has risk for drug related changes in mental status as well.

DEMENTIA

Dementia, a loss of intellectual capacity with attendant personality change, occurs when a critical mass of cerebral neurons are lost. The etiology of Alzheimer's dementia is unknown. Pathologic brain specimens show neurofibrillary tangles and senile plaques, but brain biopsy is rarely performed for diagnostic reasons. The diagnosis is made by the history of a slowly progressive decline in memory

Table 12.26.
Laboratory Evaluation of Dementia

CBC
Chemistry profile, glucose, creatinine, electrolytes, calcium, liver functions
Thyroid-stimulating hormone
VDRL[a]
CT or MRI of brain (unless diagnosis of Alzheimer's disease is certain)[a]
Vitamin B_{12} level[a]
Erythrocyte sedimentation rate[a]
Serum drug levels (ilicit or prescription drugs)[a]
HIV testing[a]
PPD testing[a]
CSF examination[a]

Workup of dementia focuses on diagnosing treatable or curable causes. PPD, purified protein derivative.
[a] Selected patients only.

and intellectual function in an older patient who has a nonfocal neurologic examination and no likely causative underlying disease. Always confirm the history with a family member. The memory loss occurs over months to years. Acute memory loss is not likely to be Alzheimer's. Memory loss is seen early and affects recent or short term memory, sparing remote memory. A patient will often be able to recite details of childhood but will not remember what he or she ate that day or who the president is. The patient is seen as "forgetful" early on, but the memory impairment will progress such that he or she forgets how to get home from the store, to turn the stove off, or to eat.

Although researchers have identified markers for Alzheimer's disease, these are not readily available. Imaging studies show cortical atrophy and enlarged ventricles. Complete blood count, chemistry profile, VDRL, thyroid functions, and possibly vitamin B_{12} levels should be checked to look for treatable causes (Table 12.26).

Memory worsens with normal aging. The Folstein mini-mental status examination (see Chapter 7) is used to assess intellectual functioning. and can be repeated serially to gauge decline in mentation.

Dementia can be secondary to several small, lacunar strokes. These strokes are seen most often in diabetic and/or hypertensive patients. The presentation of multiinfarct dementia may be the same as Alzheimer's, but imaging studies would show infarcts.

Drugs. Many drugs can cause dementia or delirium. A "rule of thumb" is to always consider drugs in the differential diagnosis, regardless of the patient's age or socioeconomic status. Prescription drugs (Table 12.27) such as opiates, steroids, major tranquilizers, lithium, barbiturates, and digoxin can be causative. Among illicit drugs the list includes cocaine and its relatives, heroin, marijuana, phencyclidine (PEP), lysergic acid derivative (LSD), amphetamines, and glue. History of drug use obtained from the patient and companions and a high degree of suspicion are necessary to make this diagnosis. Concentrations of specific drugs can be checked in the serum or urine for confirmation.

By far the most common drug that causes change in mental status is alcohol. Alcohol can often be recognized by its characteristic smell on the breath. Blood concentrations are readily available. The inebriated patient is not likely to complain about altered mental status, but the clinician is likely to note it during the examination. Alcohol users are at high risk of head injury and intracranial bleeding. Any focal signs on neurologic examination should be evaluated by CT or MRI imaging.

Infection. Although infections of the CNS are always dangerous, the most common infection, meningoencephalitis, usually presents with headache and preserved mental status. Mental status declines if the infection progresses untreated. If a patient with severe headache, fever, and altered mental status is seen, he or she should have diagnostic lumbar puncture. Blood and CSF should be sent for culture and sensitivity. Antibiotic therapy should be instituted immediately depending on the result of the Gram stain of the CSF. The most common bacterial causes of meningitis in immunocompetent adults are *Neisseria meningitis* and *Streptococcus pneumoniae*. Besides the appearance of Gram-negative rods or Gram-positive diplococci on staining, the CSF should reveal polymorphonuclear leukocytes. The CSF in viral meningitis should show a predominance of lymphocytes and no bacteria.

Tuberculosis of the CNS can present with a change in mental status over weeks to months. Past history of tuberculosis is a risk factor, as is HIV disease. A patient who has this type of relatively rapid mental status change will often have a normal CT or MRI of the head and should have lumbar puncture. The CSF may show acid fast organisms and should be cultured; it will show white blood cells, predominantly lymphocytes.

Tertiary syphilis can cause mental status change that worsens over months to years. Serum VDRL and fluorescent treponemal antibody testing are not diagnostic of CNS infection. Although not highly specific in the serum, VDRL positivity in the CSF is a fairly specific test for CNS syphilis.

Table 12.27.
Drugs Associated with Psychomotor Impairment and Schizophrenic-Like and Manic Reactions

Psychomotor Impairment

Psychotherapeutic: antipsychotics (phenothiazine, butyrophenones), antidepressives (tricyclics, monoamine oxidase inhibitors, second-generation drugs), mood stabilizers (lithium, carbamazepine), antianxiety agents (benzodiazepines), hypnosedatives (barbiturates, nonbarbiturates)

Antihistamine, antimotion sickness: most common antihistamines are sedating; astemizole and terfenadine may be exceptions

Narcotic-analgesic: morphine, codeine, pentazocine, dextropropoxyphene

"Social": alcohol, marijuana, hallucinogens, cocaine, amphetamines

Miscellaneous: methyldopa, clonidine, indomethacine, any drug that primarily produces other psychiatric syndromes

Schizophrenic-Like Reactions

Social: phencyclidine, LSD, and others; sympathomimetics (amphetamines, phenmetrazine, diethylpropion, Khat); cannabis

Dopaminomimetic: levodopa, bromocriptine, baclofen, ketamine, bupropion

Anti-inflammatory: indomethacin, sulindac

Corticosteroid: many, rare

Cardiac: procainamide, lignocaine (lidocaine), tocainide, propranolol (also withdrawal), withdrawal-clonidine

Anticonvulsant: phenytoin, primidone, carbamazepine

Miscellaneous: fenfluramine, methysergide, disulfiram, procainamide, carbimazole, isoniazid, anabolic steroids

Manic Reactions

Dopaminomimetic: levodopa, bromocriptine, metoclopramide

Sympathomimetic: phenylephrine, theophylline, yohimbine, reserpine (withdrawal)

Antidepressant: tricyclics (also withdrawal); monoamine oxidase inhibitors (also withdrawal); second-generation-amoxapine, trazodone, fluoxetine, alprazolam, buproprion

Gastrointestinal: cimetidine

Corticosteroid: prednisolone, others

Miscellaneous: fenfluramine, antimalarials, muscle relaxants, metrizamide, carbamazepine indomethacin, AZT (azidothymidine), intravenous penicillin

From Hollister LE. Psychiatric disorders. In: Melmon KL, Morrelli HF, Hoffman BB, et al. Melmon and Morrelli's clinical pharmacology: basic principles in therapeutics. New York: McGraw-Hill, 1992:376–377.

Patients with AIDS are at risk for opportunistic CNS infections, such as toxoplasmosis and *Cryptococcus.* CSF should be examined accordingly (i.e., staining with India ink to diagnose *Cryptococcus*). The virus itself appears to infect neurons and cause an AIDS related dementia. This is, however, a diagnosis of exclusion.

Septicemia can cause change in intellect. The mentation should normalize as the underlying infection is treated. In general, if a patient's mental status change is mild and felt to be proportional to the degree of systemic infection, a CNS infection workup need not be done.

Toxins. Heavy metals and organophosphates are two toxins that can cause changes in mental status. Lead poisoning occurs in adults who work with lead, such as contractors or individuals who, during remodeling, destroy walls laden with lead-based paint. High concentrations of lead are found in the drinking water of many older houses. Other symptoms of lead poisoning include headache, peripheral neuropathy, ataxia, and abdominal pain. Anemia and elevated creatinine are found on labo-

ratory workup as well as an elevated lead level of $>10~\mu g/dl$.

Vaporized mercury is absorbed in the lungs of persons who have occupational exposure. Mercury salts (found in topical medicines) and organic mercury (found in paints, cosmetics, fungicides, and wood preservatives) are absorbed via the skin or gastrointestinal tract. The symptoms of toxicity are memory loss, insomnia, delirium, anorexia, and weight loss. Diagnosis is based on history of exposure, compatible findings on physical examination, and blood levels of $>3.5~\mu g/dl$.

Organophosphates, common in insecticides, can cause confusion, restlessness, and convulsions along with nausea, vomiting, abdominal cramps, sweating, salivation, and miosis. Diagnosis is based on history and physical examination.

Trauma/Bleeding. Head trauma is a cause of acute or subacute change in mental status. Patients with concussion or frank intracranial bleeding secondary to trauma can be confused and forgetful. A patient who has head trauma and symptoms or findings out of proportion to the apparent damage should have an imaging study to search for bleeding. A serious type of bleed, subarachnoid hemorrhage, can present as worsening confusion and headache hours or days after head trauma. Imaging studies miss a small number of subarachnoid hemorrhages. If subarachnoid hemorrhage is suspected and an imaging study shows no bleeding, lumbar puncture should be performed to look for blood in the CSF.

Patients who fall, particularly the elderly, alcoholics, and those on anticoagulant medications, are at risk for subdural hematoma. Usually associated with slower bleeding than the subarachnoid hemorrhage, symptoms of altered mentation often with headache and focal neurologic findings that occur over days to weeks warrant imaging studies. Strokes, hemorrhagic or ischemic, can cause change in mental status. Strokes are discussed in detail under "Stroke and Transient Ischemic Attack."

Psychiatric Illness. Depression and psychosis can cause changes in mental status. In adults, a past history of psychiatric illness will be the clue to a current diagnosis, as will a normal physical examination.

Cancer. Primary CNS tumors, such as astrocytoma or glioma, are uncommon causes of dementia. Lymphoma and metastatic cancers that are more common may cause symptoms secondary to increased intracranial pressure or to destruction of neurons. Past history of cancer or current unexplained weight loss may be diagnostic clues. The physical examination will often show a focal neurologic deficit. Imaging followed by biopsy of the primary tumor is indicated.

Metabolic Causes. Many diseases, if severe or poorly controlled, can cause changes in mental status. This group of commonly seen diseases accounts for a significant percentage of patients who have a loss of intellect. Pulmonary or cardiac disease or anemia lead to hypoxemia or hypotension. Inflammatory diseases such as giant cell arteritis or systemic lupus erythematosus can directly affect neurons or cause alterations in circulation or emboli. Liver and renal failure cause buildup of substances that are toxic to the CNS. Hyper- or hypothyroidism and diabetes complicated by hyper- or hypoglycemia can also change mentation. In malnutrition or alcoholism, deficits of thiamine or vitamin B_{12} can also be causative.

PRIMARY NEUROLOGIC DISEASE

Seizures can cause altered mental status that persists throughout the postictal period. Anticonvulsants can sometimes cause alterations as well. Parkinson's disease, multiple sclerosis, and Huntington's chorea are three of the many primary neurological diseases that can cause changes in mental status. The diagnoses are usually detected based on abnormal neurologic examination and abnormal imaging studies. Parkinson's disease is discussed under "Parkinson's Disease."

Hydrocephalus can cause symptoms from increased intracranial pressure. In older patients with normal pressure hydrocephalus (NPH), the symptoms do not appear to be pressure related. The diagnosis of NPH is based on dementia, gait abnormality, incontinence, and finding hydrocephalus without evidence of increased pressure on imaging.

DELIRIUM

Delirium is an acute disorder of mentation characterized by agitation, extreme excitability, and hallucinations. The patient has abnormal attention and is confused. Delirium is common in hospitalized patients, drug users, and persons with psychiatric illness but can be caused by infections, toxins, trauma, metabolic causes, or primary neurologic disease. Drugs also cause delirium (Table 12.28). Complete blood count and chemistry profile should be checked. Drug levels, blood gas analysis, cultures, and thyroid studies should be sent if indicated. Lumbar puncture and EEG may be helpful in selected patients.

Management

The clinician looks for treatable or curable causes of dementia and delirium. The workup for delirium and dementia of recent onset is performed in the inpatient setting. The management recommendations in this section will focus on chronically dementing processes that do not require hospitalization.

DEMENTIA

There is no cure for Alzheimer's or multiinfarct dementia. Pharmacologic therapy with tetrahydroaminoacridine, an acetylcholinesterase inhibitor, may slow the progress of symptoms for a short time. Multiinfarct dementia can be stabilized by treatment of the underlying disease.

Demented patients need supervision. Often this is provided by a family member, but private caregivers can be hired or the patient may have access to a day care facility. The patient and family may participate in Alzheimer's support groups for psy-

Table 12.28.
Drugs Associated with Delirium

Anticholinergic: atropine family (atropine, hyoscine (scopolamine)); antihistamines (diphenhydramine, dimenhydrinante); mydriatics (cyclopentolate)
Antidepressant: tricyclics, e.g., imipramine, amitriptyline
Antiparkinsonian: conventional, e.g., trihexiphenidyl, benztropine; newer, e.g., levodopa, amantadine, bromocriptine
Gastrointestinal: cimetidine, ranitidine, famotidine (especially in elderly); metoclopramide
Social: withdrawal from alcohol, sedative-hypnotic; use of hallucinogens, cannabis, nitrous oxide
Narcotic: dextropropoxphene, pentazocine
Cardiac: antiarrhythmics, e.g., disopyramide, lignocaine (lidocaine), procainamide; positive inotropics, e.g., digitalis preparations; antihypertensives, e.g., clonidine, propranolol; others, e.g., theophylline, captopril, calcium-channel blockers
Anti-infective: penicillins, cephalosporins

From Hollister LE. Psychiatric disorders. In: Melmon KL, Morrelli HF, Hoffman BB, et al. Melmon and Morrelli's clinical pharmacology: basic principles in therapeutics. New York: McGraw-Hill, 1992: 376.

chological and social aid. Legal intervention, such as assignment of power of attorney, should be anticipated early by the clinician so that the patient is involved in decision making.

Patients may have reversal of sleep patterns that can be trying for the family. Judicious use of benzodiazepines, such as temazepam, may help establish a normal sleep cycle. Agitation may be treated by low dose haloperidol. Any drug, but especially drugs with CNS effects, can alter mental status. Be aware of the risk of instituting any new drug therapy to a patient with altered mental status.

Drugs. Management of drug induced change in mental status is to discontinue the offending drug. If the drug is necessary, decrease the dose to the lowest effective amount. Users of illicit drugs should be referred to drug treatment programs. Of particular note it is reasonable to give alcoholics 100 mg thiamine parenterally to treat Wernicke-Korsakoff's syndrome, (confusion, ataxia, and ophthalmoplegia from thiamine deficiency).

Infections. The patient should be hospitalized unless a mild aseptic or viral meningitis has been diagnosed. In that case, pain management is

necessary. The provider must be assured that the patient will not be alone for a few days until there is an improvement in symptoms. Treatment of bacterial meningitis should begin immediately in the office if medications are available. Penicillin G, 4 million units intravenously, is reasonable initial coverage for *S. pneumoniae* and *N. meningitis.*

Toxins. Treatment of poisoning is usually done in the hospital. Lead is treated with chelating agents: ethylenediamine tetraacetic acid (EDTA) or penicillamine. Mercury is treated with dimercaprol or penicillamine: emesis is induced if the toxin was ingested. For organophosphates, atropine and/or 2 pralidoxime can be used, but neither is effective for CNS symptoms. Consult a poison control center for specific recommendations.

Psychiatric Illness. Depression often can be treated in the outpatient setting. Please read Chapter 23 for details.

Other Causes. The other causes detailed under "Differential Diagnosis" will likely be treated in the hospital by treating the underlying illness or with the guidance of a specialist.

ILLUSTRATIVE CASES WITH SELF-ASSESSMENT QUESTIONS AND ANSWERS

Case 1

J. G. is a 47-year-old gardener with confusion, sweating, and vomiting that his wife noted today after work. He has no significant medical illnesses. Family history is positive for dementia in his grandmother.

QUESTION: *What diagnosis is least likely?*

a. Head trauma
b. Alzheimer's dementia
c. Organophosphate poisoning
d. Bacterial meningitis

ANSWER: *b. Alzheimer's dementia is characterized by a gradual onset of symptoms. The other three diagnoses cause symptoms quickly.*

Case 2

H. G. is a 73-year-old retired banker. Her daughter is concerned about her forgetfulness. Over the past several months the police have had to bring her home because she gets lost while walking in the neighborhood. The family has noted that she has gotten "less focused" over the past few years. Physical examination is normal.

QUESTION: *What tests are indicated?*

a. Complete blood count
b. Chemistry panel
c. VDRL
d. Thyroid functions

ANSWER: *All of these tests are indicated. A more thorough history is also indicated, particularly regarding her past medical history, family history, and use of alcohol, drugs, or medications.*

PARKINSON'S DISEASE

In the ambulatory care setting, the most common movement disorder treated is Parkinson's disease. First described in 1817 by James Parkinson, Parkinson's disease (idiopathic parkinsonism or paralysis agitans) is a neurodegenerative disease usually presenting in mid to late adulthood and characterized by tremor at rest, rigidity, and bradykinesia and frequently associated with depression and cognitive impairment. Before the era of drug therapy, Parkinson's disease led to severe disability for 80% of patients within 10 years. Although the pathophysiology of the disease remains poorly understood, the introduction of levodopa provided symptomatic relief for many Parkinson's patients, and recent refinements of treatment that may slow disease progression promise to improve long term quality of life for these patients.

Pathophysiologic Correlation

Parkinson's disease is a neurodegenerative condition affecting the nigrostriatal dopaminergic pathway. Characteristically there is a loss of the melanin-containing nerve cells in the substantia nigra in the brainstem, which terminate in the caudate nucleus and putamen, although other nuclei may be affected as well. In addition, neuronal loss is accompanied by intracytoplasmic hyalin inclusions that were initially described in 1913 by F. H. Lewy, called Lewy bodies. Degeneration of these cells results in depletion of the neurotransmitter dopamine in the caudate and putamen and an imbalance between dopaminergic and cholinergic influences.

Use of the drug MPTP (an analog of meperidine) by intravenous drug users has provided much information on the pathophysiology of Parkinson's disease. These patients develop the clinical manifestations of Parkinson's disease because the drug selectively destroys the neurons of the substantia nigra through effects on monoamine oxidase B and inhibition of the mitochondrial respiratory pathway. Pathologically there is no formation of Lewy bodies with the use of MPTP, and only the cells of the substantia nigra are affected.

Clinical and Laboratory Evaluation

Parkinson's disease is diagnosed on the basis of history and physical examination. Laboratory testing is useful only to eliminate other diagnoses.

HISTORY

The relevant history in a patient with a parkinsonian disorder should include the age of onset (typically two-thirds of patients have the onset of Parkinson's disease after the age of 50) and address the duration and progression of symptoms. Typically patients will describe a slowly progressive course over months to years, initially noting only muscle stiffness and aching. The possibility of exposure to toxins should be addressed, including illicit drugs and medications. History of an infectious source such as encephalitis and disturbances of consciousness or of ocular function should be obtained. A family history of dementing illnesses or of hereditary disorders must also be considered.

Nonmotor manifestations occur frequently in Parkinson's disease, although diagnosis cannot be made until motor findings are present. Sensory disturbances such as pain, numbness, or tingling occur commonly. Decreased sense of smell occurs in greater than 75% of patients, and depression may also develop. Autonomic findings such as urinary problems, impotence, and constipation are also common. Dementia has also been associated with Parkinson's disease.

PHYSICAL EXAMINATION

Although in its fully developed form Parkinson's disease does not provide a clinical diagnostic dilemma, in its initial stages its presentation may be quite variable. In the early stages, resting tremor may be the only finding, although it is estimated to be absent in 20% of patients and may initially be present asymmetrically. Tremor is usually most apparent in the hands ("pill-rolling tremor") but may occur in the lips and tongue, neck muscles, legs, and trunk. Patients may present with aching pain in the back and limbs and may typically exhibit hypokinesia and muscle stiffness. Cogwheel rigidity is most often noted in the elbows and wrists on physical exam. The classic "masked facies" of Parkinson's disease is in part due to decreased blinking of the eyes and immobility of the facial musculature. All movements are slowed. The stooped posture and loss of movements of postural adjustment contribute to the classical festinating gait, in which the patient's initially slow, shuffling gait progresses with increasing rapidity. Turns are usually accomplished slowly and en bloc. The neurological examination, in addition to the findings above, reveals normal deep tendon reflexes and may reveal dementia in up to one-third of all patients. An extensive neurological examination should be performed, because the findings of cerebellar, corticospinal, or lower motor neuron dysfunction may indicate alternative diagnoses.

LABORATORY EVALUATION

There is no blood marker for Parkinson's disease. The workup may include an imaging study (CT scan or MRI) to evaluate possible mass lesions or infarction that may mimic the Parkinsonian state.

Differential Diagnosis

The diagnosis of a patient with the classic triad of tremor, rigidity, and bradykinesia is usually quite clear; however, it may become more complicated if any of these features is not present. The criteria for diagnosis of Parkinson's disease include at least 1 year of two of these signs, as well as responsiveness to levodopa treatment for at least 1 year (note, however, that other parkinsonian syndromes may show a response to levodopa as well). New criteria for clinically possible, probable, and definite idiopathic Parkinson's disease are listed in Table 12.29. Although the disorders listed in Table 12.30 may all present with parkinsonian symptoms, a careful history and physical examination can eliminate most of these disorders. A history of exposure to toxins or drugs listed in Table 12.30 is sufficient to exclude the diagnosis of Parkinson's disease, and often removal of the offending agent will reverse

the disease symptoms. Physical examination revealing oculomotor findings, focal upper or lower motor neuron dysfunction, or cerebellar disease would point to other multisystem degenerative diseases or cerebral infarctions, which may mimic Parkinson's disease.

Management

Once the diagnosis of Parkinson's disease is established, the decision of whether to begin pharmacotherapy must be made. The goals of treatment are to enhance the quality of life, not necessarily to return to the patient's previous level of function. Symptomatic therapy alone has been shown to improve quality of life and morbidity, but there is evidence that treatment with levodopa over long periods results in fluctuations in motor response and dyskinesias. Although traditionally treatment has focused on alleviating symptoms, there have been recent studies which suggest that monoamine oxidase B inhibition may be involved in halting disease progression, and research on the role of oxidative injury to the evolution of Parkinson's disease is continuing. These studies have provided a new direction in which pharmacotherapy, by delaying disease progression, may improve and extend a patient's functional life. The classes of medications offering symptomatic relief are the anticholinergic agents and amantadine, levodopa, and the dopamine agonists.

ANTICHOLINERGIC AGENTS AND AMANTADINE

The anticholinergic drugs (trihexyphenidyl and benztropine) are antagonists at the muscarinic receptors in the striatum. They act to restore the balance between dopaminergic and acetylcholinergic influences. Usually they provide some relief of tremor but not of rigidity or bradykinesia. Their use is limited by side effects (dry mouth, urinary retention, constipation, difficulties with ocular accommodation, impairment of memory, and confusion). Amantadine, initially used as an antiviral agent, is similar to the anticholinergic agents but also improves the bradykinesia and rigidity. The side effects are also similar to the anticholinergics but also include pedal edema and livedo reticularis.

LEVODOPA

Levodopa is the most effective agent available for the symptomatic treatment of Parkinson's disease. As a precursor of dopamine, it is decarboxylated

Table 12.29.
Criteria for Clinically Possible, Probable, and Definite Idiopathic Parkinsonism

Clinically Possible	Clinically Probable	Clinically Definite
	Either	**Either**
Any one of	Any two of	Any three of
Rest tremor	Rest tremor	Rest tremor
Rigidity	Rigidity	Rigidity
Bradykinesia	Bradykinesia	Bradykinesia
	Impaired postural reflexes	Impaired postural reflexes
	Or	**Or**
	One of the first three displaying asymmetry	Any two of the above four with one of the first three displaying asymmetry

From Calne DB. Initiating treatment for idiopathic parkinsonism. Neurology 1994;44(suppl 6):16–22.

throughout the body and can act on all dopamine receptors. The decarboxylation of levodopa to dopamine outside the blood-brain barrier results in side effects (most notably nausea and vomiting) that are reduced with the concomitant administration of a peripheral decarboxylase inhibitor (carbidopa or benserazide). In the United States, combinations of levodopa and carbidopa are marketed as Sinemet (levodopa-benserazide combinations are available outside the United States as Madopar). The available combinations of levodopa-carbidopa are 100 mg levodopa/25 mg carbidopa (Sinemet 100/25) or 250 mg levodopa/25 mg carbidopa (Sinemet 250/25) for those patients requiring larger doses of levodopa. Because carbidopa and benserazide are noncompetitive inhibitors of the decarboxylase, there is no need to increase the dosing of these agents. Motor fluctuations occurring after prolonged intermittent treatment with levodopa eventually affect most Parkinson's disease patients. Newer controlled-release preparations (such as Sinemet CR), which provide increased steady state concentrations of levodopa with fewer fluctuations of plasma concentration, may serve to alleviate some dyskinesia associated with long term levodopa use. Note that controlled release preparations have approximately 70% of the bioavailability of the standard preparations and therefore require an increase in dosage.

The appropriate time for initiation of levodopa treatment is determined by clinical judgment. Because there is a decline in its effectiveness in many patients with prolonged use, therapy traditionally has been delayed; although it now appears that beginning therapy early in the symptomatic disease may decrease mortality. Levodopa is particularly effective for bradykinesia and rigidity but has significant side effects. Initially, nausea and hypoten-

sion are the most common problems. With prolonged treatment, motor fluctuations (including early morning akinesia, "wearing off" phenomena at the end of the dosing interval, and erratic "on-off" oscillations with dystonia and sensory, autonomic, and psychiatric symptoms) can occur, making the therapy for advanced Parkinson's disease extremely challenging.

SYNTHETIC DOPAMINE AGONISTS

These agents act directly on the dopamine receptors. Bromocriptine and pergolide are available throughout the world, and lisuride is available in Europe. They are efficacious in reduction of symptoms, although patients usually do not respond as well to the dopamine agonists as they do to levodopa. The plasma half-lives of these agents are all greater than that of levodopa; 5 mg bromocriptine, 0.5 mg pergolide, 0.5 mg lisuride, and 100 mg levodopa combined with a decarboxylase inhibitor are all approximately equivalent dosages.

NEUROPROTECTIVE TREATMENT

The oxidative injury, or free-radical hypothesis of the pathogenesis of Parkinson's disease, has led to the use of selegiline (deprenyl), a monoamine oxidase B inhibitor, as an antiparkinsonian agent. Although selegiline has some symptomatic action, it may serve a neuroprotective function by decreasing the rate of neuronal death and delaying the progression of Parkinson's disease. The most common side effect is insomnia, but hallucinations and confusion may occur as well. When used concurrently with levodopa, it can increase both the therapeutic effects as well as the side effects of levodopa.

Table 12.30.
Some Causes of Parkinsonism

Idiopathic parkinsonism (Parkinson's disease)

Infectious and postinfectious
Postencephalitis lethargica (von Economo's disease)
Other viral encephalitides

Toxins
Manganese
Carbon monoxide
Carbon disulfide
Cyanide
Methanol
MPTP and its analogs

Pharmacologic agents
Neuroleptics (blockers of postsynaptic dopamine receptors)
Reserpine, tetrabenazine (presynaptic dopamine depletors)
Alpha-methyl-paratyrosine (inhibitor of dopamine synthesis)
Alpha-methyldopa
Lithium
Aminodarone
Phenelzine
Meperidine
Amphotericin B
Cephaloridine
Diltiazem
Ethanol
Procaine

Multisystem atrophies
Striatonigral degeneration
Progressive supranuclear palsy
Olivopontine cerebellar atrophy
Shy-Drager syndrome

Other degenerative diseases
Primary pallidal atrophy of Hunt
Idiopathic dystonia-parkinsonism
Corticobasal ganglionic degeneration
Hemiatrophy-hemiparkinsonism
PD-ALS-dementia complex of the Western Pacific
"Senile" parkinsonism
Alzheimer's and Pick's diseases
Creutzfeldt-Jacob disease
Gerstmann-Straussler-Scheinker disease
Rett syndrome
Neuroacanthocytosis syndrome

Other CNS disorders
Hydrocephalus (normal pressure, high pressure)
Multiple cerebral infarction (including lacunar states, Binswanger's disease, amyloid angiopathy)
Brain tumors, arteriovenous malformations
Posttraumatic encephalopathy
Electrical injury
Subdural hematoma

Table 12.30. (*continued*)

Metabolic conditions
Disorders of calcium metabolism (parathyroid hormone disorders) with or without basal ganglia calcifications
Chronic hepatocerebral degeneration

Hereditary disorders
Wilson's disease
Huntington's disease (rigid variant)
Hallervorden-Spatz disease
Spinocerebellarnigral degeneration
Joseph (Azorean) disease
Parkinsonism with depression and alveolar hypoventilation

From Koller WC. How accurately can Parkinson's disease be diagnosed? Neurology 1992;42(suppl):6–16.

PHARMACOLOGIC TREATMENT

There are many schools of thought regarding the appropriate treatment for the different stages of Parkinson's disease. The initial use of selegiline is advocated by some neurologists for the possible protective action it may provide. It remains unclear whether the use of levodopa in the early stages of Parkinson's disease should be withheld because of the potential for future mobility and dyskinesia problems with long term use. Because of this, some neurologists choose to use synthetic agonists initially, even though they are less efficacious, to postpone the use of levodopa. Others delay the use of any pharmacologic therapy until the later stages of the disease.

Once the decision to begin levodopa-carbidopa therapy has been made, low dose controlled-release preparations should be used four times daily after meals. With progression of the disease, the dosage of levodopa should be increased to maintain the patient's functional status. Addition of an artificial dopamine agonist may take place when the levodopa dose approaches approximately 600 mg to decrease side effects of higher doses. Management of patients with progressive disease or adverse reactions is much more complicated and may require alterations in the dosage of the offending medication or the addition of other agents.

Side effects of treatment with levodopa and the dopamine agonists initially include hypotension, which may be treated by taking the medication after meals and by increasing salt and fluid ingestion, and nausea. In refractory cases of hypotension, the use of mineralocorticoids (such as fludrocortisone) or alpha-adrenergic agonists (such as midodrine) may be necessary. Long term complications such as dyskinesias, mobility fluctuations, and psychiatric disturbances are more difficult to manage. Motor disturbances may require decreasing the levodopa dose while increasing the dose of the dopamine agonist. Psychiatric manifestations may begin as nightmares and progress to psychosis and may be improved by decreasing the dose of the synthetic dopamine agonist or by stopping the nighttime dose. Neuroleptics should not be used because they produce exacerbations of the underlying disease.

NONPHARMACOLOGIC THERAPY

Most importantly the patient and the patient's family must have an ongoing therapeutic relationship with the health care provider. They must be well educated about the disease and the need for open communication and must understand the need for frequent alterations of medications to manage the changing symptoms of the disease. Physical therapy may also provide improved quality of life for the patient, as can psychologic intervention.

CURRENT RESEARCH

Recent studies into the transplantation of fetal tissue as a potential treatment for Parkinson's disease have been encouraging. Other surgical procedures are also being explored, as are new approaches to alternative routes of medication administration. Additionally newer pharmacologic agents are being evaluated that may offer protective effects, longer half-lives, or improved management of dyskinesias.

ILLUSTRATIVE CASES WITH SELF-ASSESSMENT QUESTIONS AND ANSWERS

Case 1

A 68-year-old white man comes to your office for a routine physical examination. He has a history of diet-controlled diabetes mellitus and of hypertension and has been using reserpine with good control of his blood pressure. His wife has noticed that the patient has been "slowing down" and has been having some difficulty rising from a seated position for the past 7–8 months. The patient describes only some aches and pains in his shoulders and back each morning that have not limited his activities, and he is otherwise feeling well. You notice a resting tremor of his arms while he is speaking.

QUESTION: *Can the diagnosis of Parkinson's disease be made in this patient?*

ANSWER: *Although the symptoms are suggestive of Parkinson's disease, this diagnosis cannot be made at this time for several reasons. The duration of symptoms in this patient is <1 year, the duration necessary for diagnosis. Other diagnoses must be eliminated, most notably the possibility of reserpine-induced parkinsonian symptoms. Once these criteria are met, a diagnosis of probable Parkinson's disease may be made.*

QUESTION: *How would you manage this patient?*

ANSWER: *Of greatest importance will be the ongoing support he will receive from his family and primary care provider. Once alternative diagnoses have been eliminated (initially by withdrawing the drug) and the diagnosis of probable Parkinson's disease has been made, the education of the patient and his family should be the first treatment modality employed. The efficacy of pharmacotherapy at this time can be argued. Traditional treatment for symptomatic relief would not be involved unless the patient had worsening symptoms and a deterioration of status, because there is no conclusive evidence that treatment is beneficial before symptoms start to affect the patient's life.*

REFERENCES

Headache

1. Kroenke K, Mandgelsdorff D. Common symptoms in ambulatory care: incidence, evaluation, therapy, and outcome. Am J Med 1989;86:262–266.
2. Rapoport AM. Update on severe headache with a migraine focus. Neurology 1994;44(suppl 3):S5.
3. Osterhaus JT, Gutterman DL, Plachetka JR. Health care resources and lost labor costs of migraine headache in the United States. PharmacoEconomics 1992;2:67–76.
4. Dhopesh V, Anwar P, Herring C, et al. A retrospective assessment of emergency department patients with complaints of headache. Headache 1979;19:37–42.

5. Leicht MJ. Nontraumatic headache in the emergency department. Ann Emerg Med 1980;9:404–409.
6. Stang PE, Osterhaus JY. Impact of migraine in the United States: data from the National Health Interview Survey. Headache 1993;33:29–35.
7. Kawamura J, Meyer JS. Headaches due to cerebrovascular disease. Med Clin North Am 1991;75:617–630.
8. Silberstein SD, Lipton RB. Overview of diagnosis and treatment of migraine. Neurology 1994; 44(suppl 7):S6–S16.
9. Ferrari MD. Treatment of migraine attacks with sumatriptan. N Engl J Med 1991;325:316–321.
10. Mathew NT. Cluster headache. Neurology 1992: 42(suppl 2):22–31.

Stroke and Transient Ischemic Attack

11. Biller J. Medical management of acute cerebral ischemia. Neurol Clin 1992;10:63–85.
12. Hazzard W, Andres R, Bierman E, Blass J. Principles of geriatric medicine and gerontology. New York: McGraw-Hill, 1990:926.
13. Collins R, Peto R, MacMahon S, et al. Blood pressure, stroke and coronary heart disease. Short-term reductions in blood pressure, overview of randomised drug trials in their epidemiological contest. Lancet 1990;335:827–838.
14. Shinton R, Beevers G. Meta-analysis of relation between cigarette smoking and stroke. Br Med J 1989; 298:789–794.
15. Putman SF, Adams HP Jr. Usefulness of heparin in initial management of patients with recent transient ischemic attacks. Arch Neurol 1985;42:960–962.
16. Guberman A. An introduction to clinical neurology. Boston: Little, Brown, 1994:394.
17. Scheinberg P. Transient ischemic attacks: an update. J Neurol Sci 1991;101:133–140.
18. Gent M, Blakely JA, Easton JD, Ellis DJ, et al. The Canadian American Ticlopidine Study (CATS) in thromboembolic stroke. Lancet:1989;i:1215–1220.
19. Hass WK, Easton JD, Adams HP Jr, et al. A randomized trial comparing ticlopidine hydrochloride with aspirin for the prevention of stroke in high-risk patients. N Engl J Med 1989;321:501–507.
20. Feinberg WM, Albers GW, Barnett HJM, et al. Guidelines for the management of transient ischemic attacks. Stroke 1994;25:1320–1335.
21. European Atrial Fibrillation Trial Study Group. Secondary prevention in non-rheumatic atrial fibrillation after transient ischaemic attack or minor stroke. Lancet 1993;342:1255–1262.
22. Lorish, T. Stroke rehabilitation. Clin Geriatric Med 1993;94:705–715.
23. North American Symptomatic Carotid Endarterectomy Trial Collaborators. Beneficial effects of carotid endarterectomy in symptomatic patients with high grade carotid stenosis. N Engl J Med 1991;325: 445–453.
24. European Carotid Surgery Trialists' Collaborative Group. MRC European Carotid Surgery Trial: interim results for symptomatic patients with severe (70–99%) or with mild (29%) carotid stenosis. Lancet 1991;337:1235–1243.

SUGGESTED READINGS

Headache

Cady RK, Fox AW, eds. Treating the headache patient. New York: Dekker, 1995.

Olesen J, Tfelt-Hansen P, Welch KMA, eds. The headaches. New York: Raven, 1993.

Raskin NH. Headache, 2nd ed. New York: Churchill Livingstone, 1988.

Saper JR. Clinician's manual on headache. Princeton NJ: Science Press, 1995.

Tollison CD, Kunkel RS, eds. Headache: diagnosis and treatment. Baltimore: Williams & Wilkins, 1993.

Dizziness

Reilly, Brendan M. Practical strategies in outpatient medicine, 2nd edition. Philadelphia: Saunders, 1991:162–236.

Weiner WJ, Goetz CG, eds. Neurology for the non-neurologist. 2nd ed. Philadelphia: Lippincott, 1989:174–186.

Stroke and Transient Ischemic Attack

Biller J. Medical management of acute cerebral ischemia. Neurol Clin 1992;10:63–85.

Feinberg WM, Albers GW, Barnett HJM, et al. Guidelines for the management of transient ischemic attacks. Stroke 1994;25:1320–1335.

Scheinberg P. Transient ischemic attacks: an update. J Neurol Sci 1991;101:133–140.

Seizures

Adams RD, Victor M. Epilepsy and other seizure disorders. In: Adams RD, Victor M, eds. Principles of neurology. New York: McGraw-Hill, 1993:273–299.

Hauser WA. Seizure disorders: the changes with age. Epilepsia 1992;33(suppl 4):S6–S14.

Tettenborn B, Kramer G. Total patient care in epilepsy. Epilepsia 1992;33(suppl 1):S28–S32.

Wilder BJ. The treatment of epilepsy: an overview of clinical practices. Neurol 1995;45(suppl 2):S7–S11.

Abnormal Mental Status: Dementia and Delirium

Barry PB. Medical evaluation of the demented patient. Med Clin North Am 1994;78:779–784.

Ciarfield AM. Reversible dementias: do they reverse? Ann Intern Med 1988;109:476–486.

Parkinson's Disease

Koller WC. How accurately can Parkinson's disease be diagnosed? Neurology 1992;42(suppl):6–16.

Calne DB. Initiating treatment for idiopathic parkinsonism. Neurology 1994;44(suppl 6):19–22.

Poewe WH. Clinical aspects of motor fluctuations in Parkinson's disease. Neurology 1994;44(suppl 6): 6–9.

Calne DB. Treatment of Parkinson's disease. N Engl J Med 1993;329:1021–1027.

chapter 13

CARDIOLOGY
Cynthia M. Chong, Paul Marantz, and Lisa M. Rucker

CHEST PAIN

Chest pain can be the presenting symptom of abnormality of any organ in or around the thorax. Diseases of the heart, stomach and esophagus, lungs, breast, bones and joints, skin, and nerves feature chest pain as a prominent symptom. The diagnostic evaluation and management of the common causes of chest pain will be reviewed in this section.

Pathophysiologic Correlation

A review of the innervation of the organs of the chest can be useful to the clinician trying to uncover the cause of a patient's pain. At the location of each spinal nerve is a dorsal ganglion. Two types of nerve cells emanate from these ganglia (Fig. 13.1). The visceral nerve cells convey pain impulses from the organs along autonomic nerves. This type of pain is perceived as vague and poorly localized, although it may be severe. The clinician must carefully question the patient to locate its source and define associated symptoms to secure the diagnosis.

Somatic nerve cells convey pain impulses along spinal nerves. Somatic cells supply the skin and organs positioned close to the skin as well as the parietal pleura and parietal peritoneum. Pain transmitted by these nerve cells is perceived as distinct (sharp, stabbing) and localized.

Because visceral and somatic nerve cells share dorsal root ganglia, pain transmitted by the visceral route may be referred to the related somatic locus (dermatome). An example is the patient who experiences left arm pain during a myocardial infarction.

Clinical and Laboratory Evaluation

A detailed history will uncover the diagnosis of the chest pain in most cases. The physical examination is confirmatory in some cases and useless in others. Laboratory evaluation is used to confirm the diagnosis or to determine the severity or extent of disease once the diagnosis is made.

HISTORY

Decisions about further testing and treatment will often be based solely on the patient's story. Questions regarding the quality of the pain aid in determining which organ system is involved. Questions about the time course of the pain are essential. When the patient first felt the pain and how often the pain has recurred help to define the chronicity of the pain. A patient who describes dull, gripping substernal pain intermittently for the past 30 years is less likely to have angina than one who has had the same pain for the last 30 days. The duration of the pain is particularly helpful in distinguishing angina from nonangina. Pain that lasts 1 second or more than 30 minutes is not likely to be anginal in nature. A pain that is worsening over time is likely to be more serious than one that is stable.

Location of the pain can be useful diagnostically. If the patient can point to the site of the pain with one finger and state "This is the spot that hurts," the pain is likely to be somatic. Additionally, pain tends to manifest near its source. Pain from esophagitis will be in the midline; pain from a pleural infarction involving the right middle lobe will be in the right chest. Pain of myocardial ischemia classically radiates from the substernal area to the left shoulder, jaw, or ear.

The circumstances of the pain episode can be elicited by asking, what makes the pain begin? what makes it stop? is the pain reproducible? Patients frequently note that they have some control over their pain episodes. A patient who feels burning substernal pain when napping postprandially and takes antacids for relief probably has a gastrointestinal disorder. The presence of associated symptoms

163

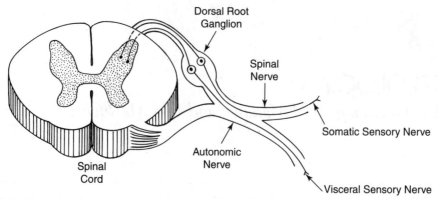

Figure 13.1. Visceral and somatic pain pathways. Note that cell bodies of visceral and somatic sensory nerve cells reside in the dorsal root ganglion. Visceral pain may be transmitted in the ganglion (or referred) to the dermatome supplied by the somatic nerve.

can help to secure the diagnosis. Sharp chest pain in the patient with productive cough and high fever indicates pneumonia. Chest pain that is squeezing in nature, is accompanied by dyspnea and sweating, and occurs with exercise in a 50-year-old man suggests the diagnosis of angina.

The patient's past medical history, family history, and social and drug histories are important to obtain. A history of a parent's death from myocardial infarction is a risk factor for heart disease in the offspring. A past history of esophagitis, ulcer, myocardial infarction, or pulmonary embolus increases a patient's risk for recurrent disease. Smokers are at risk for ulcer, myocardial infarction, and lung disease; drinkers are at risk for esophagitis and ulcer.

PHYSICAL EXAMINATION

The physical examination can confirm the diagnosis of some conditions, such as pneumonia and costochondritis. The examination is generally not helpful in the diagnosis of angina and esophagitis. Given the many potential causes of chest pain the clinician must pay particular attention to the following eight areas when evaluating the patient with chest pain.

General Appearance. Note the appearance of the patient. Is he or she uncomfortable? Is the patient sweaty? Can the patient give the history without having to stop because of pain or dyspnea? Patients who have costochondral pain usually appear well: patients who have cardiac or pleural pain appeal ill.

Vital Signs. Note pulse (rate and regularity) and respiration (rate and effort). Fever is often present with infection or with myocardial infarction. Blood pressure can be high in patients with severe pain or preexisting hypertension. The pressure will be low in extremely ill patients.

Neck Examination. Examine the veins of the neck. Distension of the veins is seen in heart failure. The carotid artery is the most reliable place to check a pulse and to determine the volume of the pulse. A bounding pulse is found in aortic insufficiency or infection. The clinician should check the thyroid gland next. Hyperthyroidism can cause angina to worsen.

Pulmonary Examination. The examiner should inspect, palpate, percuss, and then auscultate the chest. Hyperresonance on percussion may alert the clinician to the presence of pneumothorax. Increased fremitus, dullness on percussion, and inspiratory rales suggest consolidating pneumonia. Palpation of the chest wall may reproduce musculoskeletal pain.

Cardiac Examination. The cardiac examination begins without the use of the stethoscope. The clinician palpates the precordium and locates the point of maximal cardiac impulse. A normal point is found at the fifth intercostal space at the midclavicular line. A diffuse or displaced point is abnormal and is often found in cardiac disease. The clinician listens carefully to identify the rhythms of S1 and S2 and then concentrates on listening for gallops, clicks, murmurs, and other sounds. A gallop is a low pitched sound that occurs during rapid atrial filling (S3) or after atrial contraction (S4). Gallops

(Fig. 13.2) indicate noncompliance of the ventricle and are often found in patients with hypertension or congestive heart failure.

A murmur is a sound produced by turbulent blood flow in the heart. If a murmur is present, it is imperative to know if it is heard during systole or diastole or both and if it radiates. The intensity and pitch must be noted, as well as the duration of the murmur.

Examination of the peripheral pulses can reveal useful information. Absent or diminished pulses in the extremities are found in patients with widespread atherosclerosis. New absence of leg pulses, particularly when arm pulses are normal, suggests aortic dissection.

Abdominal Examination. The epigastrium should be palpated for masses and tenderness. Some patients equate the epigastrium with the chest because it is so high in the abdomen. The rest of the abdomen should then be palpated, because disease of other intraabdominal organs can cause chest pain.

Back and Local Neurological Examination. The back should be palpated for tenderness. Range of motion and sensation then are evaluated. The skin is briefly viewed.

Mental Status. The mood of the patient should be noted. The level of concern about his or her pain can be helpful diagnostically; few patients with pleuritic chest pain are unworried about their pain, whereas many patients with mild esophagitis mention their pain as an afterthought.

LABORATORY EVALUATION

Few tests are helpful in the initial diagnosis of chest pain. In general, the test results confirm a diagnosis or define the extent or severity of disease. If heart disease is suspected, order an electrocardiogram (ECG). A normal ECG does not eliminate heart disease, but it gives information about electrical conduction, arrhythmias, chamber hypertrophies, and past infarction. Order a chest x-ray if pulmonary or skeletal abnormality is suspected. If the patient has obvious dyspnea, evaluate his or her oxygenation by ordering an arterial blood gas or oximetry.

Several specialized tests warrant review in this section because of the frequency of their use in the further evaluation of chest pain. Upper gastrointestinal endoscopy is ordered to confirm the diagnosis of esophagitis, gastritis, peptic ulcer disease, and tumor of the stomach or esophagus. Endoscopic biopsies are useful for defining whether a lesion is infectious, inflammatory, or neoplastic.

The most widely utilized cardiac test in the evaluation of angina is the exercise stress test (EST). The patient, while monitored by ECG, walks on a treadmill at a speed and incline that increases gradually. He or she exercises until 85% of the predicted maximum heart rate ($220 - \text{age} \times 85\%$) has been reached, he or she has angina, or there is another indication to stop, such as ST elevation on the ECG or severe leg cramps. The EST has several indications:

To evaluate exercise tolerance in a stable patient;
To determine prognosis after myocardial infarction;
To determine severity of disease;
To aid in diagnosis of angina.

The test is not indicated for patients with unstable angina, those with symptomatic or "tight" aortic stenosis, or those who have abnormal baseline ECGs for whom interpretation of exercise induced ECG changes would be unreliable. The patient must also be physically able to exercise. Exercise parameters associated with an adverse prognosis and/or multivessel coronary artery disease are listed in Table 13.1.

Two important studies defined the prognostic value of the stress test. The Coronary Artery Surgery Study (1) showed that patients who could not

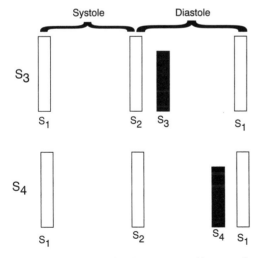

Figure 13.2. Timing of gallops in normal heart cycle. An S_4 gallop of atrial filling is heard just before S_1. An S_3 gallop of ventricular filling is heard just after S_2 (From Willms JL, Schneiderman H, Algranati PS. Physical diagnosis: bedside evaluation of diagnosis and function. Baltimore: Williams & Wilkins, 1994:292).

Table 13.1.

Exercise Parameters Associated with an Adverse Prognosis and/or Multivessel Coronary Artery Disease

Duration of symptom-limiting exercise (<6METS)

Failure to increase systolic blood pressure to ≥120 mmHg or sustain decrease ≥10 mmHg or below rest levels during progressive exercise

ST segment depression of ≥2 mm, downsloping ST segment, starting at <6 METS, involving ≥5 leads persisting ≥5 minutes to recovery

Exercise-induced ST segment elevation (aortic valve replacement excluded)

Angina pectoris during exercise

Reproducible sustained (>30 sec) or symptomatic ventricular tachycardia

From Chaitman B. Exercise stress testing. In: Braunwald E, ed. Heart disease: a textbook of cardiovascular medicine, 4th ed. Philadelphia: Saunders, 1992:168.

exercise past Bruce Stage 1 (usually the first 3 minutes of exercise) and developed ST depression of +1 mm had a much greater 1-year mortality rate (5% vs. 1%) than patients able to exercise to Stage III without ST depression. Before hospital discharge, postmyocardial infarction patients able to exercise >4 METS (a measure of oxygen consumption) had a much lower rate of new myocardial infarction or death at 1 year than those who could not—2% vs. 18% (2).

The EST is useful diagnostically and is cost effective when there is a reasonable pretest probability of coronary arterial disease but when the symptoms are not entirely consistent with typical angina. The test is not likely to be useful diagnostically or to be cost effective when the pretest probability of angina is low because the chance of a false-positive result becomes too great. The test also is not useful diagnostically when the pretest probability of angina is high because the chance of a false-negative result becomes too great.

In a nuclear medicine stress test, thallium, a potassium analog, is injected after a standard EST. Cardiac scans after exercise and at rest are compared. The appearance of a cold defect at stress that disappears at rest is suggestive of ischemia. A cold defect at stress and rest may be a scar. This test is indicated in patients who have abnormal baseline ECGs or suspected false-positive or false-negative ESTs.

In an adenosine or Persantine thallium stress test, the injection of these potent coronary dilators will aid in defining a relative cold spot on thallium scan. This test is useful for patients who cannot walk sufficiently well to do an EST. It is the most expensive noninvasive cardiac test discussed here.

Echocardiography is a safe and noninvasive test that is used to give information about cardiac valves, chamber size, wall thickness, and ventricular function. Stress echocardiography can be used to evaluate dynamic ventricular wall dysfunction.

Cardiac catheterization with angiography is the gold standard for evaluation of coronary arterial disease. Complications of this invasive test, such as arrhythmia and dye-induced renal failure, are serious but uncommon. This test is done as part of a preprocedure (preangioplasty or precoronary artery bypass) evaluation and has limited use in the diagnosis of angina. Angiography is indicated for patients with unstable angina who fail medical therapy or who have noninvasive stress tests that are strongly positive for ischemia. Catheterization and arteriography are helpful in that they identify several subgroups of patients with angina (Table 13.2) and can thus be used to dictate therapy.

Table 13.2.

Patients with Angina: Subgroups Identified by Cardiac Catheterization and Angiography

Patients with left main coronary artery disease—the most life-threatening form of the disease—in whom urgent surgery is indicated

Patients with multivessel obstructive disease without a clear "culprit" lesion and who are not suitable for angioplasty

Patients with left ventricular dysfunction and multivessel disease who should have revascularization to improve long-term survival

A small number of patients (about 10% of all patients with unstable angina) with no demonstrable coronary arterial disease in whom the prognosis appears to be excellent with medical management and in whom no further surgical consideration is necessary; in some of these patients, coronary spasm is responsible for the angina

Patients with single-vessel or double-vessel disease with a discrete narrow proximal lesion (e.g., "culprit" lesion) amenable to percutaneous transluminal angioplasty

Patients with diffuse distal coronary artery disease unsuitable for angioplasty or bypass grafting

From Rutherford JD, Braunwald E. Chronic ischemic heart disease. In: Braunwald E, ed. Heart disease: a textbook of cardiovascular medicine, 4th ed. Philadelphia: Saunders, 1992:1339.

Table 13.3.
Differential Diagnosis of Chest Pain

Musculoskeletal	Psychological
Muscle strain	Depression
Costochondritis	Anxiety
Arthritis	Hyperventilation
Rib fracture	Cardiac neurosis
Cardiac	Malingering
Angina, stable and un-	**Gastrointestinal**
stable	Esophageal spasm
Myocardial infarction	Esophagitis
Angina, vasospastic	Gastritis
Pericarditis	Peptic ulcer
Mitral valve prolapse	Cholecystitis
Aortic dissection	Cancer
Cocaine ingestion	
Aortic stenosis	**Breast**
	Cyclical pain
Pulmonary	Infection
Bronchitis	Tumor
Asthma	
Pneumonia	**Neurologic**
Pleurisy	Nerve root compression
Pulmonary embolus	Shingles
Pneumothorax	

Differential Diagnosis

Chest pain can be caused by myriad underlying conditions. It is essential that the clinician make the correct diagnosis of chest pain for reasons of patient safety, psychological well-being, and cost. The differential diagnoses are listed by system in Table 13.3. Only the most common or most serious diagnoses will be reviewed here.

MUSCULOSKELETAL CHEST PAIN

The typical history for musculoskeletal chest pain is trauma or overuse of the chest muscles. Patients often have well defined localized areas of tenderness that when palpated reproduce their pain. Some chest wall maneuvers (Fig. 13.3) may help to elicit pain. Common diagnoses are muscle strain, costochondritis, arthritis, and rib fracture. Musculoskeletal pain is extremely common among young people with chest pain.

CARDIAC CHEST PAIN

Cardiac pain is highly prevalent in older adults. The clinician must differentiate angina from other cardiac causes of pain. Cardiac causes of chest pain can be deadly, as in myocardial infarction, or merely bothersome, as in mitral valve prolapse.

Angina Pectoris. In coronary arterial disease there is a fixed obstruction in any or all of the three arteries supplying the myocardium. The fixed obstruction, sometimes accompanied by dynamic obstruction caused by arterial spasm, impairs the blood flow to the myocardium. In angina pectoris this blood flow is adequate when the heart is at rest but is insufficient for the further demands of stressors such as tachycardia, increased force of ventricular contraction, and elevated arterial resistance. When blood flow is inadequate, the myocardium becomes ischemic, triggering the neurochemical responses that the patient experiences as pain.

Ischemic cardiac pain is highly prevalent and its course deadly. In the Framingham study, the most common manifestation of coronary arterial disease in men was myocardial infarction (45%) and in women was angina (32%) (3). The diagnosis of angina is made by history. There are atypical presentations of angina. Patients may complain only of jaw pain or dyspnea, or they may have no symptoms whatsoever. Although angina pectoris can present in various ways, it is helpful to have an understanding of typical angina. Answers to our series of questions from patients with and without typical angina pectoris are given in Table 13.4. If the patient's pain is consistent with angina, the physician must consider the patient's risk factors for coronary arterial disease. The risk factors are male gender, advanced age, positive family history, hypertension, diabetes mellitus, hypercholesterolemia, and smoking.

Mortality rate and coronary heart disease mortality rate was assessed over 6 years in 361,662 men in the MRFIT trial (4). Both total mortality and cardiac mortality increased as serum cholesterol or diastolic blood pressure increased (Fig. 13.4). The Coronary Artery Surgery Study showed an increased 5-year mortality rate of 22% in smokers versus 15% in nonsmokers. Most of this increased mortality was due to sudden death or myocardial infarction (5).

Unstable Angina/Myocardial Infarction. A patient who presents with anginal-type symptoms that are more severe or more frequent than usual, that occur at rest, and that last longer than usual (e.g., >15 minutes) may have unstable angina or myocardial infarction. Such a patient should be hospitalized for further evaluation.

Aortic Valve Stenosis. Chest pain is one of the three cardinal symptoms of aortic stenosis. The two other symptoms are palpitation and syncope. The pain is typical for angina and occurs when

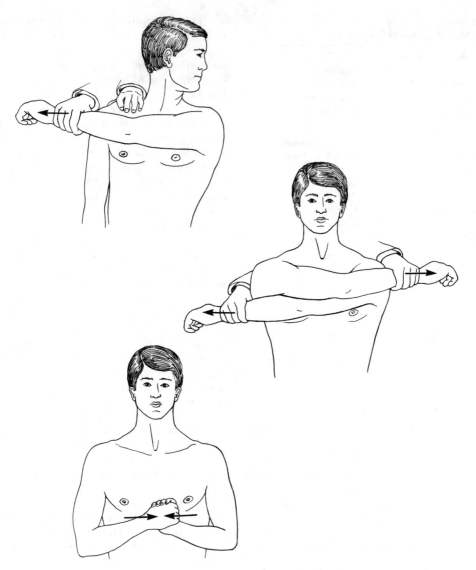

Figure 13.3. These maneuvers are used to reproduce chest wall pain (adapted from Reilly BM. Practical strategies in outpatient medicine, 2nd ed. Philadelphia: Saunders, 1991:456).

blood flow into the muscular wall of the left ventricle is impaired because of the extremely high pressure the ventricle must produce to pump blood past the "tight" aortic valve. Diagnosis is made by cardiac auscultation (hearing a systolic ejection murmur that radiates to the carotid artery) and noting delayed and low-volume pulses. Echocardiography confirms the diagnosis.

Vasospastic Angina. Anginal type chest pain that occurs almost exclusively at rest, is usually not precipitated by exertion or emotional stress, and is

associated with ST segment elevation on the ECG is known as Prinzmetal's or vasospastic angina. This type of angina is caused by arterial spasm. Definitive diagnosis can be made by injection of ergonovine during cardiac angiography, which reproduces ECG changes and symptoms.

Pericarditis. Pericarditis is typically a viral disease that presents as a respirophasic burning chest pain in a young person. The patient may have a friction rub—a scratchy sounding rub that may be heard in systole, diastole, or both. The pain

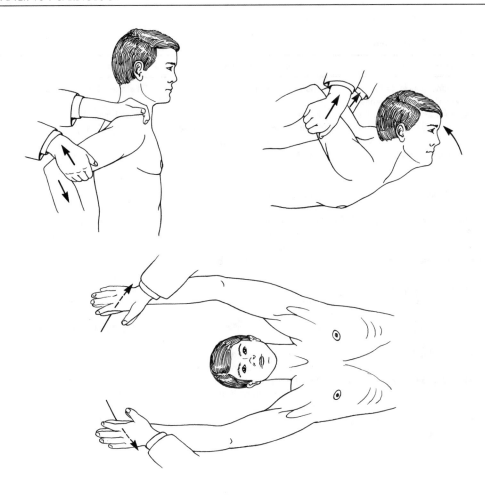

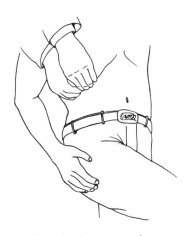

Figure 13.3.—*continued*

Table 13.4.
Medical History of Chest Pain

Historical Questions	Responses Typical of Angina	Responses Not Typical of Angina
What is the time course of the pain? When did it first begin?	"The pain began weeks ago."	"It started 5 years ago."
How long does each episode last?	"It lasts 5 minutes at a time. I didn't come in sooner because I thought it would go away."	"It lasts from 1 second to constantly all day."
How often does it happen?	"I go to the store three or four times a week. That is when I get the pain."	"I have it every couple of months."
How does it feel?	"It feels like pressure, like I can't catch my breath."	"It is like a knife."
Where does it hurt? Does it radiate?	"It aches around the breast bone (or neck, jaw, ear) and then the left shoulder."	"It moves down my leg."
Are there associated symptoms?	"I get sweaty, short of breath, and nauseous."	"I get it after I burp—my mouth tastes like vomit."
What makes a pain episode start? Is it reproducible?	"It happens every time I walk three blocks to the store."	"Sometimes nothing does it. I got it while watching TV today. I was in a 10-mile Walkathon yesterday and felt fine. I get it when I bend over."
What makes it stop?	"I have to sit down and rest. It goes away in a few minutes."	"I take a walk and I feel better."
Is it worsening in severity or frequency?	"No, it happens as often now and feels the same as it did a month ago."	"It is bad, but it was worse 2 years ago."
What are the family, past medical, social, and drug histories?	"My father died when he was 50 from a heart attack."	"I am young and lift weights at the gym from time to time."

tends to be positional. The ECG may show tachycardia, PR segment depression, and/or widespread ST elevations. The patient may develop pleuritic pain caused by inflammation of the parietal pleura.

Mitral Valve Prolapse. Mitral valve prolapse may be seen in up to one-third of young women. Symptomatic patients present with a syndrome of anxiety, atypical chest pain, and palpitations. A mitral click and/or a mitral regurgitant murmur is heard on auscultation.

Aortic Dissection. Aortic dissection is a tear in the lining of the aorta that allows blood to leak into the arterial wall or beyond. It is not a common outpatient problem, but one that the physician must never misdiagnose. The chest pain of dissection is often described as tearing in nature and may be located anteriorly or posteriorly. The patient may have hypertension, a new diastolic murmur, and arterial pulses that are diminished distal to the dissection. CXR may show widening of the mediastinum. If aortic dissection is strongly sus-

pected, further diagnostic testing (e.g., CT scan, transesophageal echocardiography, angiography) must be performed immediately.

Cocaine Ingestion. Cocaine ingestion can cause anginal-type chest pain. The clinician must always be on the lookout for substance abuse and its effects. Consider cocaine ingestion if the patient is nervous, tachycardiac, and has dilated pupils.

PULMONARY CHEST PAIN

The chest pain of pulmonary disease varies depending on the site of involvement. In general, processes involving the pleura will be localized, exquisitely painful, and respirophasic. Processes involving the parenchyma will be less well localized and less painful. In patients with cough or signs and symptoms of infection, the diagnoses of bronchitis, asthma, pneumonia, and pleurisy must be considered. A patient with dyspnea and with risk factors should be evaluated for pulmonary embolus. A young healthy man with abrupt onset of chest pain

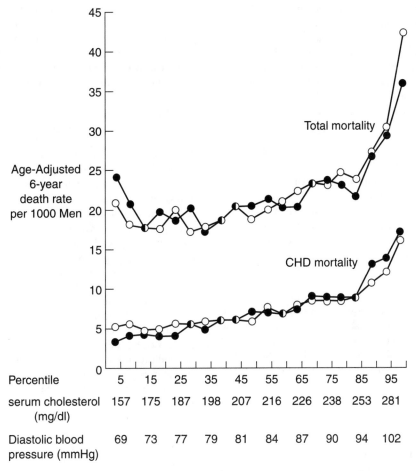

Figure 13.4.   Age adjusted cardiac mortality and total mortality rate in 361,662 men according to serum cholesterol (*solid circles*) or DBP (*open circles*) percentiles. CHD, coronary heart disease (modified from Martin MJ, et al. Serum cholesterol, blood pressure, and mortality: implications from a cohort of 361,662 men. Lancet 1986;2:935).

and dyspnea may be suffering from spontaneous pneumothorax. Please refer to chapter 15 for more details.

PSYCHOLOGICAL CHEST PAIN

Patients who have depression or significant anxiety may focus on mild chest pains and interpret these pains as severe. A patient may hyperventilate and experience chest pain. Some patients have cardiac neurosis, and others are malingerers.

GASTROINTESTINAL CHEST PAIN

Under normal circumstances, the esophagus is the only gastrointestinal organ in the chest. Esophageal spasm and esophagitis each can cause chest pain.

The pain can be similar to angina but tends to be related to eating and drinking and not to exercise.

Esophageal Spasm.   Esophageal spasm causes a gripping pain that may be associated with dyspnea. The pain is precipitated by eating, often by food or drink that is extremely hot or cold. The pain is midline and corresponds to the portion of the esophagus that is in spasm.

Diagnosing spasm is difficult, often relying on the history and the absence of abnormality on cardiac testing and endoscopy.

Esophagitis.   Acid reflux from the stomach via an incompetent lower esophageal sphincter will damage the epithelial lining of the esophagus. The resultant esophagitis will manifest as a burning or boring pain, usually in the epigastrium or lower chest. Symptoms worsen under conditions that increase intraabdominal pressure (wearing tight waisted clothing or eating a large meal), decrease the tone of the sphincter muscle (caffeine), or directly irritate the exposed esophageal mucosa or interfere with its ability to heal (alcohol). Esophagitis is confirmed by endoscopy. Endoscopic biopsies can be sent for pathologic or microbiologic testing if a tumor or infection is suspected.

REFERRED CHEST PAIN

Although the only intrathoracic gastrointestinal organ is the esophagus, several organs of the gastrointestinal tract cause chest pain when inflamed. Among these are the stomach (ulcers, tumors), gallbladder, pancreas, and liver. Please refer to chapter 16 for details.

Management

After accurately diagnosing the cause of chest pain, the clinician then must devise a plan to treat the pain. In this section management of angina will be covered in detail. Musculoskeletal pain and pulmonary pain are covered in other chapters of this book.

MUSCULOSKELETAL CHEST PAIN

If the specific cause is elicited, the physician should advise the patient to refrain from that activity. Pain relief can often be accomplished by the use of local heat and acetaminophen or nonsteroidal anti-inflammatory agents. The pain of a simple rib fracture is managed the same way.

CARDIAC CHEST PAIN

Angina. There are four aspects to the management of angina. The first is to modify the cardiac risk factors—help the patient to stop smoking and control hypercholesterolemia, diabetes, and hypertension. Risk factor improvement is extremely cost effective. A doctor is a teacher and must educate his or her patient! Local hospital and national organizations such as the American Cancer Society also offer information and group sessions to assist interested patients.

A simple and effective first-step therapy is to determine how far the patient can walk and then to devise an exercise prescription. Results of EST are useful for determining a patient's exercise capacity. The exercise prescription should explicitly state how far and how often the patient should walk. Results of EST are useful for determining a patient's exercise capacity. An example of an exercise prescription is "walk two blocks 5 days this week—add an additional block each week." The patient should stretch muscles for 5 minutes before and after exercise. Tell the patient to stop exercising if chest pain or severe fatigue is felt. At the very least, encourage the patient to move around as much as possible.

The second aspect of management is to give psychological support. Angina pectoris can be frightening. For many individuals the diagnosis is their first confrontation with their own mortality.

The third aspect of management is to medicate. There are three classes of antianginal drugs: nitrates, beta-blockers, and calcium channel blockers.

Nitrates. Nitrates increase myocardial perfusion by dilating coronary arteries. They also dilate veins and peripheral arteries, decreasing preload and afterload, respectively, and thereby reducing myocardial oxygen demand. The nitrates can be given by many routes and are available in short-acting and long-acting preparations. If a patient has angina infrequently, sublingual nitroglycerin 0.4 mg can be taken as needed. This same dosage can be used for the patient who takes daily antianginal medication but has breakthrough angina. Sublingual nitroglycerin works quickly, usually relieving pain in minutes and can be repeated every 5 minutes up to a total of three doses. If anginal pain is not relieved after three doses of sublingual nitroglycerin, the patient should be instructed to go to the hospital because a myocardial infarction might be occurring.

Longer acting nitrate preparations are available in oral, transdermal, and sublingual forms. Dosage regimens vary, depending on the specific brand. Isosorbide dinitrate is usually prescribed in dosages of 5–30 mg two to four times daily orally or sublingually. A typical dosage of isosorbide mononitrate is 20 mg orally twice daily. Transdermal ointments have faster onset than patches but are messier to use. A usual dosage of nitroglycerin ointment is 1/2" to 2" daily. Easy to use nitroglycerin patches are dosed at 0.1–0.6 mg/hour daily. If any nitroglycerin preparation is given for 24 hours, without a drug free period of 10 hours, tolerance (loss of effectiveness) may occur (6). Therefore nitrates are usually administered during the daytime and are discontinued at night. Adverse effects include headache and hypotension.

Beta-Blockers. Stimulation of beta-receptors increases heart rate and strengthens the force of ventricular muscle contraction. Drugs that competitively block the beta-adrenergic receptors in the heart act by decreasing the heart rate and the force of ventricular muscle contraction, thereby decreasing the heart's metabolic demand. Usual doses of beta-blockers for the control of angina are

- Propranolol—80–320 mg total two to four times daily or once daily in extended release formulation;
- Metoprolol—50–400 mg total twice daily;
- Atenolol—50–100 mg once daily.

Propranolol has been shown to reduce mortality of patients after myocardial infarction. Compared with placebo, 1-year mortality was reduced 39%, and 2-year mortality was reduced 26% in the beta-blocker heart attack trial (7). Other beta-blockers have shown favorable reductions in mortality in the peri-infarction period.

Beta receptors are found in many sites other than the heart. In the lung, beta$_2$ stimulation causes dilation of airways. Blockage of beta$_2$ receptors in the airways can lead to symptomatic bronchospasm and asthma. At low doses, beta$_1$ selective blockers (e.g., metoprolol and atenolol) do not impair forced expiratory volume as much as nonselective beta-blockers (e.g., propranolol).

Beta$_2$ stimulation causes arteriolar dilation. With beta-blockade, arteriolar resistance increases, but this effect is brief. Nevertheless beta-blockers should be used carefully in patients with severe peripheral arterial disease. Because beta-blockers compete for binding sites with sympathetic hormones, beta-blockers should be avoided if sympathetic effect is essential. Some patients with dilated cardiomyopathy rely on sympathetic stimulation to maintain their cardiac output. In addition, in hypoglycemia sympathetic stimulation not only leads to glycogenolysis and increased blood glucose but is responsible for the symptoms of tachycardia, sweating, and nervousness that the patient may feel. For these reasons, beta-blockers should be avoided in tightly controlled diabetics. Beta-blockers also tend to decrease high density lipoprotein cholesterol and increase serum triglycerides.

As a class, beta-blockers are excellent antihypertensive agents. They are used to treat some supraventricular tachycardias and are useful in migraine prophylaxis. Because of the risk of sudden uncontested adrenergic effect, these drugs should not be discontinued suddenly. Their use should be tapered off over several days.

Calcium Channel Blockers. Calcium channels are in all muscles—smooth, cardiac, and striated. There are different types of calcium channels, but their overall function is to allow calcium flux across the cell membrane, triggering muscle contraction. The calcium channel blockers prevent or weaken muscle contraction in the arteries, thereby causing arterial dilation in both peripheral and cardiac systems. Of the three oldest drugs in this class, nifedipine is the most potent dilator. Verapamil and diltiazem have the added advantage of slowing sinoatrial and atrioventricular (AV) node conduction. Nifedipine does not affect AV conduction. Typical antianginal doses of the three drugs are listed here:

- Nifedipine 30–90 mg total dose daily given twice or once daily in extended release formulation;
- Diltiazem 90–270 mg total dose daily given twice or once daily in extended release formulation;
- Verapamil 120–360 mg total dose daily given twice or once daily in extended release formulation.

Calcium blockers do not alter cholesterol levels and are well tolerated. All three are effective antihypertensive agents. Bothersome side effects include constipation with verapamil and peripheral edema with nifedipine.

The choice of medication depends on the patient's concomitant conditions and frequency of symptoms. In general, opt for the fewest medications possible. If a patient has angina infrequently, drugs may not need to be taken daily. Sublingual nitroglycerin, taken as needed, may be the best treatment. A patient who is hypertensive and who had a myocardial infarction 6 months ago should be treated with a beta-blocker unless otherwise contraindicated. If a single drug is ineffective, combinations of drugs may help to maximize antianginal effects. See Table 13.5 for a listing of suggested drugs for treatment of angina in patients with concomitant conditions.

The daily use of aspirin is becoming popular as a preventative for myocardial infarction. Although it is efficacious in unstable angina and myocardial infarction, it is not considered an antianginal drug. In the Physician's Health Study, a study of long term prophylactic use of aspirin by physicians, evaluation of a subset of doctors with stable angina showed that aspirin takers had fewer myocardial infarctions but more strokes than predicted (8).

The fourth aspect to the management of angina is to refer for angioplasty or coronary artery bypass grafting when symptoms are not controlled by medication or when diagnostic/prognostic testing is consistent with serious disease. The CASS study showed that for patients with angina or recent myocardial infarction, 10-year survival was not significantly different in medical versus surgical groups—69 versus 66%. However, in patients with ejection fractions of 35–50%, survival rates favored surgical treatment 79 versus 61% (9). CASS registry studies showed that of surgically treated patients, those with decreased ventricular function and severe angina who underwent three-vessel bypass grafting benefitted the most (10).

Other Cardiac Chest Pain. Patients with unstable angina/myocardial infarction or aortic dissection should be hospitalized immediately. Patients with vasospastic angina should receive intensive therapy with nitrates or calcium channel blockers for control of vasospasm. Patients with aortic stenosis can be treated with drugs that decrease the force of ventricular contraction. They should be referred to a cardiologist if symptoms worsen or if the valve area is <0.75 cm².

The stable pericarditis patient without arrhythmia can be followed closely as an outpatient. Nonsteroidal anti-inflammatory agents are helpful for control of inflammation. For mitral valve prolapse, treatment may be supportive only or may include pharmacologic therapy to suppress symptomatic atrial arrhythmias. The data are not conclusive regarding the need for subacute bacterial endocarditis prophylaxis before surgical procedures.

PULMONARY CHEST PAIN

The physician should treat the underlying cause, as detailed in Chapter 15.

PSYCHOLOGICAL CHEST PAIN

After assessing mental status, the physician may reassure the patient, attempt to treat the underlying problem, or refer the patient to a mental health specialist. Please refer to chapter 23 for details.

GASTROINTESTINAL CHEST PAIN

As the diagnostic methods for esophageal diseases are different from other chest diseases, so are the treatments. For mild symptoms, antacid therapy may be sufficient. More specific therapy is included when antacids fail to control symptoms.

Esophageal Spasm. Avoidance of precipitating factors is sufficient treatment for some patients. Others will respond to nitrates or antacids. Reassurance that the pain is not due to heart attack can be helpful.

Esophagitis. For reflux esophagitis, first employ nonpharmacological therapy such as elevating

Table 13.5.
Suggested Drugs for Treatment of Angina in Patients with Concomitant Conditions

High blood pressure	Beta-blockers, calcium channel blockers
Recent myocardial infarction	Beta-blockers
Peripheral arterial disease	Calcium channel blockers, nitrates
Elderly	Calcium channel blockers, nitrates
Hyperlipidemia	Calcium channel blockers, nitrates
PVCs	Beta-blockers
Supraventricular tachycardia	Beta-blockers, verapamil/diltiazem
Hypertropic myopathy	Beta-blockers, verapamil/diltiazem
Dilated myopathy	Nifedipine, nitrates
Asthma	Calcium channel blockers, nitrates
Impotence	Calcium channel blockers, nitrates
Diabetes	Calcium channel blockers, nitrates
Peripheral edema	Beta-blockers, verapamil/diltiazem
Anxiety	Beta-blockers
Tremor	Beta-blockers
Depression	Calcium channel blockers, nitrates
Migraine	Beta-blockers, verapamil
Chronic constipation	Beta-blockers, diltiazem/nifedipine, nitrates

Note these drugs are listed by class, alphabetically, and not in order of preference.

the head of the bed on bed blocks; wearing loose-waisted clothing; avoiding cigarettes, alcohol, chocolate, and coffee; losing weight; eating small meals; and not eating or drinking before bedtime. If symptoms persist, the physician can prescribe half strength antacids as needed, histamine (H_2) receptor antagonists (cimetidine 300 mg four times daily or ranitidine 150 mg twice daily), metoclopramide 10 mg four times daily, or cisapride 10 mg four times daily to promote quick transit through the gastrointestinal tract. Omeprazole, a drug that may suppress gastric acid production better than the histamine receptor blockers, can be prescribed at a dose of 20 mg daily for 4–8 weeks. If the esophagitis is infectious, specific antibiotic therapy should be instituted.

ILLUSTRATIVE CASES WITH SELF-ASSESSMENT QUESTIONS AND ANSWERS

Case 1

G.P. is a 54-year-old man who works as a school custodian. He has had intermittent chest pain for 2 months. The pain is vague in nature, aching, and associated with dyspnea and sweating. He gets it every time he mows the lawn or climbs two flights of stairs. The pain lasts 5–7 minutes, but he can sit and rest for a few minutes and feel ready to continue.

QUESTION: *What is the most likely diagnoses?*

a. Psychogenic pain
b. Typical angina
c. Peptic ulcer disease
d. Costochondritis

ANSWER: b. *The description, duration, associated symptoms, reproducibility, and relieving factors are all consistent with angina.*

QUESTION: *What diagnostic test is indicated?*

a. EST
b. Echocardiagram
c. Catheterization
d. None of these

ANSWER: d. *None of these are indicated for diagnosis, although they may be considered for prognosis or to determine therapy. An ECG is indicated.*

Case 2

W.P. is a 36-year-old secretary who has had chest pain. It hurts over her upper left chest and is more painful if she rubs it. She has noted that the pain is worse when she does heavy lifting at work or when she babysits her 11-month-old niece.

QUESTION: What is your diagnosis?

a. Musculoskeletal pain
b. Angina

c. Esophageal spasm
d. Mitral valve prolapse

ANSWER: a. *The pain has the description and localization of chest wall pain. Because she is a young woman, she is less likely to have angina.*

Case 3

S.F. is a 57-year-old professional housekeeper who has had 7 months of left parasternal chest pain. The pain is dull and takes her breath away. It occurs two to three times daily when she is doing heavy housework and never occurs at rest. She can walk three blocks without symptoms. The pain is relieved by resting a few minutes or by belching. She has a 17-year history of type II diabetes mellitus and is 8 years postmenopausal. She has peripheral venous disease and 2+ ankle edema. Her ECG is normal. Her current medications include NPH insulin 45 units subcutaneously daily and ibuprofen as needed for aches and pains. Based on this brief history, an EST is obtained. It shows 2-mm ST segment depressions after 6 minutes of exercise. She develops her usual symptoms.

QUESTION: *What treatment would you recommend?*

a. Nitroglycerin 0.4 mg as needed
b. Propranolol 40 mg by mouth four times daily
c. Nifedipine 10 mg by mouth twice daily
d. Diltiazem 30 mg by mouth four times daily

ANSWER: d. *She has symptoms two to three times daily so should be medicated on a regular basis. Propranolol is not the first choice in diabetics. Nifedipine may lower her blood pressure and cause peripheral edema. Diltiazem extended release has the advantage of easy compliance.*

ARRHYTHMIAS

Pathophysiologic Correlation

All myocardial cells can initiate or conduct an electrical impulse. The normal electrical conduction of

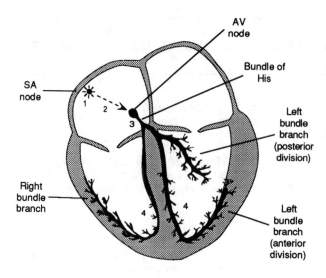

Figure 13.5. Electrical conduction of the heart. Normal electrical impulse begins at the sinoatrial node and travels across the atria to the AV node and down the bundle of His. Impulse then progresses down the left and right bundles and ultimately proceeds to the Purkinje fibers. When an electrical impulse originates at the AV node (above *dotted line*), QRS will be narrow. When the impulse originates distally, QRS complex will be wide (from Lilly LS. Pathophysiology of heart disease. Philadelphia: Lea & Febiger, 1993:61).

the heart commences at the sinoatrial node in the atrium and then radiates via the atria to the AV node. From the AV node, the electrical impulse passes to the ventricle via the bundle of His and finally via the Purkinje fibers (Fig. 13.5). Normal conduction on ECG is illustrated in Figure 13.6. Conditions such as ischemia, hypoxemia, lung disease, electrolyte abnormalities, fibrosis, infection, or inflammation that alter the normal electrochemical properties of myocardial cells can cause abnormal conduction and arrhythmia. Certain medications, drugs or alcohol, fatigue, and stress can also cause arrhythmia.

Arrhythmias may be divided into three broad types according to the nature of the underlying conduction disorder. The electrical impulse may follow the normal pathway but at an abnormal rate; it may originate from an ectopic site, or it may be blocked somewhere along the pathway. If conduction is blocked, the impulse will either extinguish or proceed more slowly along the usual pathway, sometimes depolarizing retrogradely and causing a fast, short-circuited kind of conduction called reentry (Fig. 13.7).

In normal sinus rhythm, there is an orderly de-

polarization of atria and ventricles leading to efficient propulsion of blood. In arrhythmia, symptoms often are related to the beating sensation created by the abnormal rate or rhythm. More worrisome and dangerous symptoms are due to hypo-

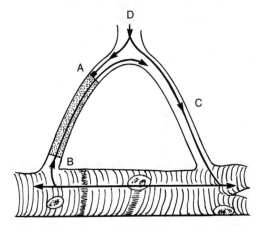

Figure 13.7. Reentry. This model depicts a branch of the conduction system (D) dividing into two terminal branches conducting an electrical impulse to cardiac muscle. Normal conduction proceeds down the right terminal branch at C. Antegrade conduction down the left branch is blocked at A because of a depressed segment of tissue (*shaded area*). Conduction proceeds from the right branch, through muscle and retrogradely to the left branch at B. Retrograde impulse may be blocked, but if the depressed tissue is not in its refractory state, the impulse may be propagated up the left branch and back down the right branch over and over again (adapted from Schmitt FO, Erlanger J. Directional differences in the conduction of the impulse through heart muscle and their possible relation to extra systolic and fibrillary contractions. Am J Physiol 1928;87:341).

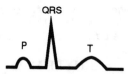

Figure 13.6. Normal ECG. P-wave corresponds to atrial depolarization. QRS complex corresponds to ventricular depolarization. T-wave corresponds to ventricular repolarization (from Lilly LS. Pathophysiology of heart disease. Philadelphia: Lea & Febiger, 1993:61–62).

tension and hypoperfusion. Hypoperfusion may be caused by tachyarrhythmias, which decrease stroke volume and bradyarrhythmias, which decrease heart rate.

Clinical and Laboratory Evaluation

The history and physical examination may be diagnostic, particularly if the arrhythmia is present on examination. The patient's symptoms are of great importance, because the symptom rather than the type of arrhythmia may dictate further evaluation and therapy. Laboratory testing is ordered for all patients who have worrisome symptoms.

HISTORY

The patient should be asked to describe his or her symptoms, including chest pain, respiratory difficulty, syncope, or presyncope. The onset and resolution and the rate and regularity of the palpitations must be determined. Information about heart or lung disease, medications, and the use of drugs, alcohol, and tobacco must be obtained.

PHYSICAL EXAMINATION

The examination should focus on the pulse, auscultation of the heart, and examination of the chest. The carotid pulses are the most reliable pulses to check. A bounding, regular pulse can be noted in patients with sinus tachycardia or bradycardia or paroxysmal supraventricular tachycardia. An early pulse beat that occurs in the midst of an otherwise normal pulse is the hallmark of atrial or ventricular premature contractions. An irregular pulse is found in atrial fibrillation.

The chest examination is reviewed elsewhere in this book. Examine carefully for signs of ischemia, failure, valvular disease, and pulmonary disease. Arrhythmias are more likely to be found if these conditions exist.

LABORATORY EVALUATION

An ECG and rhythm strip should be ordered first. The ECG will be needed to identify the arrhythmia and also to screen for other signs of pathology that can lead to arrhythmia, such as ST elevation in acute infarction or tall peaked T waves in hyperkalemia. If arrhythmia is not documented by ECG, a 24-hour Holter monitor can be ordered. General laboratory evaluation of arrhythmia should include electrolytes (to check potassium, magnesium, calcium, acid/base status), complete blood count, and thyroid functions. Drug levels such as cocaine or quinidine should be sent if indicated. Examination

of arterial blood gases should be considered if hypoxemia or acid/base abnormalities are suspected.

Differential Diagnosis

This section describes the arrhythmias commonly diagnosed in the outpatient setting. Illustrative ECGs are included for most diagnoses.

ATRIAL ARRHYTHMIAS

Atrial arrhythmias have one common ECG finding: the QRS complexes look normal because the pathway for ventricular depolarization is intact. Any condition listed under "Pathophysiologic Correlation" can cause atrial arrhythmia. In addition, caffeine, smoking, and anxiety may trigger atrial arrhythmia.

Sinus Tachycardia and Sinus Bradycardia. Sinus rhythm at a rate of >100 beats/minute, known as sinus tachycardia, is usually caused by systemic factors such as pain, anxiety, hypoxemia, hypovolemia, or anemia (Fig. 13.8).

Sinus rhythm at a rate of <60 beats per minute, known as sinus bradycardia, is often caused by drugs, such as beta-blockers or verapamil. It may also be seen in well-conditioned athletes (Fig. 13.9).

Atrial Premature Contractions. Atrial premature contractions are early ectopic beats originating at an atrial site other than the sinoatrial node. The associated P-wave on the ECG appears different from the normal P-wave. Atrial premature contractions can be present in healthy patients (Fig. 13.10).

Paroxysmal Supraventricular Tachycardia. Paroxysmal supraventricular tachycardia is characterized by sudden onset of a rapid, regular tachycardia followed by an equally sudden cessation of the tachycardia. This reentry arrhythmia is initiated by an atrial premature contraction.

Atrial Fibrillation. Atrial fibrillation is characterized by chaotic, rapid (up to 400 beats/minute) atrial depolarization. It is commonly seen in patients who have mitral stenosis, cardiomyopathy, or thyrotoxicosis. Because of disorganized depolarization of the atrium and the AV node, the atrial myocardium does not contract, and the ventricular rhythm is irregular. The ECG is devoid of P-waves, and the QRS complexes are irregularly timed (Fig. 13.11).

Bradycardia-Tachycardia Syndrome. This arrhythmia is characterized by recurrent atrial tachyarrhythmias in patients with underlying bradycardia. The patient may have symptoms of hypoperfusion from the fast and/or slow compo-

Tachycardia (sinus)

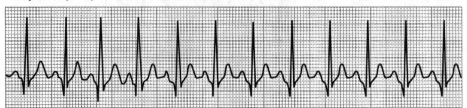

Figure 13.8. Sinus tachycardia. A P-wave precedes each narrow QRS complex. Rate is 140 beats/minute. Each 5-mm box equals 0.2 seconds (From Willis MC. Medical terminology: the language of health care. Baltimore: Williams & Wilkins, 1996:292).

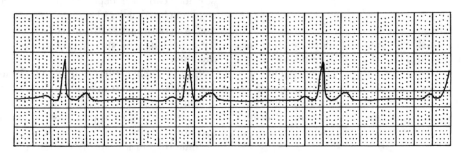

Figure 13.9. Sinus bradycardia. P-QRS-T is normal in configuration, but the rate is only 56 beats/minute.

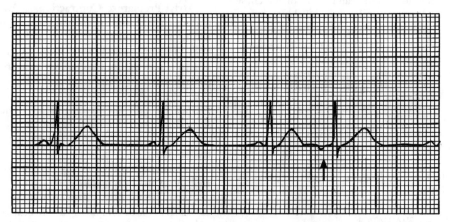

Figure 13.10. Atrial premature contraction. Note that this early beat is preceded by an abnormal P-wave (*arrow*) (From Berstein D, Shelov SP. Pediatrics. Baltimore: Williams & Wilkins, 1996:358).

nent. Fibrosis of the conduction system is often found on pathologic examination.

AV NODAL ARRHYTHMIA

The type of AV block most commonly seen in the outpatient setting is the first degree AV block. The ECG demonstrates a prolonged P-R interval

(>0.2–0.24 msec.) This can be caused by disease or drugs (Fig. 13.12).

VENTRICULAR ARRHYTHMIAS

Ventricular arrhythmias are characterized by QRS complexes that appear bizarre because the ventricle does not depolarize via the usual pathway. Because

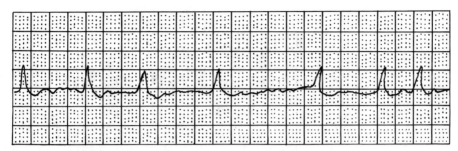

Figure 13.11. Atrial fibrillation. Note absence of P-waves and irregular timing of QRS complexes. (These QRS complexes are wide. Usually they would be narrow.)

the depolarization is initiated in the ventricle, no P-wave is seen.

Premature Ventricular Contractions. Premature ventricular contractions (early beats of ventricular origin (PVC)) can be caused by any factor listed under "Pathophysiologic Correlation" and can also be seen in healthy patients. ECG characteristics of a PVC are as follow: (*a*) QRS duration is >0.12 msec (wide QRS); (*b*) main QRS axis is often opposite that seen in a normally depolarizing ventricle (e.g., if QRS is usually positive or upright, it will be negative); (*c*) T-wave axis is usually opposite the QRS axis of the PVC; (*d*) there is a "compensatory pause" after the PVC (distance from the R-wave of the beat before PVC to the R-wave of the beat after the PVC will be exactly twice the distance between the R-waves of two consecutive normally conducted beats); (*e*) PVC is not preceded by a P-wave (Fig. 13.13). In the general ambulatory setting, PVCs are unlikely to progress to a hemodynamically compromising dangerous rhythm.

Ventricular Tachycardias. Ventricular tachycardia is present if there are three consecutive beats of ventricular origin at a rate of >100 beats/minute. These episodes may be asymptomatic;

however, if prolonged, they may cause hypoperfusion and even death (Fig. 13.14).

BUNDLE BRANCH BLOCK

Bundle branch block is a conduction defect, not a rhythm disorder. It usually does not cause symptoms itself but is a fairly common ECG finding. Conduction down one of the interventricular bundles is slowed relative to the other, resulting in a widened "rabbit ears" QRS on ECG. Rabbit ears in lead V_1, V_2 are consistent with right bundle branch block (Fig. 13.15); rabbit ears in lead V_5, V_6 are consistent with left bundle branch block (Fig. 13.16).

Management

The treatment of arrhythmia depends on the extent of symptomatology and the cause and degree of the underlying disease. All antiarrhythmic drugs have serious potential side effects.

ATRIAL ARRHYTHMIAS

Sinus Tachycardia and Sinus Bradycardia. The cause of the abnormal rate should be investi-

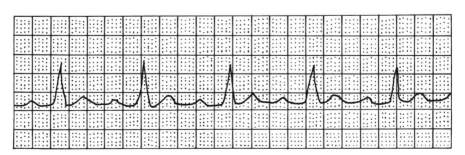

Figure 13.12. First degree AV block. P-R interval (time from the start of the P-wave to the start of the QRS complex) is more than 0.2 seconds.

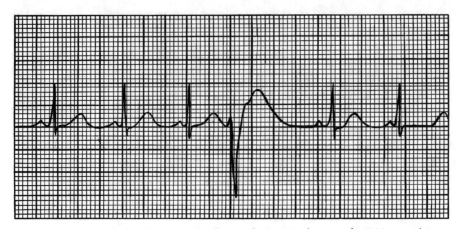

Figure 13.13. Premature ventricular contraction. PVC (*arrow*) has a QRS duration of >0.12 seconds; its main QRS axis is opposite that seen in the normally conducted beat; T-wave axis is opposite the QRS axis, and there is a compensatory pause. (From Berstein D, Shelor SP. Pediatrics. Baltimore: Williams & Wilkins, 1996:359.)

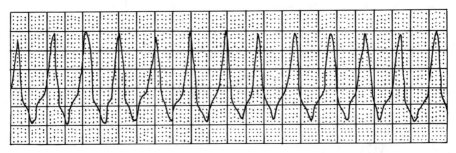

Figure 13.14. Ventricular tachycardia. These bizarre beats, each with a QRS duration of >0.12 seconds, occur here at a rate of about 150 beats/minute.

gated. For the patient who is asymptomatic and has no evidence of underlying illness, no treatment is indicated. For sinus tachycardia, encourage the patient to get lots of rest and avoid alcohol, tobacco, decongestants and antihistamines, caffeine, and illicit drugs. Check thyroid function tests if hyperthyroidism is suspected. For the patient who is bradycardic and symptomatic, a careful review of medications is indicated with discontinuation of any offending agents (e.g., beta-blockers or verapamil).

Atrial Premature Contractions. Atrial premature contractions are not likely to progress to a dangerous arrhythmia. They can be found in healthy patients. In general, patients can be reassured that their palpitations are not life-threatening and require no treatment. However, atrial prema-

ture contractions may be more prevalent in patients with cardiac, pulmonary, or thyroid disease, so these areas must be carefully addressed on physical examination.

Paroxysmal Supraventricular Tachycardia. Because this arrhythmia tends to be sporadic, an effective treatment is to teach patients to perform the Valsalva maneuver when they feel the arrhythmia. If this fails (assuming no evidence of carotid arterial disease), the physician can then attempt carotid sinus massage. Either intervention should increase vagal tone and "break" the cycle of reentry.

Atrial Fibrillation. Evaluation and treatment of the patient with atrial fibrillation deserve special emphasis because of the high incidence of treatable serious underlying disease, decisions regarding

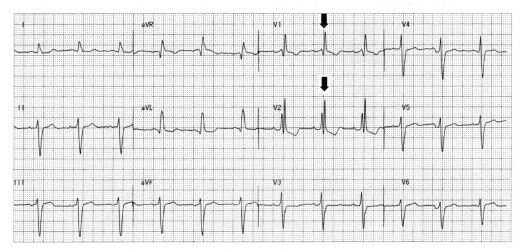

Figure 13.15. Right bundle branch block. Note "rabbit ears" (*arrows*) in V_1 and V_2. QRS duration is >0.12 seconds.

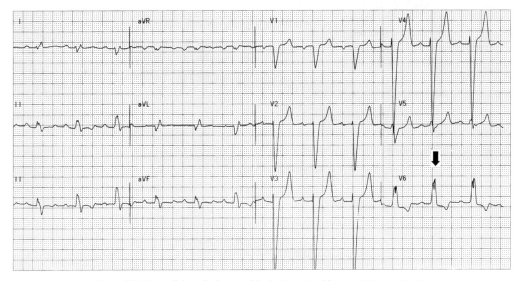

Figure 13.16. Left bundle branch block. Note "rabbit ears" (*arrow*) in V_6.

treatment of the arrhythmia and institution of pro-phylactic anticoagulation, and the long term, close follow-up that often is necessary.

Evaluate the patient for valvular disease, ische-mic disease, cardiomyopathy, and thyrotoxicosis. Unless the patient's ventricular rate is already slow or normal, he or she will require medication. Di-goxin 0.125–0.25 mg daily, verapamil 80 mg three times daily, or a beta-blocker can be given initially to slow the ventricular rate. These drugs may con-vert the rhythm to normal sinus rhythm. Type IA antiarrhythmics such as quinidine and procainam-ide may chemically convert atrial fibrillation to nor-mal sinus rhythm. If chemical cardioversion fails, electrical cardioversion should be tried. Anticoagu-lation with warfarin should be established before attempting any method of cardioversion. An at-tempt to convert the rhythm to normal sinus rhythm is indicated unless the atrial fibrillation has been present for many months, the left atrium is enlarged (>5 cm), or the patient has failed previous attempts at cardioversion, in which case the conversion attempt is unlikely to succeed.

Because the atria do not contract normally, there is a risk of local clot formation and arterial embolism. The Framingham study reported the incidence of stroke in 5184 male and female patients without valvular heart disease followed for 30 years. The proportion of stroke increased with age, from 6.7% of patients 50–59 years to 36.2% of patients age 80 and older (11). The Stroke Prevention in Atrial Fibrillation study showed that warfarin or aspirin significantly decreased the risk of stroke and transient ischemic attack when compared with placebo (12). The choice of drug for prevention of stroke is controversial. Most recent studies favor warfarin at doses sufficient to raise prothrombin INR to 2–3. Once stable, prothrombin times are checked monthly. Anticoagulation should be continued for the remainder of the patient's life unless contraindications develop.

Certain groups of patients with atrial fibrillation appear to be at higher risk for stroke or transient ischemic attack. Patients with past history of embolism, with valvular heart disease, or with dilated or hypertrophic cardiomyopathy should be anticoagulated in some fashion. Patients who have atrial fibrillation and also suffer from hypertension, coronary arterial disease, or diabetes may benefit from anticoagulation. Patients should be anticoagulated 3 weeks before cardioversion and 2–4 weeks after a successful attempt. Elderly patients with atrial fibrillation should be anticoagulated cautiously because of the risk of intercranial hemorrhage. Patients with atrial fibrillation unassociated with risk factors do not necessarily require anticoagulation (13).

Bradycardia-Tachycardia Syndrome. If the patient has sequelae of hypoperfusion, the physi-cian must diagnose whether the fast and/or slow arrhythmia is causing the symptoms. A 24-hour Holter monitor can be helpful in diagnosing this arrhythmia. Digoxin 0.25–0.25 mg daily, verapamil 80 mg three times daily, or a beta-blocker should be prescribed to control the fast rhythm. Insertion of a pacemaker may be required for the slow rhythm.

NODAL ARRHYTHMIA

First degree AV block is asymptomatic and requires no treatment.

VENTRICULAR ARRHYTHMIAS

Ventricular arrhythmias are a marker for underlying cardiac disease. A reasonable first line therapy for ventricular arrhythmia is to treat the underlying disease. The Cardiac Arrhythmia Suppression Trial (CAST) showed that antiarrhythmic therapy does not reduce the long term risk of sudden death in postinfarction patients who have PVCs or short episodes of ventricular tachycardia (14). In addition, antiarrhythmic drugs may cause arrhythmia. Since publication of the CAST study, the trend has been to initiate treatment of ventricular arrhythmia while the seriously symptomatic patient is hospitalized.

PVCs are not treated. For the patient who is symptomatic and already on antiarrhythmics, a 24-hour Holter monitor can be ordered. Patients who have failed conventional treatment, or who have life threatening symptoms, should be considered for programmed electrical stimulation study.

BUNDLE BRANCH BLOCK

Bundle branch block is not likely to progress to a dangerous arrhythmia. It is, however, a marker underlying cardiac disease. The patient with bundle branch block should be evaluated for cardiac disease.

ILLUSTRATIVE CASES WITH SELF-ASSESSMENT QUESTIONS AND ANSWERS

Case 1

A 65-year-old woman with mitral stenosis and 3 years of atrial fibrillation moves to your city. She feels well. Her only medication is digoxin 0.125 mg daily. Her physical examination reveals only mitral stenosis and atrial fibrillation. Her heart rate is 76 beats/minute.

QUESTION: *What is your first priority?*

a. Order echocardiogram
b. Begin anticoagulation
c. Order 24-hour Holter monitor
d. Test thyroid function

ANSWER: b. *The correct answer is to begin anticoagulation, because she has significant risk of stroke. Echocardiography would be useful to determine degree of mitral stenosis; it would not aid in decisions about cardioversion because the atrial fibrillation is chronic. A 24-hour Holter monitor would show whether she has periods of normal rhythm or of fast ventricular rate but overall would not change your management. Thyroid function testing should be considered, but it is not the first priority.*

Case 2

A 72-year-old man with known angina had a 24-hour Holter monitor placed because he complained of palpitations. The monitor revealed four episodes of ventricular tachycardia, rate 140 beats/min, during exercise.

QUESTION: *Should you start antiarrhythmic therapy?*

ANSWER: *No. Because of the risks associated with antiarrhythmics, therapy is usually reserved for patients with dangerous or life-threatening symptoms. An evaluation of his underlying disease and adjustment of his antianginal regimen would be warranted.*

Case 3

A 45-year-old healthy woman describes episodes of "heart pounding" every time she argues with her teenaged son. She denies chest pain or syncope.

QUESTION: *What other information is important for you to obtain?*

a. History of smoking
b. History of alcohol use
c. History of caffeine intake
d. History of her methods for coping with stress
e. All of the above

ANSWER: e. *The answer is all of the above. This would be an excellent opportunity to discuss lifestyle modification.*

HYPERTENSION

Hypertension affects approximately 50 million Americans. It is a major risk factor for the number one cause of death in the United States, cardiovascular disease. Worldwide, as the average lifespan is increasing in developed countries, hypertension is becoming more prevalent.

Hypertension is a condition that exists when measured blood pressure consistently exceeds an arbitrary value (usually 140/90) (Table 13.6). Well over 90% of patients diagnosed as hypertensive have idiopathic essential hypertension; the remaining patients have hypertension that is second-

Table 13.6.
Classification of Blood Pressure for Adults Aged 18 Years and Older

Category	Systolic (mmHg)	Diastolic (mmHg)
Normal[a]	<130	<85
High normal	130–139	85–89
Hypertension[b]		
Stage 1 (mild)	140–159	90–99
Stage 2 (moderate)	160–179	100–109
Stage 3 (severe)	180–209	110–119
Stage 4 (very severe)	≥210	>220

Patients are not taking antihypertensive drugs and are not acutely ill. When systolic and diastolic pressures fall into different categories, the higher category should be selected to classify the individual's blood pressure status. For instance, 160/92 mmHg should be classified as stage 2, and 180/120 mmHg should be classified as stage 4. Isolated systolic hypertension is defined as a systolic blood pressure of >140 mmHg and diastolic blood pressure of <90 mmHg and staged appropriately (e.g., 170/85 mmHg is defined as stage 2 isolated systolic hypertension). In addition to classifying stages of hypertension on the basis of average blood pressure levels, the clinician should specify presence or absence of target-organ disease and additional risk factors. For example, a patient with diabetes and a blood pressure of 142/94 mmHg, plus left ventricular hypertrophy, should be classified as having "stage 1 hypertension with target-organ disease (left ventricular hypertrophy) and with another major risk factor (diabetes)." This specificity is important for risk classification and management.
[a]Optimal blood pressure with respect to cardiovascular risk is <120 mmHg systolic and <80 mmHg diastolic. However, unusually low readings should be evaluated for clinical significance.
[b]Based on the average of two or more readings taken at each of two or more visits after an initial screening.
From Anonymous. The fifth report of the joint national committee on detection, evaluation, and treatment of high blood pressure. Bethesda MD: National Institutes of Health, 1994;4 (NIH publication no. 93-1088).

ary to a specific disease. The reason it is important to identify and treat patients with this condition is that individuals with high blood pressure are at increased risk of stroke, myocardial infarction, and kidney failure. This risk can be attenuated by treatment.

Pathophysiologic Correlation

A consideration of the pathophysiology of hypertension involves a review of the normal physiology of blood pressure, a presentation of epidemiological evidence of the long term effect of hypertension, and a discussion of the clinical trials that demonstrate the benefits of antihypertensive treatment.

PHYSIOLOGY OF BLOOD PRESSURE

Under normal conditions, the blood circulates through the arterial system under pressure sufficient to perfuse the tissues. This pressure is a function of cardiac output and peripheral vascular resistance. Cardiac output is in turn related to intravascular volume, heart rate, and myocardial function. Peripheral vascular resistance is modulated by a wide range of physiologic factors, including the sympathetic and parasympathetic nervous systems and higher centers in the nervous system; hormonal factors, such as circulating norepinephrine, insulin, vasopressin, and renin and angiotensin; and locally released mediators such as adenosine and prostaglandins.

Beta-adrenergic receptors are found in many locations. B_1 receptors are found in the myocardium, and B_2 receptors are found in the arterioles. Stimulation of B_1 receptors will lead to increases in heart rate and in force of ventricular contraction; stimulation of B_2 receptors leads to increased arteriolar resistance.

Calcium channels are ubiquitous in the muscle cells of the body. Stimulation of calcium influx at the calcium channels leads to increases in both the force of ventricular contraction and in peripheral vascular resistance and may lead to a faster heart rate.

The renin-angiotensin system is the third physiological entity that influences blood pressure. If the juxtaglomerular apparatus in the kidney senses that blood pressure is too low, it releases renin, which ultimately is metabolized to angiotensin II, causing vasoconstriction and increased vascular resistance. Angiotensin II also stimulates aldosterone production, causing sodium retention and increased intravascular volume.

Consideration of the factors that regulate blood pressure will guide a reasonable approach to pharmacotherapy and a rational search for secondary causes of hypertension, such as renovascular disease or renal parenchymal disease. In general, medications that slow heart rate (such as beta-blockers and calcium channel blockers) or medications that decrease the force of ventricular contraction (again beta-blockers or calcium channel blockers) will cause a lowering of blood pressure. Likewise, drugs that lower peripheral vascular resistance, such as diuretics, angiotensin converting enzyme (ACE) inhibitors, calcium channel blockers, and alpha-blockers, will lower blood pressure.

EPIDEMIOLOGY OF HYPERTENSION

Since the turn of the century, when Korotkov discovered that blood pressure could be measured indirectly, clinical pathologic correlations were observed between marked elevations of blood pressure and such abnormalities as left ventricular hypertrophy, nephrosclerosis, and stroke. The consequences of more subtle blood pressure elevations, however, evolve over many years, and the associated consequences could not be appreciated until the development of sophisticated observational epidemiological studies.

The most important of these studies was the Framingham Heart Study (15), a prospective long-term cohort study designed to determine the risk factors for the development of cardiovascular disease. Data from Framingham clearly demonstrated that individuals with high blood pressure had a higher incidence of stroke and heart attack when compared with those with lower blood pressure. Importantly this increased risk with higher blood pressure was a continuous effect, with no physiologic cut point. That is, at every level of blood pressure, a lower blood pressure was associated with a lower risk of cardiovascular disease. Epidemiological data do not support any particular level of blood pressure as indicating hypertension but rather suggest an equivalent improvement in risk of cardiovascular disease by lowering diastolic blood pressure (DBP) from 100 to 90, from 90 to 80, or from 80 to 70.

Because clinical action requires a chosen cut point for defining hypertension, this choice must be guided by public health concerns, a useful distinction between relative and absolute risk, and evidence from clinical trials. On a public health basis, a cut point should be selected that does not commit, say, two-thirds of the population to begin potentially lifelong treatment yet identifies a sufficient proportion of the population at risk to materially reduce the incidence of cardiovascular disease.

Absolute risk reduction shows that, for a constant relative risk reduction, a greater proportion of individuals are likely to benefit if they start from a position of higher risk. Thus a cut point should identify a population at high enough risk to be likely to achieve significant benefit. Analysis of risk has relevance when considering special subgroups of patients such as women, diabetics, or patients with multiple risk factors. These subgroups will be discussed further in the section labelled special considerations.

CLINICAL TRIALS IN HYPERTENSION

In hypertension trials, the evidence advocating lowering of blood pressure has been quite consistent. Large trials in the United States (Hypertension Detection and Follow-up Program (HDFP)) (16), Great Britain (Medical Research Council (MRC) trial) (17), and Australia (18) all demonstrated significant reductions in the risk of stroke for patients with mild hypertension treated with diuretics and/or beta-blockers. The benefits of these drugs in preventing heart attack are less dramatic; however, they are consistently demonstrated and in meta-analysis (19) are shown to be statistically significant. In summary, meta-analysis suggests that successful drug therapy of patients with mild hypertension, maintained over a 5-year period, is associated with a 42% reduction in the risk of stroke and a 14% reduction in the risk of heart attack. Although there was some variability in these trials regarding the definition of mild hypertension, the largest trial used a DBP range of 90–104 mmHg, lending support to the clinical usefulness of this range in determining the need for treatment.

Clinical and Laboratory Evaluation

The history and physical examination can give information about the consequences and severity of hypertension. In addition, certain findings can alert the clinician to secondary causes of hypertension. Laboratory evaluation aids in identification of consequences and causes.

HISTORY

Hypertension is usually asymptomatic. It is important to obtain information about target-organ disease (cardiac, cerebral, renal, peripheral vascular,

ocular) during history taking (Table 13.7). Diseased target organs are seen in more serious hypertension. The clinician should question the patient about consequences of hypertension such as headaches, vision loss, chest pain, claudication, and neurologic defects. Questions about past or current renal disease are important in assessing causes or consequences of hypertension. Although patients with hypertension will state that they can tell when their pressure is up (e.g., noting headache or anxiety), they are usually wrong—they cannot tell what their pressure is. Most patients must be disabused of that notion, because this belief can be a barrier to compliance with a regimen of antihypertensive medication. The few patients who can sense elevations in their pressure can benefit therapeutically. These patients might be particularly likely to succeed with relaxation techniques to control blood pressure.

Relevant history in newly diagnosed hypertension focuses on the other cardiovascular disease risk factors: smoking, hypercholesterolemia, diabetes, and family history of heart disease. The presence of multiple risk factors helps the clinician to estimate cardiac prognosis. Patients often offer a family his-

Table 13.7.
Manifestations of Target-Organ Disease

Organ System	Manifestations
Cardiac	Clinical, electrocardiographic, or radiologic evidence of coronary artery disease, left ventricular hypertrophy or "strain" by electrocardiography or left ventricular hypertrophy by echocardiography, left ventricular dysfunction or cardiac failure
Cerebrovascular	Transient ischemic attack or stroke
Peripheral vascular	Absence of one or more major pulses in extremities (except for dorsalis pedis) with or without intermittent claudication, aneurysm
Renal	Serum creatinine >130 μmol/l (1.5 mg/dl), proteinuria (1+ or greater), microalbuminuria
Retinopathy	Hemorrhages or exudates, with or without papilledema

From Anonymous. The fifth report of the joint national committee on detection, evaluation, and treatment of high blood pressure (JNC-V). Bethesda MD: National Institutes of Health, 1994;5 (NIH publication no. 93-1088).

tory of hypertension, but given the high prevalence of hypertension, it is probably not relevant. Absence of a family history of hypertension may be a relevant clue that secondary hypertension is present. It is important to determine if the patient is taking any medications, notably steroids or estrogen, that may increase blood pressure. Cocaine and its derivatives cause temporary elevations of blood pressure. Information about the patient's weight, exercise habits, and dietary practices must be obtained. A history of weight loss with episodes of sweating, tachycardia, and orthostatic hypotension suggests the diagnosis of pheochromocytoma.

For patients with a known prior history of hypertension, it is important to determine its duration, the medications used, side effects from treatment, and the presence of any complications.

PHYSICAL EXAMINATION

The examination should focus on signs of hypertensive complications or potential secondary causes of hypertension. Correct measurement of blood pressure is essential to assure accurate diagnosis. Examination of specific target-organ systems such as the eye, heart, and neurologic systems is essential.

General Appearance. The general appearance of the patient should be noted. For instance, the patient may have the moon facies, central obesity, and buffalo hump suggestive of Cushing's syndrome. The patient's age should be noted (a first diagnosis of essential hypertension is less common in children, teens, and the elderly). Does the patient appear to be in pain? Systolic blood pressure rises in response to pain.

Vital Signs. An elevated pulse may suggest autonomic dysfunction or pheochromocytoma. Bradycardia is most commonly seen in patients already treated with beta-blockers. The most important part of the physical examination is a careful measurement of the blood pressure. Choose a cuff of appropriate size. A normal size cuff on an obese or a thin arm will give an inaccurate measurement. On the initial visit, the pressure should be measured in both arms. A consistent difference may be seen in patients with the rare vascular anomaly, coarctation of the aorta, leading to a lower blood pressure in the left arm. Blood pressure is measured at equilibrium with the patient seated, standing, and supine (after at least 2 minutes in each position): orthostatic hypotension is seen in pheochromocytoma or with some treatments; postural changes are common in the elderly with autonomic dysfunc-

tion. On subsequent visits the clinician should measure the blood pressure in a consistent manner, usually while the patient is seated and by using the arm with the higher pressure.

The standard recording of the blood pressure requires that disappearance of sound (Korotkoff phase V) be used as the DBP and that the average measurement be recorded. Hypertension is only diagnosed in a patient with persistently elevated blood pressure on three occasions (or fewer, if there are signs and symptoms of target-organ damage).

The anxiety of being examined can cause "white coat hypertension." Blood pressure rises in response to exercise and stress. Skilled clinicians allow the patient to relax before assessing blood pressure. Blood pressure can fall from hypertensive to normotensive ranges in a few minutes as the patient relaxes.

Eye. Classification of the presence or severity of background retinopathy can help to assess the duration of hypertension. The types of retinopathy range from arteriolar narrowing to hemorrhages to papilledema. Hypertensive retinal changes can suggest severe or longstanding hypertension. In the most severe cases (with DBP usually >130 mmHg), the presence of papilledema indicates a diagnosis of malignant hypertension, a syndrome of life-threatening urgency that requires immediate in-hospital treatment. Conversely the absence of papilledema and of other end-organ signs (new heart failure, unstable angina, acute renal failure, or encephalopathy) in a patient with severe hypertension (DBP >115 mmHg) is *not* an emergency. In fact, although severe hypertension without these other findings has been described and treated as an "urgency," it is unclear whether the risk outweighs the benefit of urgent treatment. In such cases, the health care provider may be "treating" his or her own discomfort.

Neck. The thyroid gland and the carotid arteries should be carefully examined. Thyroid disease is sometimes invoked as a cause of hypertension. Hyperthyroidism is not a cause of hypertension. Hypothyroidism may be associated with a rise in blood pressure, which is rarely substantial enough to lead to a diagnosis of hypertension. The presence of carotid bruits may suggest atherosclerotic disease and may indicate an increased risk of stroke.

Heart. Signs of left ventricular hypertrophy should be sought: a left ventricular lift or an S4. A diffuse or laterally displaced point of maximal impulse, or an S3, are uncommon in uncomplicated hypertension. If these signs are related to hypertension, they are usually seen in patients with later stage hypertensive cardiomyopathy or those who have had prior myocardial infarctions. Heart murmurs should be listened for carefully, because the presence of valvular lesions may determine a specific therapeutic approach. A blowing diastolic murmur heard at the left sternal border suggests aortic valvular insufficiency. A harsh systolic murmur heard in the back may suggest coarctation of the aorta, especially if encountered in a patient with reduced femoral pulses.

Abdomen. Auscultation of the upper quadrants or flanks should evaluate for a possible renal artery stenosis; the bruit should have both systolic and diastolic components. A large palpable aorta suggests the diagnosis of aneurysm. A palpable kidney may suggest polycystic kidney disease or tumor.

Peripheral Pulses. The symmetry, force, and presence of the pulses of the extremities should be noted. Absent or asymmetrical pulses suggest vascular obstruction. Bounding pulses may be found in patients with aortic valvular insufficiency, a cause of systolic hypertension.

Neurologic. A brief neurologic exam, noting mental status, deep tendon reflexes, and function of the motor, sensory, and cerebellar systems, is mandatory. Mental status abnormalities can be due to reversible cerebral vascular insufficiency, stroke, or intracerebral hypertension with edema. Focal motor, sensory, or cerebellar findings suggest serious localized effects of hypertension, such as stroke.

LABORATORY EVALUATION

The appropriate laboratory evaluation should assess electrolytes, glucose, blood urea nitrogen/creatinine, urine, and serum lipids and include ECG and (perhaps) chest x-ray. Serum potassium should always be checked; a low value may indicate hyperaldosteronism. Renal dysfunction or abnormal urinalysis may be a clue to renal causes of hypertension. If serum creatinine is elevated, sonography or pyelography should be done to further evaluate the structure and/or function of the kidneys. Red blood cell casts and proteinuria indicate glomerulonephritis. Hyperglycemia may indicate concomitant diabetes or the effect of medication, and serum lipid elevation may identify patients with hypercholesterolemia. Patients who have diabetes or hypercholesterolemia may benefit from more aggressive blood pressure treatment because of their higher cardiovascular risk. Likewise the presence of left ventricular hypertrophy on ECG, while of very low sensitivity, is highly specific and identifies a subgroup with more significant hypertension and at increased risk for cardiovascular disease. The ECG should be evaluated for evidence of myocardial infarction. Chest x-ray may show cardiac enlargement or rib notching (associated with coarctation of the aorta). Laboratory evaluation of secondary hypertension is outlined in Table 13.8 (22).

Differential Diagnosis

Once the physician has established a diagnosis of hypertension, a study of the initial history, physical examination, and laboratory evaluation may provide clues to possible underlying causes of hypertension. About 95% of hypertension is essential hypertension. About 2–3% of cases are due to renal disease (parenchymal or renovascular); 1 to 2% of cases are induced by oral contraceptive use; the rest are due to such causes as primary aldosteronism, Cushing's syndrome, steroid use, pheochromocytoma, and coarctation of the aorta. As a general

Table 13.8.
Workup of Secondary Hypertension

Diagnosis	Initial	Additional
Chronic renal disease	Urinalysis, serum creatinine, sonography	Isotopic renogram, renal biopsy
Renovascular disease	Plasma renin before and 1 hour after 25 mg captopril	Aortogram, isotopic renogram 1 hour after captopril
Aortic coarctation	Blood pressure in legs	Aortogram
Primary aldosteronism	Plasma potassium, plasma renin-to-aldosterone ratio	Urinary potassium, plasma or urinary aldosterone after saline load
Cushing's syndrome	Morning plasma cortisol after 1 mg desamethasone at bedtime	Urinary cortisol after variable doses of dexamethasone
Pheochromocytoma	Spot urine testing for metanephrine	Urinary and plasma catecholamines, basal and after 0.3 mg clonidine

From Kaplan NN. Establishing control of refractory hypertension. Hosp Prac 1994;29:92.

principle, given the low probability of secondary hypertension, there is a high risk of false positive tests in patients undergoing workup. Thus workup should be reserved for those patients in whom initial evaluation suggests a possible underlying cause or those who do not respond to treatment. Table 13.8 outlines the suggested workup of secondary hypertension.

Management

The Fifth Report of the Joint National Committee on Detection, Evaluation, and Treatment of High Blood Pressure (JNC V) in Table 13.9 lists the recommended frequency of follow-up based on initial blood pressure reading. Treatment focuses initially on lifestyle changes. Pharmacological intervention begins when lifestyle changes are not sufficiently effective.

NONPHARMACOLOGIC THERAPY

Nonpharmacologic therapy of hypertension is the first step of intervention, particularly in patients with mild hypertension. Although the effect of these interventions is usually minimal (either because of noncompliance or limitations of the therapy itself), there is little chance of iatrogenic insult, providing an appealing first-line treatment. Non-

pharmacologic treatment includes weight reduction, exercise, reduction of alcohol intake, increased potassium and calcium intake, and dietary sodium restriction. The last of these is the most frequently prescribed, although data on its efficacy are inconsistent.

Sodium Restriction. Although it is true that populations with low-sodium diets have, on average, lower blood pressures, these cross-cultural comparisons are confounded by other variables. Indeed these same populations with low sodium intake and low blood pressure have high mortality rates, and countries with high sodium intake and high average blood pressure (such as the United States and Japan) have low mortality rates. On an individual basis, some patients will experience a reduction in blood pressure with sodium restriction but by no means will all. In fact, some will experience a rise in blood pressure, probably through activation of the renin-angiotensin system. In general, sodium restriction is most likely to be effective in highly motivated patients able to achieve significant reduction of sodium intake (<1 g dietary sodium/day) and particularly in low-renin hypertensives, who are generally more volume sensitive.

Other Dietary Interventions. Obese patients should be counseled to lose weight. Obese hypertensives achieve better blood pressure control as they lose weight. Patients should reduce alcohol intake. Simple dietary recommendations to increase potassium and calcium intake (e.g., drink more orange juice and eat yogurt) can improve blood pressure.

Exercise. Exercise can be an important therapy. Hypertensives who regularly exercise aerobically have lower blood pressures than those who do not. Isometric exercise, such as weight lifting, should be avoided.

Risk Factor Modification. Other items to consider under the rubric of nonpharmacologic therapy are smoking cessation and modification of dietary fat intake to reduce the serum cholesterol. Although neither of these measures is directly related to blood pressure per se, since the goal of antihypertensive therapy is to improve the cardiovascular risk profile, these major risk factors should also be addressed as part of the comprehensive care of the patient.

Table 13.9.
Recommendations for Follow-up Based on Initial Set of Blood Pressure Measurements for Adults

Systolic (mmHg)	Diastolic (mmHg)	Recommended Follow-up[a]
<130	<85	Recheck in 2 years
130–139	85–89	Recheck in 1 year[b]
140–159	90–99	Confirm within 2 months
160–179	100–109	Evaluate or refer to source of care within 1 month
180–209	110–119	Evaluate or refer to source of care within 1 week
≥219	≥129	Evaluate or refer to source of care immediately

If the systolic and diastolic categories are different, follow recommendation for the shorter follow-up (e.g., 160/85 mmHg should be evaluated or referred to source of care within 1 month).
[a]Scheduling of follow-up should be modified by reliable information about past blood pressure measurements, other cardiovascular risk factors, or target-organ disease.
[b]Consider providing advice about lifestyle modifications.
From Anonymous. The fifth report of the joint national committee on detection, evaluation, and treatment of high blood pressure (JNC-V). Bethesda MD: National Institutes of Health, 1994;6. (NIH publication no. 93-1088).

PHARMACOLOGIC TREATMENT

For patients with sustained hypertension after repeated measures, despite appropriate counseling about nonpharmacologic approaches, the clinician must next choose whom to treat with drugs and which drugs to use. The recommendation for treatment is based largely on the blood pressure, although individualized assessment is appropriate. In general, anyone with sustained DBP of >100 mmHg should receive medication; most with DBP of >90 mmHg will receive medication. Within the mild range of 90–100 (called "Stage 1" by the JNC-V), however, some clinicians opt for a period of watchful waiting, especially in patients without other risk factors and with no evidence of target organ damage. This approach is supported by observations from clinical trials where many mild hypertensives treated with placebo reached normotensive levels and had generally good outcomes.

The old-fashioned stepped-care approach was phased out some years back and replaced by a long list of potential first-line agents. This list included diuretics, beta-blockers, ACE inhibitors, calcium channel blockers, and alpha-blockers. Although this long list was appealing to some (particularly to representatives of the pharmaceutical industry), it was confusing to many.

Diuretics and Beta-Blockers. With the publication of JNC-V, the approach has been streamlined and made more rational. Although drugs from any of the above classes can be used as initial monotherapy, most would be reserved for situations with special indications. In the absence of specific indications for other drugs, two classes of agents should be used first: diuretics and beta-blockers. The rationale for this approach is simple: although it is reasonable to suppose that any agent that lowers blood pressure could prevent cardiovascular disease, only diuretics and beta-blockers have been shown in large, randomized, double-blind, placebo-controlled trials to prevent heart attack and stroke. It is therefore questionable, both clinically and ethically, to choose an unproven drug of potential value when proven alternatives exist that are safe, well-tolerated, inexpensive, and effective. Diuretics are administered once daily. Symptomatic adverse drug reactions are uncommon; however, hypokalemia is commonly seen. Dietary potassium supplementation with oranges or bananas or administration of triamterene can normalize serum potassium. Beta-blockers are administered once or twice daily. They may cause fatigue and impotence. Beta-blockers should be avoided for patients who have asthma, dilated cardiomyopathy, severe peripheral vascular disease, or high grade heart block.

Other Drugs. In many situations, the patient's overall health and the presence of concomitant disease justify initial monotherapy with an ACE inhibitor (e.g., diabetes or heart failure) or a calcium-channel blocker (e.g., angina pectoris or hypertrophic cardiomyopathy). In addition, many situations call for these drugs or an alpha-blocker to replace a diuretic and/or beta-blocker when they are ineffective or poorly tolerated (see Table 13.10 for a listing of suggested starting doses of first-line agents). ACE inhibitors are well tolerated, and many are administered once daily. They can cause hyperkalemia. Calcium-channel blockers have varied effects, depending on the specific one chosen. They can decrease peripheral resistance and force of ventricular contraction. Calcium channel blockers can slow heart rate. Verapamil slows heart rate and decreases the force of ventricular contraction much more than does nifedipine. However, nifedipine is a more potent peripheral dilator. Diltiazem has effects that fall between those of verapamil and nifedipine. Further, these other first-line drugs, as well as the second-line drugs (central alpha-2 agonists (e.g., clonidine), peripheral adrenergic antagonists (e.g., reserpine), or direct vasodilators (e.g., hydralazine)) may be added to a regimen when adequate control of the blood pressure is not achieved (see Fig. 13.17 for the treatment algorithm recommended in JNC-V).

SPECIAL CONSIDERATIONS

Treatment decisions in certain subgroups of patients may require special consideration (Table 13.11). These groups include women, blacks, el-

Table 13.10.
Suggested Initial Doses of Antihypertensives

Diuretics	
Hydrochlorothiazide	25 mg qd
Chlorthalidone	25 mg qd
Beta-blockers	
Propranolol	80 mg bid
Metroprolol	50 mg qd
Atenolol	50 mg qd
Alpha-blockers	
Prazosin	1 mg tid
Alpha- and beta-blockers	
Labetalol	400 mg bid
Calcium channel blockers	
Verapamil	80 mg bid
Diltiazem	60 mg tid
Nifedipine	10 mg tid
ACE inhibitors	
Captopril	50 mg bid
Enalapril	5 mg qd

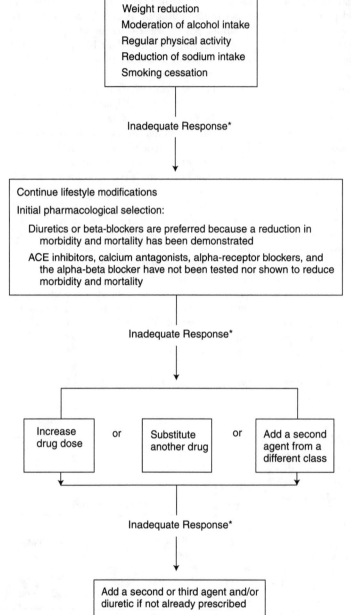

Figure 13.17. Treatment algorithm recommended in JNC-V. *Response means the goal of blood pressure is achieved or patient is making considerable progress toward goal (from Fifth report of the joint national committee on detection, evaluation, and treatment of high blood pressure (JNC-V). Bethesda MD: National Heart, Lung, and Blood Institute, 1994;16 (NIH publication no. 93–1088)).

derly, diabetics, and pregnant women. A review of therapies for these groups follow.

Women. The most important consideration for the clinician treating women with hypertension is the recognition that data to support specific recommendations in women are generally lacking. Although many clinical trials have excluded women, the largest (HDFP and MRC) had a large proportion of female subjects. Neither demonstrated a significant benefit from therapy for women by post hoc subgroup analysis. In the HDFP, all sex and race subgroups showed some overall reduction in mortality with stepped-care treatment with one exception: White women had a slight (2.7%) increase

Table 13.11.
Individualized Choices of Therapy

Coexisting Condition	Diuretic	Beta-blocker	Alpha-blocker	Calcium blocker	ACE
Older age	++	±	+	+	+
Black race	++	±	+	+	±
Coronary disease	±	++	+	++	+
Postmyocardial infarction	+	++	+	±	++
Congestive failure	++	−	+	−	++
Cerebrovascular disease	+	+	±	++	+
Renal insufficiency	++	±	+	++	++
Diabetes	−	−	++	+	++
Dyslipidemia	−	−	++	+	++
Asthma or chronic obstructive pulmonary disease	+	−	+	++	+

++Preferred, +suitable, ±usually not preferred, −usually contraindicated.
From Kaplan NM. Treatment of hypertension; drug therapy. In Kaplan NM, ed. Clinical hypertension, 6th ed. Baltimore: Williams & Wilkins, 1994:255.

in mortality. This difference was not statistically significant. In the British MRC trial, the all-cause mortality was lower among actively treated men (157 versus 181 deaths) but higher among actively treated women (91 versus 72 deaths). Neither of these differences was significant, but the difference between the sexes was statistically significant ($P < 0.05$).

Thus it may be that young, hypertensive women would be less likely than men to benefit from intervention. Because all drugs carry some risk, the minimal potential harm of antihypertensive therapy may be magnified in the setting of lower potential benefit. However, no study has been specifically designed to answer the questions of treatment efficacy for women. Therefore the failure to demonstrate unequivocal benefit by post hoc subgroup analysis does not mean that drug therapy is not of benefit. Although further study of this question is needed, it is reasonable at present to extrapolate findings in men to guide therapeutic decisions in women.

Blacks. The prevalence of hypertension is higher in blacks than in whites, and the consequences of hypertension generally more severe. Particularly, African-American patients are at increased risk for renal failure, left ventricular hypertrophy, and stroke. The increased incidence of renal disease is particularly striking. Although the overall incidence of coronary artery disease may be the same or lower in hypertensive blacks myocardial infarctions tend to occur at an earlier age. Thus there is compelling reason to be especially diligent with black patients in detecting and treating hypertension.

Although group-based recommendations do not apply to all individuals, they can serve as generalizations to guide clinical decision making. On a population basis, there is a greater prevalence of low-renin hypertension in blacks than in whites. This would predict that, as a first-line agent, a diuretic or calcium-channel blocker is more likely to be effective than a beta-blocker or ACE inhibitor. In fact, this prediction has been substantiated in clinical trials.

Elderly. There had been some question in the past regarding the value of antihypertensive therapy in elderly hypertensives, particularly in those with isolated systolic hypertension. In recent years, several studies have been published that demonstrate the efficacy of such treatment. These studies include the Systolic Hypertension in the Elderly Program (SHEP) (20), Swedish Trial in Old Patients with Hypertension (STOP-Hypertension) (21), and the British MRC trial (22). All show efficacy of treatment, particularly with respect to stroke prevention.

With respect to choice of antihypertensive drugs, the greater prevalence of low-renin hypertension would suggest a preference for diuretic-based regimens. Again the effectiveness of diuretics was borne out in the trials mentioned above, particularly the MRC trial, where those treated with diuretics had significant reductions in all cardiovascular disease outcomes, whereas those treated with beta-blockers did not.

Diabetics. In recent years, data have emerged that make the treatment of hypertensive diabetics a special case. Specifically, studies have shown that the development and progression of renal disease can be significantly delayed by blood pressure reduction, particularly by using ACE inhibitors. More recently, it has been shown that even normotensive diabetics enjoy a reduced rate of nephropathy when treated with ACE inhibitors (23). Although the ideal blood pressure is not established for most hypertensives, the data support the notion that diabetics should have their blood pressure more aggressively lowered than nondiabetics.

Pregnant Women. Methyldopa and hydralazine are the safest antihypertensives for use in pregnant women. Neither drug negatively affects organogenesis or the outcome of pregnancy. The suggested starting dose of methyldopa is 250 mg two or three times daily.

GOALS OF TREATMENT

General goals of treatment include informing the patient about the risk of hypertension and the benefits of its treatment, discussing reduction of other cardiovascular risks, and providing treatment in a manner that interferes as little as possible with the patient's lifestyle. The ideal treatment regimen is one that the patient can afford, can take as directed, can tolerate, and is effective. Specific goals of treatment are harder to come by. There is some debate about what level of blood pressure should be set as a treatment target. Some have argued that physicians should aim for the lowest level of blood pressure that can be achieved without causing symptoms. This theory has been challenged recently because it rests on the flawed assumption that blood pressure reduction is cost free. Although observational epidemiological evidence shows that a higher blood pressure, at any level, is linked to an increased risk of cardiovascular disease, the observational data in treated hypertensive males with evidence of ischemia or left ventricular hypertrophy have shown a J-shaped curve to describe the relationship between attained DBP and risk of myocardial infarction (Fig. 13.18). Coronary blood flow decreases as diastolic filling pressures to the diseased left ven-

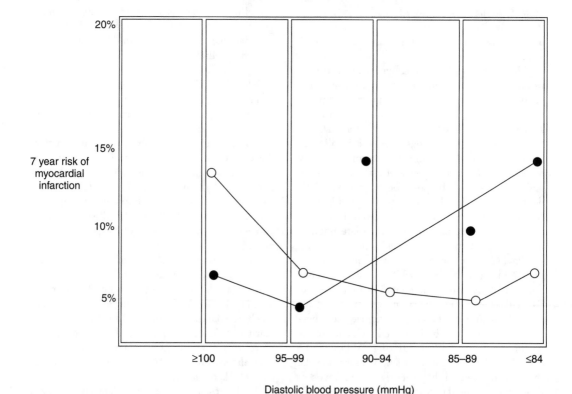

Figure 13.18. Seven-year risk of first myocardial infarction by category of blood pressure after 1 year of treatment in men with normal ECG (*open circles*) versus ECG showing hypertrophy or ischemia (*solid circles*) (from Linblad U, Rastam L, Ryden L, et al. Control of blood pressure and risk of first acute myocardial infarction: Skaraborg hypertension project. Br Med J 1994:308, 681–685).

tricle decrease. Thus although it may be true that "lower is better" in the natural state, this adage may not apply to patients whose blood pressure is artificially manipulated by drugs. However, no study yet has been specifically designed to determine the blood pressure goal of treatment; such a trial is underway. Until those results are available, clinicians might well view a dramatic blood pressure fall with treatment as cause for further scrutiny and not just a striking success. An appropriate goal of treatment may be to aim for a DBP of 80–85 mmHg or about 15 mmHg below baseline DBP. Fewer data are available to discuss systolic blood pressure goals.

ILLUSTRATIVE CASES WITH SELF-ASSESSMENT QUESTIONS AND ANSWERS

Case 1

A 45-year-old black man comes to your office for a preemployment physical examination. He has not had a physical examination for about 15 years. He has two brothers who are hypertensive. He is asymptomatic. His BP is 156/104.

QUESTION: *Which of the following historical questions should be asked?*

a. Do you smoke?
b. Do you exercise?
c. Do you drink alcohol?
d. What are your dietary practices?
e. All of the above.

ANSWER: e. *Each question is important, because each has a bearing on his hypertension, cardiovascular risk, or both. Lifestyle changes are the least risky interventions in treatment of hypertension.*

QUESTION: *What drug would you choose for initial therapy?*

a. Hydrochlorothiazide
b. Propranolol
c. Verapamil
d. Captopril
e. Other

ANSWER: e. *The answer is other. It would be essential to confirm the diagnosis of hypertension by repeated measurement of the blood pressure. If the diagnosis was confirmed, hydrochlorothiazide would be the best choice: diuretics and beta-blockers are the drugs of first choice unless an-other class is specifically indicated; and diuretics are more likely to be effective in blacks.*

Case 2

A 35-year-old white woman comes to your office because she has a headache. Her blood pressure is 212/118, and she has a systolic and diastolic bruit in the left flank.

QUESTION: *What is the likely diagnosis?*

a. Essential hypertension
b. Renovascular hypertension
c. Glomerulonephritis
d. Pheochromocytoma

ANSWER: b. *The answer is renovascular hypertension. Although essential hypertension is the most common type of hypertension in this age group, renal bruits suggest diagnosis of renovascular hypertension.*

Case 3

A 48-year-old Hispanic man has been taking propranolol 80 mg twice daily for 2 months. His blood pressure decreased from a pretreatment level of 192/108 to 178/102.

QUESTION: *What are your treatment options?*

a. Increase dosage of propranolol.
b. Discontinue propranolol and start hydrochlorothiazide.
c. Continue propranolol and add another drug.

d. Review his compliance with medications and lifestyle modification.

e. Any of the above.

ANSWER: e. *The answer is any of the above. The first step intervention is to review his compliance with medications and lifestyle modification. However, any of the listed options are appropriate.*

Case 4

A 62-year-old woman returns to your office to have her blood pressure checked. She feels tired. She forgot her medication today. Her blood pressure is 230/122. She has no papilledema but does have her usual S4 gallup on cardiac examination. Her neurologic examination is normal.

QUESTION: *Should she be admitted for emergency treatment of "malignant" hypertension?*

ANSWER: *No. Malignant hypertension, requiring emergency treatment, is defined by the presence of papilledema on physical examination, often accompanied by marked mental status change, acute heart failure, unstable angina, or acute renal failure. If untreated, malignant hypertension could quickly progress to death. Severe hypertension in and of itself does not equal malignant hypertension.*

EDEMA OF LOWER EXTREMITIES

Almost everyone will experience leg edema at some time. There are many causes, some benign, others less so. At the very least, edema of the lower extremities is unsightly and uncomfortable. Edema is the presence of excess interstitial fluid usually accompanied by increased total body fluid and weight. Whether the edema is localized or generalized depends on its cause and/or mechanism. This discussion will be confined to edema of the lower extremity; see Chapters 15–17 for a discussion of edema not confined to the lower extremities.

Pathophysiologic Correlation

Extracellular fluid is approximately one-third of the body's total fluid. Of the extracellular fluid, 25% is in the vascular space and 75% in the interstitium. At the capillary level, fluid moving between vascular and interstitial spaces is balanced by forces known as Starling forces. In short, the vascular hydrostatic pressure and the colloid oncotic pressure of the interstitial space at the arterial end of the capillary bed combine to move fluid into the interstitium. At the venous end, the colloid oncotic pressure of the vascular space and the hydrostatic pressure of the interstitium move fluid back into the vascular space. The forces moving fluid into the interstitium are greater than those returning fluid into the vascular space, resulting in some fluid remaining in the interstitium. This excess interstitial fluid is returned via the lymphatics through the thoracic duct to the vascular space, resulting in a steady state. Figure 13.19 summarizes the Starling forces.

When there is a perturbation of the Starling forces, damage to the integrity of the capillary epithelium increasing capillary permeability, blockage of venous return, or obstruction of the lymphatics, there is greater movement of fluid into the interstitium and/or diminished movement of fluid out of the interstitium. Excess interstitial fluid accumulates as edema.

Normal calf muscles alternately contract and relax during lower extremity exercise such as walking or cycling and act as an external compression pump on the leg veins. Coupled with one-way valves in the veins, this promotes return of fluid to the heart. Any condition that decreases calf activity would contribute to venous pooling and hence edema. Examples are prolonged standing or sitting or immobilization. These mechanisms, singly or in combination, underlie the many causes of lower extremity edema.

Clinical and Laboratory Evaluation

HISTORY

Patients complain of swelling, puffiness, weight gain, tightness of shoes, or tightness and tenderness of the skin or flesh. The onset may have been insidious or sudden. The relation of the edema to body position, time of day, activity level, or menstrual cycle must be elicited. It is essential to get a complete medical history, including medications, chemical exposure, alcohol intake, and a review of systems to clarify the cause of the edema and its possible relationship to other diseases. The patient should be questioned about risks for venous thromboembolism as outlined in Table 13.12.

PHYSICAL EXAMINATION

Findings include increased weight, puffiness, and pitting (indentation) (Fig. 13.20) of the affected

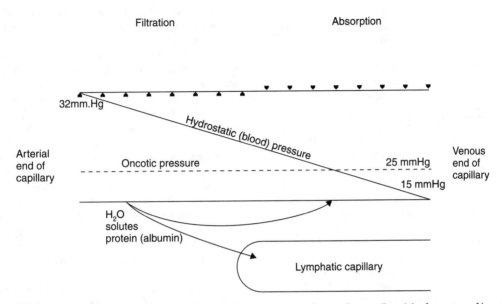

Figure 13.19. Factors responsible for filtration and absorption across the capillary wall and the formation of lymph. Tissue pressure = 0.

area with pressure and tenderness. The skin may be tense and glistening, thickened, erythematous, or hyperpigmented or show peau d'orange changes.

Edema accumulates in dependent areas of the body such as the feet and ankles and is obvious on examination. Presence of varicosities, a palpable venous cord, Homan's sign (tenderness of the calf with abrupt dorsiflexion of the foot), and stasis skin changes suggest venous disease. Warmth and redness are present with infection. Unilateral swelling suggests a local phenomenon, whereas bilateral edema suggests a systemic problem.

The physical examination could also show jugular vein distention, an S3 gallop, pulmonary rales, hepatomegaly, and hepatojugular reflux in patients with heart failure. Cardiac murmurs of valvular disease could be auscultated. Jaundice, ascites, hepatomegaly, palmar erythema, or a caput medusa suggest hepatic insufficiency. Hyperreflexia, tachycardia, diaphoresis, exophthalmus, lid lag, and tremor are seen in hyperthyroidism.

Table 13.12.
Risk Factors for Venous Thromboembolism

Surgery and other trauma
Previous thromboembolism
Prolonged immobility and paralysis
Malignancy
Congestive heart failure
Obesity
Advanced age (>40)
Pregnancy and puerperium
Varicose veins
Oral contraceptives (?)
Hypercoagulability

From Mammen EF. Pathogenesis of venous thrombosis. Chest 1992;102(suppl 6):640S–644S.

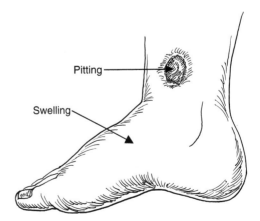

Figure 13.20. Pitting and puffiness found during physical examination of patient with edema.

LABORATORY EVALUATION

Laboratory tests are directed toward evaluating systemic or local causes of edema.

- *Cardiac evaluation:* chest x-ray and nuclear ejection fraction if ventricular failure is suspected; echocardiography if ventricular failure or valvular disease is suspected;
- *Blood chemistry:* helps evaluate renal and hepatic function; identifies hypoalbuminemia; thyroid studies if myxedema is being considered;
- *Urine chemistry:* dipstick for albumin or spot or 24-hour collection for albumin, creatinine, or sodium if a renal cause is suspected;
- *Venous studies:* impedance plethysmography, B mode real-time ultrasonography, Doppler, iodine-125 fibrinogen scans, and venography to evaluate for deep venous thromboses;
- *Arterial studies:* Doppler and angiograms if arterial insufficiency is suspected;
- *Lymphatic studies:* radioisotope lymphangiograms if lymphatic obstruction is suspected;
- *CT or MRI:* more useful in evaluating secondary causes, e.g., a pelvic mass.

Differential Diagnosis

SYSTEMIC

Cardiovascular, renal, and hepatic diseases are the major systemic causes of edema.

Cardiovascular. Heart failure—right-sided, and biventricular—is the most common cardiovascular cause of edema. It is characterized by impaired forward flow of blood, decreased renal perfusion, reflexive sodium and water retention to improve heart pump performance and renal perfusion, and increased ventricular end diastolic, venous, and capillary pressures. These contribute toward shifting the Starling forces in favor of fluid movement into the interstitium. In addition, the rise in systemic venous pressure with right-sided failure is transmitted to the thoracic duct, discouraging lymph flow back into the systemic circulation. This is yet another factor favoring interstitial fluid accumulation. Valvular heart disease impedes the forward flow of blood, increases venous pressures, and can lead to ventricular failure and edema.

Renal. Renal causes of edema include renal insufficiency, nephritis, and nephrotic syndrome. Their characteristics include oliguria, albuminuria, and sodium and water retention. There may be an antecedent history of strep throat, antibiotic use,

hypertension, or diabetes. The etiology of the renal pathology may be unclear. Please see "Renal Disorders" in Chapter 18.

Hepatic. Lower extremity edema can be seen in hepatic failure. Impaired hepatic synthetic ability leads to hypoalbuminemia. The decrease in the vascular colloid oncotic pressure promotes movement of fluid into the interstitium (Starling forces) and compensatory renal uptake of sodium to maintain intravascular volume. Additionally, increased portal pressures contribute to increased renal sodium uptake, increasing the total body fluid volume. See Chapter 16 for further discussion.

Sepsis. One consequence of overwhelming sepsis is toxin mediated injury to the capillary walls. The massive fluid shift out of the vascular space allowed by the increased capillary permeability results in hypotension, anasarca, and the adult respiratory distress syndrome.

Nutrition. Severe protein malnutrition seen in starvation and wasting states such as advanced cancer or AIDS can cause edema. Thiamine deficiency (beriberi) as seen in alcoholics causes peripheral vasodilation and increased sodium and water retention and hence edema.

Enteropathy. Protein losing enteropathies are associated with many conditions such as gastric or colonic cancer, ulcerative colitis, congestive heart failure, and intestinal sprue. The supernormal gastrointestinal loss of protein causes hypoalbuminemia and peripheral edema.

Drugs. Medications listed in Table 13.13

Table 13.13.
Drugs That May Cause Edema of Leg

| **Antihypertensive drugs** |
| Methyldopa |
| Clonidine hydrochloride |
| Nifedipine |
| Guanethidine sulfate |
| Hydralazine hydrochloride |
| Minoxidil |
| **Hormones** |
| Testosterone |
| Corticosteroids |
| Progesterone |
| Estrogen |
| **Others** |
| Phenylbutazone |
| Monoamine oxidase inhibitors |

From Young J. The swollen leg: clinical significance and differential diagnosis. Cardiol Clin 1991;9:3, 443–456.

cause vasodilation and/or sodium and fluid retention and may result in edema. Many are commonly prescribed, so the medication history should not be overlooked.

Myxedema. Pretibial myxedema is rare in patients with Grave's disease.

Idiopathic. In idiopathic edema, there are periodic episodes of edema. Women are almost exclusively affected. There is a characteristic transient increase in abdominal girth and a large diurnal fluctuation in weight associated with standing for several hours. It is most prominent just before the menses and improves with progesterone administration. There is a possible hormonal effect on capillary permeability, movement of fluid into the interstitium, and renal retention of salt and water to compensate for the decreased intravascular volume.

LOCAL

Physiologic Edema. Physiologic edema is the most common cause of lower extremity edema. Prolonged sitting or standing results in venous pooling in the lower extremity in almost everyone. There is no pumping action of the calf to promote venous return. This is exacerbated by excessive sodium intake, hot weather, and wearing constricting clothing such as knee high nylon stockings, which lack graduated compression and impede venous return from the lower extremities.

Venous Disorders. Chronic venous insufficiency is the most common cause of unilateral leg edema. Valves of the deep and perforating veins of the leg are damaged, perhaps by an unrecognized thrombosis, and are incompetent. The venous hydrostatic pressure rises and fluid remains in the interstitium, forming edema. Initially, the edema is soft and pitting, and there may be dependent rubor (redness of the skin caused by venous pooling, relieved by leg elevation). However, after several years of constant edema, induration and fibrotic changes take place, and the edema becomes firmer. Stasis dermatitis (hyperpigmentation, dryness, and thinning), cellulitis, and stasis ulceration develop.

In contrast, varicose veins are tortuous dilatations of superficial veins that pose little venous compromise of the lower extremity. Common causes are obesity and pregnancy. Occasionally there is no obvious cause. These vessels are unsightly and tender, can thrombose, and contribute to mild leg edema.

Deep venous thrombosis is clinically significant because pelvic and femoral thrombi are the source of most emboli that travel to the lungs. Pulmonary emboli lead to significant morbidity and mortality. Therefore timely recognition and treatment of a deep venous thrombosis is imperative. Deep venous thrombosis is an acute event. Edema caused by a thrombus develops rapidly over 48–72 hours. A carefully taken history may reveal a predisposing condition for thrombosis (Table 13.14). On physical examination, the leg is warm, red, soft, and pitting. Other physical findings that may be present are prominent superficial veins, tenderness, low grade fever (to 38.2°C), palpable venous cord in the popliteal fossa, and Homan's sign. Only 20–30% of clinically suspected deep vein thromboses are proven by venous studies. When there is a high likelihood of or confirmation of deep venous thrombosis, prompt hospitalization is necessary to begin thrombolytic therapy.

The venous studies include impedance plethysmography, B-mode real time ultrasonography, Doppler, iodine-125 fibrinogen scans, and venograms. Briefly, impedance plethysmography measures the change in electrical resistance (impedance) in the leg in response to venous occlusion by a blood pressure cuff. The established norms would be deviated from if there is a thrombus. Real-time ultrasound creates an image of the vasculature. Doppler ultrasound looks at frequency changes in reflected ultrasound waves that are proportional to the velocity of the blood flow. A fibrinogen scan uses a radioactive tracer that is incorporated into a newly formed thrombus. A contrast venogram visualizes the vessels and looks for an intraluminal filling defect. Serial examinations and/or combined noninvasive studies may be utilized before venography.

Pregnancy, massive obesity, and pelvic masses (e.g., a tumor) can compress the inferior vena cava. This obstructs venous return, increases venous pressure below the point of obstruction, and encourages edema formation.

Arterial Disease. Severe ischemia from arterial occlusion in the extremity may result in swelling. Atherosclerosis may cause pain of gradual or insidious onset. There is usually a history of calf claudication (exercise induced pain) that improved after an exercise program because of formation of collateral circulation and then progressed to rest pain when continued arterial narrowing overwhelmed the collateral's ability to maintain tissue perfusion. The history may also reveal risk factors for atherosclerosis: diabetes, hypertension, hypercholesterolemia, and cigarette smoking. Pain is a major complaint and is relieved by keeping the

Table 13.14.
Characteristics of Diagnostic Tests for Deep Venous Thrombosis

Diagnostic Test	Sensitivity (Proximal Thrombi)	Sensitivity (Distal Thrombi)	Specificity	Comments
Contrast venography	++++	+++	+++ to ++++[a]	Gold standard for diagnosis but false-positive or false-negative results occur; most expensive
Impedance plethysmography	+++	+	+++[b]	Least expensive; has been evaluated for serial testing of patients with calf thrombi
Venous Doppler	++ to +++	++	++[b]	Usually performed in conjunction with either impedance plethysmography or ultrasound; most subjective test
B-mode ultrasonography	+++ to ++++	++	+++ to ++++[b]	Often combined with Doppler analysis as a duplex study
Iodine-125-labeled fibrinogen scan	+	++++	++++[c]	Availability may be limited; useful in patients with recurrent disease

[a]Combined specificity for proximal and distal thrombi.
[b]Specificity for proximal thrombi.
[c]Specificity for distal thrombi.
From Zamorsky MA. Advances in the prevention, diagnosis, and treatment of deep venous thrombosis. Am Fam Physician 1993;47:457–469.

extremity in a dependent position. Sudden onset of severe ischemic leg pain is caused by acute arterial occlusion from trauma, thrombosis, or embolism. In longstanding arterial insufficiency, the limb may have ischemic ulcers, atrophic skin, loss of hair, and delayed capillary filling in the toes. In acute occlusion, the limb may be pale, dusky or cyanotic, cool to touch, pulseless, and tender. Hospitalization is necessary with signs of occlusion.

Lymphedema. Lymphedema is caused by the accumulation of lymphatic fluid through disruption of its drainage. With increased duration, the swelling progresses from soft and pitting to firm and nonpitting. Its reduction with bedrest also diminishes with duration. There is a primary congenital form with malformation of the lymph vessels. Women are affected more often than men. Secondary causes are commonly cancer (ovarian, lymphoma, prostate, bladder, testis, or skin) that either invade or obstruct the lymphatics. Filiarisis is common in tropical climates.

Infection. Cellulitis can be the cause of lower extremity swelling or may be a complication of edema. Cellulitis of the lower extremity is characterized by sudden red-hot painful swelling. There are signs of septicemia: fever, chills, malaise, nausea, anorexia, headache. Lymphadenopathy and lymphangitis commonly accompany cellulitis. Common portals of entry for bacteria are wounds, ulcers, fissures between toes caused by fungal infections, and hangnails. Gram-positive skin flora are usually responsible; anaerobic or Gram-negative bacteria may also be present. Fungi are rarely involved.

Lipedema. Lipedema is a common condition involving symmetric bilateral deposits of fat from the waist to the ankles. This is exclusively found in women and may be familial. The lower extremity may be painless or mildly tender. There is no true edema present, and there is no pitting. The foot is never affected.

Trauma. Burns, frostbite, surgical manipulation of the leg disrupting lymph flow, and a ruptured Baker's cyst can cause lower extremity swelling.

Hypersensitivity Reaction. In a hypersensitivity reaction the immune response damages the capillary endothelium. The resultant increased capillary permeability allows fluid to shift into the interstitial space to form an inflammatory edema. This is localized, nonpitting, red, warm, and tender.

Management

General measures in edema management include salt restriction, leg elevation, bedrest, judicious use of diuretics, and use of graduated compression stockings. Clothing that constricts circulation should be avoided. Examples are regular knee length stockings, garters, trousers with tight elastic ankles, and elastic (Ace) bandages to the knees. Specific exceptions and approaches are discussed below. Intermittent external leg compression devices have been promoted by some for edema management, but these devices confine patients to bed, are uncomfortable, generally are disliked by patients, are expensive, and are not clearly superior. Their role must be established.

SYSTEMIC

Systemic causes of edema require directed systemic treatment in addition to the general measures discussed above. Congestive heart failure is further managed with vasodilators such as the angiotensin-converting enzyme inhibitors, nifedipine and hydralazine, and digoxin. Renal causes may require corticosteroids and dialysis. Potassium sparing diuretics should be avoided. The edema of hepatic insufficiency is managed with spironolactone and paracentesis. Removal of the ascites improves lower extremity venous return and hence lower extremity edema. Refer to Chapters 15–17 for further discussion. Other directed treatments include thyroid hormone replacement, discontinuation of offending medications, appropriate antibiotics in sepsis, nutritional support with high quality proteins and vitamins, and treatment of the associated illness in protein losing enteropathies.

LOCAL

Management strategies for local causes of edema are also varied. Venous insufficiency is mainly managed with the general measures discussed above. Stasis dermatitis requires application of moisturizers to relieve the dryness and prevent breaks that would invite infection and ulceration. Attention to minor skin conditions like insect bites, abrasions, tinea infection, and eczema is necessary to prevent cellulitis. Surgical removal or embolization of varicosities help the patient's appearance and ameliorate the tenderness. Venous thromboses are initially treated in the hospital with intravenous heparin, and then a switch to oral warfarin is made to maintain the prothrombin time at 1.3–1.5 times control or 14–18 seconds. Warfarin is continued for 3–6 months for an initial thrombotic event, 12 months for a recurrent event, and indefinitely for

any ongoing risk for thrombosis. Inferior vena cava constriction can be ameliorated by weight loss, tumor resection or reduction with radiation, or chemotherapy and paracentesis in ascites. A pregnant woman can ease pressure on the inferior vena cava from the gravid uterus by lying on her side. Delivery resolves the condition.

Calf claudication is treated by asking the patient to walk to the point of pain and then a little further before resting. This encourages formation of collateral vessels. Pentoxyfilline (Trental) allows the red blood cell to become more deformable and traverse stenotic arterioles more easily. Although not superior to exercise in increasing exercise tolerance, pentoxyfilline is an alternative. Ischemia is treated by keeping the limb in a dependent position and when severe revascularization with a bypass graft or angioplasty, particularly of single, proximal lesions. Leg compression and elevation further compromise arterial circulation, increase the symptoms, and are to be avoided. Mild lymphedema can be improved with leg elevation. However, lymphatic invasion in cancers and filiarisis are difficult to manage unless the underlying disorder can be addressed.

Antibiotics are directed toward the organisms causing cellulitis. Dicloxacillin, first generation cephalosporins such as cephalexin, and erythromycin are good choices to cover staphylococci and streptococci, the usual culprits. However, in diabetics, responsible bacteria may be Gram-positive, Gram-negative, anaerobic, or mixed. Broader spectrum antibiotics such as first and second generation cephalosporins or ciprofloxacin should be considered. Antifungal therapy may be necessary in immunocompromised patients, e.g., HIV positive and recent recipients of chemotherapy, immunomodulating drugs, and corticosteroids. If ulcers are present, they should be debrided to viable tissue. Warm compresses are an adjunct and decrease the swelling by increasing circulation and resorption of the edema. If possible, oral antibiotics and outpatient management should be considered. However, patients who have poor peripheral circulation, are immunocompromised or frail, present with signs of sepsis, or have failed an oral regimen must be hospitalized.

Weight loss is necessary to reduce the fatty deposits in lipedema. Edema caused by trauma such as burns resolves with its healing; amputation may be necessary in severe frostbite. Hypersensitivity reactions are treated with anti-inflammatory agents including corticosteroids if necessary.

ILLUSTRATIVE CASE WITH SELF-ASSESSMENT QUESTIONS AND ANSWERS

Case 1

L.S. is a 34-year-old woman seated on the examining table complaining of right lower extremity pain and swelling for 2 days. You learn that she has multiple sclerosis that has progressed since the birth of her child 5 weeks ago and that she now uses a powered mobility device to get around. L.S. tells you she always had a little leg swelling that went away after sleep and did not really bother her, but this is different. She recently restarted oral contraceptives. The physical examination reveals pitting edema to just above the knee, and the leg is warm, erythematous, with moderate popliteal tenderness. There are varicosities of both legs. A venous cord is not appreciated. Attempts to elicit Homan's sign result in sustained clonus and discomfort. L.S. has 1+ lower extremity strength and cannot stand.

QUESTION: *What is the likely diagnosis?*

ANSWER: *A deep venous thrombosis.*

QUESTION: *What supports this diagnosis?*

ANSWER: *L.S. has multiple risks: immobilization, recently postpartum, oral contraceptive use, and varicosities. Physical findings are consistent with a deep venous thrombosis. The lack of a palpable cord and difficulty assessing Homan's sign do not eliminate deep venous thrombosis.*

QUESTION: *The noninvasive vascular lab closes at 4:30 PM. It is now 5:00. What do you advise L.S. to do?*

ANSWER: *There is a high risk of deep venous thrombosis that is consistent with her clinical course and physical examination. Hospitalization and initiation of heparin while awaiting venous studies are advisable.*

REFERENCES

Chest Pain

1. Weiner DA, et al. Prognostic importance of a clinical profile and exercise test in medically treated patients with coronary artery disease. J Am Coll Cardiol 1984;3:772–779.
2. Madsen EB, et al. Production of functional capacity and use of testing for predicting risk after myocardial infarction. J Cardiol 1988;56:839–845.
3. Kannel WB. Some lesions in cardiovascular epidemiology from Framingham. Am J Cardiol 1976;37:269–282.
4. Martin MJJ, et al. Serum cholesterol, blood pressure, and mortality: implications from a cohort of 361,662 men. Lancet 1986;2:933–936.
5. Vlietstra RE. Effect of cigarette smoking on survival of patients with angiographically documented coronary artery disease. Report from CASS registry. JAMA 1986;255:1023–1027.
6. Elkayam U. Tolerance to organic nitrates. Ann Intern Med 1991;114:667–677.
7. Beta Blocker Heart Attack Trial Research Group. A randomized trial of propranolol in patients with acute myocardial infarction. 1. Mortality results. JAMA 1982;247:1707–1714.
8. Ridker PM, et al. Low-dose aspirin therapy for chronic stable angina. A randomized clinical trial. Ann Intern Med 1991;114:835–839.
9. Alderman EL, et al. Ten-year follow-up of survival and myocardial infarction in the randomized Coronary Artery Surgery Study. Circulation 1990;82:1629–1646.
10. Bell MR, et al. Effect of completeness of revascularization on long-term outcome of patients with three-vessel disease undergoing coronary artery bypass surgery: a report from the Coronary Artery Surgery Study (CASS) registry. Circulation 1992;86:446.

Arrhythmias

11. Wolf PA, Abbot RD, Kannel WB. Atrial fibrillation: a major contributor to stroke in the elderly. The Framingham study. Arch Intern Med 1987;47:1561.
12. Stroke Prevention in Atrial Fibrillation Study. Final results. Circulation 1991;84:527.
13. Dunn M, Alexander J, deSilva R, et al. Antithrombotic therapy in atrial fibrillation. Chest 1989;95(suppl):118S.
14. Echt DS, Liebson PR, Mitchell LB, et al. Mortality and morbidity in patients receiving encainide, flecainide, and moricizine: the Cardiac Arrhythmia Suppression Trial. N Engl J Med 1991;324:781.

Hypertension

15. Kannel WB. Some lessons in cardiovascular epidemiology from Framingham. Am J Cardiol 1976;37:269–282.
16. Hypertension Detection and Follow-up Program

Cooperative Group. Five-year findings of the hypertension detection and follow-up program. I. Reduction of mortality in persons with high blood pressure, including mild hypertension. II. Mortality by race, sex, and age. JAMA 1979;242:2562–2577.

17. MRC Working Party. MRC trial of treatment of mild hypertension: principal results. Br Med J 1985;291:97–104.

18. The Management Committee. The Australian therapeutic trial in mild hypertension. Lancet 1980; 1:1261–1267.

19. Collins R, Peto R, MacMahon S, et al. Blood pressure, stroke, and coronary heart disease. Part 2, short-term reductions in blood pressure: overview of randomized drug trials in their epidemiological context. Lancet 1990;335:827–838.

20. SHEP Cooperative Research Group. Prevention of stroke by antihypertensive drug treatment in older persons with isolated systolic hypertension. Final results of the systolic hypertension in the elderly program (SHEP). JAMA 1991;265:3255–3264.

21. Dahlof B, Lindholm LH, Hansson L, et al. Morbidity and mortality in the Swedish trial in old patients with hypertension (STOP-Hypertension). Lancet 1991; 338:1281–1285.

22. MRC working party. Medical research council trial of treatment of hypertension in older adults: principal results. Br Med J 1992;304:405–412.

23. Ravid M, Savin H, Jutrin I, et al. Long-term stabilizing effect of angiotensin-converting enzyme inhibition on plasma creatinine and on proteinuria in normotensive type II diabetic patients. Ann Intern Med 1993;118:577–581.

SUGGESTED READINGS

Arrhythmias

Albers GW. Atrial fibrillation and stroke. Three new studies, three remaining questions. Arch Intern Med 1994;154:1443–1448.

Atrial Fibrillation Investigators. Risk factors for stroke and efficacy of antithrombotic treatment in atrial fibrillation: analysis of pooled data from five randomized controlled trials. Arch Intern Med 1994;154:1449–1457.

Ukani ZA, Ezekowitz MD. Contemporary management of atrial fibrillation. Med Clin North Am 1995;79:1135–1152.

Edema of Lower Extremities

Ciocon JO, Fernandez BB, Ciocon DG. Leg edema: clinical clues to differential diagnosis. Geriatrics 1993;48:34–40.

Young J. The swollen leg: clinical significance and differential diagnosis. Cardiol Clin 1991;9:3, 443–456.

Zamorsky MA. Advances in the prevention, diagnosis, and treatment of deep venous thrombosis. Am Fam Physician 1993;47:457–469.

chapter 14

HEMATOLOGY
Fabio Volterra

ANEMIA

In the medical office practice the discovery of anemia in a patient may lead to a diagnostic challenge. Remember that anemia is a clinical sign of an underlying pathological state. Anemia occurs when the need for red blood cells (RBC) exceeds the ability of the bone marrow to produce them. The erythrocyte mass measured by the hematocrit decreases compared with standard values.

Many factors had to be considered when the normal limits of the hemogram were established as standard reference for a heterogeneous adult population: age, sex, lifestyle (e.g., living at high altitude or smoking), and others. The major difference, which is that between sexes, is related to the higher androgen stimulation of the erythroid compartment in men, accounting for an average 2–4 g/dl of higher hemoglobin in the male population. The normal values are derived from a heterogeneous population of healthy individuals (Table 14.1).

This section will focus on the most common causes of anemia encountered in the outpatient setting: thalassemia, sickle cell anemia, iron deficiency anemia, anemia of chronic disease, and megaloblastic anemias.

Pathophysiologic Correlation

Hematopoiesis in the adult occurs in the bone marrow. The richest areas of production are found in the vertebrae (especially thoracic and lumbar), pelvic bones, ribs, and sternum. The hematopoietic compartment equally shares space with fat cells, but it is expandable; under stressful conditions the marrow in almost every bone could be used to produce erythrocytes.

Pluripotent stem cells are the earliest hematopoietic cells recognizable in the marrow. They give rise to more mature forms and become committed to one cell lineage, either erythroid or myeloid. Normally the myeloid-to-erythroid ratio is maintained at 3–5 : 1.

Erythrocyte production, like every other hematopoietic differentiation process, is under the influence of local growth factors released in the bone marrow microenvironment by different cells. Erythropoietin is one of the most extensively studied. It is a hormone glycoprotein produced by the kidney. It mainly stimulates growth and differentiation toward erythroblasts.

Morphologically, the erythroblast is the most immature erythroid cell that can be recognized in a stained bone marrow slide. During the maturation stages it will transform into a basophilic normoblast, a polychromatophilic normoblast and lastly into the orthochromic normoblast. This last, incapable of self dividing, will expel the nucleus and reach the circulation as a reticulocyte (Fig. 14.1). The normal reticulocyte count is between 0.5 and 2% of the total erythrocyte number. In homeostatic conditions the number of erythrocytes is maintained at a constant level. The number of RBC, aged or injured, removed from the circulation or lost, will equal the production (on average 5 × 10,000 cells/μl blood). The average lifespan of a RBC is 120 days. For comparison the granulocytes have an intravascular half-life of 6–12 hours, whereas the platelets survive 7–10 days in the circulation. RBC turnover can be measured, for diagnostic purposes, after having been labeled with radioactive substances.

Clinical and Laboratory Evaluation

Anemia is commonly discovered during a routine medical examination. A thorough history and physical examination must be combined with laboratory data to evaluate the anemia. Common causes of anemia frequently are not primary hematological

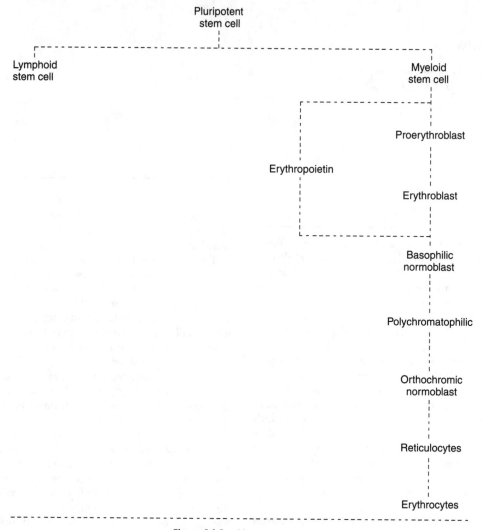

Figure 14.1. Hematopoiesis.

disorders (i.e., bleeding, iron or vitamin deficiency, etc); hence the evaluation is initially global. The data gathered will then focus the search.

HISTORY

Signs and symptoms of anemia are related to the rapidity of the patient's RBC decline and the cardiovascular status. A chronic hemorrhage with a loss of only a small quantity of RBC in a young adult may manifest with subtle symptoms of fatigue and weakness, whereas the rapid loss of a large quantity will produce sudden onset of tachycardia, postural hypotension, and skin and mucosal pallor.

Fatigue, lassitude, and malaise are nonspecific symptoms, but they occur frequently. When the anemia develops slowly the patient may not have noticed a decrease in exercise tolerance. Weight loss should alert the clinician to the possibility of illnesses such as neoplasm, tuberculosis, etc. Fever is frequently encountered in chronic inflammatory diseases and infections but also in leukemia, lymphomas, and neoplasms. Chills may be a symptom of hemolysis. Weakness can be localized to certain areas, as in pernicious anemia or multiple myeloma, or can be generalized as in cancer victims.

More specific symptoms such as headache, vertigo, and tinnitus are encountered in severe ane-

Table 14.1.
Normal Red Cell and Platelet Values in Adults

	Men	Women
Red cell count ($\times$1 million/μl)	4.5–6	4–5.5
Hematocrit (%)	40–50	37–46
Hemoglobin (g/dl)	14–16.5	12–15
MCV (fl)	80–97	80–97
MCH (pg)	28–32	28–32
MCHC (g/dl)	32–35	32–35
Platelet count ($\times$1 thousand/mm^3)	150–400	150–400
Reticulocyte count (%)	0.5–1.8	0.5–2

Reticulocyte index = Retic% $\times$ (hematocrit observed/hematocrit normal) $\times$ 0.5.

mias. Paresthesia, anosmia, or soreness of the tongue may be related to pernicious anemia. Patients, especially those with underlying cardiovascular disease, can present with palpitations, dyspnea on exertion, congestive heart failure, and angina. Interestingly, dysphagia could be a symptom of iron deficiency anemia when associated with severe mucosal atrophy. Patients with sickle cell disease can suffer severe attacks of priapism, whereas impotence may be secondary to pernicious anemia. A complaint of menorrhagia should alert the physician to the possibility of iron deficiency anemia. Bone and arthritic pain are frequent complaints in patients with sickle cell anemia, but they also occur with multiple myeloma or carcinoma metastatic to the bone.

The patient's family history must be investigated, particularly if one suspects the presence of a hemoglobinopathy. Often a patient may recall a relative who required chronic transfusion. A history of gallstones or jaundice should alert the practitioner to the possibility of hemolytic disorders. Gender and race are also important because some genetic disorders occur only in certain populations (i.e., thalassemia and hereditary spherocytosis). The history of hereditary disorders should prompt genetic counseling and family planning for the patient and the spouse.

PHYSICAL EXAMINATION

The physical examination should focus on organs or organ systems that are specifically involved in hematological diseases.

Lymph Nodes and Spleen. The most accessible lymph node chains are the cervical, axillary, epitrochlear and inguinal. Palpable nodes in the above areas or an inguinal node of >2 cm are associated with inflammatory or neoplastic processes. The nodes should be palpated with the fingertips using a circular motion and progressive pressure. Measurements can be facilitated with calipers or small rulers. The location and size of any enlarged lymph node should be recorded.

The spleen may enlarge under different conditions. It follows a typical pattern: the inferior pole usually moves downward and medially. A proper spleen examination is, needless to say, important. Palpation should start from the lower left upper quadrant rather medially and move cranially and laterally toward the left costal margin.

Skin and Appendages. Skin pallor or jaundice are found in anemic patients. These are not very specific signs because numerous conditions may influence skin color (i.e., amount of skin pigment, alteration in capillary blood flow, or temperature extremes). Inspection of the palmar creases has been used for many years to detect anemic conditions. They are normally red-pink, unless the hemoglobin is ≤7 g/dl. Unfortunately, this too can be unreliable: palmar erythema of liver disease may mask the pallor of a concurrent anemia. The nails may show koilonychia (spoon shape deformities) or longitudinal ridges. These are rarely seen now but are very specific for severe iron deficiency anemia. Ulcers of the lower extremities or the presence of healed scars are commonly found in patients with sickle cell anemia, reflecting the microangiopathy.

Mucous Membranes. Inspection of the mucous membranes for detection of pallor is more reliable than inspection of the skin. Additionally, the tongue may lose the papillae and appear smooth in iron deficiency or pernicious anemia.

Gastrointestinal Tract. Rectal examination with a stool test for occult blood should be performed in every anemic patient, particularly those with iron deficiency anemia. The stools are routinely tested after three consecutive bowel movements to increase sensitivity.

Genitourinary Tract. Female patients should receive a pelvic examination to search for possible sources of bleeding (e.g., polyp, endometriosis, neoplasm, and so forth).

Nervous System. Paresthesia and peripheral neuropathy are associated with vitamin B_{12} deficiency, myeloma, leukemia, and lymphoma. Sensory, proprioception, and gait evaluations must be performed studiously (Table 14.2).

Table 14.2.
Common Symptoms and Signs in Anemic Patients

History
Fatigue, lassitude, malaise
Decreased exercise tolerance, weakness, palpitations
Weight loss
Fever, chills
Headache, vertigo, tinnitus
Bleeding
Dysphagia
Multiple pregnancies
Bone, arthritic pain
Alcoholism
Malnutrition

Family history
Anemia
Recurrent transfusion
Recurrent cholelithiasis
Splenectomy
Jaundice

Physical examination
Lymphadenopathy
Splenomegaly, hepatomegaly
Positive stool test for occult blood
Koilonychia
Pallor, jaundice
Tachycardia, new heart murmur
Paresthesia, gait disturbances, psychosis

LABORATORY EVALUATION

Included in the complete blood count (CBC) are the RBC indexes, i.e., mean corpuscular volume (MCV), mean corpuscular hemoglobin, and mean corpuscular hemoglobin concentration. MCV is a measure of the average RBC volume. Sometimes it is erroneously elevated in the presence of hyperglycemia or RBC clumping in the presence of cold agglutinins. The mean corpuscular hemoglobin represents the amount of hemoglobin per cell; the mean corpuscular hemoglobin concentration expresses the percentage of concentration of hemoglobin in the cell. For practical purposes, only the MCV has been proven useful for the evaluation of anemias. The red cell distribution width measures the heterogenicity of the RBC population or degree of anisocytosis. It is derived from the distribution of the MCVs of the RBCs; the higher red cell distribution widths reflect greater cell size variance. It is used to distinguish between two conditions that share a low MCV, i.e., iron deficiency, where the presence of anisocytosis is one of its hallmarks, and thalassemia minor that is characterized by a more homogeneous cell size.

It is important to assess if the anemia is due to an increased loss or to a decreased production of RBC. The reticulocyte count is helpful to distinguish between the two; it is usually elevated in the presence of blood loss or hemolysis. Occasionally the reticulocyte count is inappropriately higher than expected for the degree of anemia because of an earlier release of the cells from the bone marrow. A correction formula, the reticulocyte index, was introduced to provide a more accurate estimate of the erythropoietic activity. The morphological examination of the peripheral smear is part of the routine evaluation. The clinician should be able to recognize the most common characteristics, e.g., RBCs of abnormal size and/or shape, as in thalassemia, or inclusion bodies such as basophilic stippling and Howell-Jolly bodies.

A practical diagnostic approach is to classify anemic patients according to the MCV into normocytic, microcytic, and macrocytic categories. These categories can be further subclassified by the red cell distribution width or degree of anisocytosis (Table 14.3).

In conclusion the initial evaluation of the anemic patient should include a routine history and physical examination, a CBC, and tests to detect occult bleeding (i.e., stool and urine).

Differential Diagnosis

HEMOGLOBINOPATHIES

Hemoglobinopathies are a group of disorders characterized by abnormal synthesis, function, or structure of the hemoglobin. Thalassemia and sickle cell anemia are the most common.

Thalassemia. Thalassemia, from the Greek word for the sea, was once considered a disease of the Mediterranean population. Subsequently it was discovered in other tropical and subtropical areas where malaria was endemic. The condition gave a survival advantage to the heterozygote carriers. Porphyrin iron and the protein globin are the main components of the hemoglobin molecule. Abnormalities in either will cause a diminished hemoglobin content in the erythrocyte, resulting in hypochromic microcytic anemia.

Thalassemia is characterized by an altered synthesis of the globin chains. Beta-thalassemia major (or the homozygous disease) is seldom encountered in an adult outpatient clinic. This is a devastating illness that begins in childhood and rarely allows survival beyond the second decade of life. Seemingly alpha-thalassemia in the homozygous form, where no alpha-chains are produced, causes hy-

Table 14.3.
Classification of Anemic Patients by MCV and RDW

	Red Cell Distribution Width (RDW)	
	High	Normal-Low
MCV <80 (microcytosis)	Iron deficiency Sickle or beta-thalassemia HbH	Alpha- or beta-thalassemia ACD
MCV 80–100 (normocytosis)	Sickle cell anemia HbS, HbC Sideroblastic anemia Extramedullary erythropoiesis	Normal ACD HbA-, HbS
MCV >100 (macrocytosis)	Pernicious anemia Cold agglutinin disease	Myelodysplastic syndrome

MCV, mean corpuscular volume; ACD, anemia of chronic disease.

drops fetalis and early death of the affected individual.

In the adult, the main hemoglobin (namely HbA) contains two alpha- and two beta-globin chains. Although the alpha-globin appears in the early embryogenesis and remains there until adulthood, there are different beta-like globin chains that alternate during fetal development. Besides the HbA (two alpha- and two beta-globin), the adult RBC contains also 1–2% of hemoglobin A_2 (where the two beta-chains are substituted by two delta-chains). In the normal individual the globin synthesis is in a constant balance. The globin subunits (alpha-, beta-, delta-) are assembled in the cell to form the hemoglobin tetramer.

Alpha-Thalassemia. Alpha-thalassemia (Table 14.4) arises from an altered production of the alpha-globin. In most cases this is the result of gene deletion during egg or sperm formation. Some patients with alpha-thalassemia have one missing gene. About 30% of black Africans have this anomaly. There are four different phenotypes characterized by the number of missing genes; the severity of the disease is proportional to the number of the alpha-genes deleted. When one gene is missing, there are no detectable hematological abnormalities, except that the MCV may be low, and the patient is a silent carrier. This anomaly could be detected by the Southern blot technique. If two of the four genes are missing, there will be microcytosis, hypochromia, and anemia.

HbH results from a severe deficiency of alpha-globin. It occurs when only one alpha-globin gene is present. The lack of an adequate amount of alpha-globin creates tetramers of beta-globin (i.e., HbH). Owing to its instability, these tetramers precipitate within the cell. They are visible as Heinz bodies

on a Wright stain and produce hemolytic anemia with secondary splenomegaly. The condition is common in populations of Southeast Asia but is rare in the black populations of Africa.

The absence of alpha-genes produces hydrops fetalis, which is characterized by a nonfunctional hemoglobin. The fetus is severely hypoxic and is stillborn or dies soon after birth.

Most of the common adult forms of alpha-thal minor encountered in an outpatient medical clinic have no abnormal hemoglobin detectable by electrophoresis. More sensitive and specific tests, such as globin synthesis studies or gene mapping analysis, are not always available and are expensive for the patient and the community. Because the syndrome has no clinical consequences for the carrier, the diagnosis should be pursued only in a prenatal prevention program.

Beta-Thalassemia. Beta-thalassemia results from impaired beta-globin chain synthesis. The disease can be divided in two major groups: one in which the synthesis of beta-globin occurs but the amount is markedly reduced and the other where a nonsense mutation produces an unstable, unviable beta-globin.

Although beta-chains can self-associate to form tetramers (as HbH), the alpha-globin cannot. In patients with beta-thal, other beta-like chains will form, and this is reflected by an increasing amount of HbA_2 (if delta-globins) or HbF (if gamma-globins). The decreased synthesis of beta-globin chains leads to an excess of alpha-globin chains. These will precipitate within the erythrocyte (Heinz bodies), causing decreased pliability and consequently damaging the cell membrane. There is a decreased amount of hemoglobin per cell, reflected by a low MCV and mean corpuscular hemo-

Table 14.4.
Alpha-Thalassemia

Genotype	Phenotype
AA/AA	Normal
AA/A –	Silent carrier
	No abnormalities or low MCV
Diagnosis: Southern blot or HbA/HbB synthesis (decreased ratio)	
AA/– – (common in Asian) or A –/A – (common in African, Mediterranean, and Asian people)	Alpha-thalassemia minor
	Anemia
	Low MCV
– –/A – (common in Asian)	HbH disease
	Hemolytic anemia
	Splenomegaly
	Reticulocytosis
Excess of beta-chains precipitates inside the erythrocyte as Heinz bodies	
– –/– –	Hydrops fetalis
Absence of alpha-globin, nonfunctional hemoglobin with high oxygen affinity, cannot release oxygen to tissues; death by hypoxia	

globin. Thus the red cell has a shorter survival time in circulation. Additionally, abnormal erythroid cells are destroyed in the bone marrow before release into circulation—hence erythropoiesis is ineffective. Anemia is usually severe in the homozygous beta-thal, with a marked increase in erythropoietin level that in turn produces activation of erythropoiesis within the bone marrow as well as outside (i.e., liver, spleen).

The most common types encountered in an adult medical clinic are the beta-thalassemia minor syndromes (Table 14.5). They must be recognized because often they must be differentiated from iron deficiency anemia or anemia of chronic disease. Unfortunately, sometimes these conditions are concurrent. The patients often present with mild anemia, reticulocytosis, and a mild increase in indirect bilirubin; the HbA_2 is usually increased (about 5%); and occasionally the HbF may be elevated. The iron stores are normal. Of note, when iron deficiency is present, HbA_2 may be normal or decreased because low iron suppresses its production. Generally patients with thal minor do not experience the clinical sequelae of the homozygous type.

The diagnosis of thal minor is often obtained by routine history, especially the family history, and standard hematological tests. When the diagnosis is unclear (as in some cases of alpha-thal where hemoglobin electrophoresis could be normal or in iron deficiency anemia concurrent with beta-thal minor where HbA_2 may be normal), there are more specific but expensive tests that can be performed. They include measurements of the rate of globin chain synthesis, intracellular distribution of HbF or the structural analysis of the hemoglobin variants. Southern blotting, a technique to detect changes in the genome, is also a useful test for the diagnosis of alpha-thalassemia or in difficult cases of beta-thalassemia; it should be restricted to the research laboratory only. In most cases, a diagnosis of thalas-

Table 14.5.
Beta-Thalassemia Trait

Symptoms and signs: none
Laboratory data: Low hemoglobin   Low MCV
                 Increased indirect bilirubin   Reticulocytosis
                 Increased HbA$_2$ or HbF[a]
                 Iron studies normal
Peripheral blood smear: poikilocytosis, microcytosis, RBC stippling
Therapy: none (must be differentiated from iron deficiency), prenatal counseling (molecular techniques)

[a]If iron deficiency is present HbA$_2$ may be normal because the lack of iron suppresses HbA$_2$ production.
MCV, mean corpuscular volume.

semia should be pursued for prenatal screening and genetic counseling. Finally, thalassemia must be differentiated from iron deficiency anemia or the anemia of chronic disease. An accurate diagnosis may help to reduce future tests or unjustified therapies.

Sickle Cell Anemia. The disease results from substitution of the amino acid valine for glutamic acid at the sixth position of the beta-globin chain. The abnormal hemoglobin, called HbS, changes its configuration under hypoxic conditions. The molecule polymerizes into a rigid structure in the RBC with consequent less pliability, membrane damage, and dehydration. Clinical manifestations of the disease are consequences of the microinfarcts caused by the sickled RBCs.

Although sickle cell diseases refer to disorders in which sickling is the most important manifestations (i.e., sickle cell beta-thalassemia, sickle cell HbC disease, etc.), sickle cell anemia indicates the homozygous state for the sickle cell gene (sickle cell disease). This last is the most severe; it has a poor quality of life and a shorter survival.

About 8% of African-Americans have the sickle cell trait as a result of the survival advantage from malaria in the heterozygous population (HbS trait). When the thalassemia gene and the sickle cell gene concur in the same individual (sickle thalassemia), the clinical manifestations are less severe because of a decreased production of HbS and more soluble hemoglobin tetramers.

The life of a sickle cell anemia patient is characterized by periods of relative well-being alternating with various types of crisis. These are classified as painful crisis, hemolytic crisis, infarct crisis, sequestration crisis, and megaloblastic and aplastic crises.

The microvascular disease produces damage to several different organs. Splenomegaly occurs in early childhood, but the spleen slowly "shrinks" and is usually not palpable in the adult. Sickle cell patients have a nonfunctioning spleen with im-

paired immune response, especially to encapsulated bacteria (pneumococcus, *Haemophilus*). Hepatomegaly and jaundice are also common; intrahepatic cholestasis is a rare but serious complication. More than half of the adult population has bilirubin stones. Bone abnormalities are common because of the hyperplastic bone marrow and the multiple infarcts. Osteomyelitis, often from *Salmonella* infection, and necrosis of the head of the femur typically occur in these patients. Pulmonary infarctions may occur, sometimes because of fat emboli departing from the necrotic bone marrow. Retinal vessel obstruction may lead to blindness.

The kidneys cannot concentrate urine. This defect occurs also in patients with the sickle cell trait. Hematuria is often present, and renal papillary necrosis is a serious complication. Priapism often requires surgical decompression. Chronic leg ulcers, especially around the ankles, are common.

Patients with sickle cell anemia have hematocrits in the range of 15–30%. The MCV is typically normal and the reticulocyte count always elevated (except during aplastic crisis). The presence of sickle cell is documented by the sickling test where RBCs are suspended in a hypoxic environment to produce sickled forms. Hemoglobin electrophoresis may be required to confirm the diagnosis or to eliminate concurrent hemoglobinopathies (i.e., HbS thalassemia).

IRON DEFICIENCY ANEMIA

Iron deficiency ensues when the amount in the body is not sufficient to provide for the normal metabolism of the iron-containing molecules (hemoglobin, enzymes, etc). In Western countries it is commonly seen as the consequence of blood loss in adults or insufficient iron intake in children and pregnant or menstruating women. The body utilizes iron to catalyze redox reactions. These are under rigid control because of the potential cellular damage that they may cause (i.e., peroxidation of lipid membrane). To control its reactivity, iron is commonly chelated to a protein.

In the average adult 1 mg of iron is lost daily from cell sloughing in the gastrointestinal and genitourinary tracts or skin. Women may lose up to 2 mg/day during menstruation and even more during pregnancy. The loss is usually replaced by dietary intake. The duodenum and the upper jejunum are the predominant sites of iron absorption. Normally only 10% of the elemental iron is absorbed, but it may increase to four-fold if iron is needed. Ferrous iron is better absorbed than ferric, but organic iron is the best source because its absorption is pH independent, making meat the preferred dietary source. Tannin (found in tea) decreases iron absorption by preventing its uptake, whereas citrate and ascorbate, as weak chelators, increase the rate of absorption. Other conditions such as achlorhydria, pernicious anemia, celiac sprue, and Crohn's disease will cause a decrease in iron absorption.

Once released into the circulation, iron is bound to transferrin—two atoms for each molecule. Under normal circumstances two-thirds of the binding sites are available (this constitutes the total iron binding capacity). Ferrokinetic studies revealed that iron is removed from the circulation by tissues; 80% is removed by the bone marrow alone to be used for the synthesis of new heme. Transferrin binds to specific membrane receptors on the peripheral tissue, and it is internalized in an acidic vesicle. The low pH allows the release of iron into the cytosol where it will be utilized by different organelles for synthesis or storage. The transferrin molecule is then recycled to the membrane and into the circulation to bind more iron. The intracellular released iron is believed to be the biologically active form, although most of it will enter a large ferritin molecule for storage purposes. The ferritin molecule can be described as a hollow shell where iron enters through pores and is stored. The metabolic fate of ferritin includes aggregation of different molecules or endophagocytosis by lysosomes to form hemosiderin, which precipitates as an insoluble compound in the cell. Hemosiderin (which contains degraded proteins, lipid, and iron) is at one end of the metabolic pathway of iron; when needed, iron can then be mobilized and reused. Ferritin is also actively secreted in the circulation, although there is some leakage from necrotic cells. Measurement of plasma ferritin strongly correlates with tissue iron stores, although many conditions may alter its level (e.g., inflammation, infections, tumors, hemodialysis, or chronic liver disease).

Etiology. The most common causes of iron deficiency are (a) hemorrhage and pregnancy, (b) conditions that produce decreased intestinal absorption, and (c) inadequate dietary intake. Once a history of multiple pregnancies or heavy menstrual bleeding has been excluded, the patient must receive a thorough evaluation of the gastrointestinal and genitourinary tracts to detect possible sources of bleeding. Other conditions, such as chronic hemoptysis (e.g., patients with bronchiectasis) or chronic intravascular hemolysis (where iron is lost in the urine) should also be considered. Nonsteroidal anti-inflammatory drugs may cause chronic gastrointestinal bleeding, resulting in iron deficiency anemia. This is especially common in the elderly.

Diagnosis. Two definite stages precede the development of anemia of iron deficiency. Initially, when iron stores in the bone marrow are depleted, the serum iron level and the hemogram may still be normal. This stage is diagnosed only by bone marrow examination of the iron stores. It should be strongly suspected when the history is consistent with blood loss (e.g., multiple pregnancies, etc.). Then as the deficit worsens, the serum iron decreases and the total iron binding capacity increases, but the hemogram may still be normal.

Iron deficiency anemia is the final stage, characterized by decreased hemoglobin and hematocrit, low MCV, microcytosis, and hypochromia. The lack of iron may affect other cells and cause some typical abnormalities, such as koilonychia (spooning of the nails) or Plummer-Vinson syndrome (postcrycoid web). They are both signs of severe iron deficiency but are rarely seen today. Another typical manifestation of iron deficiency is pica, an unexplainable craving for ice, starch, or clay. Angular stomatitis and/or glossitis are more frequently seen. Iron deficiency anemia is associated with thrombocytosis (platelet <400,000). The most accurate diagnosis of iron deficiency would require demonstration of decreased or absent tissue iron stores in the liver or the bone marrow. This last is preferred because of easier and safer access. Unfortunately biopsies are inconvenient as well as expensive, and they are indicated only when indirect measurements fail to provide a clear diagnosis.

Serum iron is typically low, but it is not specific. Transferrin saturation is a commonly used method to evaluate iron stores indirectly. Values of <13% are highly diagnostic for iron deficiency. Unfortunately conditions such as chronic infections, malignant neoplasm, or inflammatory processes will alter both transferrin and plasma iron levels, decreasing the sensitivity of the test.

Plasma ferritin may also be used as a measure of iron stores. It has been found to be a powerful test for the diagnosis of iron deficiency anemia. The plasma ferritin level is also affected by chronic infections or inflammation, but, unlike iron, it usually increases. The red cell distribution width is usually high, reflecting anisocytosis and helping to differentiate iron deficiency anemia from thalassemia and anemia of chronic disease, although recent studies have criticized its validity. The MCV is characteristically low when iron deficiency anemia is in an advanced stage.

The free erythrocyte protoporphyrin level is a highly specific and sensitive test, but it is not readily available. Measurement of the circulating transferrin receptors is a fairly new method for the diagnosis of iron deficiency; it should be considered only in selected cases.

ANEMIA OF CHRONIC DISEASE

Anemia of chronic disease is one of the most frustrating diseases to diagnose because of the lack of any specific tests. The diagnosis is often made by exclusion. It was more common in the preantibiotic era. The anemia is generally mild to moderate, with the hematocrit in the range of 21–33%; the patient is rarely symptomatic. Typically it occurs in patients with chronic inflammatory diseases or neoplasms.

Etiology. Interestingly, much research and theory have been produced, but there is no clear mechanism to explain the disease. It is known, for example, that the average lifespan of the erythrocyte is shortened, that the bone marrow production is impaired because it cannot compensate for the degree of anemia, and that the iron metabolism is disturbed, as reflected by a low serum iron.

Among several mechanisms proposed, the lactoferrin theory (lactoferrin production is increased during inflammatory states) of interference with iron metabolism gained some popularity, although it has been challenged by many. More recently, it has been found that cytokines may inhibit erythropoietin, but again studies have been contradictory because some found normal erythropoietin levels, whereas others found decreased levels.

Diagnosis. Patients with anemia of chronic disease have a hematocrit in the range of 21–33%, and they are often asymptomatic. The hemogram shows normal or decreased MCV and mean corpuscular hemoglobin concentration, although it is generally described as a normocytic, normochromic anemia. Typically, there is a low iron concentration and a moderately low transferrin with a high saturation ratio. The ferritin level is high, reflecting its role as an acute phase protein.

As stated earlier, the diagnosis of anemia of chronic disease is largely by exclusion. Other conditions must be considered, such as drug induced bone marrow suppression, renal disease, bone marrow infiltration by neoplastic cells, chronic blood loss as in gastritis or peptic ulcer disease, nonsteroidal anti-inflammatory drug use, or iron malabsorption. When in doubt, a therapeutic trial of iron should be instituted. The diagnosis requires the presence of a chronic infection, inflammation, or a neoplastic disorder, although sometimes these cannot be found.

MEGALOBLASTIC ANEMIAS

Megaloblastic anemias are a group of disorders characterized by impaired DNA synthesis. A preliminary distinction should be made between megaloblastic anemia and macrocytosis with or without anemia. The condition of macrocytosis is characterized by an increased MCV with or without anemia, but the erythropoietic cells do not show megaloblastic changes. Some causes of macrocytosis are listed in Table 14.6. In megaloblastic anemia the erythropoietic cells show megaloblastic changes. The peripheral blood smear shows hypersegmented polymorphonucleocytes (>5 lobes/nucleus) and macroovalocytes.

Pathophysiology. Folic acid and vitamin B_{12} are cofactors for the pyrimidine synthesis of DNA. Their deficiency alters the synthesis of DNA, which slows cellular duplication. Abnormal amounts of DNA and proteins are produced, leading to the morphologic changes of megaloblastosis. Most cells in the body are affected, becoming enlarged, deformed, and dysfunctional.

Folic acid is provided mostly by vegetables, whereas B_{12} is found in animal products. The minimum daily requirement is approximately 150 μg folate and 1–2 μg vitamin B_{12}. Folate deficiency

Table 14.6.
Different Causes of Macrocytosis

Alcoholism	Aplastic anemia
Hypothyroidism	Liver disease
Myelodysplastic syndrome	Hydroxyurea
Neoplasia	Cold agglutinin
Copper deficiency	Pregnancy
Acquired sideroblastic anemia	

usually develops after 4 months of a folate deficient diet, whereas up to 4 years are required to develop vitamin B_{12} deficiency if it is not supplied by the diet. Both folate and vitamin B_{12} are actively absorbed in the gastrointestinal tract: folate in the proximal small bowel and vitamin B_{12} in the terminal ileum (upon binding to the intrinsic factor in the antrum of the stomach).

Etiology. Folate deficiency is caused by decreased intake or increased requirements. Dietary deficiency is most commonly seen in the elderly, alcohol abusers, and hemodialysis patients or when absorption is impaired in conditions such as tropical and nontropical sprue. Increased requirement of folate may occur during pregnancy and situations with increased cell turnover such as exfoliative dermatitis (i.e., psoriasis) or hemolytic anemia.

Vitamin B_{12} deficiency can be secondary to decreased intake, as in a strict vegetarian diet, but more frequently is from impaired gastric or intestinal absorption. Pernicious anemia, the postgastrectomy states, and Zollinger-Ellison syndrome are some of the gastric causes. Disease or resection of the terminal ileum (as in Crohn's disease) is the most common intestinal cause.

Other conditions affecting vitamin B_{12} absorption include the blind loop syndrome, parasites (fish tapeworm), and pancreatic insufficiency. Megaloblastic anemia may also develop in patients receiving antifolate or antimetabolite therapy (i.e., methotrexate, trimethoprim-sulfamethoxazole, fluorouracil, hydroxyurea, citarabine, zidovudine (AZT), suffering collagen vascular disease or human immunodeficiency virus (HIV) infection, or taking medication for seizure disorder (i.e., phenytoin, phenobarbital).

Diagnosis. Symptoms include weakness, palpitations, fatigue, dyspnea, slight jaundice (caused by increased bilirubin from ineffective erythropoiesis), and glossitis. Serum lactate dehydrogenase is usually elevated, differentiating megaloblastic from nonmegaloblastic anemias. Folate deficiency can be easily distinguished from vitamin B_{12} deficiency by the absence of neurological symptoms, a history consistent with folate deficiency, the response to exogenous folic acid, and the low folate level. Serum folate concentration varies with dietary intake, alcohol ingestion, or starvation; tissue folate concentration, measured as red cell folate, provides a better assessment of the folate level.

Typical of vitamin B_{12} deficiency is a neurological syndrome that causes paresthesias, disturbances of proprioception, progressive dementia, and psy-

chosis. These abnormalities may precede the anemia and all the hematological anomalies. For this reason it is always good practice to check the serum vitamin B_{12} level in any patient with neurological complaints.

Management

HEMOGLOBINOPATHIES

Thalassemias. Alpha- and beta-thalassemia minor may represent a diagnostic challenge, but they are benign disorders that do not require any specific treatment.

Sickle Cell Anemia. Sickle cell crisis should be treated in the hospital. The role of the clinician in the treatment of the patient between crises is to focus on the diagnosis and the supportive management of the chronic complications as they arise. The patient should be advised to maintain an adequate hydration, especially in the hot weather or during heavy manual labor. The management of pain in patients with sickle cell anemia can be difficult. Like many patients with chronic and or recurrent pain there is a risk of addiction to analgesics. In addiction, high doses of narcotics depress the respiratory center, causing decreased oxygenation and worsening sickling. Because it is impossible to quantify the pain each person experiences, it is safe to administer the dose that obtains the most adequate pain relief. The search for a cure produced several promising but still experimental modalities such as bone marrow transplant, use of antisickling agents, and administration of drugs that increase fetal hemoglobin.

Patients with sickle cell trait do not experience the same clinical course. The blood count is normal, and except for the renal complications mentioned it is a benign condition.

IRON DEFICIENCY ANEMIA

There is a general consensus that iron in combination with other vitamins or minerals is no better than iron alone. Ferrous sulfate is the most widely used preparation but can cause gastrointestinal discomfort, constipation, or bloating. Ferrous gluconate is better tolerated. Some clinicians add ascorbic acid to increase absorption, generally 500 mg three times a day. It may take 3–6 months or more to correct iron deficiency. The patient should be followed with monthly CBC and reticulocyte counts. Once the anemia has been corrected it will be necessary to continue iron treatment for a few more months to replenish its stores. If the anemia is not corrected after a few months of therapy, other etiologies must be considered, including a reassessment of possible blood loss.

ANEMIA OF CHRONIC DISEASE

It is not necessary to treat anemia of chronic disease because the anemia is usually mild and the patient asymptomatic; every effort should be taken to treat the underlying disease. The administration of erythropoietin has been proposed for patients with a low serum level, but it should be considered investigational. When the diagnosis is uncertain a trial of iron followed by monthly CBC and reticulocyte count is justified. When the anemia is severe, a transfusion of packed RBC may become necessary.

MEGALOBLASTIC ANEMIAS

The treatment for folate or vitamin B_{12} deficiency is replacement therapy. Folate is usually given orally at doses of 1–5 mg/day; folinic acid is used parenterally in severe cases at doses of 3–6 mg/day. Vitamin B_{12} is commonly given parenterally, as in pernicious anemia where it is the treatment of choice. The usual schedule in severe deficiency consists of daily intramuscular injections of 1000 μg for 1–2 weeks followed by weekly injections of the same dose until the anemia has resolved.

The maintenance therapy includes a monthly injection of 1000 μg. Patients with dietary cobalamin deficiency or in whom intramuscular injection is contraindicated (i.e., hemophilia) will benefit from oral therapy.

ILLUSTRATIVE CASES WITH SELF-ASSESSMENT QUESTIONS AND ANSWERS

Case 1

A 35-year-old Korean woman comes to the office complaining of progressive fatigue and weakness for about 2 years. Her medical history is unrevealing. She has two children ages 4 and 3 and two brothers in apparent good health. Her mother was told she was anemic and had two miscarriages; her father is in good health but was rejected as blood donor several times. She is pale; her pulse is 105, and she has a 3/6 systolic ejection murmur. The hemogram shows

Hemoglobin 7.2 g/dl
Reticulocyte count 1% (corrected)
Hematocrit 21.5%
MCV 67
Red cell distribution width 21

QUESTION: *Based on this information what is the most likely diagnosis?*

a. Iron deficiency anemia
b. Beta-thalassemia
c. Anemia of chronic disease
d. Alpha-thalassemia minor
e. Iron deficiency anemia in a silent carrier of alpha thal.

ANSWER: a. *Although this is a possible answer, it is not complete.* **b.** *The relative recent onset*

of symptoms and the normal reticulocyte count make this diagnosis unlikely. **c.** *No history of chronic disease, and the anemia is too severe.* **d.** *Alpha-thalassemia minor is again unlikely because of the low hemoglobin, high red cell distribution width, and normal reticulocyte count.* **e.** *The patient has iron deficiency anemia and is also a silent carrier of alpha-thalassemia. Her mother has HbH disease (genotype – A/– -) whereas the father has alpha-thalassemia minor (genotype A – /A -).*

Case 2

A 68-year-old African-American woman comes to the office because of severe pain in her left wrist of 2 weeks duration. She tells you that she has had chronic arthritic pain for many years. Physical examination reveals ulnar deviation of the metacarpophalangeal joints.

QUESTION: *Which of the following findings would not apply to this patient?*

a. Decreased serum erythropoietin
b. Elevated serum ferritin
c. Low serum iron
d. Low transferrin saturation
e. Microcytosis

ANSWER: *All of the above are common findings in patients with anemia of chronic disease except d, which is a typical finding in iron deficiency.*

Case 3

A 30-year-old intravenous drug user infected with HIV comes to your clinic complaining of generalized weakness and "body pain." He is taking only AZT. The physical examination is normal.

Laboratory data:
White blood cell count 5200
Hemoglobin 11
Hematocrit 32.5%
MCV 105
Platelets 130,000
Red cell distribution width 13
Reticulocyte count 0.1%

QUESTION: *The most likely cause of the patient's hematological abnormalities is _____.*

a. HIV induced hemolytic anemia
b. Cobalamin deficiency
c. AZT toxicity
d. Non-Hodgkin's lymphoma
e. Toxoplasmosis

ANSWER: a. *Weakness, myalgia, and anemia with macrocytosis are common side effects seen*

in patient on AZT. These symptoms usually resolve once the drug is discontinued. If the hemogram does not normalize another diagnosis should be pursued.

COAGULATION DISORDERS

Pathophysiologic Correlation

The evaluation of a patient with a hemostatic disorder requires a good understanding of the coagulation system (see Table 14.7).

Hemostasis refers to the process that prevents bleeding after an injury to a blood vessel. This system, when not regulated properly, may cause thrombosis or emboli. The mechanism depends on the proper interaction between platelet, plasma coagulation factors, and the exposed injured vessel wall. Under normal circumstances the body can control small vessel hemorrhages, and even a more severe trauma may not cause major problems if the hemostatic mechanism functions correctly. Obviously trauma to a large artery or vein will require a more aggressive intervention, such as pressure on the site of injury, vessel ligation, or sutures.

The hemostatic process is usually divided into primary and secondary hemostasis to better explain the complex interactions occurring after a vessel injury. It should be emphasized that much of the currently available information about hemostasis is

Table 14.7.
Disorders of Hemostasis

Platelet Disorders (Primary)	Vascular Disorders	Blood Coagulation Disorders (Secondary)
Quantitative platelet disorders	Nonthrombocytopenic purpura	Congenital
Thrombocytopenia	Hereditary telangiectasia	Hemophilia
Increased destruction		von Willebrand's disease
Decreased production		Acquired
Sequestration		Vitamin K deficiency
Thrombocytosis		Nephrotic syndrome
Qualitative platelet disorders		Amyloidosis
Congenital		Circulating anticoagulant
Disorders of adhesion		Diffuse intravascular coagulation
Disorders of aggregation		
Disorders of secretion		
Acquired		
Myeloproliferative disorders		
Liver disease		
Diffuse intravascular coagulation		
Uremia		
Drug		
Antiplatelet antibody		

Table 14.8.
Clinical Differences in Primary and Secondary Hemostasis

	Platelet Disorder (Primary)	Plasma Protein Defects (Secondary)
Usual types of complaints	Skin; mucous membrane (gastrointestinal, genitourinary)	"Deep" joint, muscle, retro-peritoneal
Bleeding occurrences	Immediate	Delayed after trauma
Family history	Usually negative or autosomal dominant	Mostly positive, cross-linked or autosomal
Physical examination	Petechiae, ecchymosis	Hematoma, hemarthrosis
Therapy	Local pressure may be effective; rapid response to treatment	Local pressure not effective, prolonged systemic therapy often necessary

a result of in vitro laboratory study. In the actual in vivo process different hemostatic interactions may happen at the same time or in other sequences.

PRIMARY HEMOSTASIS

Primary hemostasis refers to the platelet plug formation as it occurs at the site of injury. The reaction is triggered by the collagen exposed from the subendothelium, causing platelet adhesion, activation, and aggregation. This process is activated seconds after the injury and is completed in a few minutes. The von Willebrand factor is one component involved in this phase. The bleeding time is the test that studies primary hemostasis.

SECONDARY HEMOSTASIS

Secondary hemostasis describes the complex interactions that occur among plasma proteins to form the fibrin clot around the platelet plug. The process is strongly related to thrombin formation and modulated by interactions with fibrinolytic proteins. It requires minutes to be completed (Table 14.8).

Clinical and Laboratory Evaluation

In the medical office the evaluation of the hemostatic process commonly occurs in two settings: the patient describes episodes of spontaneous or excessive traumatic bleeding or as preoperative screening before a surgical procedure. A good history and physical examination may help establish the correct diagnosis, but the laboratory evaluation is more important.

Table 14.9.
Evaluation of the Bleeding Patient (History)

Bleeding at multiple sites and on multiple occasions suggests a systemic coagulopathy
Example: life-long history of easy bruising or bleeding suggests a congenital coagulopathy (e.g., a factor deficiency)
Response to common stresses
Dental extraction, laceration, menses, labor and delivery
Example: von Willebrand's disease, minor factor deficiency
Family history
Bleeding in males only (hemophilia)
Bleeding in both sexes—von Willebrand's disease (factor XI deficiency)
Drugs
Inquire about all medications including over-the counter drugs that patients often overlook; remember the most common drugs affecting the platelets are aspirin and nonsteroidal anti-inflammatories.

HISTORY

The patient's history may contain several elements that can give a clue to the diagnosis (Table 14.9). The suspicion of a systemic coagulopathy should arise when bleeding occurs at multiple sites and on several occasions without any history of trauma. A family history of bleeding disorders must be investigated, especially in men because hemophilia accounts for most congenital coagulopathies. History of excessive bleeding in response to common stressful situations (e. g., menstruation, labor and delivery, surgical procedures, dental extraction, or trauma) should alert the practitioner about a possible coagulopathy in a patient with no signs or symptoms of spontaneous bleeding. An accurate history of all medications and drugs taken is essential, specifically those affecting the platelets (aspirin, antibiotics, Coumadin, nonsteroidal anti-inflammatory drugs, alcohol). Questions should also include over-the-counter drugs because many patients, particularly the elderly, do not know about adverse reactions.

From the history one should be able to distinguish between a defect involving the platelet or the plasma coagulation system. The bleeding caused by an abnormality of secondary hemostasis, for example, often occurs hours or days after trauma or surgery and mostly in joint spaces, muscles, subcutaneous areas, or body cavities. Local pressure may slow the hemorrhage, but it generally recurs once it is removed. When the defect involves primary hemostasis, bleeding immediately follows the trauma or surgery. The hemorrhage is mostly localized to skin or mucous membranes; it can be well controlled with local pressure, and it does not recur once the pressure is removed. Any bleeding should be investigated for the possible source even in the presence of an underlying coagulopathy (e.g., polyp or ulcer if gastrointestinal bleeding).

PHYSICAL EXAMINATION

The evaluation of the skin and mucous membranes may reveal the presence of petechiae or purpura (Table 14.10). Petechiae are red or brown round

Table 14.10.
Physical Examination of the Bleeding Patient

Joints
Deformities of large weight-bearing joints
Acute hemarthroses (think of severe plasma coagulation disorder)
Organomegaly
Enlarged spleen
Platelet sequestration
Hepatomegaly
Vitamin K-dependent factor deficiency
Low fibrinogen—dysfibrinogenemia
Skin
Petechiae (do not blanch with pressure)
Low platelet (look in dependent areas)
Ecchymoses
Platelet dysfunction
Hematomas
Platelet dysfunction
Telangeltasias (blanch with pressure)
Hereditary disorders

spots, generally 1–2 mm in diameter, arising from microvessel hemorrhages into the skin. They are not raised and do not blanch on pressure. These lesions commonly occur in areas of high venous pressure, e.g., lower extremities (or in the lumbosacral area if the patient is bedridden). Purpura refers to coalescent petechiae, and petechiae are also a sign of thrombocytopenia. Ecchymoses are large subcutaneous collections of blood consequent to leakage from small vessels. They are often secondary to traumas. When palpable they are called hematomas. It is important to recognize these lesions and be able to differentiate them from others such as telangiectasia (secondary to vascular abnormalities), because the latter may cause bleeding in several sites but is not secondary to a hemostatic disorder. Hemarthrosis is a common manifestation of hemophilia that often requires hospitalization. Its recurrence eventually results in joint deformities.

The spleen should be carefully evaluated (see "Anemia") because it may enlarge in many neoplastic, infective, or other disorders (e.g., liver cirrhosis), resulting in thrombocytopenia.

LABORATORY EVALUATION

There are few screening tests used to diagnose bleeding disorders (Table 14.11). Platelet count and bleeding time assess the primary hemostatic system. Prothrombin time (PT), activated partial thromboplastin time (aPTT), and thrombin time are the screening tests for the plasma coagulation functions (secondary hemostasis). These tests will be described under "Differential Diagnosis."

Differential Diagnosis

When the bleeding history is unclear or an abnormal test is discovered, it is important to make the correct diagnosis so the appropriate therapy can be instituted and the risk of surgery or possible trauma minimized.

DISORDERS OF PRIMARY HEMOSTASIS

Platelet disorders are divided into quantitative and qualitative (Table 14.7). The platelet is part of the cytoplasm of the megakaryocyte. The different stages of thrombopoiesis are under the influence of several cytokines that provide stimuli for the maturation of the stem cell to the megakaryocyte. Platelets are constantly produced; the average survival is 8–10 days. Two-thirds of the platelets are in circulation, and one-third is in the spleen. Under stressful conditions the spleen will "squeeze out"

Table 14.11.
Laboratory Evaluation of the Bleeding Patient

Platelet Disorders (Primary Hemostasis)			
Platelet count			
Bleeding time			
Platelet function tests			
von Willebrand's assays			

Plasma Protein Deficiencies (Secondary Hemostasis)			
Test	Technique	Mechanism Tested	Abnormal Value
PT	Mix citrate test plasma with a source of tissue factor (rabbit brain extract) Ca^{2+} and phospholipid	Measures factors in extrinsic and common pathways	Liver disease, DIC, defect in vitamin-K dependent factors, warfarin therapy
aPTT	Mix citrate test plasma with an activator of factor XII (kaolin) Ca^{2+} and phospholipid	Measures factors in intrinsic and common pathways	Deficits in contact factors, DIC, deficiencies in factors XII, XI, and IX; to monitor heparin therapy, hemophilia, von Willebrand's disease, circulating anticoagulants
TT	Diluted thrombin is added to citrated test plasma	Measures conversion of fibrinogen to fibrin (sensitive test × screen fibrogen and detect inhibitors)	Abnormal fibrogen (qualitative-quantitative) DIC, fibrin split product, substance interference with fibrin formation (heparin)
Inhibitor screen	50 : 50 mix of normal and test plasma when initial screening showed prolonged PT or PTT	Measures presence of an inhibitor (usually an antibody)	Failure to correct implies presence of the inhibitor of coagulation
Factor assays	Mix test plasma with specific factor-deficient plasmas and plotting activity (fibrin generation times) against a standard curve	Measures level of individual factors	

DIC, diffuse intravascular clotting.

the remaining platelets into the circulation, and the production may increase up to 10-fold. Platelet function can be divided into four phases: adhesion, aggregation, secretion, and clot formation.

The adhesion phase allows the platelets to anchor and spread to the injured vessel. It involves among other proteins the von Willebrand factor (vWF).

Platelet aggregation contributes to the formation of the hemostatic plug. This phase is modulated by specific substances that potentiate the reaction (agonists), e.g., thromboxane and prostaglandin. Aspirin and other nonsteroidal anti-inflammatory drugs inhibit the formation of these agonists that act on the precursor arachidonic acid.

The secretory phase that follows allows excretion of the platelet granules. These contain numerous factors involved in the clot formation.

The last phase, clot retraction, requires factor XIII or fibrin stabilizing factor. Its absence makes the clot soft and inflexible and therefore unstable (bleeding time).

It is difficult to predict what platelet count will be associated with significant clinical bleeding. Most of the experience derives from patients with acute leukemia where it is known that the lower the platelet count, the higher the risk of significant hemorrhage. The normal platelet count is between 150,000 and 450,000 platelets/ml^3. No clinical bleeding usually occurs when the platelet count is above 100,000 per ml^3 and the bleeding time also is normal. With a platelet count below 100,000 but above 50,000/ml^3 the patient may undergo minor surgical procedures, but if the bleeding time is prolonged, significant hemorrhage may occur after severe trauma. When the count is between 50,000 and 20,000 platelets/ml^3 the patient may experience easy bruising, menorrhagia, or bleeding even after minor surgery, but major fatal hemorrhages are unusual. A platelet count of <20,000/ml^3 is associated with a high incidence of spontaneous bleeding (i.e., intracranial, gastrointestinal), and prophylactic platelet transfusion is often necessary.

Quantitative Platelet Disorders. Quantitative platelet disorders (i.e., thrombocytopenia and thrombocytosis) can be divided according to the kinetic derangement.

Thrombocytopenia can occur as consequence of decreased or faulty production, increased destruction, or sequestration and loss of platelets. Decreased production is often secondary to drugs, toxins, or ionizing radiation that specifically targets the megakaryocyte (alcohol, cimetidine, thiazide diuretics, phenytoin, viral infections, radiotherapy, etc.). Aplastic anemia, myelofibrosis, cobalamin and folate deficiency, leukemia, and neoplastic infiltration of the bone marrow are also responsible for decreased production of platelets. It is therefore important to take an accurate history regarding drug exposure, viral illnesses, nutritional deficiencies, alcohol intake, etc.

Thrombocytopenia secondary to increased platelet destruction can be congenital or acquired and immune or nonimmune mediated. Viral and bacterial infection are among the causes of nonimmune thrombocytopenia. Gram-positive and -negative bacteria have been associated with increased platelet destruction by toxin production; common viruses, such as herpes simplex virus, cytomegalovirus, Epstein-Barr virus, mumps, and varicella may produce thrombocytopenia during the acute phase, and sometimes a low platelet count may last up to 2 months afterward. Disseminated intravascular coagulation, a serious complication of sepsis or cancer, causes platelet destruction by a nonimmune mechanism. Patients with aortic valve stenosis or prosthetic heart valves may have thrombocytopenia caused by an increased destruction from the mechanical trauma of the turbulent blood flow. Thrombotic thrombocytopenic purpura and its pediatric variant, the hemolytic uremic syndrome, are rare and complex disorders of unclear etiology with a high mortality rate.

In the medical clinic immune thrombocytopenia is frequently discovered in asymptomatic individuals during a routine examination. Sometimes the patient may seek medical attention because of petechiae, gingival bleeding, or epistaxis.

Idiopathic Thrombocytopenic Purpura. Idiopathic thrombocytopenic purpura (ITP) can be divided into acute and chronic forms. The acute ITP occurs usually during childhood. It is often preceded by a history of infection, generally viral. The abrupt onset is followed by a complete resolution in about 80% of the cases.

Chronic ITP typically occurs in adults (peak age 20–50), seldom resolves spontaneously, is a disease prevalent in women (3 : 1), and rarely strikes blacks. The etiology of the adult form of ITP is unclear. A history of infection is rare, and in 80–90% of the patients platelet associated immunoglobulin (Ig) is elevated. The platelet half-life is decreased. They are mainly destroyed in the spleen, but the liver and other sites of the reticuloendothelial system may be involved in severe cases. Occasionally active bleeding with a higher platelet count has been associated with an autoantibody that interferes with platelet function, complicating the clinical outcome.

Symptoms and signs of ITP vary greatly. Often the patient is asymptomatic; sometimes there is a longstanding history of easy bruising, recurrent epistaxis, or menorrhagia. Bleeding into mucous membranes or gastrointestinal or genitourinary tracts indicates severe thrombocytopenia and the need for emergency therapy. The potential for intracranial bleeding warrants careful neurological monitoring. The spleen is rarely palpable, and the presence of splenomegaly should argue against ITP as a primary diagnosis.

The diagnosis of ITP is one of exclusion because there are no specific tests. Platelet associated Ig is elevated in 90% of patients, but this is not a specific test. The peripheral blood smear shows decreased platelets with a predominance of larger forms.

Secondary ITP defines disorders associated with ITP as it occurs in patients with systemic lupus, HIV infection, lymphoproliferative disorders, or thyrotoxicosis. Useful diagnostic tests include CBC, antinuclear antibody, serum protein electrophoresis, quantitative immunoglobulins, liver enzymes, and thyroid function assays.

Thrombocytopenia complicating systemic lupus erythematosus occurs in about 20% of patients; the platelet count seldom goes below 50,000 platelets/ml^3; splenomegaly is a common finding; and bleeding complications are rare.

HIV Associated Thrombocytopenia. HIV associated thrombocytopenia has been described at all stages of infection. An immune mediated mechanism is believed to be the etiology, although many other factors can contribute to the low platelet count, including impaired platelet production, concurrent infections, or drug toxicity.

Drug Induced Immunologic Thrombocytopenia. Drug induced immunologic thrombocytopenia can be produced by many drugs. The most common and extensively studied are quinidine, quinine, and heparin. Quinine and quinidine can cause immune mediated thrombocytopenia in days to weeks of exposure; the frequency is about one in 1000 patients taking these drugs, and it is not dose related.

Heparin induced thrombocytopenia is not commonly seen in the outpatient population but is an important complication in hospitalized patients. There are two separate syndromes, a benign mild thrombocytopenia that is not immune mediated and a more severe immune mediated syndrome caused by an antibody of the IgG class induced by heparin. This last occurs rarely, is more frequent with the bovine type and is dose related (higher risk at higher doses). Paradoxically the more severe form produces thromboembolic complications such as strokes, pulmonary emboli, and myocardial infarction.

Thrombocytopenia Secondary to Sequestration in the Reticuloendothelial System. Hepatic and/or splenic sequestration are common occurrences in patients with liver disease (especially liver cirrhosis with portal hypertension) and any condition causing functional hypersplenism. The thrombocytopenia is rarely severe enough to cause hemorrhages. Splenectomy is rarely indicated.

Qualitative Platelet Disorders. Qualitative platelet disorders should be suspected when a patient with a normal platelet count has symptoms of unusual bleeding and/or a prolonged bleeding time. These abnormalities can be congenital or acquired. Petechiae are not seen in these disorders, but the most common complaints are epistaxis, increased bleeding after a dental or surgical procedure, and menorrhagia. The bleeding time is prolonged in all these disorders; therefore more specialized tests are necessary to make the diagnosis.

Congenital Qualitative Platelet Disorders. Congenital qualitative platelet disorders are divided according to what phase of the platelet function is affected (e.g., adhesion, aggregation, secretion, and procoagulant activity). Most often these disorders are diagnosed by a hematologist.

Acquired Qualitative Platelet Disorders. Hematologic disorders such as chronic myelocytic leukemia, myelofibrosis, polycythemia vera, acute leukemia, and the dysproteinemia of multiple myelomas have all been associated with bleeding diathesis secondary to platelet dysfunction. The platelets of uremic patients, for reasons still unclear, do not function properly. This is reflected by an abnormal bleeding time.

Drug Induced Platelet Disorders. Drug induced platelet disorders are quite common in clinical practice. Aspirin inhibits the enzyme cyclooxygenase in an irreversible manner so that the abnormality persists for the lifespan of the platelet. Nonsteroidal anti-inflammatory drugs also inactivate the same enzyme, but the effect is reversible and limited only to the time of drug exposure. The bleeding time is increased because of the blocking of the aggregation phase.

Thrombocytosis and Thrombocythemia. Thrombocytosis refers to an elevated platelet count secondary to other disease conditions (platelet $>400,000/ml^3$). It is distinguished from thrombocythemia or primary thrombocytosis, a group of myeloproliferative disorders (polycythemia vera, chronic myelogenous leukemia, primary thrombocytemia, agnogenic myeloid metaplasia) (Table 14.12).

Elevated platelet count is usually asymptomatic, but complications may occur when the count is >1 million platelets/ml^3, especially in the elderly. As opposed to thrombocytemia, no bleeding abnormalities occur in thrombocytosis; the blood cell morphology is normal, and there is no splenomegaly.

DISORDERS OF SECONDARY HEMOSTASIS

Once the platelet plug is formed, different plasma proteins interact to form the fibrin clot that stabilizes and replaces platelets (Table 14.13). These plasma proteins, the coagulation factors, circulate as inactive forms (called zymogens) and are activated into serine proteases by two different pathways. Factor V and factor VIII are exceptions because they have no enzymatic property and act as cofactors with their proper substrate (Fig. 14.2). The extrinsic pathway is initiated by tissue factors, whereas the intrinsic pathway is activated by surface contact.

The coagulation cascade is a simplified version of the in vivo reaction, and understanding is limited by the difficulties in reproducing this process in the laboratory. It is known that the endothelial surface is key as substrate and modulator in the

Table 14.12.
Common Causes of Platelet Elevation

Thrombocythemia (primary thrombocytosis)
Myeloproliferative disorders
  Polycythemia vera
  Chronic myelogenous leukemia
  Primary thrombocythemia
  Agnogenic myeloid metaplasia
Thrombocytosis (secondary or reactive thrombocytosis)
Chronic inflammatory states
  Tuberculosis
  Rheumatoid arthritis
  Hepatic cirrhosis
  Osteomyelitis
  Acute rheumatic fever
  Sarcoidosis
  Ulcerative colitis
  Regional enteritis
Acute hemorrhages
Iron deficiency
  Chronic blood loss
  Dietary deficiency
Recovery from acute infection
Malignancy
  Epithelial carcinomas
  Lymphomas
"Rebound"
  Bone marrow recovery after myelosuppressive
    drugs, alcohol
Physiological response to exercise
Surgery (post-op)

coagulation process. Both the intrinsic and extrinsic pathways lead to the activation of factor X. Activated factor X together with activated factor V, calcium, and phospholipids forms the prothrombinase complex that converts prothrombin to thrombin. This last acts on the fibrinogen molecule, modifying it into the insoluble fibrin.

Congenital Disorders of Blood Coagulation. Congenital disorders of blood coagulation factors (i.e., hemophilia, von Willebrand's disease) are relatively rare diseases often discovered in childhood. Most patients are under specialized care and should be treated only by an experienced physician. The routine laboratory evaluation of the plasma coagulation proteins includes the prothrombin time, aPTT, thrombin time, fibrinogen titer, inhibitor screen, and factors assays (see Tables 14.11 and 14.14).

Prothrombin Time. In testing the prothrombin time, the patient's plasma is mixed with rabbit brain extract (as source of tissue factor), phospholipids, and calcium. The prothrombin time measures factors in the extrinsic pathway including factors V, VII, and X, fibrinogen, and prothrombin. The test is used as the initial screening for acquired or congenital coagulation disorders and to monitor therapy with vitamin K antagonists.

Warfarin therapy is monitored following the ratio between the patient's prothrombin time versus a reference control. The World Health Organi-

Table 14.13.
Plasma Coagulation Factors

Name	Half-life	Calcium as Co-factor	Vitamin K Dependent	Comments
Factor XII (Hageman factor)	40–50 hr	no	no	
Prekallikrein	35 hr	no	no	contact factors
High Molecular weight, kininogen	6 days	no	no	
Factor XI	60–80 hr	no	no	
Factor X	24–48 hr	yes	yes	
Factor IX (Christmas factor)	20–24 hr	yes	yes	
Factor VIII	9–18 hr	no	no	
Factor VII	1.5–6 hr	yes	no	shortest half-life
Factor V	12–14 hr	yes	no	synthesized in liver
II (Prothrombin)	1–3 days	yes	yes	
I Fibrinogen	3–4 days	no	no	synthesized in liver
von Willebrand factor	24 hr	no	no	synthesized in endothelium and megacaryocytes

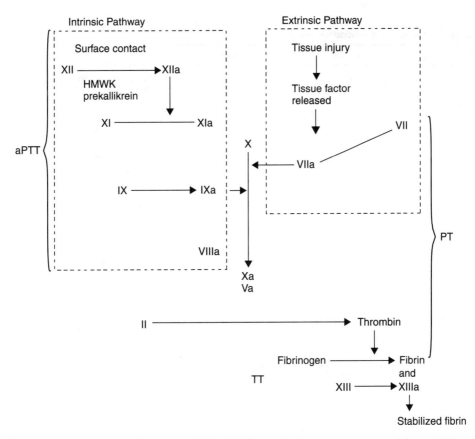

Figure 14.2. Coagulation cascade. HMWK, high molecular weight kininogen; a, activated form; aPTT, activated partial thromboplastin time; PT, prothrombin time; TT, thrombin time.

zation international reference thromboplastin was created to correct the differences in sensitivity among the numerous laboratory kits of tissue thromboplastin for prothrombin time assay. Results from these kits are compared with the standard reference. The international normalization ratio (INR) defines the relation between any new lot of thromboplastin and the World Health Organization international reference thromboplastin. Manufacturers usually include a conversion table to the equivalent INR. The therapeutic ranges for anticoagulation therapy are therefore expressed also as "recommended INR" (Table 14.15).

Prolonged prothrombin time occurs commonly in patients with vitamin K deficiency or liver disease or undergoing Coumadin therapy. The abnormality reflects deficiency in factors V, VII, and X, prothrombin or fibrinogen level below 100 mg/dl.

Activated Partial Thromboplastin Time. The aPTT test screens factors in the intrinsic and common pathways (XII, XI, X, IX, VIII, V, prothrombin, fibrinogen) and is commonly used to detect factor deficiencies, circulating anticoagulant (lupus-like), and to monitor heparin therapy. The test does not screen factors VII and XIII.

Thrombin Time. Thrombin time is the time required to form a clot when diluted thrombin is added to citrated plasma. The test is prolonged in the presence of qualitative or quantitative fibrinogen abnormalities, substances interfering with fibrin formation, fibrinogen split products, or heparin.

Inhibitor Screen. When the prothrombin time and/or aPTT are abnormal it is standard practice to perform an inhibitor screen. The patient's plasma is mixed with an equal volume of normal plasma (50 : 50 mix). Correction of the abnormality

Table 14.14.
Clinical Application of Some Laboratory Test Results

Abnormal Test(s)	Normal Test	Bleeding	Differential Diagnosis
PT	aPTT	+ −	Factor VII deficiency
			Warfarin
			Liver disease
			Vitamin K deficiency
		−	Deficit in factor XII
			Deficit in factor prekallikrein
			Deficit in HMWK
			Inhibitor (no correction with mix study)
aPTT	PT		Heparin
		+	Deficit in factor VIII (hemophilia A,B)
			Deficit in factor IX
			Deficit in factor XI
			Heparin
PT and aPTT		+ −	Factor II, V, and X deficiencies
			Vitamin K deficiency
			Liver disease
			DIC
			Massive transfusion (dilution)
Thrombin time	PT and aPTT	+ −	Hypofibrinogenemia
			Excess of heparin
			Dysfibrinogenemia
			FSP (DIC)

HMWK, high molecular weight kininogen; DIC, diffuse intravascular clotting; FSP, fibrin split products.

Table 14.15.
Recommended Therapeutic Ranges for Oral Anticoagulant Therapy Expressed in INR

Clinical Situation	Recommended INR
Prophylaxis high risk surgery	2.0–2.5
Prophylaxis DVT/PE (hip surgery)	2.0–3.0
DVT or PE Initial Treatment	2.0–3.0
Prevention of systemic embolism (patients with valvular heart disease, Postmyocardial infarction, atrial fibrillation organic heart valve)	2.0–3.0
Mechanical prosthetic heart valves or atrial fibrillation with systemic embolism or recurrent systemic embolism	3.0–4.5

DVT = deep venous thrombosis. PE = pulmonary embolism.

occurs in the presence of a factor deficiency, whereas failure to correct indicates the presence of a coagulation factor inhibitor, usually an antibody.

Acquired Disorders of Blood Coagulation. Acquired disorders of blood coagulation are more often encountered in an outpatient clinic. These may occur by different mechanisms, includ-ing vitamin K deficiency, liver disease, defibrination syndromes, circulating anticoagulant, and ne-phrotic syndrome. The most common ones are discussed here.

Vitamin K Deficiency. The body absorbs vita-min K mostly from green leafy vegetables and intes-tinal bacteria. It is not stored in the body. A vitamin K deficiency may develop in normal individuals in 1 or 2 weeks.

The vitamins act as a cofactor in the gamma-carboxylation of the glutamil residues during the synthesis of clotting factor zymogens in the liver. Factors VII, X, and IX and prothrombin (factor II) require vitamin K as a cofactor for their synthesis. They are all synthesized in the liver. Vitamin K deficiency occurs in malabsorption syndromes, poor dietary and intake, prolonged antibiotic use, causing sterilization of the intestinal tract and bile salt deficiency.

The diagnosis is based on the history and an abnormal prothrombin time-aPTT, but it is only proved by correction of the tests after administra-tion of vitamin K, usually within 12–24 hours.

Liver Disease. The liver synthesizes all the co-agulation factors except factor VIII. Diseases affect-ing the liver parenchyma can alter the synthesis of vitamin K dependent as well as other factors. Prolonged prothrombin time is considered a poor prognostic factor in patients with liver disease because it implies severe functional impairment. If correction of prothrombin time does not occur with 24 hours of vitamin K supplement, other etiologies besides terminal liver disease should be considered, such as dysfibrinogenemia, disseminated intravascular coagulation, etc. Bleeding abnormalities are corrected only by administration of fresh frozen plasma.

Acquired Anticoagulants. The development of acquired anticoagulants occurs commonly in patients affected by hemophilia, von Willebrand's disease, or other factor deficiencies as a natural response to the antigenic stimulation of multiple transfusions. Bleeding can be severe.

The most common cause of prolonged aPTT in asymptomatic patients is the presence of the "lupus anticoagulant." This is an antibody that arises from a dysfunctional immune system in patients with systemic lupus erythematosus or other autoimmune disorders, but it is also seen in patients with lymphoproliferative diseases, plasma cell disorders, AIDS, or in association with certain drugs. Failure to correct an abnormal aPTT with a 50:50 mixed dilution strongly implies the presence of an inhibitor.

The lupus anticoagulants are usually antibodies (IgG or IgM) against phospholipid or other coagulation proteins. It occurs in about 5–15% of patients with systemic lupus erythematosus or other conditions. The antibody produces a prolonged aPTT, but it is not associated with abnormal bleeding, stressing the differences between an in vitro test and the in vivo consequences. Paradoxically, the presence of the lupus anticoagulant has been associated with thrombotic episodes.

THROMBOSIS

Three major factors are involved in the pathophysiology of venous thrombosis: altered blood flow, abnormalities in the endothelium, and alteration of the clotting factors (Virchow triad).

Several regulatory and protective mechanisms physiologically limit the extension of the thrombus formation. Blood flow removes coagulation factors from the thrombus site but, more importantly, inhibits the thrombin action locally and decreases its production. These are crucial regulatory mechanisms.

Substances that locally inhibit the thrombus formation include antithrombin III, proteins C and S,

plasminogen activator factors, prostaglandin, and endothelial relaxation factors such as nitrous oxide.

Antithrombin III action is strongly enhanced by binding of heparin. Congenital abnormalities or deficiencies of this factor cause venous thrombosis. The congenital deficiency is an autosomal dominant disorder that occurs mostly before the age of 50 and accounts for about 3% of all venous thrombosis. An acquired form of antithrombin III deficiency occurs in patients with liver disease or nephrotic syndrome.

The most sensitive and specific test for the diagnosis of thromboembolic events is angiography. However, because of its cost, complications, and availability, other less invasive and expensive tests are used as an initial evaluation. These tests are less sensitive and specific and include plethysmography, duplex Doppler or echo Doppler.

Management

DISORDERS OF PRIMARY HEMOSTASIS

Disorders of primary hemostasis are important to recognize because the appropriate therapy may increase the survival rate to 80% and also because platelet transfusion is generally contraindicated.

Idiopathic Thrombocytopenic Purpura. The decision to treat ITP is based on the severity of the illness. Asymptomatic individuals with low platelet counts or normal bleeding time may not require therapy and could be followed regularly. The thrombocytopenic patient with symptomatic life threatening hemorrhage (i.e., intracranial) should be hospitalized and treated with platelet transfusion and high dose intravenous IgG concurrent with glucocorticoids.

Patients who require surgery or have mucosal bleeding can benefit from intravenous Ig (at doses of 400 mg/kg/day for 5 days) or intramuscular anti-D Ig, which is less expensive but only possible if the patient is Rh-positive. When chronic treatment is required steroids are used first. The most common regimen includes prednisone at a dose of 1 mg/kg. It may take days to weeks before the platelet count starts to rise. Once a satisfactory platelet count is reached and the patient is clinically stable, attempts should be made to decrease the steroids to the minimum effective dosage. This strategy is necessary to minimize the numerous side effects associated with glucocorticoids. If no improvement is noted after 2–3 weeks, splenectomy will result in a cure or long-term remission in about 60% of the patients. When these two modalities fail, alternative therapies with danazol, vincristine, colchicine, or splenic radiotherapy (especially in the elderly population) may be useful in selected cases.

For unclear reasons, about two-thirds of these patients with secondary ITP will respond to danazol (400–800 mg/day). Corticosteroids used judiciously in this population are reserved for treatment failures.

HIV Associated Thrombocytopenia. Treatment of the immune mediated form of HIV associated thrombocytopenia with AZT increases the platelet count in few cases. Corticosteroids should be used with caution because of the high incidence of opportunistic infection (most commonly oral candidiasis). Intravenous Ig and anti-D serum produces transient remission. Splenectomy remains the best option with long and sustained remissions and less morbidity, although an increased risk of septicemia is present.

Drug Induced Immunologic Thrombocytopenia. The drugs causing drug induced immunologic thrombocytopenia should be discontinued immediately. Severe or life threatening cases may benefit from high dose intravenous Ig with platelet transfusion; steroids have not shown any benefit. Platelet transfusions are strongly contraindicated. Heparin should be discontinued.

Hematologic Disorders. The pathogenesis of hematologic disorders involves different mechanisms. The therapy should target the primary disorder. Dialysis corrects the bleeding tendency in uremia. Deamino-8-D-arginine vasopressin infusion is the recommended treatment, although its effect is short lived. Platelet transfusion is not indicated because the platelets acquire the same host defect. Estrogen has been found to decrease the bleeding time in some studies. These drugs should be avoided in patients with platelet abnormalities.

Thrombocytosis and Thrombocythemia. The benign and often transient nature of thrombocytosis usually does not require treatment. Occasionally symptomatic patients can be treated with apheresis.

DISORDERS OF SECONDARY HEMOSTASIS

Treatment of underlying disease is the cornerstone of therapy. Vitamin K deficiency is the most common malady requiring treatment. In vitamin K deficiency, the vitamin is generally administered orally, but absorption is erratic. For very sick patients the intravenous route is preferred. Intramuscular injection can cause hematomas in patients with coagulopathy and is usually contraindicated.

THROMBOSIS

The treatment includes plasma infusion in patients undergoing surgery or on heparin therapy for thrombosis. An antithrombin III concentrate is under investigation.

The therapy in patients with recurrent thrombosis is long term oral anticoagulants. Remember and recognize the occurrence of skin necrosis in patients with heterozygous protein C deficiency when placed on Coumadin therapy.

The prevention and treatment of thrombosis include strategies aimed at different phases of thrombus formation. These include inhibition of platelet deposition, interference with fibrin formation, and thrombolysis. The main anticoagulant drugs are heparin, vitamin K antagonists (Coumadin), antiplatelet agents, and thrombolytic agents.

Heparin. Heparin is a cofactor for antithrombin III. Once the complex is formed, the inhibitory reaction of proteases is enhanced several times. Heparin has a half-life of 1–2 hours. It is administered subcutaneously or intravenously by bolus or continuous infusion. For the initial treatment of deep vein thrombosis or pulmonary embolism, the heparin dose is adjusted to an aPTT of 1.5–2.0 times the control, usually 50–80 seconds. The infusion is preferred to bolus because it requires less heparin and it is associated with fewer bleeding complications. Before a patient is started on heparin, a baseline platelet count should be obtained, and it should be repeated after 5 days or if bleeding occurs to monitor the risk of heparin associated thrombocytopenia. An excess of heparin is counteracted by the administration of protamine sulfate.

Recently low molecular weight heparin has been introduced into clinical practice with the advantage of a longer half-life and lower incidence of bleeding complications.

Aspirin. Aspirin irreversibly inhibits the platelet cyclooxygenase. The effect lasts for the entire lifespan of the exposed platelet (7–9 days). The most commonly used doses are 81 or 325 mg/day. Aspirin does not cause bleeding at these dosages unless there is an underlying bleeding diathesis (e.g., as in uremia).

Aspirin has been found to be worse than warfarin but better than placebo in patients with nonvalvular atrial fibrillation and is a good alternative for young patients who do not want to experience the side effects of warfarin.

In doses of 1300 mg/day aspirin reduced the incidence of stroke and death compared with a placebo group in a Canadian study and, for unclear reasons, with the male population (5). Because of the high incidence of gastrointestinal discomfort with high doses, low dose aspirin was studied. A few studies proved the efficacy of low dose aspirin (75–300 mg/day) in reducing the incidence of recurrent stroke or myocardial infarction in patients with coronary artery disease, although this benefit was unclear for transient ischemic attacks (6–8).

Aspirin is recommended after coronary artery bypass surgery in a dose of 325 mg/day starting a few hours after the operation and continuing for 1 year.

Aspirin prolongs the bleeding time and may cause increased bleeding during surgical procedures. For this reason it is usually discontinued 1 week before an operation. Only platelet transfusion will correct bleeding defects secondary to aspirin ingestion.

Dipyridamole.   Dipyridamole is a platelet inhibitor whose action seems to involve the metabolism of cyclic adenosine monophosphatase. It is also a coronary vasodilator. The drug has been found effective in conjunction with Coumadin in preventing postoperative thromboembolism after artificial heart valve replacement.

Dipyridamole has not been found useful, alone or in combination with aspirin, in the treatment of coronary artery or cerebrovascular disease (5, 9). The dose ranges from 75 to 100 mg four times a day.

Ticlopidine.   Ticlopidine is a relatively new antiplatelet drug. The mechanism of action has not been completely discovered. Ticlopidine does not affect the cyclooxygenase pathway or the cyclic adenosine monophosphatase metabolism. The drug apparently causes inhibition of both platelet aggregation and granule release, which is dose and time dependent. Its maximal effect occurs in 24–48 hours. It is irreversible and disappears within 1 week after the drug is discontinued. The bleeding time can be prolonged two- to five-fold.

The Ticlopidine Aspirin Stroke Study randomized about 3000 patients with transient ischemic attack or minor stroke to one of the two drugs. Ticlopidine was found more effective in reducing the incidence of death and nonfatal stroke (10).

In the Canadian American Ticlopidine Study the drug was compared with placebo and was found to be useful in the secondary prevention of stroke (11). Side effects such as reversible bone marrow

suppression (neutropenia), diarrhea, and skin rash, together with the cost, are negative aspects of this drug when compared with aspirin. The usual dose is 250 mg twice a day. A monthly CBC should be obtained in the first 3 months of therapy.

Warfarin.   The family of the coumarin drugs, such as warfarin, compete with vitamin K for a common receptor site. The lack of vitamin K or the presence of warfarin impairs the carboxylation of the vitamin K-dependent clotting factors (factors II, VII, IX, and X), resulting in nonfunctional proteins. The prothrombin time is the test that more closely reflects the therapeutic activity of warfarin, and, as mentioned previously, the optimal therapeutic range for anticoagulant is expressed in INR (Table 14.15).

Warfarin has been found effective in preventing thromboembolic events in patients with nonvalvular atrial fibrillation. The benefits are more pronounced in older populations, although benefits are unclear in patients older than 75 years. The drug is also recommended for 6 months after placement of a bioprosthetic valve, but if the patient has atrial fibrillation warfarin should be continued indefinitely. Patients with mechanical prosthetic heart valves are also placed on lifelong warfarin therapy.

Aspirin should never be prescribed to a patient on warfarin. The physician must also be aware of the potential drug interactions that warfarin may cause (i.e., barbiturates induce microsomal activation and increase the metabolism of warfarin, consequently diminishing the anticoagulant effect). The dose of warfarin is generally titrated to the recommended INR. It is common practice to start to anticoagulate a patient with a daily dose of 10 mg orally for 3 days and follow the prothrombin time and the INR on a regular basis until a steady state is achieved.

ANTICOAGULANT DURING PREGNANCY

Warfarin is contraindicated in pregnancy; therefore heparin should be used in these patients. Patients with prosthetic heart valves, atrial fibrillation with documented systemic embolisms, deep vein thrombosis, or pulmonary embolism on warfarin therapy should be switched to heparin when pregnancy is diagnosed.

Subcutaneous heparin is injected every 12 hours and the dose adjusted to maintain an aPTT 1.5–2 times control measured 6 hours after the injection. Heparin therapy has been found useful in patients with recurrent spontaneous abortion associated with antiphospholipid antibodies.

THROMBOSIS ASSOCIATED WITH CANCER

The association between cancer and thromboembolism was first observed by Trousseau more than a century ago. Numerous factors are responsible, and among them surgery, radiotherapy and chemotherapy are important.

Systemic anticoagulants such as heparin or warfarin are less effective in cancer patients and are associated with an increased risk of hemorrhages.

When there are no known contraindications, heparin followed by warfarin is still the recommended approach. However, the placement of a mechanical filter (Greenfield filter) is more often advocated by some authors.

PERIOPERATIVE PATIENTS

The perioperative patient should be screened to predict and prevent possible hemostatic or thrombotic problems (e.g., deep vein thrombosis) related to surgery. A practical approach is described in Table 14.16.

If the patient is already on an anticoagulant it is wise to discontinue it in a timely fashion. When aspirin is used it should be stopped 7–10 days before surgery, whereas if the patient is on a nonsteroidal anti-inflammatory drug, the drug should be discontinued 1 or 2 days before the operation.

Ticlopidine has a longer half-life, and its use must be discontinued 10–14 days before. The patient taking dipyridamole or heparin can safely stop the medication the day before because of the short half-life. Sometimes heparin, in low doses, is used during surgery as deep vein thrombosis prophylaxis.

Coumadin is frequently used as long term therapy, and the practitioner is often asked to withhold it before surgical procedures. For minor dental surgery and even cataract surgery, warfarin is safely continued. However, most of the time it must be discontinued to allow a safe surgical procedure. There is no clear or definite data regarding the optimal time to discontinue warfarin. A recent study partially addressed these issues (11). Patients on warfarin with an INR of 2.0–3.0 and on a steady-state required an average of 96–115 hours (four doses) discontinuation to achieve an INR of 1.2, which is considered safe for surgery. Patients with an INR of >3.0 or elderly patients required more time.

Table 14.16.
Practical Approach to Screen for Hemostasis in Perioperative Patients

Why Screen?
Predict and prevent bleeding problems related to surgery
Assess risk for deep vein thrombosis and/or pulmonary embolism

History—What to Ask
Do you bleed a long time after minor cuts or trauma?
   If yes, how old were you when this began and, how long has it occurred?
Do you develop large bruises with no good reason?
Did you bleed for a long time after a dental procedure?
Did you ever have an operation? Did you have any bleeding problems during or after surgery? Were you transfused with a blood product?
Do you drink alcohol? If yes, how much?
What medications do you take?
   Any over-the-counter drugs?
   What medicines have you taken in the past 5–7 days?
Any family member with a bleeding problem?

Physical Examination
Look for petechiae, ecchymosis, joint deformities (weight bearing joints)

Laboratory—What Tests to Order
Minor surgery and negative history—no screening tests needed
Major surgery and negative history—prothrombin time, aPTT, platelet count
Major surgery and questionable or positive history—prothrombin time, aPTT, platelet count, bleeding time

ILLUSTRATIVE CASES WITH SELF-ASSESSMENT QUESTIONS AND ANSWERS

Case 1

An 82-year-old man comes to the office complaining of fatigue and weight loss. He has a history of hypertension, non-insulin dependent diabetes mellitus and peptic ulcer disease; 6 weeks before this visit he underwent partial gastrectomy for a bleeding ulcer. His medications include glyburide, chlorthalidone, ranitidine, and enalapril. The physical examination revealed an underweight elderly man with no petechiae or ecchymosis and no mucosal bleeding. He had normal vital signs, no orthostatic changes, and no abnormal findings. The laboratory evaluation showed

White blood cell count 6500
Platelets 24,000
aPTT 33 (35) (control 35)
Hemoglobin 12.5
Hematocrit 35.7
SMA 20 normal
MCV 85
Prothrombin time 12.4 (control 11.3)

QUESTION: *Based on this information what would you do?*

a. Transfer the patient immediately to the emergency room for platelet transfusion.
b. Send a blood specimen for platelet activated Ig test.
c. Get a more detailed history and review the peripheral blood smear.
d. Perform a bone marrow aspiration and biopsy to eliminate leukemia.

ANSWER: c. *In this patient a history of new drug exposure, over-the-counter medication, and quinine use (tonic water) should be obtained. Ranitidine more frequently than enalapril or chlorthalidone has been associated with thrombocytopenia that generally resolves after discontinuation of the offending drug. The drugs should be withheld and the platelet count monitored, perhaps while he is hospitalized.*

There is no need to send the patient for an emergency platelet transfusion because he is not acutely bleeding.

The platelet associated Ig test is used to diagnose immune thrombocytopenia. Because the test is nonspecific it should not be ordered for screening purposes.

Case 2

A 55-year-old man that you have followed in the clinic for the past 6 months comes for preoperative medical clearance. The patient is a salesperson who frequently travels overseas by airplane. He had an episode of deep vein thrombosis 4 months ago that required hospitalization, and he has hypertension; otherwise he still enjoys jogging a few miles twice a week. He does not smoke or drink. The surgery is an elective cholecystectomy scheduled in 3 weeks. He is on a steady dose of warfarin, and his last prothrombin time was 21 (11.4) with an INR of 2.7. He is also taking hydrochlorothiazide.

QUESTION: *What would you advise?*

a. Monitor the prothrombin time daily for the next 3 weeks, adjusting the warfarin to an INR of 1.2.
b. Stop warfarin 1 week before surgery and monitor the prothrombin time and the INR. Start subcutaneous heparin when the INR is < 2.
c. Place an inferior vena cava filter (Greenfield filter).

ANSWER: b. *Although there are no well published guidelines or studies addressing this issue, it is common practice to discontinue warfarin at least 1 week before surgery and to continue anticoagulation with subcutaneous heparin. This patient seems to be well controlled on warfarin and at low to moderate risk for surgery. A Greenfield filter would be indicated for high risk patients, e.g., patients with recurrent pulmonary embolisms from deep vein thrombosis.*

Case 3

A 67-year-old woman returns to your clinic 1 week after hospital discharge. She was treated for osteomyelitis with intravenous antibiotics and released on oral medications. She said that it took longer than normal to stop a small cut on her finger from bleeding. She denies hematemesis, melena, or mucosal bleeding. Her medical problems also include chronic angina pectoris, diabetes mellitus, and hiatal hernia.

She is taking insulin, a calcium channel blocker, an antacid, and the prescribed antibiotic. The physical examination reveals an obese woman of her stated age with no petechiae and no ecchymosis. Bowel sounds were decreased, and the remaining examination was benign. The laboratory tests are as follow:

White blood cell count 12,000
Fibrinogen 300
Hemoglobin 11.0
Prothrombin time 19.6 (10.3)
Hematocrit 32.7
aPTT 32.2 (31.7)
MCV 101
SMA 20 normal
Platelets 300,000

QUESTION: *What is the likely cause of prolonged prothrombin time in this patient?*

a. Chronic osteomyelitis with disseminated intravascular coagulation
b. Diabetes mellitus with gastroparesis
c. Pernicious anemia
d. Vitamin malabsorption from prolonged antibiotic use

ANSWER: d. *Vitamin malabsorption is a common complication of antibiotic therapy. Abnormalities in the clotting factor became more frequent because of the introduction of the third generation cephalosporin.*

REFERENCES

Anemia

1. Massey AC. Microcytic anemia. Differential diagnosis and management of iron deficiency anemia. Med Clin North Am 1992;76:549–566 (review).
2. Fuchs D, et al. Immune activation and the anemia associated with chronic inflammatory disorders. Eur J Haematol 1991;46:65–70 (review).
3. Bailey LB. Folate status assessment. J Nutr 1990;120(suppl 11):1508–1511.
4. Metz J. Cobalamin deficiency and the pathogenesis of nervous systemic disease. Ann Rev Nutr 1992;12:59–79.

Coagulation Disorders

5. Canadian Cooperative Study Group. A randomized trial of aspirin and sulfinpyrazone in threatened stroke. N Engl J Med 1978;299:53–59.
6. Levy M. Aspirin use in patients with major upper gastrointestinal bleeding and peptic-ulcer disease. N Engl J Med 1974;290:1158–1162.
7. Bornstein NM, Karepov VG, et al. Failure of aspirin treatment after stroke. Stroke 1994;25:275–277.
8. Dyken ML. Controversies in stroke: past and present. The Williis lecture. Stroke 1993;24:1251–1258.
9. Gent M, Blakely JA, Hachinski V, et al. A secondary prevention, randomized trial of sulocitidil in patients with a recent history of thromboembolic stroke. Stroke 1985;16:416–424.
10. Hass WK, Easton JD, Adams HP Jr, et al. A randomized trial comparing ticlopidine hydrochloride with aspirin for the prevention of stroke in high risk patients. N Engl J Med 1989;321:501–507.
11. White RH, McKittrick T, et al. Temporary discontinuation of warfarin therapy: changes in the International Normalized Ration. Ann Intern Med 1995;122:40–42.

SUGGESTED READINGS

Anemia

Damon LE. Anemia of chronic disease in the aged: diagnosis and treatment. Geriatrics 1992;47:47–54, 57.

Ferguson BS, et al. Serum transferrin receptors distinguishes the anemia of chronic disease from iron deficiency. J Lab Clin Med 1992;119:385–390.

Guyatt GH, et al. Laboratory diagnosis of iron deficiency anemia: an overview. J Gen Intern Med 1992;7:145–153.

Kazazian HH. The thalassemia syndrome. Molecular basis and prenatal diagnosis in 1990. Semin Hematol 1990;27:206–228.

Mohler ER Jr. Iron deficiency and anemia of chronic disease. Clues to differentiating these conditions. Postgrad Med 1992;92:123–128.

Coagulation Disorders

EAFT (European Atrial Fibrillation Trial) Study Group. Secondary prevention in non-rheumatic atrial fibrillation after transient ischaemic attack or minor stroke. Lancet 1993;342:1255–1262.

Fihn SD, McDonell M, Martin D, et al. Risk factors for complications of chronic anticoagulation: a multicenter study. Ann Intern Med 1993;118:511–520.

Sinha RK, Kelton JG. Current controversies concerning the measurement of platelet-associated IgG. Transfusion Med Rev 1990;4:121–135.

Stroke Prevention in Atrial Fibrillation Investigators. Predictors of thromboembolism in atrial fibrillation. I. Clinical features of patients at risk. Ann Intern Med 1992;16:1–5.

Stroke Prevention in Atrial Fibrillation Investigators. Stroke prevention in atrial fibrillation study: final results. Circulation 1991;84:527–539.

Stroke Prevention in Atrial Fibrillation Investigators. Warfarin versus aspirin for prevention of thromboembolism in Atrial Fibrillation II Study. Lancet 1994;343:687–691.

chapter 15

PULMONARY MEDICINE

Cynthia M. Chong, Lori A. Lemberg, and Christine Oman

COUGH

Cough commonly brings patients to medical attention. Patients may present with sudden severe symptoms caused by the self-limiting common cold or they may be unaware of the chronic cough heralding terminal lung cancer. Although infection, whether minor or serious, usually induces acute cough, uncovering the etiology of chronic cough can be a challenging medical problem.

This section reviews the major causes of acute and chronic cough, noting the features of the history and physical exam that lead to the correct diagnosis. Discussion of management will focus on the proper role of nonspecific cough remedies and the decision whether to hospitalize a patient with pneumonia. Finally some cases illustrate the diagnostic challenge of chronic cough.

Pathophysiologic Correlation

Cough protects air exchange by removing foreign material from the bronchial tree, trachea, and larynx. When the respiratory mucociliary clearance mechanism cannot remove the irritant, because of excess mucus and debris or impaired ciliary motility, the patient coughs. People normally cough several times each day, unobtrusively swallowing material displaced into the pharynx; fewer coughs occur at night, especially in the deeper sleep stages. The same mechanisms initiate and effect both pathologic and normal cough.

Cough receptors are stimulated to initiate cough. Located throughout the larynx, trachea, bronchi, and bronchioles, they concentrate at areas such as bifurcations of the bronchi, where foreign particles precipitate out of the airstream. The ear canals, paranasal sinuses, pericardium, and diaphragm, among other sites, also contain cough receptors. Infections (e.g., the common cold) can up-

regulate cough receptors, leaving the patient highly sensitive to cough stimulation for several weeks. Cough receptors appear similar yet distinct from receptors initiating bronchoconstriction; cough often exacerbates bronchoconstriction and vice versa, but each can be experimentally induced while blocking the other.

Most sensory stimulation from cough receptors travels via the vagus nerve, although other cranial nerves and the phrenic nerve convey sensory data from the nonpulmonary sites they innervate. The cough center, whose role is unclear, rests in the medulla and regulates the cough reflex. The vagus, among other efferent nerves that control the diaphragm, the intracostal and abdominal muscles, and the musculature of the upper airways, carries the impulse to initiate the cough. Impaired nerve or muscle function diminishes the power of cough, increasing the risk of infection and aspiration.

A cough begins with deep inspiration. Closure of the glottis follows; then the thoracic muscles contract to increase pleural pressure and compress the airways. When the glottis opens, air rushes out at tremendous velocity along compressed airways. Turbulence and high shear forces propel foreign material and sputum up and into the pharynx. A cough is audible as the larynx and trachea vibrate.

Cough is thus a normal defense against abnormal irritants, infection, or overproduction of pulmonary secretions; suppressing this protective mechanism can be harmful. Irritants include cigarette smoke, foreign bodies, caustic gases, gastric acid in patients with reflux, secretions from the sinuses in patients with sinusitis, and compression from tumors. Depending on the host, infections run the gamut of viruses, bacteria, fungi, and parasites. The copious sputum produced by patients with chronic bronchitis or bronchiectasis must be cleared by coughing.

Several anatomic points bear emphasis in discussing cough. The path through the trachea to the right mainstem bronchus is relatively straight; aspirated material preferentially travels to the right lung. Arising from the third cervical nerve (C3), the phrenic nerve innervates the diaphragm. Irritation of the diaphragm causes referred pain to the ipsilateral shoulder via other branches of C3. Finally, because the esophageal and tracheal outlets are located together, patients aspirate refluxed gastric acids and surreptitiously swallow sputum.

Clinical and Laboratory Evaluation

The clinical approach to the coughing patient has two goals. The clinician must first discern the etiology of the cough, and then, in patients with a pulmonary infection, determine the severity of the illness to select inpatient or outpatient treatment. In most cases, the diagnosis emerges during a careful history.

HISTORY

Patients may visit their health care provider complaining of cough, or, particularly with patients who cough on a daily basis, the provider may notice the cough first, through simple observation or during the review of systems. Patients with chronic cough eventually seek medical care because they feel the cough is a sign of "something wrong"; in addition, they may fear cancer, tuberculosis, or AIDS or suffer from complications of coughing (e.g., loss of sleep, musculoskeletal pain, or stress incontinence).

Time Course. The distinction between acute cough and chronic cough is important because the etiologies are different. Because increased cough stimulation persists for several weeks after acute viral upper respiratory infection, acute and chronic coughs are not easily distinguished by counting the number of days or weeks of coughing. An acute cough from upper respiratory infection or foreign body inhalation usually has a rapid, well-defined onset. The patient with chronic cough can rarely define the onset.

After understanding the initiation of coughing, inquire about the progression of severity of the cough. A mild cough that later worsens and becomes productive of purulent sputum characterizes pneumonia or bronchitis superimposed on a viral upper respiratory infection. A chronic, familiar smoker's cough that changes character or frequency alerts the physician to lung cancer. An acute, disruptive cough that later becomes milder

and less frequent suggests an acute upper respiratory infection with lingering hypersensitivity to cough stimulation. Diurnal variations in the cough or exacerbation with certain activities suggest diagnoses such as postnasal drip (nighttime, early morning), cardiac failure (lying flat), or exercise-induced asthma.

Associated Symptoms. Any fever associated with the cough suggests an infectious cause; cough with fever and a shaking chill is the classic presentation of pneumococcal pneumonia. Upper respiratory symptoms such as nasal stuffiness, ear pain and pressure, sore throat, headache, and conjunctivitis also suggest infection as the source of the cough. Chronic upper respiratory symptoms may reveal sinusitis to be the cause. A history of wheezing is important since cough is a major symptom of asthma; in contrast, occasional patients without underlying asthma wheeze only during acute bronchitis. Gastrointestinal symptoms that accompany cough can be helpful. Whereas the force of coughing can induce nausea, regurgitation, and even abdominal pain from muscular strain, symptoms such as diarrhea and vomiting suggest viral infection or Legionnaire's disease. Chronic reflux or aspiration may be the cause of cough in patients with dyspepsia. Elderly patients with pneumococcal pneumonia may present with prominent abdominal symptoms and minimal cough.

Inquire about chest pain, and pursue this inquiry until certain of the character, location, exacerbating factors, and duration of this important symptom. A patient with angina and cough may have cardiac failure worsened by ongoing ischemia. Pleuritic chest pain is located laterally or posteriorly, can radiate to the shoulder, and is intensified by deep respiration. The patient attains greatest comfort by leaning away from the painful region. Tracheobronchitis often causes a raw pain located in the upper substernal region. Musculoskeletal pain frequently complicates coughing. Dyspnea experienced by the patient is important to elucidate, for this implies hypoxemia and reveals a more serious illness. Constitutional symptoms such as weight loss and night sweats are ominous signs of tuberculosis or cancer.

Patient Characteristics. Some diseases afflict certain patients; conversely, the characteristics of the patient determine how a given disease will present. Moreover, morbidity and mortality from pneumonia depend upon such variables as the patient's age and underlying medical problems. Cardiac disease, when present, complicates the course of any acute infection. Chronic pulmonary patients who develop viral upper respiratory infection are in danger of superimposed pneumonia; abnormalities on their chest x-rays and arterial blood gases are sometimes difficult to ascribe either to the acute or the underlying disease. Various opportunistic organisms infect immunocompromised patients, causing pneumonia. Alcoholic patients are the traditional victims of lung abscess and tuberculosis. Time spent in jails, homeless shelters, or urban emergency rooms can also expose the patient to tuberculosis. Travel and occupational histories often reveal the cause of a puzzling case of cough. Review all medications: angiotensin-converting enzyme inhibitors cause cough, and patients frequently use over-the-counter remedies or leftover antibiotics before seeking medical care.

Nature of the Cough.   Cough can be deep or shallow and throat-clearing. Coughs occur singly or in paroxysms. Sputum, when produced, is the most important feature of cough; however, the patient may swallow it unawares. Sputum color, as reported by the patient, is pertinent; bacterial infection is least likely to cause clear or white sputum and most likely to cause green. Changes in sputum color and consistency provide clues to the progression of the illness. Patients with chronic bronchitis produce significant amounts of sputum, and those with bronchiectasis may produce a cup a day or more.

PHYSICAL EXAMINATION

Talking exacerbates most coughs, so the clinician's observations of the patient during the history help to reveal the cause. Chronic cough, in rare instances, has psychogenic causes, and these patients do not cough spontaneously during the interview. Observe the level of distress the patient exhibits. Does dyspnea interfere with normal speech? Does the patient appear fatigued from cough interrupting sleep? Mental status changes, especially in elderly patients, alert the clinician to serious infection or hypoxemia. Note any generalized rashes, such as those from varicella. A patient wearing ill-fitting clothes may have had recent weight loss. Finally note the package of cigarettes in a breast pocket, the staining of fingers and teeth, and the odor of stale cigarettes, all of which indicate the heavy smoker.

Vital Signs.   Fever signals an infectious cause of cough. Tachycardia may parallel fever or may be a sign of hypoxemia. Count respirations and record the rate accurately. Do not write "20" in the chart to indicate a normal-appearing respira-

tory rate. Any adult requiring 20 breaths each minute is tachypneic.

Head and Neck Examination.   During the head and neck examination, search for evidence of upper respiratory infection and sinusitis. Conjunctival injection, periorbital swelling, nasal mucosal edema, pharyngitis, and otitis all suggest viral infection or rhinosinusitis as the etiology of cough. Note dentition, and then check the oral mucosa, especially in a tobacco smoker or chewer, for evidence of oral cancer. Assess the jugular veins for distention; in addition, palpate the anterior and posterior cervical lymph nodes for isolated or generalized swelling. Thrush and diffuse posterior lymphadenopathy are signs of immunocompromise that should not be overlooked.

Pulmonary Examination.   Examine the lungs by first observing respiration. Is deep respiration painful? Does the patient have increased anterior-posterior chest diameter suggestive of chronic pulmonary disease? Note use of accessory respiratory muscles and the position of greatest comfort that the patient instinctively assumes. Percussion dullness signals consolidation or effusion. Auscultate for rales, rhonchi, and wheezes. Wheezes are pathognomonic for bronchoconstriction. Rales are heard when terminal bronchioles and alveoli, closed because of atelectasis, fluid, or interstitial fibrosis, open during inspiration. Air passing through congested larger airways creates rhonchi. Clarify the cause of regional abnormal breath sounds by checking for fremitus: hold the side of your hand to the chest wall and ask the patient to say "ninety-nine." Consolidation enhances vibration; effusions muffle vibration. Elicit egophony by having the patient say "eee" while you auscultate; consolidation changes the sound from "eee" to "aay." Table 15.1 lists common patterns of lung sounds and their causes.

Cardiac Examination.   Heart failure leads to pulmonary congestion, which induces cough. Assess the patient for heart failure by examining the heart for enlargement, gallops, murmurs, and rubs. Examine the legs for edema and the hands for clubbing or cyanosis.

LABORATORY EVALUATION

Thoughtful selection of laboratory testing in the patient with cough can lead quickly to the diagnosis. Chronic cough is particularly challenging because the wide range of etiologies could lead the patient to have numerous invasive tests. Selection of a laboratory test based on a careful history will be the most fruitful and cost-effective.

Table 15.1.
Chest Physical Examination Findings of Common Cardiopulmonary Conditions

	Wheezes	Rhonchi	Rales	Fremitus	Egophony	Percussion
Asthma	Present	Present				
Consolidation	Possible	Possible	Present	Increased	Present	Dullness
Effusion			Present at top of fluid	Decreased	Absent	Dullness
Bronchitis	Possible	Present	Possible in chronic bronchitis	Absent	Absent	Normal, increased in chronic bronchitis
CHF	Possible, "cardiac asthma"		Present			

Evaluation of Sputum. To determine the pathogen in a patient coughing up sputum, the single most valuable test is the Gram stain. Aggressively obtain a sample from any patient admitting to sputum production. The desired material is from the lungs, not the mouth; coach the patient to cough deeply and expectorate directly into the container. On the slide, search for areas of polymorphonuclear white blood cells (polys) free of squamous epithelial cells (these come from the mouth); look for organisms among the polys. The predominant bacteria is the likely pathogen. Equally helpful, the absence of bacteria identifies noninfectious inflammation, or infection with viral or atypical organisms. Multiple organisms, including rods and cocci, suggest pulmonary abscess.

Chest Radiography. Chest x-rays are mandatory in smokers with any change in the pattern of cough, because these patients are at high risk for malignancy. A study of patients, mostly current or former smokers, presenting to a Veterans Administration hospital walk-in clinic revealed that chest x-ray yielded a diagnosis in 35% of patients with cough (1). Common findings were either infiltrates or signs of congestive heart failure; although physical examination might have identified these problems, over 10% of chest x-rays disclosed a new nodule or mass.

In the patient with clinical signs of pneumonia, chest x-ray confirms the diagnosis, determines the extent of pulmonary involvement, excludes the presence of effusions, and documents a starting point from which the course is followed. Furthermore, the pattern of the infiltrate may be a clue to the etiology.

Oxygenation. Hypoxemia occurs with severe disease and will dictate inpatient management. Pulse oximetry is a simple method of determining arterial oxygen saturation. *Pneumocystis carinii* pneumonia, for instance, can cause profound resting hypoxemia; milder cases produce only exercise

induced hypoxemia. Arterial blood gases, although painful and expensive, yield vital information about carbon dioxide retention and help guide the management of chronic pulmonary patients.

White Blood Cell Count. Elevated in both bacterial and viral infections, the white blood cell count is more useful for monitoring established infection than for making the diagnosis. A low white blood cell count in a patient with pneumonia is an ominous sign; it could be depressed from a preexisting immunocompromise or from acute overwhelming infection. Either circumstance heralds a complicated course.

Serologic Testing. Certain causes of cough are diagnosed by serologic tests. Often requiring paired acute and convalescent samples, most of these assays are used only for retrospective diagnosis. In contrast, during influenza epidemics, serologic testing identifies the viral strain and aids in containing the epidemic. Serum tests for mycoplasma, Legionella, and chlamydia are available.

Tests for Mycobacterial Infection. Patients with normal immune defenses who have been exposed to tuberculosis will develop induration at the site of intradermal injection of purified protein derivative (PPD). A positive PPD does not prove that the cough is from active tuberculosis. Characteristic chest x-ray findings confirm the suspicion, as does identification of the *Mycobacterium* in an acid-fast stain of sputum, but definitive diagnosis awaits positive cultures of the slowly growing *M. tuberculosis*. Simultaneous planting of *Candida*, tetanus, or mumps antigens in the skin assesses the immune response; if anergy testing yields no induration, indicating the patient is immunocompromised, then tuberculosis cannot be excluded on the basis of the PPD test.

Pulmonary Function Tests. Pulmonary function tests (PFT) often reveal the cause of chronic cough. Patients with classic asthma have diminished expiratory flow responsive to bronchodilators; for patients with cough-variant asthma, a methacholine challenge inducing wheezing and decreased expiratory flow is diagnostic. Restrictive diseases such as pulmonary fibrosis can cause cough and are diagnosed with PFTs. PFTs are also used to evaluate patients with chronic obstructive pulmonary disease (COPD).

Invasive Testing. Bronchoscopy and bronchioalveolar lavage, in patients with poorly responsive or recurrent pneumonia or in patients who are immunocompromised and at risk for unusual pathogens, allow collection of biopsies and uncontaminated bronchial secretions for examination. Routine use of these procedures in patients with chronic cough has not proven fruitful (2, 3). In stubborn cases of cough that are suspected of being caused by reflux or recurrent aspiration, ambulatory esophageal pH monitoring can be attempted. An ENT evaluation with fiberoptic laryngoscopy can exclude laryngeal disease in a patient with chronic cough.

Differential Diagnosis

The common causes of cough fall into two groups: infectious and noninfectious. Pulmonary infections generally cause cough of acute onset, and cough from other causes has a less well-defined onset. The most usual cause of cough is the common cold; the most life-threatening cause of cough, after sudden foreign body aspiration, is pneumonia.

COMMON COLD

Caused by various antigenically distinct viruses, colds frequently afflict patients of all age groups. Cough may be the chief complaint, but the patient typically has accompanying low grade fever, rhinitis, conjunctival injection, sore throat, and malaise. Residual persistent cough frequently follows an acute cold; this is caused by increased sensitivity of the cough receptors and may last for several weeks. Common colds may lead to sinusitis, which also causes cough. Cough from sinusitis, however, is accompanied by symptoms of chronic nasal sinus congestion.

BRONCHITIS

Whereas pneumonia is infection of the air-exchanging segments of the pulmonary system, bronchitis affects the air-conducting structures. A patient with bronchitis will not have high fever, rigors, signs of consolidation on chest exam, or radiographic infiltrates. Bronchitis can be acute or

chronic. Smoker's cough will be considered here as well.

Acute Bronchitis. Most organisms causing acute bronchitis can also cause pneumonia and are discussed under "Pneumonia." The patient has a milder illness: patients frequently have fever only at the onset, or a persistent low-grade fever, and are not hypoxemic but will have prominent cough. Associated symptoms suggesting atypical pathogens or viral infection are common. Examination of the lungs should only reveal rhonchi. If they are heard, asking the patient to cough usually clears them. Occasional patients without an antecedent history of asthma will wheeze in response to bronchial inflammation. Chest x-ray should be obtained in patients who have other abnormal lung sounds or in whom rhonchi and wheezes are localized to a single lung field. A sputum Gram stain may disclose the organism. Unless the acute illness is superimposed on chronic bronchitis or other serious pulmonary or cardiac disease, patients will be managed at home.

Chronic Bronchitis. Along with emphysema, chronic bronchitis is a condition of longstanding pulmonary damage, usually brought on by cigarette smoking. Patients with chronic bronchitis have cough and sputum production for 3 months over 2 years. The disease predisposes patients to other pulmonary infections since the symptoms are caused by a pulmonary clearance mechanism that is chronically overwhelmed. PFTs reveal an obstructive pattern.

Smoker's Cough. Although meeting criteria for chronic bronchitis, a patient with smoker's cough nevertheless has similarly impaired mucociliary clearance from tobacco smoking. To cure the condition, the patient must stop smoking. Many patients state that their cough worsens when they stop smoking, and although this is often true, it is a temporary sign that clearance mechanisms are regaining their power. Any change in the cough pattern or frequency or sputum character in a patient with smoker's cough requires a chest x-ray to exclude lung cancer.

PNEUMONIA

Pneumonia is infection of the lower respiratory tract and can be diffuse or confined to a single lobe of the lung. Pneumonia can have myriad causes; many of the same organisms cause both pneumonia and bronchitis. However, patients with pneumonia are more ill than those with bronchitis, display clinical and radiographic evidence of interstitial or airspace disease, and are in danger of hypoxemia from involvement of air-exchanging pulmonary surfaces. Fatal pneumonia more often strikes the elderly, patients with serious underlying illnesses, and patients infected with Legionella, Pneumocystis, or Gram-negative rods. Features of the clinical presentation are not reliable indicators of the cause, but sputum Gram stain may reveal the pathogen.

Bacterial Pneumonia. The most common community-acquired bacterial cause of pneumonia is the pneumococcus. Classic symptoms develop suddenly, with a single shaking chill and cough productive of rusty sputum, but many patients lack these features. Pneumococcal pneumonia forms lobar consolidation on physical exam and on chest x-ray (Fig. 15.1) and may be complicated by effusion. Other bacterial causes are *Haemophilus influenzae* (especially in smokers), staphylococcus (classically complicating influenza), Klebsiella (especially in alcoholics), and other strep organisms in patients with poor dentition or endocarditis. Patients acquiring pneumonia while in the hospital or while residing in a nursing home may be infected with resistant Gram-negative rods. For any case of bacterial pneumonia, Gram stain of the sputum is the

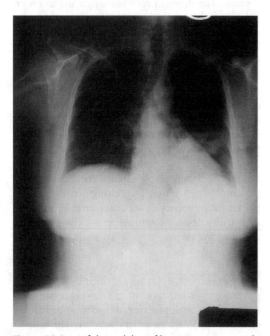

Figure 15.1. Left lower lobe infiltrate in a patient with acute fever and cough. Note that the posterior location of the infiltrate preserves the left heart border.

single most important diagnostic test, showing numerous polys and a predominant organism.

Atypical Pneumonia. Rather than the abrupt onset and lobar consolidation characteristic of pneumococcal infection, atypical organisms more often cause progressive disease with diffuse pulmonary involvement. Frequently these illnesses begin with upper respiratory symptoms; cough comes later. Sputum Gram stain shows polys but no organisms. Clinical distinction between the more common atypical pneumonias, mycoplasma and chlamydia, and viral pneumonia is difficult because none have unique identifying features (Table 15.2); the high prevalence of these organisms in community-acquired pneumonia dictates treatment with antibiotics to which they are sensitive. Atypical pneumonias are stubborn and may require more than 2 weeks of treatment and a long convalescence, but most patients are safely managed as outpatients.

Mycoplasma pneumoniae attaches to respiratory mucosa, sets up an inflammatory response, and interferes with mucociliary function. It is prevalent among young adults and lingers, causing prominent fatigue and a nonproductive cough. Occasional patients develop hypoxemia and require hospitalization. Additional symptoms include sore throat, fever, headache, and earache from bullous myringitis. Mycoplasma is diagnosed with serologic tests for cold agglutinins and for mycoplasma antibodies and by identifying mycoplasmas in the sputum with fluorescent antibody testing or culture.

Chlamydia pneumoniae, originally termed TWAR, is a more recently described cause of outpatient pneumonia. The chlamydiae are pathogens that multiply intracellularly and then cause the cell to rupture, releasing more organisms. *C. pneumoniae* has affinity for the respiratory tract. Whereas *C. psittaci* is an unusual cause of atypical pneumonia that is acquired from infected birds, *C. pneumoniae* seems to be passed from person to person, albeit with incomplete penetrance and long incubation times. The illness usually is progressive, with upper respiratory symptoms, including pharyngitis, preceding pneumonia. Identifying chlamydia antigens in throat cultures confirms the diagnosis. Serological tests can be used, with high IgM or IgG titers implying current infection.

Legionnaire's disease first caused an outbreak of fatal pneumonia at a convention of legionnaires in Philadelphia in the 1970s. The responsible organism, *L. pneumophila*, normally multiplies in water, and the cooling system of the hotel was the source. Since then, other institutions' water

Table 15.2.
Clinical Presentation of Patients with Chlamydia, Mycoplasma, and Viral Pneumonias

Characteristic	Organism		
	C. pneumoniae (n = 14)	*M. pneumoniae* (n = 17)	Viral[a] (n = 17)
History of fever	4 (29)	8 (47)	6 (35)
Headache	8 (57)	11 (65)	9 (53)
Cough	14 (100)	16 (94)	17 (100)
Sore throat	10 (71)	7 (41)	7 (41)
Hoarseness	2 (14)	0	0
Temperature >37.8°C	2 (14)	5 (29)	2 (12)
Pharyngeal erythema	11 (79)	14 (82)	12 (71)
Sinus tenderness to percussion	5 (36)	0	1 (6)
Abnormal breath sounds	13 (93)	16 (94)	15 (88)
Leukocytes >10,000/mm^2	2 (15)[b]	6 (35)	3 (19)[c]
Sedimentation rate >15 mm/hour	11 (85)[b]	15 (88)	9 (56)[c]

From Thom DH, Grayson JT. Infections with *Chlamydia pneumoniae* strain TWAR. Clin Chest Med 1991;12:245–256.
[a]The viral infections consisted of 10 cases of influenza A, four of influenza B, one of respiratory syncytial virus, and two of adenovirus.
[b]Based on 13 cases.
[c]Based on 16 cases.

supplies have caused smaller outbreaks. Sporadic cases also occur, and the bacteria can cause mild self-limited infection (Pontiac fever). Legionnaire's disease is most severe in smokers and patients with other chronic illnesses. Gastrointestinal symptoms often accompany the pneumonia, but their absence does not reliably exclude the disease. Multilobar involvement is a clue to this infection, and patients will often be profoundly ill, with high fevers, lethargy, and hyponatremia. The organism can be cultured from sputum, or fluorescent tests of sputum or bronchoalveolar lavage fluid can be performed and urine tested for Legionella antigens. None of these diagnostic methods has reliable sensitivity. This disease is managed in the hospital.

Viral Pneumonia. The common cold is the most common cause of cough but does not cause pneumonia. Influenza causes pneumonia predominately in infants, in the elderly or immunocompromised, or in patients with chronic illnesses such as diabetes. It also predisposes the patient to bacterial pneumonia such as *Staph. aureus.* Usually seen during epidemics, influenzal pneumonia begins with the typical flu symptoms of high fever and myalgias that progress to prostration, cough, and hypoxemia. Diagnosis is made by isolating the virus from the throat, nose, or bronchoscopy samples. Serological testing identifies the strain of virus, helping to contain epidemics.

Chickenpox in adults may progress to varicella pneumonia. Although rarely seen in children with chickenpox, this complication can be fatal in adults. Adult patients with chickenpox who have dyspnea or cough require a chest x-ray to exclude pneumonia. Other viral causes of pneumonia are adenovirus and cytomegalovirus, which can both be serious in immunocompromised patients. Viral illnesses predispose the patient with chronic lung disease to superimposed bacterial pneumonia.

***Pneumocystis carinii* Pneumonia.** A defining illness of AIDS, *P. carinii* pneumonia has decreased in frequency since the widespread prophylactic treatment of patients with low T-cell counts. The onset is often dramatic with profound dyspnea, but patients with milder cases present with cough or mild shortness of breath. Because patients may not know that they are infected with human immunodeficiency virus (HIV), this illness should be considered in all patients with pneumonia. The chest x-ray may be normal, reveal interstitial infiltrates, or show severe diffuse airspace involvement. Serum lactate dehydrogenase is usually high. Pulse oximetry reveals hypoxemia, although brief exercise may be necessary in the less acutely ill patient to elicit this finding.

Tuberculosis. In previous eras, tuberculosis was a leading cause of cough. It became infrequent but has now enjoyed a resurgence, especially in urban areas. Covered in detail elsewhere later in this chapter, it should be considered in patients with chronic cough, especially when accompanied by night sweats, weight loss, and fever.

Aspiration Pneumonia. Aspirating small amounts of saliva is a normal occurrence, with normal respiratory defenses easily managing the volume and bacterial challenge. Aspiration pneumonia can develop, however, after large volumes are inhaled, for instance during a seizure, or if the bacterial load is particularly heavy, as in patients with poor dentition. This disease classically affects an alcoholic patient with poor dentition who passes out and aspirates infected saliva, developing a right upper lobe pneumonia. The pneumonia can organize into a lung abscess, producing purulent, malodorous sputum; Gram staining reveals a multitude of organisms.

CAUSES OF CHRONIC COUGH

Numerous problems cause patients to cough for several weeks. Smokers and former smokers frequently suffer from smoker's cough and chronic bronchitis. In any patient with a recent upper respiratory infection, hypersensitivity of the cough receptors can persist for up to 8 weeks and should be considered as the cause of a lingering cough. Cough in patients who are immunocompromised is often caused by indolent opportunistic infections. Many patients take angiotensin-converting enzyme inhibitors, and a major side effect of this class of drugs is cough. Patients with cardiac disease must be evaluated for worsened heart failure causing cough. Furthermore, cough in one patient may have multiple causes, so incomplete resolution of cough that is treated based on historical findings should prompt consideration of additional causes.

Rhinosinusitis. The most common cause of chronic cough is postnasal drip from rhinosinusitis, and evaluation and treatment for this problem are recommended as the initial step for most patients with chronic cough. Evidence for this problem includes any of the features of sinusitis (see Chapter 11): repeated throat-clearing, increased coughing at night or upon arising, and history of recent pharyngitis or cold. Because this is such a common etiology, consider empiric treatment for rhinosinusitis even in patients with other problems (e.g., asthma or gastroesophageal reflux).

Asthma. The sole feature of asthma may be cough. The clues to this diagnosis in patients without wheezing are exacerbating circumstances such as cold air, exercise, or upper respiratory infection. Routine PFTs may be normal, but exercise PFTs

or methacholine challenge are abnormal. Patients, especially children, with this presentation may with time develop classic symptoms of asthma.

Gastroesophageal Reflux. Gastroesophageal reflux can induce chronic cough by stimulation of cough receptors in the esophagus and larynx. In patients who do not complain of other symptoms of reflux or dyspepsia, the diagnosis of gastroesophageal reflux can be definitively confirmed or excluded by ambulatory esophageal pH monitoring. Empiric treatment for gastroesophageal reflux, however, is warranted in most cases where the problem is suspected.

Angiotensin-Converting Enzyme Inhibitors. Used with increasing frequency to treat various cardiac, hypertensive, and diabetic patients, angiotensin-converting enzyme inhibitors can induce cough in nearly 20% of patients (4). The cough is typically dry and persistent, begins soon after initiation of treatment or many months later, and may affect women more than men. It usually subsides within days to weeks of changing to another class of drugs. The cough may be associated with scratchy throat or nasal symptoms. The suggested mechanism for this side effect is increased sensitivity of cough receptors, probably in the larynx or other extrathoracic sites, mediated by changes in prostaglandins, bradykinins, and neurotransmitters caused by angiotensin-converting enzyme inhibition. Because these drugs are used frequently in treatment of cardiac failure, the patient should be carefully evaluated to determine whether the cough is due to worsened heart failure or to the medication.

SYMPTOM OF CHRONIC UNDERLYING DISEASES

Cough can be a symptom of tumor (lung or other), cardiac failure, or a psychiatric illness. As mentioned above, smokers with new cough should be evaluated for lung cancer with a chest x-ray. Coughing can be the result of nonpulmonary tumors irritating the diaphragm, pericardium, or pharynx and larynx. Additionally, metastatic disease to the lung can cause cough in a patient with history of cancer.

Cardiac failure can present with cough as fluid accumulates in the interstitium and alveoli of the lung. Symptoms should worsen with exercise or recumbency and may accompany angina. Cardiac evaluation and chest x-ray confirm the etiology.

Rarely, cough can be a manifestation of psychiatric illness, particularly those disorders associated with somatization. Consider this cause in patients complaining of a cough that is minor or inapparent. Depression, anxiety disorders, and somatoform disorder are common underlying problems in outpatient practice; cough serves as the means of access to medical care for the patient. Embarking on a long and invasive workup in a patient with undiagnosed psychiatric illness only reinforces somatization as a behavior and worsens the patient's sense of loss of control.

Management

Successful treatment of cough relies on the determination of the cause. For patients with infection, the pathogen must be susceptible to the antibiotic selected. For patients with pneumonia, the clinician must select inpatient or outpatient management. In the case of chronic cough, the most successful outcomes are obtained by following protocols that determine the location of the irritated cough receptors and direct treatment to eradicate the source of irritation.

COMMON COLD

Although colds are self-limited, they cause significant symptomatic distress. The patient should first use acetaminophen 650 mg orally every 4–6 hours. If additional symptomatic relief is needed, antihistamines or decongestants may be helpful, but there is no well-documented evidence of their effectiveness. Disruptive cough can be treated briefly with antitussive agents. Reassurance, rest, fluids (especially hot tea or soup), and acetaminophen are the mainstays of cold therapy.

ACUTE BRONCHITIS

Most cases of bronchitis are viral, and if there is no evidence of bacterial infection, no antibiotics should be offered. After viruses, bacteria and atypical organisms cause most community acquired upper respiratory infections; effective treatment of the patient with bronchitis covers both classes of pathogens. Oral erythromycin 250–500 mg every 6 hours for 7–10 days (or one of the newer, more expensive, but more convenient macrolides) is the first choice in treating patients with bronchitis and purulent sputum. *H. influenzae* frequently infects smokers or patients with COPD, and macrolides are likewise useful against this pathogen.

PNEUMONIA

Treatment for pneumonia is complex. A study of patients admitted to the hospital for pneumonia in 1986–1987 (5) revealed that pneumococcus, *H. influenza*, Legionella, and chlamydiae were the most frequent pathogens. Next was Gram-negative pneumonia, and *P. carinii* accounted for few cases. Current admissions to major inner city centers comprise greater numbers of cases of *P. carinii* pneumonia. Outpatient antibiotic treatment of pneumonia, undertaken only in stable patients representing a higher proportion of cases of atypical pneumonias, depends on the macrolide antibiotics, in larger doses and for longer courses than with bronchitis. For instance, oral erythromycin 500 mg every 6 hours for 10–14 days is a good choice. If, however, the sputum Gram stain reveals a preponderance of Gram-positive diplococci, the correct antibiotic is oral penicillin V, 500 mg every 6 hours for 10–14 days. Pleomorphic Gram-negative rods on sputum exam dictate the use of an antibiotic that will reliably treat *Haemophilus* flu, such as a second-generation cephalosporin or a penicillin in combination with a beta-lactamase inhibitor, e.g., Augmentin 500 mg orally every 8 hours for 10–14 days.

Inpatient treatment of patients with pneumonia is warranted when the clinical evaluation reveals altered mental status; high fever, rapid respiratory rate, tachycardia, or hypotension; any complication such as bacteremia or effusion; large derangements in laboratory values such as high or unexpectedly low white blood cell counts or electrolyte abnormalities; or acute coexisting medical problems. Prospective study has additionally identified age of >65, immunosuppression, and high-risk etiology as risks for a complicated course (6). High-risk etiology in this study included aspiration or postobstructive pneumonia, and pneumonia caused by Gram-negative rods or staphylococcus. Patients with these features are more safely managed as inpatients, as are patients who cannot tolerate oral antibiotics or who cannot return for close follow-up. Close follow-up of the patient managed at home or discharged after a short hospitalization, with careful attention to signs of deterioration, is mandatory when managing pneumonia. To confirm that an effusion is not developing, consider repeating the chest x-ray 2–3 days after the onset of the illness. After clinical resolution in 2–4 weeks, a chest x-ray should show improvement. It is important to confirm complete radiological resolution of pneumonia.

When pneumonia fails to resolve as expected, or when a patient develops repeated episodes of pneumonia involving the same lobe, the clinician must suspect an underlying disease interfering with the process of lung clearance. Slowly resolving pneumonia is usually found in elderly patients, patients with COPD, or alcoholics. The atypical pathogens are notorious for resolving slowly, with Legionella causing the longest course. Recurrent pneumonia should prompt a search for an obstructing lesion in the involved bronchus. Computed tomography (CT) scanning may reveal the lesion, but if no lesion can be distinguished on CT, bronchoscopy is required. Recurrent pneumococcal pneumonia is a criterion for the diagnosis of HIV infection.

Treatment of certain viral pneumonias can be successful. The problem with treating influenzal pneumonia is determining whether type A or B is the cause: amantadine is used in the treatment of seriously ill patients with influenza A, and ribavirin is showing promise in treating influenza B. Varicella pneumonia can be treated with acyclovir. Owing to the high fatality rate, adults with influenzal pneumonia or varicella pneumonia should be managed in the hospital.

CHRONIC COUGH

Patients with chronic cough for >3 weeks are challenging to manage. Localizing signs and symptoms revealed during a careful history and physical examination should guide initial management (Table 15.3). Because cough may have several causes in a given patient, and because cough from asthma, rhinosinusitis, and gastroesophageal reflux are prevalent, the empiric approach used by Pratter et al. (7) can resolve chronic cough in most patients without an obvious etiology or when cough fails to resolve with initial treatment (Fig. 15.2). The use of cough suppressants has a role only in cases where the cause of the cough cannot be eliminated (e.g., inoperable cancer).

SYMPTOMATIC MEDICATIONS

Suppressing cough is often the goal of the patient, but treatment of the underlying cause should be the goal of the clinician. Self-limited cough from the common cold, cough from untreatable diseases, or cough that interferes with sleep during the convalescence from a treatable illness are the few indications for nonspecific cough suppression.

Nonspecific cough remedies act on the cough receptors, the mucus layer, or the cough center. The mode of action of commonly employed cough remedies is listed in Table 15.4. Only the narcotic derivatives have consistently been proven effective in suppressing cough. Cough medications are, in the aggregate, extremely expensive, offering no permanent solution to the problem of cough. Because the purpose of cough is to clear the bronchial passages, allowing free gas exchange in the lungs, suppression of this important protective mechanism may be harmful. Specific treatment, based on careful determination of the cause, is the best approach to the patient with cough.

Table 15.3.
Directed Approach to Chronic Cough (>3 Weeks)

History and Physical Exam Reveals	Management
Tobacco use	Obtain Chest x-ray: if positive: evaluate and treat abnormality, if negative: obtain PFTs to evaluate for COPD; counsel smoking cessation
Congestive heart failure	Treat cardiac disease; be cautious with ACE inhibitors, which may cause cough
Immunosuppression	Evaluate for opportunistic infections such as pneumocystitis, tuberculosis, or atypical mycobacteria
ACE inhibitor use	Discontinue ACE inhibitors
Sinusitis or recent upper respiratory infection	Empiric treatment for sinusitis
Wheezes on physical exam or history of asthma	Trial of inhaled beta-agonists or inhaled steroids
Dyspepsia	Gastroesophageal reflux precautions and antacids
Depressed mood, anxiety, or multiple somatic symptoms	Consider mood, anxiety, or somatoform disorders

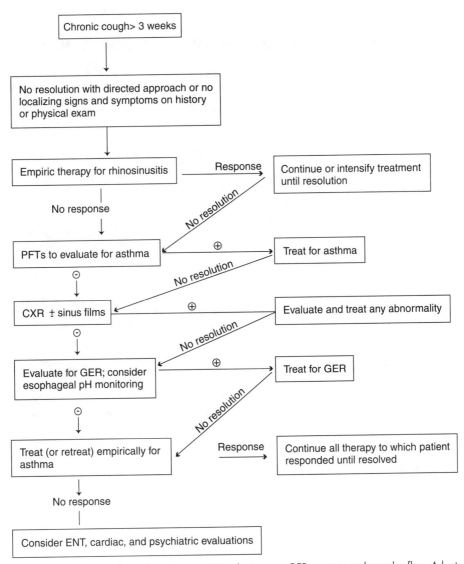

Figure 15.2. Empiric approach to chronic care. CXR, chest x-ray; GER, gastroesophageal reflux. Adapted from material presented in Pratter MR, Bartter T, Akers S, DuBois J. An algorithmic approach to chronic cough. Ann Intern Med 1993;119:977–983.

Table 15.4.
Nonspecific Cough Remedies

Remedy	Mechanism	Utility
Syrups, lozenges, and honey (active ingredient: sugar, some contain aromatic compounds)	Coating of mucous membranes interferes with cough receptor stimulation	Brief relief; sugar content makes them unwise for diabetics
Guaifenisin	Marketed as an expectorant	Studies fail to demonstrate effectiveness in recommended doses
Dextromethorphan	Suppression of the cough center	Effective by subjective and cough-counting criteria
Codeine	Suppression of cough center, narcotic with abuse potential	Effective by subjective and cough-counting criteria

ILLUSTRATIVE CASES WITH SELF-ASSESSMENT QUESTIONS AND ANSWERS

Case 1

R.I. is a 28-year-old clerical worker with no medical problems who comes to the walk-in clinic complaining of runny nose, cough, headaches, and fever for 3 days. "I feel terrible," he says, "My whole body aches, especially my chest. I feel like I'm going to die. I think I need some antibiotics. I always get them when I have a really bad cold." On examination he looks miserable. He is afebrile; his heart and lungs sound normal. His face is nontender. His speech is not nasal.

QUESTION: *What is the most likely cause of his symptoms?*

a. Bronchitis
b. Viral upper respiratory infection
c. Bacterial sinusitis
d. Pneumococcal pneumonia

ANSWER: b. *He has no fever or local sinus tenderness, and because his speech is not suggestive of obstruction bacterial sinusitis is less likely. Although he could have bronchitis, he has many upper respiratory symptoms, so this is not your leading diagnosis. He does not have pneumococcal pneumonia. His lung exam is normal, he does not appear toxic, and he has no fever.*

Case 2

B.C. is a 26-year-old investment banker who complains of "colds, colds, colds one after another," all through the winter. Her nose runs; she cannot breath through her nose at night; and she has a dry cough that is sometimes so violent she vomits. She also gets a throbbing pain along the sides of her nose (when describing this, she runs her fingers down the medial sides of her maxillary sinuses). She has tried everything; Dristan, Thera-flu, Tylenol Sinus. Right now the only things that work for her are Afrin and Nyquil and even these do not really help anymore. Her history is unremarkable except for a history of hayfever (mild, always in August) and multiple ear infections as a child.

QUESTION: *What do you think might be causing her prolonged symptoms?*

a. Sinusitis
b. Asthma
c. Viral upper respiratory tract infection
d. None of the above

ANSWER: d. *She is misusing decongestants and has rebound congestion when she tries to stop. Asthma is a possibility, but it is usually not associated with predominant symptoms of runny or stuffy nose. If she had chronic or allergic sinusitis, decongestants would usually be effective if used properly. It would be unusual for her to have colds as frequently as she indicates.*

HEMOPTYSIS

Hemoptysis, the act of coughing up blood-tinged sputum or gross blood, indicates blood loss or hemorrhage via the tracheobronchial tree. It is important to differentiate this type of bleeding from upper airway or nasopharyngeal blood loss as well as from hematemesis, the vomiting of blood from the gastrointestinal tract. There appears to be a transition in what were the common causes of hemoptysis in the 1930s–1960s and what are the most common etiologies seen today. A decrease in the incidence of tuberculosis and bronchiectasis has been reported, probably secondary to the early use of antibiotic and antituberculosis therapy, with bronchogenic carcinoma and bronchitis being cited as more common causes of hemoptysis today (8). This, however, is population dependent. A younger population, with increased incidence of HIV disease, may have an infectious etiology (e.g., tuberculosis, pneumonia) as the underlying cause, whereas an older population with a history of cigarette smoking will have a higher incidence of cancer as the underlying etiology of hemoptysis.

Pathophysiologic Correlation

Pulmonary blood flow is not evenly distributed throughout the lung parenchyma but is greatest in the dependent areas—usually the basilar regions in the upright person. These are the areas where the pulmonary arterial pressure is highest. This difference in blood distribution throughout the lung, not matched by comparable changes in ventilation, leads to large differences in defense capacities in different regions of the lung as well as differences in effective gas exchange. Local factors also affect blood flow. Alveolar hypoxia can lead to vasoconstriction, causing blood flow to be directed away from poorly ventilated regions and thus preserving perfusion-ventilation matching.

Abnormalities in the distribution and volume of blood flow may result from diseases that directly involve blood vessels (e.g., emboli, vasculitis) or cause external compression of blood vessels (e.g., tumors, cysts) or may be secondary to vasoconstriction (e.g., hypoxemia). Pulmonary blood flow is important for numerous reasons in addition to the direct benefits to the lung and the maintenance of gas exchange. It also serves as a reservoir for blood from the left ventricle of the heart and can be significant in several primary cardiac disease processes.

Hemoptysis predominantly occurs from either mucosal involvement or from direct injury to the pulmonary vasculature. Mucosal injury can range from minor inflammation and erosion to necrosis and ulceration of bronchial tissues. Common sources of this type of injury include bronchitis, bronchiectasis, tuberculosis, pneumonias, and bronchogenic carcinoma. The hemoptysis noted from these types of injuries tends to be more minor, with sputum that is blood tinged and may be recurrent. Bronchiectasis may present with more grossly bloody sputum, if the mucosal necrosis is severe. It is more common for hemoptysis to occur with inactive tuberculosis than during active disease because small blood vessels have been left unsupported and exposed by the destruction and fibrosis of the lung parenchyma. The blood vessels then dilate and rupture.

Direct involvement of the pulmonary vasculature tends to produce a much more bloody sputum or expectorate. Necrotizing pneumonias, lung abscesses, or cavitary lesions can cause disruption of a blood vessel by necrosis of the vessel wall with subsequent bleeding. *Klebsiella pneumoniae*, one of the causes of necrotizing pneumonia, may produce a thick or "currant jelly" bloody sputum in 25–50% of patients infected.

Vasculitides such as Wegener's granulomatosis and Goodpasture's syndrome may produce hemoptysis secondary to inflammatory changes to the blood vessels. Congenital vascular malformations can also exist and lead to recurrent bleeding.

Primary cardiac diseases, such as left ventricular heart failure, can also lead to frothy, pink-tinged sputum, commonly known as pulmonary edema. As discussed previously, the pulmonary vasculature acts as a reservoir for the left ventricle of the heart. When the left side of the heart begins to fail, blood "backs up" into the pulmonary vascular tree, with a subsequent increase in pulmonary capillary pressure. Once this reaches a critical level where the pulmonary vasculature can no longer compensate, vascular injury occurs and leads to extravasation of red blood cells. Mitral stenosis causes a similar picture, again by using the pulmonary vasculature to compensate for a failing left heart. As mitral stenosis progresses to become more severe, the dilated pulmonary-bronchial venous connection may rupture, leading to grossly bloody hemoptysis.

Clinical and Laboratory Evaluation

An extensive history, thorough physical examination, and laboratory data may give clues to the underlying cause of hemoptysis. Quantification of the amount of hemoptysis is not helpful in discerning the etiology of hemoptysis, and in most cases patients will undergo more invasive evaluation with fiberoptic bronchoscopy or high resolution CT scan to make a conclusive diagnosis. Despite all available tools for diagnosis, 5–15% of cases of gross hemoptysis will go undiagnosed.

HISTORY

A good history may be useful in making the correct diagnosis. As mentioned previously, it is important to differentiate hemoptysis from nasopharyngeal bleeding or hematemesis by careful history taking. One must ask if the blood is coughed up and mixed with sputum as opposed to vomiting blood mixed with food products or aspirating blood from the nose. It is not always clear from history alone, especially because this is usually a frightening experience for the patient and the clinician may need to rely on physical examination and/or analysis of the fluid to ascertain that this is, in fact, tracheobronchial blood loss. The quantity and rate of blood loss from hemoptysis will not help the clinician make the proper diagnosis. Many of the same etiologies may present with gross blood, versus blood-tinged sputum, depending on the underlying status of the patient and the lesion. It is important to identify the patient with a significant amount of blood loss, however, because this may cause potential airway compromise and is a medical emergency.

Carcinoma as Underlying Cause. One must

always be concerned that the underlying cause of the hemoptysis is carcinoma, and therefore establishing the age of the patient and a quantification of the smoking history (e.g., cigarettes) is of the utmost importance. Lung cancer is much more common in men older than 50 with a significant cigarette smoking history. Environmental or occupational exposures (e.g., asbestos, nickel, chromium, arsenic, and chlormethyl ethers) have also been associated with an increase in pulmonary tumors; thus questions concerning work history and possible exposure to any of these agents must be asked.

One must question if this is the first episode of hemoptysis or if there have been previous recurrent episodes. If this has been recurring for several years it makes the diagnosis of lung cancer much less likely, and a more likely explanation would be bronchitis or bronchiectasis. However, bronchitis tends to occur in cigarette smokers, the same population at increased risk for bronchogenic carcinoma, and an extensive evaluation must be made to exclude cancer. Bronchiectasis is characterized by permanent abnormal dilatation of one or more bronchi. Clinically it can present with chronic cough with excessive expectoration of phlegm or purulent sputum and recurrent bronchopulmonary infections with or without hemoptysis. Another cause of recurrent bleeding may be a bronchial adenoma, which is a vascular tumor. They are malignant tumors but are slow growing and locally invasive and can be cured by surgical resection.

Infectious Etiology. Questions concerning an infectious etiology must be asked. Tuberculosis may be an indolent infection, and the patient may present with complaints of hemoptysis, weight loss, and night sweats with or without fevers. A prior history of tuberculosis is also important to elicit, because hemoptysis can be common during inactive disease for reasons discussed previously. Bacterial colonization, aspergillomas or fungus balls, or scar carcinomas in the cavitary site are all possible complications of previous infection with tuberculosis and can present with hemoptysis as well. Other types of pneumonias, especially bacterial infections, tend to present with fevers and purulent sputum in addition to hemoptysis. It is important at this time to determine if the patient may be in an immunocompromised state secondary to HIV disease, chronic steroid use, or a malignancy. An increase in less common infectious etiologies would then need to be considered, including necrotizing *P. carinii* pneumonia, aspergilloma, or, once again, tuberculosis.

Other Causes. A thorough review of systems is necessary to eliminate less likely causes of hemoptysis. Easy bruising and gum bleeding while brushing one's teeth, in addition to a family history of easy bleeding, leads one to consider a bleeding dyscrasia. In the same line of questioning one must ask if the patient is on anticoagulant therapy with warfarin or aspirin. It is widely believed that if a patient presents with bleeding on anticoagulant therapy, it may be due to a lesion that has been unmasked by the medication and that an evaluation of the bleeding should be conducted (9). Liver cirrhosis, secondary to any etiology, may cause significant decrease in hepatic synthetic function, with subsequent abnormalities in the clotting factors and an increased risk of bleeding. It is rarely a source of hemoptysis, however, and usually presents as a gastrointestinal bleed. Alcohol abuse is a common cause of cirrhosis. In the active alcohol user who may aspirate while being intoxicated, lung abscesses or necrotizing pneumonias may be the consequence. If that same patient has abnormalities in liver function tests and prothrombin time, he or she may present with a significant amount of hemoptysis.

Hematuria, or blood in the urine, may lead one to consider the vasculitides, if accompanied by hemoptysis. Wegener's granulomatosis is characterized by upper respiratory tract involvement (e.g., laryngitis or sinusitis) and may be associated with hematuria and hemoptysis. Goodpasture's syndrome is also associated with recurrent pulmonary hemorrhage and hematuria. The disease seems to be more prevalent in young men, who may present with cough, mild shortness of breath, and hemoptysis. The hematuria is representative usually of a rapidly progressive glomerulonephritis.

The overall health status of the patient may be useful in reaching a diagnosis. If the patient has been immobilized for any time, or is sedentary, a risk exists for deep vein thrombosis and possible pulmonary emboli. Also, if the patient has a history of malignancy, he or she may be at increased risk of thromboembolic disease including pulmonary emboli. Hemoptysis will not occur from pulmonary emboli unless subsequent pulmonary hemorrhage or infarction results. This is a relatively uncommon event, happening only in approximately 19% of patients with angiographically proven emboli. These patients may complain of acute shortness of breath and pleuritic chest pain in addition to the hemoptysis, and they tend to appear acutely ill at presentation. Metastatic spread of cancer to the lung from a primary nonpulmonary source of cancer rarely causes hemoptysis.

Questions regarding primary cardiac or valvular diseases must be asked. A history of rheumatic fever as a child or heart murmur is important to ask when there is concern of mitral stenosis. Symptoms of congestive heart failure may be useful in the elderly patient presenting with recurrent frothy pink hemoptysis. Questions about orthopnea, paroxysmal nocturnal dyspnea, dyspnea on exertion, and pedal edema can help make the diagnosis.

PHYSICAL EXAMINATION

The physical examination should be performed in a thorough and directed manner, searching for pulmonary as well as nonpulmonary sources of the hemoptysis. One must first note the overall appearance of the patient. Does he or she appear acutely ill or in respiratory distress? Does the patient look chronically ill, or are there signs of wasting and weight loss that would make one concerned about HIV disease or an underlying malignancy?

Vital Signs. Temperature is important to note, especially if the patient has a fever, indicating a possible infectious cause of the hemoptysis. Respiratory rate and heart rate also should be measured, because tachypnea and/or tachycardia may give clues to a possible etiology. Tachypnea may occur from a primary pulmonary process, such as pneumonia, or if significant airway embarrassment has happened from any cause with a large amount of blood or fluid extravasating into the lung parenchyma. Tachycardia can accompany tachypnea in the following scenarios. If there is significant airway compromise and the patient is hemodynamically unstable, heart rate will increase. This may occur with massive pulmonary emboli with infarction. A primary cardiac etiology such as congestive heart failure will increase heart rate as well and may increase respiratory rate if pulmonary edema ensues.

Head and Neck Examination. Once the vital signs have been established, the clinician is ready to proceed. The head and neck exam may provide clues toward a diagnosis. The nose should first be examined to eliminate epistaxis as the cause of blood loss by looking in the nares for dried blood or active bleeding. It should also be noted if a saddle nose deformity of the bridge of the nose is present, suggesting Wegener's granulomatosis. Following the same line of thinking, one would look for nasal mucosa ulcerations, purulent nasal discharge, or signs of sinusitis or ear involvement. The throat should be checked for erythema, which may accompany a bronchitis or upper airway infection. The neck should be palpated for lymphadenopathy. Enlarged or multiple lymph nodes may be suggestive of tuberculosis, sarcoidosis, malignancy, or HIV disease. The neck also must be examined visually for jugular venous distention, which may indicate congestive heart failure or severe mitral stenosis with prominent venous *a* waves.

Chest Examination. The chest examination is of the utmost importance. Initially the chest wall and back should be visualized before a stethoscope or hand is laid on the patient. A barrel-chested appearance or increase in the anterior-posterior diameter can be seen with COPD and emphysematous changes of the lung. This is a common change seen among chronic smokers with an increased tendency toward recurrent bronchitis and bronchogenic carcinoma. Bruising of the chest wall may be present if blunt trauma occurred, with subsequent contusion of the lung. Auscultation of the lungs is an essential part of the physical examination. The presence of wheezing may be indicative of airway obstruction or a cardiac etiology. Parenchymal disease may manifest with rales or signs of consolidation, with bronchial breath sounds and dullness on percussion. Cardiac examination may reveal a murmur on auscultation or an S3 gallop suggestive of ventricular failure.

Abdominal Examination. Abdominal examination is important to discover any enlargement of the liver or spleen. Hepatomegaly may indicate primary liver disease, possibly from alcohol abuse, with abnormal liver function tests and coagulation defects. An enlarged liver can also be from right-sided heart failure or from cancer involving the liver, either primary or metastatic. Splenomegaly can be present in the patient from a primary hemotological disturbance or as a consequence of liver cirrhosis with portal hypertension and subsequent hypersplenism.

Extremities and Skin Examination. Finally, extremities and skin must be examined for signs of telangiectasias or easy bruising suggestive of a bleeding dyscrasia. Nails should be checked for clubbing, a selective bullous enlargement of the distal digit of a finger caused by an increase in soft tissue. The mechanism of clubbing is unclear, but it has been associated with various pulmonary etiologies, including bronchogenic carcinoma and bronchiectasis.

LABORATORY EVALUATION

Chest X-Ray. The mainstay of evaluation remains the chest x-ray. Most patients with a bronchogenic carcinoma will have an abnormal x-ray (see Fig. 15.3). Besides mass lesions, a chest film may reveal an infiltrate(s), an abscess, a cavitary lesion, hilar adenopathy, congestive heart failure, or changes consistent with mitral stenosis. If the chest x-ray is normal, other studies are warranted.

Sputum. Sputum can be analyzed by looking for an infectious etiology or atypical cells suggesting malignancy. Gram stain of sputum may reveal the presence of polymorphonuclear white cells and specific bacteria. An acid-fast stain should be performed, not only to diagnose tuberculosis but as a rough assessment of infectivity. Sputum should be cultured in the laboratory as well for bacterial, fungal, and mycobacterial infections. If tuberculosis is suspected a tuberculin skin test (PPD) should be performed if the patient has a history of a negative PPD in the past or no known previous skin test. One must remember that 7% of all adults, and 25% of adults older than 50 years, will have positive skin reactions (9). Sputum can also be sent for cytological evaluation to eliminate malignancy.

CT Scan and Flexible Fiberoptic Bronchoscopy. Both high resolution CT scan and flexible fiberoptic bronchoscopy can be valuable diagnostic tools, and the combination of the two may prove to be necessary. CT scan is superior in identifying occult neoplasms in patients with normal chest radiographs, in addition to diagnosing bronchiectasis and aspergillomas (see Figs. 15.4–15.5). Fiberoptic

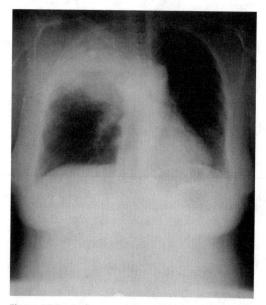

Figure 15.3 Right upper lobe is obliterated by a mass or dense consolidation.

bronchoscopy is useful with central endobronchial disease in allowing direct visualization of a lesion as well as the ability to biopsy a suspicious area or take cytological washings and brushings. It is much more sensitive than CT in demonstrating early mucosal lesions or bronchitis. Complications are rare with fiberoptic bronchoscopy, but they occur, especially in older individuals with a history of COPD or coronary artery disease, probably secondary to the hypoxia that occurs with bronchoscopy. It is probably more worthwhile to perform high resolution CT scan before bronchoscopy in that it provides invaluable information to the bronchoscopist.

Other Tests. Other tests that may be useful depend on the history and physical examination. If one suspects a bleeding disorder, a complete blood count including hematocrit and platelet count is essential as well as a prothrombin time and partial thromboplastin time. Obviously, if the patient presents with life-threatening hemoptysis and is hemodynamically unstable, a full complement of labs is necessary including a type and cross match of blood. If one suspects a vasculitis as the source of the hemoptysis, in addition to the chest x-ray one would check the blood urea nitrogen and creatinine for renal function as well as a urinalysis for red cells or red cell casts. In the case of Wegener's granulomatosis, one would send a blood test for antineutrophil cytoplasmic antibody as well. Cardiac disease could further be evaluated with echocardiogram to visualize valvular function and overall ventricular function.

Differential Diagnosis

It is useful to consider the differential diagnosis of hemoptysis by disease category (Table 15.5). Despite an extensive evaluation, a percentage of cases will remain undiagnosed, or cryptogenic, hemoptysis. Prognosis seems to be favorable in these cases, with most patients experiencing resolution of the hemoptysis within 6 months. In one study, 22% of the patients (57 patients of a total 293 patients) were classified as cryptogenic hemoptysis and followed for an average of about 42 months. Bronchogenic carcinoma was diagnosed in only two patients after 5 and 6 years of follow-up (9).

Management

The goals of therapy are threefold. The first order of business is to stop the bleeding, if it is still active. The second goal is to prevent aspiration. Most importantly, the final goal of therapy is to treat the

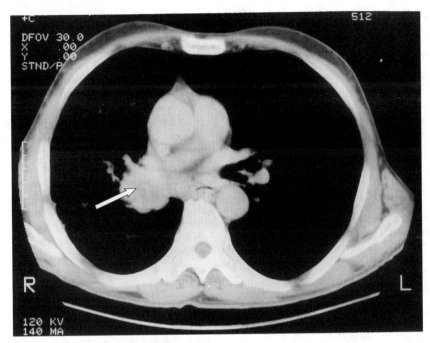

Figure 15.4. CT scan of a right hilar mass that proved
to be squamous cell carcinoma on biopsy.

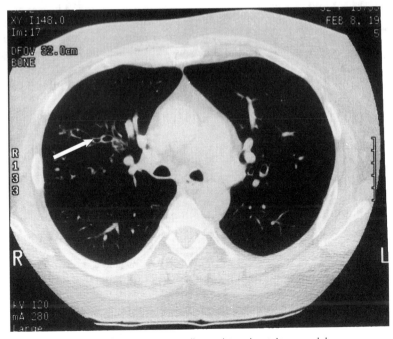

Figure 15.5. CT scan of cystic bronchiectasis, especially involving the right upper lobe.

Table 15.5.
Some Causes of Hemoptysis by Disease Category

Infectious
  Bronchial
    Bronchitis
    Bronchiectasis
  Parenchymal
    Bacterial
    Fungal
    Mycobacterial
    Parasitic

Neoplastic
  Bronchial
    Bronchogenic carcinoma
    Bronchial adenoma
    Metastasis
  Parenchymal
    Primary lung tumor
    Metastasis

Thromboembolic

Cardiac/Vascular
  Pulmonary venous hypertension
    Congestive heart failure
    Mitral stenosis
    Pulmonary venoocclusive disease
  Vascular
    Aneurysms
    Arteriovenous malformations
    Telangiectasis
    Primary pulmonary hypertension

Congenital
  Bronchial cysts
  Sequestrations

Collagen Vascular Disease/Vasculitis

Trauma
  Direct
    Blunt
    Penetrating
  Inhalation
    Acid aspiration
    Toxic gases

Miscellaneous
  Bleeding diathesis (including drug-induced)
  Hemosiderosis
  Goodpasture's syndrome
  Broncholithiasis
  Others

From Israel RH, Poe RH. Hemoptysis. Chest Med 1987;8:198.

underlying cause and prevent recurrence of hemoptysis.

Medical maneuvers may be useful in controlling hemoptysis and preventing aspiration while the work-up is being performed. In patients with scant hemoptysis, cough suppressants may be useful in controlling bleeding until a diagnosis is reached (once sputum has been collected for analysis). If more active bleeding is occurring, the patient can be placed with the responsible lung down, in the dependent position, to prevent blood from entering the airways or the second lung. In the event of massive hemoptysis, emergency therapy is required to protect the airway and find and control the bleeding as soon as possible. Surgical means must be employed at this point, including rigid bronchoscopy to try and identify the source of bleeding. The patient may need to go to the operating room for resection of the involved portion of the lung, or invasive radiographic measures may be attempted with the use of balloon catheters or Gelfoam to stop the bleeding.

A discussion of therapy for all underlying causes of hemoptysis would prove to be a major undertaking, given the large differential diagnosis. The discussion in this section will be limited to therapy for the more common pulmonary causes of hemoptysis. Pneumonia and bronchitis are discussed under "Cough."

TUBERCULOSIS

Tuberculosis has had a resurgence in the United States, in part due to the increasing population of people infected with the HIV virus. Discussion of therapy must include not only treatment of active disease but when and whom to treat with a positive PPD (tuberculin skin test). The question of who should receive preventive therapy arises. The guidelines are fairly clear: all persons age 35 or younger and persons older than 35 years with the following risk factors for the development of active tuberculosis:

- Close contact with persons with infectious tuberculosis and a PPD of ≥5 mm;
- Persons with abnormal chest radiographs consistent with fibrotic changes of old healed tuberculosis and a positive PPD of ≥5 mm;
- Persons known to be HIV positive or with risk factors for HIV disease and unknown HIV status and a positive PPD of ≥5 mm;
- Recent converters, as indicated by a positive PPD of ≥10 mm increase within 2 years;
- Active intravenous drug abusers known to be HIV negative with a PPD of ≥10 mm;
- Persons with medical conditions that place them at increased risk of developing active tuberculosis and a PPD of ≥10 mm, including

(a) Immunosuppression, either secondary to disease process (e.g., lymphoma, leukemia, congenital or acquired immunodeficiency) or secondary to medications (e.g., steroids or anticancer chemotherapy)

(b) Chronic renal failure

(c) Pulmonary silicosis

(d) Poorly controlled diabetes mellitus

(e) Postgastrectomy patients, especially those who have lost >10% of their ideal body weight or are poorly nourished

(f) Rapid weight loss cause by chronic undernutrition such as chronic peptic ulcer disease or chronic malabsorption syndrome

- Staff or residents in a group facility where development of tuberculosis could lead to potentially serious epidemiological consequences, such as staff of a newborn nursery or caregivers of patients with immunological defects, with a PPD of ≥10 mm.

In persons with a positive PPD who are 35 or older, and none of the above risk factors, tuberculosis prophylaxis is not recommended. These persons, however, should be educated in the signs and symptoms of active tuberculosis and the need to seek immediate medical attention if these occur. Isoniazid (INH) is the established therapy used for prevention. The standard dose in adults is 300 mg/day. The recommended length of treatment is 6 months unless the patient has an abnormal chest x-ray, documented HIV disease, or risk factors for HIV disease when therapy would then be given for 12 months. Pyridoxine or vitamin B_6 is given in conjunction with INH in those patients with evidence of nutritional deficiencies (e.g., alcoholics, pregnant women, or persons with an illness that predisposes to neuropathy). Healthy patients with normal diets do not require vitamin B_6. The standard dose of vitamin B_6 is 25 mg/day.

In patients exposed to known or suspected INH-resistant tuberculosis, a regimen of rifampin alone or INH plus rifampin is indicated. The dose of rifampin is 600 mg daily in adults. Therapy should be given for 9–12 months. Contraindications to INH therapy exist and include history of a past INH-induced reaction, including hepatic, skin and allergic reactions, neuropathy, and severe chronic liver disease. INH should be used with caution in pregnancy. Although no harmful effects to the fetus have been documented, it is not recommended for preventive therapy during pregnancy unless the woman is known to be HIV positive and PPD positive or a recent known PPD converter.

Standard drug therapy should be initiated for anyone with known or suspected active disease (Table 15.6). The best way to monitor therapy for pulmonary tuberculosis is sputum examination at least monthly until conversion to a negative culture. If patient's sputum cultures remain positive beyond 3 months of therapy one must be concerned about disease from drug-resistant organisms, malabsorption of the medications, or noncompliance with the drug regimen prescribed. It is important at this point to repeat drug susceptibility studies, and the patient should be enrolled in directly observed therapy, if not already done. Directly observed therapy consists of actually watching the patients take their medicine in the presence of a health care provider and is usually done on an intermittent dosing regimen in patients with drug-susceptible isolates. Therapy can be given twice a week after an initial 2-week daily treatment, or a regimen of three times a week can be used from the offset for the duration of treatment, usually continuing the four drugs throughout.

How long should a patient be treated with these medications for active tuberculosis (Tables 15.7 and 15.8)? Obviously drug regimens and length of therapy must be adjusted for culture-proven drug-resistant tuberculosis or drug intolerance (Table 15.9). Note that if a regimen is failing, two to three drugs should be added to the regimen and not one drug alone. Therapy for multidrug-resistant tuberculosis should be undertaken in consultation with an expert in the treatment of tuberculosis. Adverse reactions to the various medications were discussed in the tables, but some precautions must be discussed with the patients and known by the health care provider. INH in conjunction with daily alcohol intake increases the risk of hepatitis. Rifampin may affect the reliability of oral contraceptive pills, and other forms of contraception are advised or the dose of the pill could be increased. Rifampin also decreases the activity of methadone, and dose adjustment, usually an increase in dose of about 50%, is indicated to prevent withdrawal.

Who should be isolated? All patients with suspected or proven infectious tuberculosis should be isolated in special units for tuberculosis patients with proper ventilation, which is usually a hospital facility. Patients should not be isolated together unless specific drug resistance patterns are the same because superinfection with tuberculosis is possible. Isolation is continued until the patient shows a clinical response to therapy with resolution of

Table 15.6.
First-Line Medications for Treatment of Tuberculosis

Drug	Daily Dose	Twice Weekly Dose	Thrice Weekly Dose	Adverse Reactions
Isoniazid po or im[a]				Hepatic enzyme elevation, peripheral neuropathy, hepatitis, central nervous system effects
Child	10 mg/kg	20–40 mg/kg	15 mg/kg	
Adult	300 mg	15 mg/kg		
Maximum	300 mg	900 mg	900 mg	
Rifampin po or iv[a]				Orange discoloration of secretions and urine, hepatitis, fever, thrombocytopenia, flu-like syndrome, many drug interactions
Child	10–20 mg/kg	10–20 mg/kg	600 mg	
Adult	10 mg/kg	10 mg/kg		
Maximum	600 mg	600 mg		
Pyrazinamide po				Gastrointestinal upset, hepatotoxicity, hyperuricemia, arthralgias
Child	20–30 mg/kg	40–50 mg/kg	2.0 g (<50 kg)	
Adult	1.5 g (<50 kg)	2.5 g (<50 kg)	2.5 g (51–74 kg)	
Maximum	2 gm (51–74 kg) 2.5 g (75+ kg)	3 g (51–74 kg) 3.5 gm (75+ kg)	3.0 g (75+ kg)	
Ethambutol po				Decreased red-green discrimination, decreased visual acuity, skin rash
Child	15–25 mg/kg	30–50 mg/kg	30 mg/kg	
Adult	15–25 mg/kg	50 mg/kg		
Maximum	2.5 g			

[a]An isoniazid/rifampin combination is available in tablet form (Rifamate) containing 150 mg isoniazid and 300 mg rifampin and should be used whenever possible.
Adapted from Vasgird DR, ed. Tuberculosis at a glance. New York City Department of Health, 1993:16–17.

cough and fever and, if infected with drug-resistant tuberculosis, has three negative consecutive daily smears or, if infected with drug-susceptible tuberculosis, has sputum smears that show a decrease in the number of acid-fast bacilli organisms.

Routine follow-up in patients with a prompt bacteriological response to therapy and completion of a 6- or 9-month regimen of INH and rifampin is not necessary. Patients known to be HIV positive or with drug-resistant tuberculosis may warrant some routine surveillance after therapy is completed. All patients must be educated to seek prompt medical attention if symptoms recur.

Table 15.7.
Recommended Standard Daily Drug Regimens

INH	6 months
RIF	6 months
PZA	At least 2 months and until susceptibility results available
EMB	Until susceptibility results available

For those who are HIV negative with no other risk factors for HIV and no immunocompromising conditions.
Adapted from Vasgird DR, ed. Tuberculosis at a glance. New York City Department of Health, 1993:21.

BRONCHIECTASIS

Bronchiectasis has decreased in incidence primarily secondary to prompt antimicrobial therapy for bacterial infections and widespread vaccination against measles and pertussis. Treatment is aimed at controlling recurrent infections and providing effective drainage of secretions. When acute bacterial infections occur, antibiotic therapy should be initiated promptly with choice of antibiotic based on Gram stain of the sputum and culture whenever possible. Many times culture of the sputum will show a mixture of bacteria, with no specific pathogen identified. In patients who are not so ill that they need an inpatient setting, treatment with an oral agent (e.g., amoxicillin, ampicillin, tetracycline, trimethoprim-sulfamethoxazole, or amoxicillin with clavulanic acid) is a reasonable choice. Antibiotics should only be used for acute exacerbations of infection because prolonged and prophylactic use of antibiotics has not been proven effective in preventing recurrent infection and may promote resistance by organisms to the various antibiotics in use. Favorable responses to therapy are usually based on clinical signs of decrease and thinning of sputum production and resolution of systemic signs because sputum cultures are rarely sterilized by treatment.

Table 15.8.
Therapy Timeline for Previously Untreated Active Tuberculosis Patients

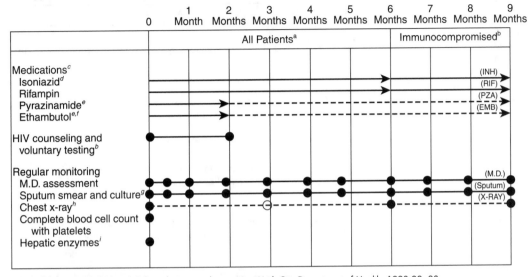

Adapted from: Vasgird DR, ed. Tuberculosis at a glance. New York City Department of Health, 1993:22–23.

[a]Pending the results of drug susceptibility testing, begin all patients on all four of the antituberculosis medications listed, unless there are absolute contraindications. Immunocompetent HIV seronegative patients should be treated for 6 months and for 3 months beyond documented culture conversion.

[b]HIV counseling and testing should be encouraged for all tuberculosis patients, ideally at the first or second clinical visit. Patients known or suspected to be immunocompromised should be treated for 9 months and for 6 months beyond documented culture conversion. Some authorities recommend longer courses of therapy for patients with extrapulmonary disease.

[c]Ideally every tuberculosis patient should receive every dose of antituberculosis medication on a program of directly observed therapy.

[d]Pyridoxine hydrochloride (vitamin B_6), 25 mg with each dose of isoniazid, may decrease peripheral neuritis and central nervous system effects. Pyridoxine should be given with isoniazid to patients who are pregnant or malnourished or use alcohol.

[e]Continue pyrazinamide until (a) at least 8 weeks of therapy have been given and (b) laboratory results document susceptibility to isoniazid and rifampin. Many authorities would continue pyrazinamide until sputum is AFB-smear negative. Ethambutol should be continued until susceptibility to isoniazid and rifampin is documented.

[f]During treatment with ethambutol, monitor visual acuity and color vision monthly.

[g]Regular monitoring of sputum AFB smears and mycobacteriology cultures is essential. If drug resistance is documented, seek expert consultation.

[h]Obtain chest x-ray after 3 months to document response to treatment if initial cultures are negative.

[i]Monitor hepatic enzymes monthly if baseline levels elevated or history of alcoholism or liver disease. At least 20% of patients will have elevated hepatic enzymes: asymptomatic elevation less than five times the upper limit of normal is not an indication to stop treatment. If patients have jaundice or symptomatic liver disease, discontinue medications immediately, and consult a specialist.

Respiratory therapy in the form of chest percussion and gravity drainage may be useful in clearing thick secretions. If bronchospasm is a component, inhaled bronchodilators may be helpful. Cigarette smoking should be strongly discouraged, and yearly influenza vaccinations should be given, as well as the vaccination against pneumococcal infection.

CARCINOMA

Hemoptysis secondary to bronchogenic carcinoma usually occurs in centrally located lesions, more commonly squamous cell carcinoma or small cell carcinoma. Squamous cell carcinoma causes hemoptysis more often because of its propensity to cavitate. Treatment of choice for nonsmall cell lung cancer, once metastatic spread has been eliminated, is surgical resection of the involved lung and surrounding lobe or total pneumonectomy for possible cure. Small cell cancer is much more difficult to treat because once detected micrometastases are usually already present, and combination chemotherapy and radiation therapy is the treatment modality of choice. Staging of lung cancer and the specifics of chemotherapy and radiation therapy are beyond the scope of this book. Bronchial adenomas were discussed under "History."

Table 15.9.
Second-Line Medications for Patients with Drug Resistance or Drug Intolerance

Drug	Daily Dose	Adverse Reaction
Streptomycin im		
Child	20–40 mg/kg	Auditory and renal toxicity, hypokalemia, hypomagnesemia
Adult	15 mg/kg	
Maximum	1 g	
Ciprofloxacin po		
Adult	750–1500 mg	Abdominal cramps, gastrointestinal upset, tremulousness, insomnia, headache, photosensitivity
Ofloxacin po		
Adult	600–800 mg	Probably similar to ciprofloxacin
Kanamycin, capreomycin im/iv		
Child	15–30 mg/kg	Auditory, vestibular and renal toxicity; hypokalemia; hypomagnesemia; eosinophilia
Adult	15 mg/kg	
Maximum	1 g	
Ethionamide po		
Child	15–20 mg/kg	Gastrointestinal upset, hepatotoxicity, hypothyroidism (especially with para-amino-salicylic acid), metallic taste
Adult	500–1000 mg	
Maximum	1 g	
Cycloserine po		
Child	15–20 mg/kg	Psychosis, seizures, headache, depression, other central nervous system effects (give vitamin B$_6$ per 50 mg/250 mg of cycloserine), rash
Adult	250–1000 mg	
Maximum	1 g	
Para-amino-salicylic acid po		
Child	150 mg/kg	Gastrointestinal disturbance, hypersensitivity, hepatotoxicity, sodium load, drug interactions
Adult	150 mg/kg	
Maximum	12 g	
Clofazimine po		
Child	50–200 mg	Orange/brown skin discoloration; gastrointestinal complaints
Adult	100–300 mg	

Medications should only be used in consultation with a physician expert in the management of drug-resistant tuberculosis. Intermittent dosing of second-line medications is not recommended. Always use two to three drugs to which the organism is likely to be susceptible. Never add one drug to a failing regimen.
Adapted from Vasgird DR, ed. Tuberculosis at a glance. New York City Department of Health, 1993:18–19.

ILLUSTRATIVE CASES WITH SELF-ASSESSMENT QUESTIONS AND ANSWERS

Case 1

A 60-year-old man comes to your office with complaints of frequent productive cough with yellow sputum that is blood-tinged. He is frightened and asks your help.

QUESTION: *What other questions would be important to ask when taking the history?*

a. Does he smoke cigarettes and, if so, for how long?
b. Occupational history?
c. Any weight loss or night sweats?
d. Any fevers or associated symptoms of runny nose, sore throat, or pleuritic chest pain?
e. All of the above.

ANSWER: *All these questions are important to establish a list of possible diagnoses.*
The patient goes on to tell you that he has smoked two packs of cigarettes per day for the past 40 years. He worked as a dock worker for 30 years, until he retired 5 years ago, and was exposed to asbestos daily. He has experienced some weight

loss and anorexia recently. He denies fevers or nightsweats.

QUESTION: *What is your differential diagnosis?*

a. Bronchogenic carcinoma
b. Bronchitis
c. Tuberculosis
d. a, b
e. All of the above

ANSWER: d. *The most likely diagnosis in a man older than 50 with a long cigarette smoking history and occupational exposure would be cancer. Weight loss and anorexia would support this. However, many of these symptoms and complaints could be seen with acute exacerbation of chronic bronchitis, with weight loss and anorexia secondary to progression of COPD. The most important aspect of this case is to recognize the possibility of cancer as an underlying cause, and to investigate fully to eliminate this diagnosis before the patient is treated for bronchitis alone.*

Case 2

A 35-year-old woman comes to see you for the first time at a neighborhood clinic. She is a former intravenous drug abuser who last used drugs in 1987 and who has a history of two hospitalizations for bacterial endocarditis. She was incarcerated in 1989 and found then to be PPD positive with a questionable cavitary lesion on chest x-ray and was treated for active tuberculosis at that time with three medications for 9 months. She complains of 6 weeks of a persistent cough with large amounts of blood, accompanied by weight loss, nightsweats, and possibly fevers— she has not used a thermometer but felt hot.

QUESTION: *What tests would you like to perform on this patient?*

a. HIV testing
b. Chest x-ray
c. Sputum for culture/AFB/fungal
d. Tuberculin skin test (PPD)/anergy panel
e. a, b, c

ANSWER: e. *She reports a history of a positive PPD in the past, so there is no gain in repeating the skin test. Because she is immunocompetent, she may mount a large and painful skin reaction. The other tests listed above would help to evalu-*

ate for an infectious etiology, which her history suggests. Her HIV status is important because if she is HIV positive with a diminished T4 helper count, she is at increased risk for opportunistic infections.

She states she was tested 3 months ago at a city clinic and is HIV negative. She denies any recent sexual contacts or repeat drug use since she received her results.

QUESTION: *What is the most likely diagnosis for this patient?*

a. Active tuberculosis
b. Inactive tuberculosis
c. Aspergilloma
d. Histoplasmosis
e. Coccidiomycosis

ANSWER: a. *Active tuberculosis. Although hemoptysis is more commonly encountered in inactive tuberculosis, given her constellation of symptoms of possible fevers, nightsweats, and weight loss, (re)activation of tuberculosis seems most likely. The other possible diagnoses are much less likely given her HIV-negative status, with the assumption that she is an immunocompetent host. Aspergilloma can be seen in a previous scar from tuberculosis but is more often seen in an immunocompromised host. She should be questioned about her travels and where she grew up, because histoplasmosis and coccidiomycosis are more common in the southeastern, mid-Atlantic, central or western United States. Again these organisms more often cause clinical illness in immunocompromised hosts.*

Case 3

A 70-year-old man, whom you have been treating for a long time, telephones and complains of recurrent, productive cough with yellowish/brownish sputum, especially in the morning, which is increasing in frequency and seems to be more bloody than previously. He is quite concerned. He has a history of cigarette smoking and several pneumonias. You ask him to come into the office. On physical examination he has a temperature of 99.1°F orally and a barrel-chested appearance with decreased breath sounds diffusely but no wheezes, rhonchi, or rales. Clubbing of the fingers is noted as well. Chest x-ray shows hyperinflated lung fields and diaphragmatic changes consistent with COPD with no acute infiltrate noted.

QUESTION: *What is the best test to diagnose bronchiectasis?*

a. Fiberoptic bronchoscopy
b. Sputum analysis for bacterial culture
c. High resolution chest CT scan
d. Rigid bronchoscopy
e. None of the above

ANSWER: c. *Before the common use of CT scan, the diagnosis of bronchiectasis was made on clinical grounds or in postmortem studies. CT scan of the chest shows dilated, peripheral airways, a fairly specific finding for bronchiectasis.*

DYSPNEA

Breathing is usually an unconscious bodily function. Dyspnea, or awareness of breathing that is unpleasant, is disturbing to patients seeking medical evaluation and treatment. Dyspnea occurs when the demand for ventilation is greater than the patient's ability to meet that demand. Dyspnea is distinct from tachypnea (rapid breathing), although they may coincide. Dyspnea accompanies physiologic conditions (exercise, stress) and a wide range of pathologic disturbances, of which approximately two-thirds are of pulmonary or cardiac origin (10). Additionally, dyspnea, like pain, is subjective and not measurable, and providers must rely on descriptions provided by patients to gauge its importance. One can easily imagine the diagnostic challenge this symptom poses!

Pathophysiologic Correlation

The body's oxygen and carbon dioxide homeostasis is maintained by an integration of the respiratory, circulatory, and central nervous systems. The respiratory system is designed for gas exchange. Air flows into the lungs during inspiration because intrathoracic negative pressure is generated by increasing the chest diameter (intercostal muscles contract and raise the ribs) and lowering the diaphragms. The lung is elastic and returns passively to its preinspiratory volume. The air is conducted by airways and bronchi, which are surrounded by smooth muscle innervated by the vagus nerve. Sympathetic stimulation of beta-receptors causes bronchodilation. Parasympathetic stimulation causes bronchoconstriction. The terminal bronchioles end in alveoli and their capillary bed, which are the units of gas exchange and the interface between the respiratory and circulatory systems.

Any disturbance, physiologic or pathologic, of these systems' functions will likely upset this homeostasis and result in dyspnea. Disorders that result in hypoxemia and cause dyspnea can be grouped anatomically into pulmonary (airways, lung, chest wall), vascular, or neuromuscular apparatus problems. They can also be viewed functionally as obstructive, restrictive, diminished diffusing capacity or ventilation/perfusion mismatch disorders. Specific disorders may be due to a single functional problem or may be mixed.

Dyspnea is a complex sensation that is not fully understood. It is different from tachypnea (rapid breathing) or hyperpnea (increased ventilation). The dyspneic patient cannot respond to the demand for ventilation, resulting in difficult, uncomfortable, or labored breathing. Changes in blood gas concentration and pH may increase the demand for ventilation. Stimulation of various peripheral sensory receptors and higher centers also contributes to dyspnea.

RESPIRATORY SYSTEM

Lung volumes, measured by spirometry, are considered in the assessment of dyspnea (Fig. 15.6). Total lung capacity is the total volume of gas present in the lungs at the end of inhalation. The volume of gas expired during complete exhalation is the vital capacity. The volume of gas remaining in the lung after maximal exhalation is the residual volume. However, after normal exhalation, the remaining volume of gas is the functional residual capacity (Fig. 15.6). The volume exhaled during a forced expiratory breath is measured at 1 second and completion, for the forced expiratory volume in 1 second (FEV-1) and forced vital capacity (FVC), respectively. Their ratio, FEV-1:FVC, if dampened to <0.7, is helpful in suggesting airways obstruction.

Obstructive Disorders. In obstructive disorders, airflow is impeded by conditions in the lumen, wall, or surrounding tissue of the airways. Lumen conditions include partial occlusion by excessive secretions or aspiration of fluids or foreign bodies. Wall conditions include contraction of bronchial smooth muscle, hypertrophy of the mucosa, and inflammation and edema of the wall. Conditions in the surrounding tissues include destruction of lung parenchyma, causing loss of radial traction on the airways that leads to airways collapse, and edema or masses that compress the airways. All effectively reduce the diameter of the airways and therefore obstruct airflow.

Restrictive Disorders. Restrictive disorders

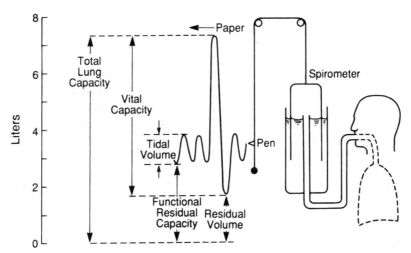

Figure 15.6. Lung volumes. From West JB. Respiratory physiology, the essentials. Baltimore: Williams & Wilkins, 1974:15.

are those in which the expansion of the lung is limited. They can be due to conditions of the lung parenchyma, pleura, chest wall, abdomen, or neuromuscular apparatus. In parenchymal conditions, the interstitium loses compliance and resists expansion. Pleural conditions cause stiffening of the pleura or introduction of excess fluid into the pleural space that in turn prevents lung expansion and/or compresses the lung parenchyma. Chest wall conditions impair chest wall excursion. Abdominal masses or huge abdomens prevent movement of the diaphragms and lung expansion. In neuromuscular conditions, degeneration of respiratory muscles or their nerve supply impair lung expansion. All compress and/or prevent the lung from expanding.

Diminished Diffusing Capacity. Diffusion is governed by Fick's law—the amount of gas that moves across a sheet of tissue is proportional to the area of the sheet and inversely proportional to its thickness. Diffusion disorders result when any disturbance prevents the diffusion of oxygen from the alveolus into the alveolar capillary. These disturbances can be due to loss of the surface area (alveolar walls) over which gas exchange occurs or an increase in the thickness of the diffusion surface (alveolar membrane). Carbon dioxide diffuses more readily than oxygen, and therefore its exchange is not usually affected by these disturbances.

Ventilation/Perfusion Mismatch Disorders. Ventilation/perfusion mismatches occur when there is ventilation of regions of the lung with little blood flow or there is poor ventilation of well perfused areas of the lung resulting in inefficient gas exchange. Regional pulmonary perfusion could be compromised by vascular occlusion or redistribution. Regional aeration compromise occurs with pulmonary parenchymal masses or infiltration. Shunts occur when some arterial blood bypasses ventilated parts of the lung as in cardiac septal defects or arterial venous malformations.

CIRCULATORY SYSTEM

The circulatory component consists of the heart, vessels, and blood and is responsible for transporting oxygen to cells and carbon dioxide away. The right ventricle pumps venous blood into the pulmonary artery, which branches to the alveolar capillary bed. Pulmonary perfusion is greater in dependent areas (the lung bases in upright posture) owing to hydrostatic pressure. Pulmonary artery vasoconstriction in areas of low alveolar partial pressure of oxygen diverts perfusion from poorly ventilated areas of the lung. Oxygen diffusing into the alveolar capillaries is bound by hemoglobin in red cells.

NERVOUS SYSTEM

The nervous system regulates the voluntary and reflexive aspects of breathing and innervates the organs involved in breathing. Table 15.10 summarizes receptors that are involved in respiration. The carotid and aortic bodies are chemoreceptors—their nerve endings sense changes in blood PaO_2 and PCO_2—and can increase respiration. There are also peripheral receptors such as the pulmonary

Table 15.10.
Receptors Contributing to Dyspnea

Mechanical
  Lung
  Respiratory muscles—intercostal, diaphragm
  Airways
Chemoreceptors
  Carotid bodies
  Aortic bodies
  Central medullary
Central nervous system
Vascular
  Right atrial mechanoreceptors
  Left atrial mechanoreceptors
  Pulmonary artery baroreceptors
  Right ventricular strain receptors

stretch receptors that alter respiratory rates in response to changes in lung compliance as in pneumothorax or effusions. Central receptors directly stimulate the medulla in response to pH and CO_2.

Clinical and Laboratory Evaluation

Careful attention to historical, physical, and laboratory findings allows the clinician to focus the search for the source of dyspnea.

HISTORY

Several key points must be addressed when obtaining the history of dyspnea.

- *Describe exactly what you feel.* Patients use many terms to describe dyspnea. Table 15.11 provides some examples. They often can differentiate dyspnea of different causes. For instance, a patient may say, "This is much more severe than running up a flight of stairs" or "This is different from my asthma attack." Patients' usage of terms may vary considerably from a clinician's, and it is essential to clarify

Table 15.11.
Phrases Commonly Used to Describe Dyspnea

Out of breath	Sighing too much
Short of breath	Fighting for breath
It's too hard to breath	Can't breathe fast enough
Can't breathe enough	Feels winded
Suffocating or smothering	Chest is tight
Wheezing	Breathing is heavy
Can't get enough air	Chest is painful
Breathing is tiring	Can't control breathing

meanings. In fact, the patient may not be describing dyspnea!

- *Are you short of breath at rest?* An affirmative response suggests more severe physiologic impairment.
- *Do you have any chest pain?* Localized chest pain raises possibilities of trauma, pneumothoraces, cardiac events, pneumonic processes, or pulmonary emboli.
- *What were you doing before and at the onset of dyspnea?* Association with exercise, sleep, coughing, or an emotional stressor leads to differing considerations.
- *Have you ever felt this way before?* Establishing an acute or chronic history changes the scope of consideration.

The history should establish duration ("lasted 10 minutes"), occurrence ("happened every day for 2 weeks"), accompanying symptoms (cough, wheezing, hemoptysis), and triggering or associated events (exercise, cold weather). The clinician must review any past medical history (cardiac or anxiety disorder), medications (beta-blockers), occupational (dust, fumes) or animal exposures, tobacco usage, and exercise history. Patients with an acute onset of dyspnea are likely to be precise with their history, whereas patients with chronic dyspnea may find it easier to describe changes.

PHYSICAL EXAMINATION

The history serves to focus the physical examination. Elevated or irregular respiratory and heart rates and hypertension accompany organic and psychogenic respiratory distress. Hypotension would suggest serious pulmonary or vascular compromise. Inspection quickly establishes skin color (cyanotic versus pink), posture (tripod versus upright), obesity or asthenia, and a general sense of distress.

The head, including the nose and oral pharynx, is examined for respiratory stridor, nasopharyngeal masses, lip cyanosis, and pursed lips. The chest is examined for symmetry, deformities, and use of accessory muscles of respiration (intercostal and neck muscles). Palpation for tenderness and crepitation helps localize areas of involvement. Percussion reveals the position of the diaphragms and hypo- or hyperresonance of the lung fields. The clinician auscultates the lungs for location, quality, and symmetry of breath sounds, wheezing, rales, rhonchi, and egophony. The cardiac exam (see Chapter 13) is an important part of evaluating a dyspneic patient. Murmurs, a displaced PMI, jugular venous distension, hepatomegaly, hepatojugular reflux, an S_3 gallop, and peripheral edema direct the clinician toward cardiac etiologies of dyspnea. The extremities may show clubbing, cyanosis, edema, venous cords, varicosities or tenderness. The neurologic exam may reveal hyper- or hyporeflexia or diminished motor strength; a psychological assessment should be performed if psychogenic causes are suspected.

LABORATORY EVALUATION

The laboratory evaluation for causes of dyspnea is imposing. The clinician must be selective and use information garnered from the history and physical examination to guide testing. The various laboratory modalities, indications, and information gathered follow.

Imaging Studies. Six imaging studies are discussed.

- Chest x-rays are essential in evaluating acute and chronic dyspnea and give information about the chest wall, diaphragms, lung parenchyma, pulmonary vasculature, heart size and configuration, pleural space, and airways. A chest x-ray is indicated if dyspnea is accompanied by abnormal lung sounds, fever, signs of fluid overload, or pain and is helpful in eliminating pathology in psychogenic causes of dyspnea.
- CT and magnetic resonance imaging are useful to provide detail in evaluating structural, parenchymal, pleural, and chest wall problems suggested by a chest x-ray. They have limited ability to visualize vascular structures and are helpful for localization of suspicious areas before thoracentesis, bronchoscopy, and needle or open biopsy.
- Echocardiograms utilize ultrasound to image the heart and can be useful if dyspnea is thought to be due to ventricular, valvular, or pericardial pathology. Consider echocardiography if the patient has signs of congestive heart failure, a murmur, or a pericardial friction rub.
- Nuclear ejection fraction studies utilize radioisotopes to evaluate ventricular function. The nuclear ejection fraction is helpful when congestive heart failure is being considered in the differential diagnosis.
- Ventilation/perfusion scans utilize radionuclides to demonstrate pulmonary ventilation and perfusion. Areas demonstrating ventilation without perfusion, or mismatches, suggest a pulmonary embolus. A ventilation/ perfusion scan should be considered if a deep vein thrombus or its risks are present. Preexisting pulmonary disease, like COPD, makes interpretation difficult.

Functional Studies. PFTs are useful if obstructive, restrictive, or diffusing capacity disorders are being considered. They provide information on lung volumes (vital capacity, residual volume, functional residual capacity, total lung capacity), flow, diffusing capacity, and response to bronchodilators. Spirometry measures the FVC and FEV-1 and can diagnose obstructive airways disease. Peak expiratory flow rates (PEFR) are useful in following the severity of asthma in an office or emergency room setting but are not specific to obstruction. They can also be diminished in neuromuscular disorders or normal or supernormal in restrictive conditions. They are not diminished if there is a cardiac problem. Inspiratory and expiratory mouth pressures at functional residual capacity can assess respiratory muscle strength. Table 15.12 summarizes PFT findings.

Cardiopulmonary exercise testing is useful in obesity, anxiety, deconditioning, and coexisting cardiac and pulmonary diseases and when PFTs are nondiagnostic. Patients perform a standard exercise stress test (e.g., treadmill, bicycle), and expired gases are analyzed for minute ventilation, oxygen consumption, and carbon dioxide production.

Blood Tests. Arterial blood gas evaluation is useful to evaluate oxygenation, hypercapnia, and acidemia in respiratory failure, metabolic acidosis with respiratory compensation, and psychogenic states. Complete blood counts should be requested in suspected cases of anemia and infection. Chemical profiles electrolyte are useful when considering metabolic acidosis.

Tissue Evaluation. Biopsy of lung parenchyma and pleura via needle aspiration, bronchoscopy, or surgery provides tissue for pathological evaluation. Biopsy can be considered for confirming neoplasm, granulomatous disease (silicosis, sarcoidosis, tuberculosis), and interstitial fibrosis.

Cytologic evaluation of sputum, pleural fluid, or bronchial lavage washings is useful if one is considering neoplasms.

Sputum examination via smears, cultures, and cytology is useful when asthma, neoplastic neoplasm, or tuberculosis and other bacterial conditions are suspected.

Mantoux Testing. Mantoux testing (PPD) should be performed when tuberculosis is being considered.

Table 15.12.
Pulmonary Function Tests and Pulmonary Disorders

Category	PFT Findings	Disorders	Additional Testing
Obstructive	FEV-1/FVC < 70%	Bronchoconstriction (acute asthma), COPD	Bronchoprovocation challenge, bronchodilator challenge
Restrictive	Decreased lung volumes	Interstitial lung disease (fibrosis) Pleural disease (effusions) Chest wall disease (kyphoscoliosis)	DLCO, CPEX Thoracentesis, pleural biopsy
		Respiratory musc. disease (polio, Guillain-Barré)	PIMAX, PEMAX
Abnormal diffusion	Decreased DLCO	Shunting (COPD, pulmonary embolus), interstitial lung disease	Ventillation/perfusion scan angiography Lung biopsy
Normal	Normal	Anemia Psychogenic (anxiety, panic disorder)	Complete blood count, Psychological evaluation,
		Deconditioning	CPEX

DLCO, carbon monoxide diffusing capacity; CPEX, cardiopulmonary exercise testing; PIMAX, inspiratory mouth pressure; PEMAX, expiratory mouth pressure.

Differential Diagnosis

As previously mentioned, the considerations when dealing with a patient with dyspnea are tremendous. It is helpful to divide the differential diagnoses into physiologic, acute, and chronic causes of dyspnea.

PHYSIOLOGIC CAUSES

Physiologic causes of dyspnea do not represent pathology. The common conditions of deconditioning, obesity, aging, and pregnancy will be discussed.

Deconditioning is common in persons with sedentary lifestyles and as people age. Most people's exercise level adjusts to their tolerance, and dyspnea is experienced only when that threshold is crossed. This may occur when there is an unexpected demand for increased activity (walking up stairs when the elevator is disabled), a sudden change in lifestyle (military training), or abrupt resumption of baseline activities after a prolonged layoff (going shopping after being bedridden for several weeks). Most situations can be identified by history taking. Cardiopulmonary exercise testing, helpful in thorny cases, will show diminished oxygen consumption and a normal electrocardiogram, and the patient will complain of lower extremity fatigue.

Moderately obese individuals often experience exertional dyspnea. Morbidly obese individuals additionally experience orthopnea and dyspnea at rest. There are multiple mechanisms at work. The fat layer over the chest wall restricts its movement.

The obese abdomen limits diaphragmatic excursion. Deconditioning contributes both to obesity and dyspnea. The increased exercise load imposed by a larger body mass is also a factor.

Dyspnea is a frequent symptom during a normal pregnancy. Dyspnea begins in the first trimester. Rest dyspnea affects about half of pregnant women by midterm and peaks between 28–31 weeks of gestation. The mechanism of the dyspnea of pregnancy is unclear, but it is thought to be a normal response to the pulmonary physiologic changes during gestation. During pregnancy, fetal and placental requirements increase oxygen consumption by 20–30%. There is a progesterone mediated increase in minute ventilation caused by increased tidal volume; the respiratory rate is unchanged. The gravid uterus raises the diaphragm and changes the configuration of the thorax. The dyspnea of pregnancy is likely due to the combination of the progesterone effect, the increased work of breathing with a changed thoracic shape, the increased body mass oxygen demand, and the anemia of pregnancy.

The aging process itself leads to alterations in respiratory physiology that can result in dyspnea in the absence of disease. Lung volumes change, and there is a progressive loss of lung function. Total lung capacity stays the same, but there is an increase in residual volume from air trapped behind collapsed airways and subsequently a decrease in vital capacity. The FVC and FEV-1 decline. There is a loss in the elastic recoil that contributes to earlier airways closure and air trapping at the bases of the lung with preservation of perfusion—a ventilation/perfusion mismatch! Diffusion capacity diminishes owing to inflammatory destruction of alveolar structures and increasing ventilation/perfusion mismatch.

ACUTE DYSPNEA

Dyspnea that has a sudden identifiable onset is generally worrisome and requires prompt attention. Table 15.13 lists causes of acute dyspnea. Of these, anxiety/hyperventilation, asthma, pulmonary edema, and pneumonia are fairly common among ambulatory patients.

Psychogenic Dyspnea. The dyspnea of anxiety or a panic attack is usually precipitated by an emotional stressor that can often be identified in the history. Some psychogenic causes of dyspnea are subtle, and the clinician or patient may fail to recognize them. The patient may also complain of numbness and tingling of the lips and fingers. In addition to tachypnea, the physical examination may be consistent with distress—tachycardia, diaphoresis, hyperreflexia—and an otherwise normal pulmonary and cardiac examination. The arterial blood gas will show a respiratory alkalosis (elevated pH with hypocapnia) and increased oxygenation. Chest x-ray and PFTs are normal. The clinician's consideration of psychogenic dyspnea is enhanced if symptoms dissipate with reassurance, distraction, or rebreathing using a paper bag. Psychiatric testing may be helpful when the stressor is not obvious

or if the patient lacks insight into the emotional issues. The clinician must suspect psychogenic dyspnea if a link to an emotional stressor is demonstrated, if the objective findings do not support the subjective complaints, and if risks for other causes of dyspnea are absent.

Asthma. Asthma is an episodic syndrome of reversible increased bronchial reactivity and therefore a cause of acute dyspnea. Asthma attacks occur acutely from isolated stimuli or more often as an intrinsic chronic inflammatory respiratory disorder. Patients have normal airways and function between attacks. The full discussion of asthma as a chronic cause of dyspnea will follow.

Acute Pulmonary Edema. Pulmonary edema occurs when backward flow of cardiac circulation causes movement of fluid from the vascular space into the interstitial, peribronchial, perivascular, and ultimately alveolar space, thereby precluding gas exchange. There is either an abrupt or progressive onset of dyspnea. Chest pain, palpitations, medication noncompliance, or dietary indiscretion may precede the dyspnea. The patient has increased respiratory and heart rates and blood pressure. There are inspiratory crackles (rales), wheezing, and a third heart sound. In acute pulmonary edema, the patient is pale and diaphoretic. Chest x-ray classically shows fluffy infiltrates in a butterfly pattern, pulmonary vascular congestion, fluid in the fissures, and Kerly B and C lines in the periphery of the lung. Pleural effusions may be present (Fig. 15.7). The arterial blood gas typically shows acidosis and hypoxemia. Hypercapnia ensues with ventilatory failure. Congestive heart failure is the most common ambulatory cause of pulmonary edema. Valvular heart disease (aortic and mitral stenosis), myocardial infarctions, and arrhythmias can also cause pulmonary edema.

Pleural Effusions. Large pleural effusions cause restriction of lung expansion and compression of lung parenchyma and can result in dyspnea. The abruptness of dyspnea depends on how rapidly the fluid accumulates and its volume. There is usually pleuritic chest pain. Dullness on percussion, decreased tactile fremitus, and diminished breath sounds to the fluid level are the characteristic physical findings. The chest x-ray shows blunting of the costal-phrenic angles and fluid layering out on decubitus views. Thoracentesis removes pleural fluid, which relieves the dyspnea and can help distinguish transudative and exudative causes to guide therapy; these characteristics are summarized in Table 15.14. Pleural effusions are commonly caused by congestive heart failure and infection.

Table 15.13.
Some Causes of Acute Dyspnea

Alveolitis
Asthma
Chest trauma
  Pneumothorax
  Rib fracture
  Pulmonary contusion
Foreign body inhalation
High altitudes
Metabolic acidosis—diabetic ketoacidosis, ingestions, sepsis
Pleural effusion
Pneumonia
Pulmonary edema
Pulmonary embolism
Smoke inhalation
Spontaneous pneumothorax

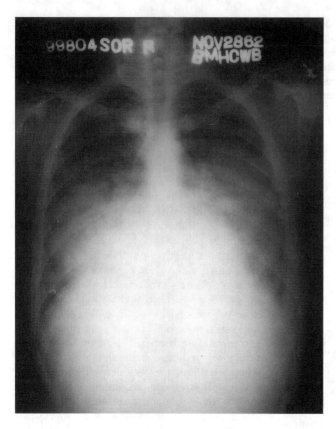

Figure 15.7. Typical radiograph of acute pulmonary edema.

Neoplasm must be considered in smokers. Other sources of pleural effusions are less common.

Pneumonia. Community acquired pneumonias such as pneumococcal and mycoplasma or *Pneumocystis* in persons with HIV can involve extensive segments of pulmonary parenchyma and compromise ventilation. This form of ventilation/perfusion mismatch results in dyspnea and is usually accompanied by signs of sepsis (see Chapter 18), pleuritic chest pain (see Chapter 13), or hemoptysis (see "Hemoptysis"). Persons with preexisting chronic lung disease, depressed consciousness or gag reflex, and the immunosuppressed are at risk for pneumonia. Pneumonia can complicate influenza and varicella.

Pulmonary Emboli. Pulmonary emboli are

Table 15.14.
Characteristics of Pleural Effusions

	Transudate	Exudate
Appearance	Clear, straw colored	Cloudy, bloody, grossly purulent
Specific gravity	<1.016	>1.016
pH	Normal	Low
White blood cells	Few lymphocytes	Many PMN or lymphs
Red blood cells	Few, unless tap is traumatic	Variable—few to grossly bloody
Glucose	Equal to serum	Decreased from serum value
Protein	<3.0 g/100 ml	>3.0 g/100 ml
Lactate dehydrogenase	Low	Increased
Clot, fibrinogen	Absent	Present
Examples	Congestive heart failure, cirrhosis, nephrosis	Infection, tuberculosis, neoplasm

relatively uncommon causes of acute dyspnea causing ventilation/perfusion mismatch. They are important because of potential mortality if unrecognized and untreated. Microscopic pulmonary emboli are readily filtered by the lung and pose few problems; larger emboli obstruct pulmonary perfusion. Risk factors for pulmonary emboli are cardiomegaly, congestive heart failure, venous disease of the lower extremities, carcinoma, oral contraceptives, recent pelvic or lower extremity surgery, and prolonged immobilization. These conditions allow for development of stasis, vascular intimal injury, or a hypercoagulable state, the prerequisites for clot formation. Fractured bones could be the source of fat emboli.

Patients usually present with abrupt onset of dyspnea. Few have pleuritic chest pain. Arterial blood gas shows hypoxemia, hypocapnia, and acidemia. Serum chemistry after several hours to days may reveal increased lactate dehydrogenase, serum glutamic-oxaloacetic acid, and bilirubin reflecting tissue demise. Chest x-ray may be normal or show pleural effusions. The ventilation/perfusion scan shows a mismatch—ventilation in areas sans perfusion (Fig. 15.8)—but can be inconclusive. The pulmonary angiogram is the "gold standard" in demonstrating an obstructing lesion. Clinicians should consider pulmonary emboli in high risk settings.

Other Causes. Other causes of acute dyspnea include chest trauma, which should be considered if there is a suggestive history. Spontaneous pneumothorax is uncommon but should be considered if there is a history of acute exacerbation of emphysema or asthma, endometriosis, or Marfan's syndrome. A chest x-ray can show fractured ribs, a pneumothorax, or a hemothorax. Dyspnea also results acutely from conditions that increase oxygen demand such as thyrotoxicosis and fever. Smoke inhalation causes breathlessness by decreasing blood oxygenation and inflaming the airways. Carbon monoxide inhalation is characterized by dizziness, breathlessness, and rapid loss of consciousness. Decreased ambient oxygen concentration in high altitude environments creates problems for the unacclimated who have not compensated with a secondary polycythemia. Metabolic acidosis such as diabetic ketoacidosis, sepsis, renal insufficiency, or ingestion can also result in dyspnea.

CHRONIC DYSPNEA

Chronic dyspnea is a common ambulatory respiratory complaint with many causes that are listed in Table 15.15. The patient's history is essential in considering these causes. Whether dyspnea is the lone complaint or is accompanied by sputum production, cough, hemoptysis, orthopnea, weight loss, or paroxysmal nocturnal dyspnea is important in narrowing the differential diagnoses. The precipitation of shortness of breath is influenced by the patient's level of physical activity. Many patients become aware of shortness of breath only after unusual exertion. Likewise, patients who have experienced chronic dyspnea may curtail their activity below the threshold of dyspnea and thus avoid it. So the context of dyspnea is essential in considering its cause. Those causes of dyspnea likely to be encountered in an ambulatory care setting will be discussed below.

Pulmonary Causes. The most common chronic pulmonary disorders seen in adult ambulatory settings causing dyspnea are COPD and asthma. Primary or metastatic neoplasms are not unusual pulmonary causes of dyspnea and will be considered briefly. Other causes are rarer and can be considered in particular circumstances such as an occupation or exposure. The pulmonary causes of chronic dyspnea are listed in Table 15.15.

Chronic Obstructive Pulmonary Disease. COPD refers to the conditions of emphysema and chronic bronchitis alone or in combination. Emphysema is characterized by enlargement of alveoli with destruction of their walls and capillary bed. The small airways are narrowed, tortuous, and atrophied (Fig. 15.9). Chronic bronchitis is characterized by hypertrophy of the airway mucosa with an increase in mucous producing goblet cells. COPD most commonly affects persons with a history of cigarette smoking. The history is that of poor exercise tolerance caused by dyspnea, progression of symptoms, and exacerbation of dyspnea with common colds. A history of cough and sputum production for at least 2 months in each of 2 consecutive years identifies chronic bronchitis. Other complaints include a predilection for upper respiratory infections, palpitations, chest discomfort, and orthopnea. Palpitations arise from sinus tachycardia caused by medications or meeting oxygen demand with exercise. Less commonly, multifocal atrial tachycardia can accompany respiratory compromise.

The physical examination shows a barrel chest with lowered diaphragms and hyperresonant lung fields, wheezing, rhonchi, rales, and a prolonged expiratory phase of respiration. In advanced COPD the physical examination may show resting tachypnea and tachycardia, pursed lips, cyanosis or plethora, clubbing of the nails, and "tripoding" (patient

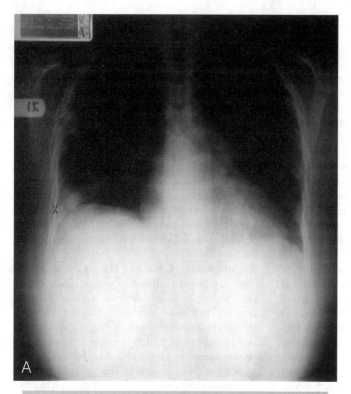

A

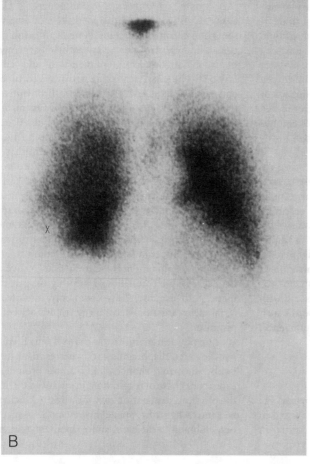

B

Figure 15.8. Characteristics of a high probability ventilation/perfusion scan and plain chest x-ray. Chest x-ray (**A**) shows two lesions (X) in the right lung that match photon deficient areas (X) in the perfusion scan (**B**) and ventilation scan (**C**). These matched defects were longstanding. Defect (Y) in the perfusion scan is not matched in the ventilation scan and is the location of the pulmonary embolus.

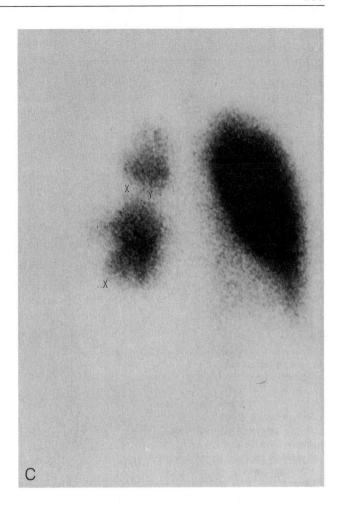

C

Figure 15.8. *(Continued).*

seated bent anteriorly and supported by both arms) (Fig. 15.10).

The chest x-ray shows enlarged, hyperaerated lung fields, lowered and flattened diaphragms, and an increased anterior to posterior diameter (Fig 15.11). Blood tests may show an increased hematocrit caused by secondary polycythemia and an increased bicarbonate from metabolic compensation for chronic respiratory acidosis driven by carbon dioxide retention. The arterial blood gas shows hypoxemia, hypercapnia, and acidemia. PFTs characteristically show decreased flow, increased lung volumes, decreased diffusing capacity, and no bronchodilator response.

Asthma. Asthma is a chronic inflammatory disorder of the airways with episodes of increased bronchial reactivity. Bronchial smooth muscle contraction, mucosal edema, and increased mucous secretion result in reversible airways obstruction. Inflammation is caused by allergens (extrinsic asthma) or nonallergic stimuli (intrinsic asthma) and leads to bronchial hyperresponsiveness and bronchoconstriction. These are reversible, and normal airways are present between attacks. Chronic asthma usually begins in childhood to young adulthood, but the first asthmatic episode may occur at any age and may pose a greater diagnostic challenge than recurrent attacks. The history is important in revealing precipitants such as allergens or irritants, an antecedent respiratory tract infection, temperature change, exercise, or an emotional event. Allergens include pollens, dust, and animal dander. Patients with allergic asthma characteristically can give a personal and/or family history of other allergic diseases such as rhinitis, urticaria, and eczema. Irritants include smoke, air pollution, insecticides, perfumes, and paint. Asthma symptoms may occur in specific environments (e.g., work, a home other than the patient's, or school) which impose an allergen or irritant that is otherwise avoided. Asthma may be precipitated by medications such as aspirin, beta-blockers (atenolol or propranolol), or sulfiting

Table 15.15.
Causes of Chronic Dyspnea

Pulmonary

Airway disease
    Upper airway obstruction—laryngeal mass, tracheal
       stenosis
    Asthma
    Chronic bronchitis
    Cystic fibrosis
Parenchymal lung disease
    Emphysema
    Interstitial lung disease—pulmonary fibrosis,
       sarcoidosis
    Neoplasms—primary or metastatic
    Pneumoconiosis—coal, silica
    Pneumonia
Pulmonary vascular disease
    Vasculitis
    Venoocclusive disease
Pleural disease
    Fibrosis
    Malignancy
Chest cavity conditions
    Deformities—kyphoscoliosis, ankylosing spondylitis,
       pectus excavatum
    Abdominal distention—obesity, pregnancy, ascites,
       masses

Cardiovascular disease

Congenital heart disease—atrial septal defect, patent
    ductus arteriosus, pulmonic stenosis
Ischemic heart disease
Left ventricular failure, biventricular failure—dilated
    cardiomyopathy
Myxoma
Pericardial disease—pericarditis, pericardial effusion
Pulmonary hypertension
Restrictive cardiomyopathy
Right-to-left shunts
Valvular disease

Neuromuscular disease

Central nervous system disorders—strokes
Myopathy and neuropathy—polio
Phrenic nerve and diaphragmatic disorders
Spinal cord disorders—acute lateral sclerosis
Systemic neuromuscular disorders—muscular dys-
    trophy

Other

Anemia
Deconditioning
Gastroesophageal reflux
Psychogenic
Thyroid disease—hyperthyroidism or hypothyroidism

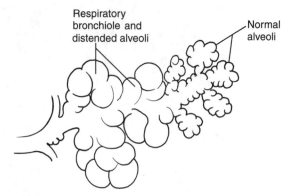

Figure 15.9. Pathological characteristics of emphysema. Destruction of the elastic elements of the terminal bronchiole and alveolar wall leads to airway collapse and air trapping during expiration.

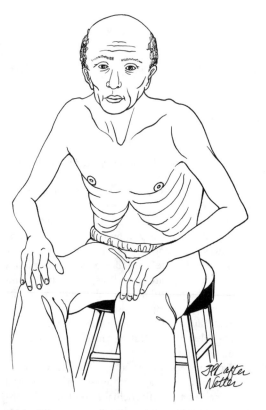

Figure 15.10. Tripod posture. Adapted from Netter F. The CIBA collection of medical illustrations. Newark: CIBA Medical, 1980;7:148.

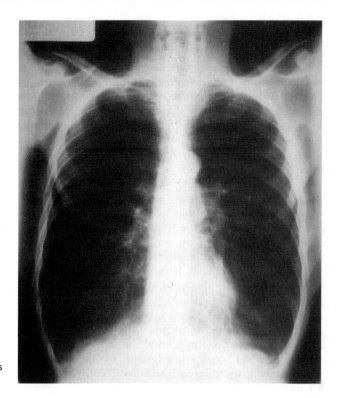

Figure 15.11. Radiographic characteristics of COPD.

agents in processed food. Therefore a medication history is essential.

At presentation, patients have symptoms of dyspnea, wheezing, chest tightness, cough, and sputum production. The patient may be febrile, especially if an upper respiratory tract infection is the precipitant. It is important to determine any precipitant and the duration of the current attack. The patient's subjective assessment of the severity of the current attack compared with previous attacks is helpful in guiding the urgency of management strategies. It is also useful to determine the course of previous attacks, need for steroids, hospitalization, or intubation, and medication compliance.

During an acute attack of asthma patients appear generally uncomfortable, anxious, or agitated and unable to talk freely. The physical examination reveals tachypnea, tachycardia, wheezing, and a prolonged expiratory phase of respiration and hyperinflation of the lungs (increased resonance). In severe cases, there may be use of the accessory muscles of respiration or retraction of the intercostal muscles, cyanosis, or a pulsus paradoxus.

Airflow measurements of PEFR and FEV-1 by peak flow meter or bedside spirometry evaluate the severity of an episode and monitor the response to

therapy; however, they are not diagnostic. Laboratory testing is characteristic but not necessary in managing most recurrent episodes of asthma. PFTs will show diminished FVC, FEV-1/FVC, and PEFR. Total lung capacity and residual volume are increased. These improve with bronchodilators. The arterial blood gas initially shows hypocapnia ($PaCO_2$ <35 mmHg), hypoxemia (PaO_2 <80 mmHg), and a respiratory alkalosis (pH >7.4). With fatigue and impending respiratory failure, normal or elevated levels of carbon dioxide and acidosis are found. An arterial blood gas should be ordered if reversal of bronchospasm is delayed or the patient indicates fatigue. The complete blood count may show eosinophilia. An elevated white count may indicate infection or follow steroid administration. After several hours, the serum chemistry shows lowered bicarbonate values indicating a metabolic compensation of the respiratory alkalosis. A chest x-ray is not always necessary but may show the hyperlucency of air trapping and patchy infiltrates indicating atelectasis behind mucous plugs. A chest x-ray should be ordered if a complicating infection or pneumothorax is being considered. Sputum examination reveals eosinophils and mucous plugs; large numbers of neutrophils suggest infection. Skin testing to allergens may be positive and direct suppressive therapy in allergen mediated asthma.

Neoplasm. Lung cancer is the second most common primary neoplasm affecting males and females. Cancers from other sites can also metastasize to the lung. A history of cigarette smoking is a major risk factor for primary lung cancer. Air pollution and occupational exposure to chromates, nickel, arsenic, asbestos, and radioactive gases also are risk factors for developing lung cancer. Early signs of lung cancer include a nonproductive cough, hemoptysis, weight loss, or rarely hoarseness. Dyspnea is usually a late sign owing to extensive parenchymal involvement, pleural effusions, or bronchial obstruction. Chest pain is another late sign caused by pleural involvement. Regional metastatic spread of the tumor causes tracheal obstruction, dysphagia, hoarseness, a Horner's syndrome, superior vena cava syndrome, and pleural effusions. A patient may first present with distant metastases to the brain, bone, and liver with seizures, bone pain, or abnormal liver function tests that prompt a diagnostic workup identifying a lung cancer as the source. Paraneoplastic syndromes may also be the presenting complaint.

In the early stages, the physical examination is often negative. Later there are signs of lobar collapse or consolidation. A chest x-ray can show a mass or infiltrating lesion but will miss small carcinomas. CT and magnetic resonance imaging scans can add detail, pinpoint location, show relationship to contiguous structures, and view lymph nodes. Therefore they are useful in confirming lesions, guiding biopsies, and staging lesions. Diagnosis is made by sputum cytology or pathological specimens obtained via bronchoscopy of central lesions, needle biopsy of peripheral lesions, or open lung biopsy. PFTs are rarely useful in making a diagnosis but will reflect the functional impairments caused by carcinoma such as a restrictive pattern with effusions or an obstructive pattern with mass effect on a large bronchus. There is no role for screening chest x-rays or sputum cytologies of the general population.

Occupational Causes. The history of chronic dyspnea includes triggers, associations, and exposures. Complaints that are associated with the work week and abate during absences from work or a history of certain occupations suggest exposure to particles (coal, silica, textile), dust, or chemicals that can cause airways disease or pneumoconiosis. The clinician's suspicions can be guided by regional economies (mining, textiles, boat building, agriculture) but must note temporally distant exposures as well. Airways disease includes byssinosis, which is bronchoconstriction after inhalation of cotton dust, and occupational asthma caused by hypersensitivity to organic dusts. Typically, dyspnea and wheezing appear after beginning work and abate overnight or after weekends. PFTs show an obstructive pattern. Pneumoconiosis refers to parenchymal lung disease caused by inhalation of inorganic particles. These particles lodge in the lung and cause fibrosis and, in silica exposure, formation of nodules as well. Patients may complain of cough and dyspnea. Chest x-ray findings of nodular, streaky markings may precede symptoms. Asbestos exposure can lead to diffuse interstitial fibrosis, carcinoma, or pleural disease. Chest x-rays find haziness, a mass, and pleural thickening and plaques, respectively. Restrictive PFT patterns are found in interstitial fibrosis and pleural disease.

Cardiac Causes. Cardiac dysfunction contributing to chronic dyspnea underscores the cardiovascular role in gas exchange. The major pathological cardiac mechanisms that impair gas exchange with resulting dyspnea are left-sided pump failure, filling or outflow obstruction, and intracardiac shunts. Congestive heart failure with left ventricular failure, valvular heart disease, and atrial septal defects as a form of intracardiac shunt will be discussed. Other cardiac causes of dyspnea are listed in Table 15.15.

Congestive Heart Failure and Left Ventricular Failure. Congestive heart failure occurs when normal cardiac hemodynamics (preload, afterload, contractility, filling volumes, or rate) are disturbed, resulting in the heart's inability to pump enough blood to oxygenate metabolizing tissues. Dyspnea is a major consequence of left ventricular failure. The most common causes of myocardial depression are ischemia, hypertension, and dilated cardiomyopathies. Dyspnea may be the sole complaint noted during myocardial ischemia. During an ischemic episode, myocyte dysfunction results in left ventricular depression that reverses with restoration of myocardial circulation. In contrast, myocytes are irreversibly damaged during myocardial infarction, leading to diminished left ventricular pumping ability. Hypertension causes increased left ventricular afterload and strain. Left ventricular hypertrophy followed by a dilated cardiomyopathy and decreased left ventricular function result. Dilated cardiomyopathies and left ventricular failure can also be caused by alcohol, viral infection, and streptococcal carditis. Congestive heart failure can also be seen with anemia, thyroid disease, and fever and as a result of medications such as beta-blockers and adriamycin.

The history usually easily reveals angina, myocardial infarctions, and hypertension. The medication history is essential. A history of an antecedent viral illness, untreated streptococcal carditis, or alcohol abuse must be sought. Dyspnea with exertion may be accompanied by dyspnea that arouses the patient from sleep (paroxysmal nocturnal dyspnea) and nocturia caused by increased venous return (preload) with recumbency. The patient also notes easy fatigue, diminished exercise tolerance, and a dry cough. In biventricular failure, dyspnea will be accompanied by complaints of peripheral edema and abdominal pain caused by a tender congested liver. The patient's history may be peppered with bouts of pulmonary edema.

The pulmonary examination reveals fluid-rales. Biventricular failure will also have jugular venous distention, hepatomegaly, and dependent edema. The chest x-ray is remarkable for vascular congestion, infiltrates, fluid in the fissures and periphery, or effusions and cardiomegaly. An echocardiogram generally shows diminished left ventricular function, cardiomegaly, and, occasionally, a pericardial effusion. The nuclear ejection fraction is usually <40% compared with 60–70% in normal individuals. Streptococcal testing is usually not helpful for distant infection. Endocardial biopsy is not routinely done but may be considered when assessing myocarditis. It shows lymphocytic, inflammatory infiltration in acute myocarditis; fibrosis and amyloid deposits may be found later.

Valvular Heart Disease. Valvular heart disease involving the mitral and aortic valves is another cause of dyspnea. Valvular heart disease causes stenosis leading to cardiac filling or outflow obstruction or regurgitation, either leading to ventricular failure. Generally, risks for valvular heart disease include rheumatic fever, endocarditis, ischemic heart disease, syphilis, and, rarely, Marfan's syndrome. A history of rheumatic fever is more prevalent in medically underserved communities and developing countries and should be suspected in patients with valvular heart disease from those backgrounds. Endocarditis should be considered in those with a history of illicit intravenous drug use. Previous rheumatic valve disease increases the risk of endocarditis, which in turn will worsen valvular disease. An echocardiogram is useful to diagnose valvular heart disease and evaluate the papillary muscles and surrounding myocardium. Major considerations will be covered below.

Mitral stenosis is usually of rheumatic origin, resulting in severe disability usually by early adulthood. Dyspnea and pulmonary edema are the principal symptoms. The physical examination is remarkable for a diastolic rumble murmur with presystolic accentuation that may be accompanied by cyanosis, an irregularly irregular pulse, a right ventricular heave, or a palpable S_1. The electrocardiogram shows atrial fibrillation with a right axis deviation and left and/or right atrial enlargement. The chest x-ray would show right and left atrial enlargement and congestive heart failure.

Mitral regurgitation is caused by rheumatic fever, ischemia, mitral valve prolapse, endocarditis, left ventricular dilation, hypertrophic cardiomyopathy, and annular calcification. Patients complain of exertional dyspnea, fatigue, and weakness. The physical is remarkable for a left ventricular lift, diminished S_1, and a loud holosystolic murmur followed by a brief diastolic murmur. The echocardiogram also shows an enlarged left atrium and a hyperdynamic left ventricle.

Aortic stenosis can be congenital, rheumatic, idiopathic, or calcific (in the elderly). The patient with aortic stenosis may be asymptomatic for years before developing dyspnea, angina, or syncope. The physical is significant for weak and delayed pulses, a carotid thrill, and a diamond shaped, harsh systolic murmur often with a thrill.

Aortic regurgitation is mainly due to rheumatic fever and less often to endocarditis and syphilis. Exertional dyspnea, palpitations, angina, and left ventricular failure are the clinical manifestations. The physical shows a wide pulse pressure, bounding pulses, nail bed capillary pulsations, an S_3, and a blowing, decrescendo diastolic murmur and a systolic murmur. Electrocardiogram and chest x-ray show left ventricular enlargement.

Atrial Septal Defects. Of the congenital heart lesions, atrial septal defects are most likely to be found in adults. Atrial septal defects are usually asymptomatic until the third or fourth decades of life but may become symptomatic during pregnancy. The major complaints are exertional dyspnea, fatigue, and palpitations. Diagnosis of an atrial septal defect presenting during pregnancy can be obscured by the physiologic dyspnea and murmurs of pregnancy. The physical is significant for a right ventricular lift, wide fixed split of S_2, and a systolic flow murmur along the sternal border. The electrocardiogram shows an incomplete right bundle branch block. Chest x-ray shows increased pulmonary vascular markings and right ventricular and pulmonary artery prominence. Doppler studies with the echocardiogram will demonstrate the atrial septal defect.

Neuromuscular Causes. Neuromuscular disturbances affect the muscles of respiration or their nerve supply and impair chest wall expansion or diaphragmatic excursion. The restrictive pattern prevents patients from taking a deep breath, and they will note exertional dyspnea. Diminished lung expansion also increases susceptibility to atelectasis, bacterial overgrowth, and infection. With disease progression, the patient will experience ventilatory failure. The physical examination is significant for shallow breathing. The chest x-ray shows small lung fields with increased lung markings from impaired inspiratory effort. Atelectasis may be present. PFTs show a reduced vital capacity, total lung capacity, inspiratory capacity, and FVC. The disease can be monitored with measurements of vital capacity over time. With vaccination against polio, neuromuscular disturbances are not a common cause of dyspnea but must be considered in unvaccinated communities. Other neuromuscular disturbances are listed in Table 15.15.

Chest Cavity Causes. Dyspnea can result from any condition that deforms or reduces the chest cavity. Conditions that deform the chest wall or distend the abdomen restrict the ability of the lung to expand. Kyphoscoliosis is a common bony deformity of the thorax caused by osteoporosis, compression fractures, bony tuberculosis, neuromuscular disease, or unknown causes. Kyphoscoliosis is commonly seen in elderly women as a result of osteoporosis. At the other extreme, idiopathic disease affects prepubescent girls. There is both backward curvature (kyphosis) and lateral curvature (scoliosis) of the spine resulting in a small chest cavity with limited rib excursion (Fig. 15.12). Respiratory failure is conferred by a stiff, restrictive chest wall. Hypoxemia is also due to the ventilation/perfusion abnormalities inherent to perfused but poorly expanded lungs. The initial complaint is exertional dyspnea. Bronchitis and pneumonia may complicate the picture. The physical examination reveals rapid, shallow breathing, the curved spine, and truncated chest cavity. Chest x-ray findings include abnormal spinal and rib configuration, small lung fields, increased markings caused by poor expansion, and atelectasis. PFTs show decreased lung volumes with a normal or increased FEV-1:FEV ratio. With progression to decompensation, hypoxemia and carbon dioxide retention will be seen on arterial blood gas.

Conditions that cause abdominal distension reduce diaphragmatic excursion and lung volumes and result in exertional dyspnea. Pregnancy and obesity were discussed under "Physiological Causes." Ascites is another cause of abdominal distension from liver disease, kidney disease, abdominal or pelvic tumors, and severe congestive heart failure with anasarca. The physical exam reveals an abdomen protuberant with a uterus, adipose tissue, fluid, or mass. Investigation is directed at the abdominal entity; further pulmonary investigation is rarely warranted. Other chest cavity conditions causing chronic dyspnea are listed in Table 15.15.

Other Causes. Dyspnea results from conditions which increase oxygen demand such as thyrotoxicosis and fever. "High output" cardiac failure's dyspnea can be seen with beriberi, anemia, or thyrotoxicosis.

Treatment

The ideal treatment of dyspnea is directed at alleviating its cause and therefore is dependent on establishing a specific diagnosis. In cases where the cause of dyspnea cannot be eliminated, therapy must be directed at compensating for the pathology. There are so many possible causes with such varied mechanisms resulting in breathlessness that it is beyond the scope of this chapter to detail all the therapeutic options. Instead, key therapeutic principles and modalities will be discussed. Management strategies for COPD, congestive heart failure, asthma, lung cancer, and valvular heart disease will follow.

GENERAL MEASURES

Vaccination against influenza and pneumococcal pneumonia are essential for persons with any pathological cause of chronic dyspnea. Their ventilatory and cardiovascular function can be further compromised by infection, leading to excessive morbidity and mortality. Weight loss should be encouraged in the obese, especially those with dyspnea caused by deconditioning or chest wall restriction. Lifestyle changes include stopping smoking, avoiding allergens, extreme temperatures, and pollution, and modifying exercise.

EXERCISE TRAINING

Exercise training is most useful in patients whose dyspnea is due to deconditioning. Exercise encourages formation of coronary collaterals and increases the threshold to dyspnea caused by coronary insufficiency. Although lung function is not improved, exercise training improves exercise tolerance in persons with COPD. Minimal goals of training are

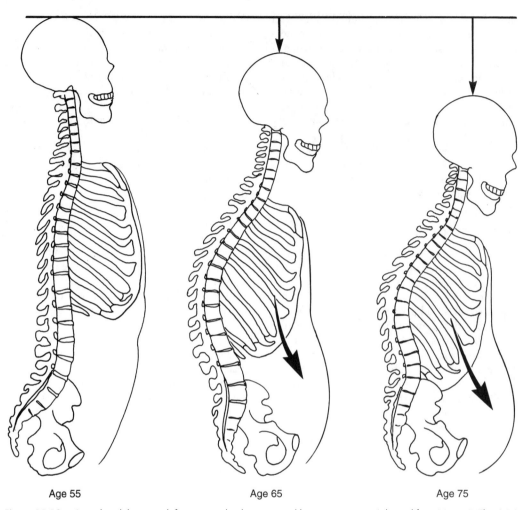

Age 55   Age 65   Age 75

Figure 15.12. Spinal and thoracic deformities in kyphosis caused by osteoporosis. Adapted from Netter F. The CIBA collection of medical illustrations. Newark: CIBA Medical, 1987;8:279.

3–5 days/week, 60% of the age adjusted maximal heart rate, and 15–30 minutes of continuous exertion (11).

BREATHING TECHNIQUES

Breathing techniques can be "discovered by" or taught to patients. Pursed lip breathing, tripod posture, and diaphragmatic breathing are simple alterations to breathing that relieve some of the compromised breathing dynamics or assist the patient's efforts to breathe. Exhaling through pursed lips increases end expiratory resistance and pressure and delays airways closure. The tidal volume is increased; the respiratory rate decreases, and alveolar ventilation is improved to slightly decrease blood carbon dioxide levels and increase oxygen saturation demonstrable by oximetry (12). In a tripod posture, the seated patient leans forward onto the supporting arms. This reduces the use of accessory muscles of respiration. In diaphragmatic breathing, the patient uses the hand to press on the upper abdomen during exhalation. This facilitates more complete exhalation. These techniques are most often seen in patients with COPD.

PULMONARY TOILET AND RESPIRATORY THERAPY

Conditions that produce excessive amounts of secretions obstruct the airway lumen and cause dyspnea. The cough reflex may be blunted if anesthesia was applied locally to the pharynx (e.g., for endoscopy or laryngoscopy), resulting in accumulation of secretions. Humidity, postural drainage, and chest percussion and coughing encourage clearing of secretions. These are most useful in bronchiectasis and can be an adjunct in pneumonia and after extubation from a ventilator. Deep breathing techniques with the aid of an incentive spirometer prevent or reverse atelectasis. These are useful after anesthesia, which results in diaphragmatic paralysis, or if a patient is splinting (breathing shallowly) after the pain of trauma or surgery.

PHARMACOLOGIC AGENTS

Pharmacologic agents are directed at reversing or ameliorating conditions that cause dyspnea. Agents that are commonly used include antibiotics, anticoagulants, bronchodilators, cardiovascular agents, corticosteroids, and psychoactive drugs.

Antibiotics. Antibiotics treat acute infections such as bronchitis and pneumonia. They can also be cycled prophylactically to decrease the pulmonary bacterial load in patients with bronchiectasis or severe chronic bronchitis and thereby decrease infections and sputum production. Amoxicillin, ampicillin, first generation cephalosporins (e.g., cefalexin), erythromycin, trimethoprim/sulfa, and tetracyclines are often used because they penetrate pulmonary tissue well and are active against likely pathogens. Second and third generation cephalosporins, azithromycin, clarithromycin, amoxicillin/clavulanic acid, and flouroquinolones are expensive alternatives that should be reserved for resistant organisms or cases where initial treatment failure could increase morbidity or mortality.

Anticoagulation. Anticoagulation treats pulmonary emboli and is used in deep vein thrombosis prophylaxis, congestive heart failure, and valvular heart disease management to prevent clot formation on akinetic ventricular walls, aneurysms, or deformed valves that could subsequently embolize to the lung or elsewhere. Intravenous heparin or oral Coumadin may be started initially, depending on the setting. Coumadin is chronically used and titrated to maintain a prothrombin time that is 1.3–1.5 times control or 14–18 seconds. Subcutaneous heparin may be used if there is a contraindication to Coumadin, as in pregnancy. Alternatively, enoxaparin, a low molecular weight heparin, can be given after hip replacement or fracture repair and after knee replacement as deep vein thrombosis prophylaxis. Monitoring of coagulation parameters is unnecessary with enoxaparin. Excessive bleeding is the major complication of anticoagulation.

Anti-Inflammatory Agents. Anti-inflammatory drugs include corticosteroids and mast cell stabilizers. Corticosteroids are potent suppressors of inflammation available in inhaled, oral, and parenteral forms. They are useful in the management of asthma, COPD, and interstitial lung diseases. Inhaled corticosteroids (triamcinolone, beclomethasone, budesonide, flunisolide) are used in maintenance airway patency in asthma and COPD. They are potent, and little is systemically absorbed; thus they are preferred over oral or parenteral forms for airways disease. Oral corticosteroids (prednisone, prednisolone) are used in management of airways disease refractory to optimum doses of inhaled bronchodilators and steroids but are indicated for interstitial processes that are not penetrated by inhaled medications. Parenteral corticosteroids are used in emergency room, operative, and acutely ill inpatient settings and are changed to oral forms when a patient has stabilized.

The systemic side effects of corticosteroids include adrenal suppression, weight gain, cataracts, glucose intolerance, osteoporosis, cardiomyopathy, psychosis, immunosuppression, and growth retardation in children and young adults. Systemically absorbed (oral or parenteral) formulations, prolonged or continuous use, and high doses lead to higher incidences of side effects. Adrenal responses to stress are suppressed for prolonged periods. Hence, "stress" doses of hydrocortisone (250 mg every 6 hours) are parenterally administered to acutely ill or operative patients who had received systemic steroids within the past year. Side effects are minimized if oral steroids are administered on alternate days. Discontinuation of chronic steroids requires the dose be tapered over weeks to months to allow adrenal recovery from suppression.

Cromolyn sodium and nedocromil stabilize mast cells and prevent their degranulation to initiate inflammation. They also have weak anti-inflammatory activity. These mast cell stabilizers are most useful in prophylaxis, especially in allergic asthma. They have no bronchodilating effect and therefore have no role in acute management. They have no side effects. Cromolyn is available in inhaler, nebulizer, and powdered forms. The powdered form often causes the patient to cough, which decreases acceptance. Nedocromil is available as an inhaler.

Bronchodilators. Bronchodilators include beta$_2$-selective adrenergic agonists, theophyllines, and atropine derivatives. Beta-agonists relax bronchial smooth muscle and are useful during acute bronchospasm or prophylactically. They are available in nebulizer, metered dose inhaler, and oral and parenteral formulations. Subcutaneous injection is generally not more effective but causes more adverse effects including tachycardia, tremor, nausea, vomiting, and headache. Angina may be precipitated. Hypokalemia can occur as well.

Older, nonselective beta-adrenergics (epinephrine, metaproterenol, isoproterenol) have greater cardiovascular side effects. Epinephrine, 0.3 ml subcutaneously, is given for acute and severe bronchospasm in emergency room or office settings for rapid effect. Patients with severe asthma are taught self-injection or use an automatic injector (epinephrine pen). Epinephrine doses must be lowered to 0.15–0.2 ml in the elderly and should be avoided in persons with a history of cardiac disease. Isoproterenol inhalers are now rarely prescribed; in the past many patients preferred its "instant" action over other beta-agonists, which contributed to its misuse.

Theophyllines are less potent bronchodilators with slower onset and are useful in chronic management. Nausea, vomiting, seizures, and arrhythmias can occur at greater than therapeutic (10–20 μg/ml) serum concentrations. Oral and parenteral forms are available. Theophylline should be loaded if given de novo.

Ipratropium, an atropine derivative, is an anticholinergic and weak bronchodilator that is useful in COPD. Although not approved for the treatment of asthma, it has been used along with beta-agonists or theophyllines in asthmatics.

Patients must be taught and monitored in proper inhaler technique. Spacers, paper bags, and various patented inhalant delivery systems (Inspireeze, Maxair Autohaler) can be used by patients who have difficulty with standard inhaler pumps.

Cardiovascular Agents. Cardiovascular agents are used to treat cardiac disorders that cause dyspnea. Congestive heart failure is treated with inotropic agents (digoxin), vasodilators to reduce afterload (angiotensin-converting enzyme inhibitors, hydralazine, nifedipine), and diuretics (furosemide) to reduce preload. Antianginal drugs (nitrates, beta-blockers, calcium channel blockers) are effective when dyspnea is an anginal equivalent. Valvular heart disease is treated medically with vasodilators to reduce afterload, diuretics to relieve congestion, and rate control agents (digoxin). These will be discussed under "Management."

Psychoactive Agents. Anxiolytics may be offered to patients whose dyspnea is due to anxiety. Panic disorders are treated with the tricyclic antidepressants imipramine and desipramine. These agents generally supplement psychotherapy and counseling.

PSYCHOLOGICAL INTERVENTION

Anxiety, depression, and panic disorders can present as dyspnea. When history and psychological testing support psychiatric causes of dyspnea, treatment must be directed toward them. Use of anxiolytics and antidepressants were discussed above. Relaxation training, behavior modification, goal setting, patient education, or psychotherapy may be appropriate

OXYGEN

Oxygen can be acutely administered to relieve hypoxia of all types of disorders except shunting. It is used in the treatment of carbon monoxide poisoning; oxygen will compete with carbon monoxide to bind with hemoglobin. Patients with chronic dyspnea and room air PaO$_2$ of <55 mmHg, typically from COPD or parenchymal lung disease, may also benefit from oxygen therapy. Caution should be exercised in patients with COPD to avoid blunting their hypoxic drive to breathe; chronic carbon dioxide retention reduces the body's ability to ventilate in response to hypercapnia. Intermittent or nocturnal administration can help patients respond to periods of increased oxygen demand, hypoventilation, and vascular redistribution. Oxygen tanks are expensive and limit a patient's mobility. Oxygen can also be concentrated from ambient air, but this method requires a power source and therefore limits a patient's mobility as well.

VENTILATORY SUPPORT

Ventilators are used when a patient can no longer adequately maintain respiration. Loss of central control of respiration (strokes, trauma), severe obstruction, and progressive parenchymal and interstitial processes are easily envisioned as requiring ventilator support. Patients with severe neuromuscular and chest cavity deformities may tire or have intermittent or progressive respiratory failure. These patients benefit from tracheostomy placement and intermittent ventilator support at night, when fatigued, or when ill. Intermittent positive airway pressure can be delivered to patients with kyphoscoliosis or other restrictive conditions to aerate collapsed lung segments.

SURGICAL INTERVENTION

Pneumonectomy or segmental resection are options in localized pulmonary neoplasms. Surgical revascularization or balloon angioplasty effectively ameliorate dyspnea caused by coronary artery obstruction. Thoracentesis removes pleural effusions and allows lung reexpansion. Pleurodesis with tetracycline or other sclerosing agents may be necessary if effusions reaccumulate. Decortication is a drastic measure if irreversible pleural fibrosis (e.g., tuberculous pleurisy) causes disabling restriction. Abdominal paracentesis removes ascitic fluid restricting lung expansion, and may be useful in managing liver disease, heart failure, or malignancies. Other surgical procedures may be directed to correcting bony deformities (Harrington rod placement in kyphoscoliosis). Transplants of donor or artificial hearts offer further longevity for a small number of patients with heart failure. Heart-lung transplants are rarely encountered but would treat pulmonary hypertension.

Management

Management of acute and chronic dyspnea is a major task of the ambulatory clinician. The various treatment modalities are discussed below as management strategies for causes of dyspnea commonly encountered in an ambulatory care setting.

CHRONIC OBSTRUCTIVE PULMONARY DISEASE

Emphysema is an irreversible condition, so therapeutic efforts are directed toward prevention and management of reversible airways obstruction and amelioration of symptoms. Vaccination against influenza and pneumococcal pneumonia, smoking cessation, and avoidance of irritants prevent further pulmonary compromise. Changes in sputum purulence, volume, and viscosity suggest bronchial infection. Antibiotics lower the intensity and duration of symptoms. Bronchodilators, including theophylline, selective beta$_2$-adrenergics, and anticholinergics improve dyspnea even if PFTs do not demonstrate bronchodilator response. Corticosteroids are useful in reducing airways inflammation. Oxygen can be administered when severe hypoxia (<55 mmHg) is present. Postural (bronchopulmonary) drainage is helpful when mucous hypersecretion is present.

CONGESTIVE HEART FAILURE

Management of congestive heart failure is directed toward

- Reversing the cause of myocardial depression;
- Reducing cardiac workload;
- Reducing congestive symptoms;
- Improving myocardial performance.

Reversing Causes of Myocardial Depression. Efforts should be made to correct underlying causes or precipitators of heart failure. These include drugs (beta-blockers, calcium channel blockers, or antiarrhythmics), ischemia, myocardial infarction, increased sodium load, arrhythmias, high output states (hyperthyroidism, fever, anemia, and pregnancy), and myocarditis. Removal of offending drugs, reduction in sodium intake, reversal of ischemia, or recovery from myocarditis or high output states should improve myocardial depression. A patient's hematocrit should be maintained above 30%.

Reducing Cardiac Workload. After congestive heart failure is identified, cardiac workload, or the effort to maintain circulation to meet the body's metabolic needs, should be reduced. Any reversible conditions precipitating failure mentioned above should be addressed. Patients should be vaccinated against influenza and pneumococcal pneumonia. Hypertension should be well controlled. The rate of ventricular contraction in atrial fibrillation should be maintained between 70 and 80 with digoxin, beta-blockers, or a pacemaker. Adequate antipyretic and analgesic administration when warranted is judicious.

Patients with congestive heart failure must modify their activity and environment to decrease cardiac work. This often means less stress and exertion—a more sedentary lifestyle, avoidance of lifting or carrying heavy loads, bed rest, and avoidance of stressful situations. The patient's home or work environment should be modified as well. Avoidance of stairs, temperature extremes, and heavy housework or labor could be achieved with elevators or single level accommodations, climate control with air conditioning, heating and dehumidification, and housekeeping assistance. "Assistive technology" is almost a part of modern living but requires some forethought in planning and acquiring appliances, electronic banking, cars with automatic transmissions and power steering, etc; rehabilitation specialists can help with the choices.

Reduction of Congestive Symptoms. Reduction of congestive symptoms from fluid overload is important in enhancing a patient's well-being. Volume expansion that follows decreased renal perfusion increases filling pressures and improves myocardial performance. However, persistent low cardiac output results in continuing fluid retention and overload. Pulmonary, peripheral, hepatic, and gut congestion result in dyspnea, skin breakdown, liver impairment and tenderness, and impairment of absorption, including medications, respectively.

Sodium restriction is a foundation of therapy. Sodium intake can be increased from dietary indiscretion or from medications. In mild congestive heart failure, dietary counseling is necessary to moderately reduce sodium intake from the usual 10 to 5 g daily. This can be achieved by refraining from adding salt, reading food content labels, avoiding canned, processed, and precooked foods such as chips, cold cuts, hot dogs, soup mixes, jarred sauces, and flavor enhancers. Fast food is to be avoided. Sodium can also be introduced with nonsteroidal anti-inflammatory drugs, antacids, or corticosteroids. More stringent sodium restriction to 2 g daily may be necessary for patients with severe decompensation but is difficult to achieve and adhere to. Moderate fluid restriction to 2 liters daily helps achieve a negative water balance and avoid hyponatremia. Diuretic agents complement sodium and fluid restriction.

Improving Myocardial Performance. Pharmacologic improvement of myocardial performance includes use of inotropic agents, diuretics, and vasodilators. Digitalis as digoxin is an oral or parenteral inotrope. Dosing should be monitored and adjusted in renal insufficiency. Hypokalemia and hypomagnesemia also increase the potential of digitalis toxicity. Frequently, digitalis and a diuretic are administered simultaneously, in which case serum potassium should be monitored and maintained in the high normal range.

Diuretics relieve congestive symptoms, decrease preload by decreasing fluid and venous return, and are vasodilators. They are listed in Table 15.16. Patients who are unresponsive to oral diuretics may benefit with intravenous administration. Remember that chronic renal insufficiency and nonsteroidal anti-inflammatory drugs, which decrease renal perfusion, reduce the response to diuretics.

Vasodilators reduce preload with venodilators and afterload with arterial dilators (Table 15.17). Venodilators increase venous capacitance, cause venous pooling, and decrease venous return to the heart, thereby reducing congestion. Arterial dilators reduce peripheral vascular resistance, hence improving forward flow of blood. Angiotensin-converting enzyme inhibitors block the formation of angiotensin II. They improve symptoms and exercise capacity, slow the progression of failure, and

may improve survival (13). Hydralazine and nitrates can be used together to decrease both preload and afterload. Flosequinan, a flouroquinolone derivative that dilates peripheral arteries and veins and may increase cardiac contractility, is available for patients intolerant or unresponsive to angiotensin-converting enzyme inhibitors.

Beta-blockers, usually avoided in patients with heart failure because of their negative inotropic effect, benefit some patients with chronic failure. Low doses of metoprolol can improve left ventricular function and symptoms in some patients with failure owing to idiopathic dilated cardiomyopathy.

Low dose dobutamine, amrinone, and nitroprusside require inpatient, monitored care and are beyond the scope of ambulatory management.

Other Therapeutic Modalities. Other therapeutic modalities can be considered under appropriate circumstances. Dialysis is useful in patients refractory to diuretics owing to renal insufficiency. Thoracentesis and paracentesis dramatically relieve pulmonary restriction. Restoration of sinus rhythm in atrial fibrillation or use of a dual chamber pacemaker preserves the "atrial kick" to ventricular filling, thereby improving hemodynamics. The rate of ventricular contraction in atrial fibrillation should be maintained between 70 and 80 with digoxin, beta-blockers, or a pacemaker. Heart transplants can be considered in young patients with only marginal response to other interventions.

ASTHMA

The management of asthma is directed at the chronic inflammatory process and bronchospasm. General measures include vaccination against influenza and pneumococcal pneumonia. Cigarette smoking should be discontinued because it is an irritant and because emphysema would possibly be superimposed.

Prevention of asthma attacks is achieved by avoidance of allergens or bronchial stimuli discussed earlier. This may mean changing jobs, giving up a pet, avoiding specific foods or medication, or reducing stressful provocations. Environmental controls such as temperature control, general housekeeping, air filtration, and laminar airflow are helpful in many cases. Using cromolyn or nedocromil can be prophylactic. Anticipatory use of bronchodilators before brief periods of exercise or cold or allergen exposure can prevent bronchoconstriction. Asthmatic patients can be taught to monitor their PEFR.

Chronic management is titrated to the severity

Table 15.16.
Diuretic Agents

Agent	Route	Typical Daily Dose (mg)
Thiazides		
Chlorthalidone	po	25–100
Hydrochlorothiazide	po	25–100
Loop diuretics		
Furosemide	po	20–80
	iv,im	10–80
Ethacrynic acid	po	25–100
	iv	50
Bumetanide	po	0.5–2
	iv	0.5–2
Potassium-sparing diuretics		
Spironolactone	po	50–200
Triamterene	po	100–200
Amiloride	po	5–10

of symptoms. Adults are offered symptomatic or maintenance adrenergics via inhalers. Inhaled corticosteroids are offered as an adjunct to adrenergics. Chronic oral corticosteroids should not be encouraged but may be offered in refractory cases. Alternate day regimens are preferred. Oral theophylline or adrenergics are less commonly prescribed now but will often be part of a regimen initiated before 1980 or because the patient cannot use inhalers (e.g., patients who are retarded or demented). Drugs that combine theophyllines with decongestants (Marax) are rarely recommended.

Once bronchospasm has begun and patients notice dyspnea or wheezing, the patient can use a beta$_2$-selective adrenergic inhaler. Fluids should be encouraged. If symptoms do not quickly abate, or are unusually severe, epinephrine can be administered subcutaneously, and adrenergic agents can be

Table 15.17.
Characteristics of Vasodilators Used for Congestive Heart Failure

Agent	Site of Action	Route	Typical Dose
ACE inhibitors			
Captopril	V = A	po	6.25–25 mg tid
Enalapril	V = A	po	5–10 mg bid
Ca^{2+} channel blockers			
Nifedipine	V < A	po	30–60 mg/day
Direct vasodilators			
Hydralazine	A	po	50–200 mg tid
Prazosin	V = A	po	1–5 mg tid
Nitrates			
Isosorbide dinitrate	V	po	10–20 mg tid
Isosorbide mononitrate	V	po	20 mg bid
Nitropaste	V	Topical	½–1 inch qhs-qid
Nitroglycerin patch	V	Topical	2.5–5 mg/24 hours

V, venous; A, arterial.

administered via nebulizer in the home by trained patients. Directing intervention against precipitants such as allergens is important. Antibiotics should be offered when purulent sputum, fever, or a pulmonary infiltrate are present. Unfortunately, viral upper respiratory infections are often a culprit for which there is no specific therapy. If severe respiratory distress persists after initiating beta-agonist or epinephrine, the patient should be managed in a treatment facility that could provide oxygen, intravenous fluids and medications, and intubation. Indications for hospitalization include an FEV-1 that is less than 30% of predicted, lack of improvement to 40% of predicted after vigorous therapy, fatigue, complicating factors (cardiac disease, pregnancy, elderly), and, obviously, impending respiratory failure.

LUNG CANCER

The management of lung cancer will not be discussed in detail, but several key points will be presented. Lung cancer is the second most common neoplasm affecting men and women. It is a rapidly growing neoplasm that is largely preventable and for which there is no cost-effective screening. Primary prevention through smoking prevention activities, smoke free environments, elimination of air pollution, and occupational safety standards is the most effective management strategy for lung cancer. Smoking cessation allows the risk of developing lung cancer to approach that of nonsmokers after 15 years.

Early detection of nonsmall cell carcinoma increases the chance of offering curative surgical resection. Therefore the pace of a workup for suspected lung cancer should be rapid. Small cell (oat cell) lesions are aggressive and usually disseminated at diagnosis and therefore require chemotherapy. If metastasis has occurred, supportive therapy involving oxygen supplementation, pain control, and control of symptoms from secondary lesions such as seizures are the management keys. Even if disease is initially felt to be localized, the overall 5-year survival is 30–50%.

VALVULAR HEART DISEASE

Management of valvular heart disease includes maximizing hemodynamic compensation, endocarditis prophylaxis, anticoagulation, and valve replacement. The clinician should also recognize situations that could exacerbate valvular heart disease. Infection, with fever and tachycardia, can compromise patients with valvular heart disease; therefore management includes vaccination against influenza and pneumococcal pneumonia, antipyretics, and appropriate fluid and antibiotic regimens. Pregnancy can also exacerbate valvular heart disease, so contraception should be advised to prevent unintended pregnancies; pregnancies in patients with valvular heart disease should be monitored for hemodynamic decompensation.

In general, the body tolerates regurgitant lesions better than stenotic lesions and may require little other than its recognition initially. Mitral stenosis is managed with rate control of the usual accompanying atrial fibrillation to allow maximal left ventricular filling. Digoxin is usually employed. Fluid overload is managed with sodium restriction and diuretics. Chronic anticoagulation is offered to patients in atrial fibrillation. Valvular commissurotomy and replacement are indicated for refractory hemodynamic compromise or valve area of <1.2 cm (11). Aortic stenosis is managed with diminished physical activity and standard congestive heart failure therapy but without reducing afterload. Valve replacement should be offered before frank left ventricular failure exists.

Regurgitant mitral valves are managed with afterload reducing agents, diuretics, and sodium restriction. Valve replacement should be offered when there is evidence of left ventricular failure but before development of severe chronic heart failure. Aortic regurgitant lesions are managed with a standard left ventricular failure regimen and valve replacement. Valve replacement should be timed soon after symptoms appear or when there is radionuclide, angiogram, or echocardiogram evidence of left ventricular dysfunction. Myocardial depressants should be avoided.

Valve replacement introduces concerns. Mechanical valves require anticoagulation, can cause lysing of red cells, and can fail. Pigskin valves do not require anticoagulation but require a larger orifice for placement.

Prosthetic valves, like damaged valves, require rheumatic fever and endocarditis prophylaxis. Rheumatic fever prophylaxis is accomplished by monthly 1.2 million unit bicillin injections or oral penicillin or erythromycin prescribed after streptococcal pharyngitis. Recommendations for endocarditis prophylaxis appear in Table 15.18.

Table 15.18.
Endocarditis Prophylaxis

Dental/oral/upper respiratory tract procedures

I. Standard regimen in patients at risk (includes those with prosthetic heart valves and other high risk patients)
    Amoxicillin 3.0 g orally 1 hour before procedure, then 1.5 g 6 hours after initial dose.[a]

For amoxicillin/penicillin-allergic patients
    Erythromycin ethylsuccinate 800 mg or erythromycin stearate 1.0 g orally 2 hours before a procedure and then half the dose 6 hours after the initial administration.[a]
                               or
    Clindamycin 300 mg orally 1 hour before a procedure and 150 mg 6 hours after initial dose.[a]

II. Alternate prophylactic regimen for dental/oral/upper respiratory tract procedures in patients at risk

A. For patients unable to take oral medications
    Ampicillin 2.0 g iv (or im) 30 minutes before procedure, then ampicillin 1.0 g iv (or im) or amoxicillin 1.5 g orally 6 hours after initial dose.[a]
                                 or

For ampicillin/amoxicillin/penicillin-allergic patients unable to take oral medications
    Cindamycin 300 mg iv 30 minutes before a procedure and 150 mg iv (or orally) 6 hours after initial dose.[a]

B. For patients considered to be at high risk who are not candidates for the standard regimen
    Ampicillin 2.0 g iv (or im) plus gentamicin 1.5 mg/kg iv followed by amoxicillin 1.5 g orally 6 hours after the initial dose. Alternatively, the parenteral regimen may be repeated 8 hours after the initial dose.[a]

For amoxicillin/ampicillin/penicillin-allergic patients considered to be at high risk
    Vancomycin 1.0 g iv administered over 1 hour, starting 1 hour before procedure. No repeat dose is necessary.[a]

Genitourinary/gastrointestinal procedures

I. Standard regimen
    Ampicillin 2.0 g iv (or im) plus gentamicin 1.5 mg/kg iv (or im) (not to exceed 80 mg) 30 minutes before procedure followed by amoxicillin 1.5 g orally 6 hours after the initial dose. Alternatively, the parenteral regimen may be repeated once 8 hours after the initial dose.[a]

For amoxicillin/ampicillin/penicillin-allergic patients
    Vancomycin 1.0 g iv administered over 1 hour plus gentamicin 1.5 mg/kg iv (or im) (not to exceed 80 mg) 1 hour before the procedure. May be repeated once 8 hours after initial dose.[b]

II. Alternate oral regimen for low risk patients
    Amoxicillin 3.0 g orally 1 hour before the procedure, then 1.5 g 6 hours after the initial dose.[b]

[a]Note antibiotic regimens used to prevent recurrences of acute rheumatic fever are inadequate for the prevention of bacterial endocarditis. In patients with markedly compromised renal function, it may be necessary to modify or omit the second dose of gentamicin or vancomycin. Intramuscular injections may be contraindicated in patients receiving anticoagulants. (From Dajani AS, Bisno AL, Chung KJ et al. Prevention of Bacterial Endocarditis Recommendations of the American Heart Association JAMA 1990;264:2919–2922).

ILLUSTRATIVE CASES WITH SELF-ASSESSMENT QUESTIONS AND ANSWERS

Case 1

M.M. is a 58-year-old woman whom you have followed for many years for COPD. She states she has had increasing shortness of breath unresponsive to her usual bronchodilator inhaler for 2 days. She has a chronic productive cough, and the sputum is now flecked with yellow. She notes chills and left subscapular pain. She last felt this way when she had pneumonia. She still smokes. Her physical exam is remarkable only for a respiratory rate of 24, a PEFR of 250, mild left sub- scapular tenderness, and occasional rales on auscultation.

QUESTION: *What is your differential diagnosis?*

ANSWER: *Exacerbation of COPD caused by acute bronchitis. Pneumonia is less likely because of her history.*

QUESTION: *What is your next step?*

ANSWER: *It is reasonable to obtain a chest x-ray. An arterial blood gas is not indicated. The chest x-ray is remarkable for increased lung markings.*

QUESTION: *She is unresponsive to several doses of albuterol via nebulizer and complains of fatigue; her arterial blood gas is unchanged from baseline. What is your next step?*

ANSWER: *Hospitalization.*

Case 2

B.E. is a 72-year-old man with COPD and mitral regurgitation. He complains of breathlessness. His physical exam is remarkable for distress, a PEFR of 170, a respiratory rate of 30, a holosystolic murmur radiating to the axilla, and fine rales on auscultation.

QUESTION: *What are you considering?*

ANSWER: *COPD and congestive heart failure. Oxygen administration and nebulized bronchodilators result in marginal improvement. The chest x-ray shows massive cardiomegaly and fluffy infiltrates.*

QUESTION: *What is your next step?*

ANSWER: *Administer a diuretic such as intravenous furosemide. B.E. improves dramatically and now recalls a deli meal with a "little" pickle and a tuna sandwich.*

QUESTION: *What medical workup and regimen would you order?*

ANSWER: *Study his left ventricular function and valves with an echocardiogram. A diuretic and an angiotensin-converting enzyme inhibitor should be added to his COPD regimen. He should receive dietary counseling to limit sodium intake.*

Case 3

D.S. is a 57-year-old woman with a 30-year history of asthma who is referred to you for workup. She experiences bouts of dyspnea after walking 20 feet and has had palpitations and chest pain intermittently over the past 2 years. You note she is jittery, and she complains she is in severe distress. Her exam is negative except for a respiratory rate of 26 and sweating; her PEFR is 320. Her medications are prednisone 30 mg daily, isoproterenol MDI as needed, metaproterenol MDI as needed, and diltiazem 30 mg four times daily.

QUESTION: *What is your differential diagnosis?*

ANSWER: *Adverse effects from medication, congestive heart failure, coronary artery disease, arrhythmias, panic disorder*

QUESTION: *What do you recommend?*

ANSWER: *Discontinue isoproterenol and metaproterenol. The medications have a high incidence of cardiovascular side effects. Your strategy is given further endorsement when D.S. reaches for inhalers to "get air" despite no evidence of bronchospasm. She admits to "spritzes" every 1–2 hours because it "gives her a lift." Previous recommendations to change medications were disregarded because "they took too long." D.S.'s steroid dose has been maintained by "patient insistence." After 1 week, D.S.'s palpitations are less, but she still notes dyspnea and chest pain with minimal walking and "out of the blue." She is less jittery but now appears anxious and is scanning the room frequently. Her respiratory rate is 28, pulse 96, PEFR 380, and lung exam benign. She admits to being scared.*

QUESTION: *Would you consider a cardiac workup?*

ANSWER: *It is reasonable to look at left ventricular function because of the patient's long-term steroid use (steroid induced cardiomyopathy) and CAD because of age. The nuclear ejection fraction is 55%. A stress test was terminated after reaching 90% of the predicted maximal heart rate because of shortness of breath; no ischemic electrocardiogram changes were noted.*

QUESTION: *Would you consider psychiatric testing?*

ANSWER: *Yes. The complaints are out of proportion to your findings. The patient is found to have a panic disorder.*

Case 4

E.W. is an 18-year-old woman who comes to your office noting severe shortness of breath since last night. She has no previous medical history, and her only medication is an oral contraceptive for the last 3 years. She looks uncomfortable, is tachypneic, is complaining of generalized chest discomfort that seems to hurt a little more in the right third intercostal space, and has faint shallow breath sounds.

QUESTION: *What differential diagnosis do you consider?*

ANSWER: *This is acute dyspnea. The patient has no medical history to narrow the considerations, so you consider a pulmonary embolus, spontaneous pneumothorax, and asthma. You refer her to the emergency room of your hospital, arrange a stat lung perfusion scan, and continue her management. In the emergency room, an arterial blood gas shows pH 7.45, PaCO2 35, and PaO2 80. The chest x-ray does not show a pneumothorax. She is whisked off to the lung scan, which shows no areas of decreased perfusion.*

QUESTION: *Can you narrow your differential diagnosis?*

ANSWER: *Pneumothorax and pulmonary embolus are unlikely. You request bedside spirometry, and her FEV-1/FVC is 65%. Asthma is your diagnosis. The patient's shallow breathing from the chest discomfort obscured the inspiratory and expiratory phase ratio and wheezing.*

Case 5

T.T. is a healthy 38-year-old man who notes a 1-week history of dry cough, bilateral chest pain, and shortness of breath. Your lung examination is normal, and he has marked tenderness of the left anterior 8th and 9th ribs and right anterolateral

6th and 7th ribs. He has been taking acetaminophen to cope with the pain.

QUESTION: *What is your differential diagnosis?*

ANSWER: *Viral or mycoplasma upper respiratory tract infection causing cough and pleuritic chest pain. At his wife's insistence, you obtain a chest x-ray that shows left lingular and right middle lobe infiltrates. You are surprised, because there was no complaint of fever, but T.T.'s use of acetaminophen for pain masked the fever.*

QUESTION: *What treatment do you offer?*

ANSWER: *The most likely causes of these infiltrates are mycoplasma and viral; mycoplasma is notable for radiographic findings worse than clinical findings. Erythromycin, azithromycin, or a tetracycline are reasonable choices.*

SUGGESTED READINGS

Cough

Kirtland SH, Winterbauer RH. Slowly resolving, chronic, and recurrent pneumonia. Clin Chest Med 1991;12:303–318.

Luby JP. Pneumonia caused by *Mycoplasma pneumoniae* infection. Clin Chest Med 1991;12:237–244.

Nguyen MLT, Yu VL. Legionella infection. Clin Chest Med 1991;12:257–268.

Rodnick JE, Gude JK. Diagnosis and antibiotic treatment of community acquired pneumonia. West J Med 1991;154:405–409.

Rubin FL, Nguyen MLT. Viral pneumonitis. Clin Chest Med 1991;12:223–235.

Thom DH, Grayston JT. Infections with *Chlamydia pneumoniae* strain TWAR. Clin Chest Med 1991;12:245–256.

Hemoptysis

Barker LR, Burton JR, Zieve PD, eds. Principles of ambulatory care medicine. Chapter 29: Tuberculosis in the Ambulatory Patient. 4th ed. Baltimore: Williams & Wilkins, 1995:348–358.

Goroll AH, May LA, Mulley Jr JB Eds. Primary Care Medicine: Office Evaluation and Management of the Adult Patient. Chapter 42: Evaluation of Hemoptysis 3rd ed. Philadelphia: Lippincott, 1995:236–239.

Israel RN and Poe RH. Hemoptysis IM: Braman SS,

guest ed. Clinics in Chest Medicine. Philadelphia: Saunders, 1987;8:197–205.

Dyspnea

Ferguson GT, Cherneiack RM. Management of chronic obstructive pulmonary disease. N Engl J Med 1993;328:1017–1022.

Kleerup EC, Tashkin DP. Outpatient treatment of adult asthma. West J Med 1995;163:49–63.

Pratter MR, Culey FJ, Dubois J, Irwin RS. Cause and evaluation of chronic dyspnea in a pulmonary disease clinic. Arch Intern Med 1989;149:2277–2282.

Schapira RM, Reinke LF. The outpatient diagnosis and management of chronic obstructive pulmonary disease: pharmacotherapy, administration of supplemental oxygen, and smoking cessation techniques. J Gen Intern Med 1995;10:40–55.

Seager LH. Congestive heart failure. Considerations for primary care physicians. Postgrad Med 1995;98:127–130, 132–134, 136–137.

REFERENCES

Cough

1. Butcher BL, Nichol KL, Parent CM. High yield of chest radiography in walk-in clinic patients with chest symptoms. J Gen Intern Med 1993;8:115–119.
2. Poe RH, Israel RH, Utel MJ, Hall WJ. Chronic cough: bronchoscopy or pulmonary function testing? Am Rev Respir Dis 1982;126:160–162.
3. Sen RP, Walsh TE. Fiberoptic bronchoscopy for refractory cough. Chest 1991;99:33–35.
4. Sebastian JL, McKinney WP, Kaufman J, Young MJ. Angiotensin-converting enzyme inhibitors and cough: prevalence in an outpatient medical clinic population. Chest 1991;99:36–39.
5. Fang GD, Fine M, Orloff J, et al. New and emerging etiologies for community-acquired pneumonia with implications for therapy: a prospective multicenter study of 359 cases. Medicine 1990;69:307–316.
6. Fine MJ, Smith DN, Singer DE. Hospitalization decision in patients with community-acquired pneumonia: a prospective cohort study. Am J Med 1990;89:713–721.
7. Pratter MR, Bartter T, Akers S, DuBois J. An algorithmic approach to chronic cough. Ann Intern Med 1993;119:977–983.

Hemoptysis

8. Johnston H, Reisz G. Changing spectrum of hemoptysis. Arch Intern Med 1989;149:1666–1668.
9. Santiago S, Tobias J, Williams AJ. A reappraisal of the causes of hemoptysis. Arch Intern Med 1987;151:2449–2451.

Dyspnea

10. Pratter MR, Curly FJ, Dubois J, Irwin RS. Sause and evaluation of chronic dyspnea in a pulmonary disease clinic. Arch Intern Med 1989;149:2277–2282.
11. American College of Sports Medicine Position Stand. The recommended quantity and quality of exercise for developing and maintaining fitness in healthy adults. Med Sci Sports 1978;10:7–10.
12. Tiep BL, Burns M, Kas D, et al. Pursed-lip breathing training using ear oximetry. Chest 1986;90:218–221.
13. SOLVD investigators. N Engl J Med 1992;327:685.

chapter 16

GASTROENTEROLOGY
Pamela Charney, Rhazib Khaund, Lisa M. Rucker, Diane Sieldecki

ABDOMINAL PAIN

Abdominal pain is a common ambulatory symptom that can develop from abdominal, chest, back, or pelvic problems. This section reviews the evaluation and management of a patient with abdominal pain. Special attention will be paid to specific gastrointestinal causes of upper abdominal pain.

Pathophysiologic Correlation

The location and contents of the abdominal cavity define possible origins of abdominal pain. The abdominal cavity is separated from the chest by the diaphragm, is anterior to the spine, and is contiguous with the pelvis. Therefore, the evaluation of acute abdominal pain must include considering acute processes both external and within the abdomen.

Within the abdominal cavity are gastrointestinal, vascular, and genitourinary structures. The upper intestinal tract (esophagus, stomach and duodenum, pancreas, and gallbladder) will be reviewed in this chapter as well as appendicitis and vascular causes of abdominal pain. Liver, colon, and renal problems will be discussed in other chapters.

Because of the extreme acidity of peptic secretions, the stomach, esophagus, and proximal duodenum have developed mechanisms to protect against mucosal erosion. The main mechanism is production of mucus that coats the epithelial surface of these organs. Other mechanisms include increasing blood flow to the epithelium in response to injury and fast replacement of damaged epithelial cells promoting rapid healing. Any process that overwhelms the protective power of the mucus (such as acid reflux into the esophagus), interrupts the epithelium *(H. pylori infection),* or affects the

blood flow to the epithelium (nonsteroidal antiinflammatory drugs) can lead to acid damage and pain. In addition, inflammation, obstruction and distension, and ischemia can also cause pain. The specific pathophysiology for each disease will be discussed in the differential diagnoses section.

Clinical and Laboratory Evaluation

A thorough history and careful physical examination are the cornerstone of clarifying where the patient's abdominal pain originates. Further evaluation frequently includes serial abdominal examinations, laboratory examinations, and sometimes other radiologic and/or endoscopic procedures.

HISTORY

During the initial interview, important history includes: the severity; location, and nature of the discomfort or pain; the natural history of the symptoms since onset; and how this compares with prior symptoms. Although the location where patients experience discomfort or pain is usually initially identified during the interview, the location should be reviewed again at the beginning of the physical.

The first priority is to determine who needs hospitalization and if immediate surgery is required. The sudden onset of severe pain may herald progressive deterioration. Examples include a ruptured appendix, an aneurysm, or an ectopic pregnancy. The associated pain increases with any movement, coughing, or straining. Patients will attempt to stay still and should be assessed promptly for impending shock.

The area of pain may relate to the structures present in the same area or may be referred. For example, left upper quadrant discomfort can be caused by splenomegaly or by constipation involving the sigmoid colon in the left lower quadrant. The pattern of how pain has evolved since its onset is also important. In appendicitis, pain initially begins periumbilically and then spreads to the right lower quadrant. Pain that originates in the periumbilical area and then radiates elsewhere can be caused by a variety of problems (Fig. 16.2).

One of the most important components of the history is focusing on the evolution of the patient's symptoms. Did the upper abdominal burning start the morning after consuming large amounts of alcohol or with the development of cough, fever, and chest pain? The time course provides another diagnostic clue.

It is critical to provide the patient with the opportunity to explain how the pain developed by using open-ended questions, such as "Would you please explain what the pain was like when it began?" Once the broad picture is understood, further details can be obtained. "How does the quality of this pain remind you of previous experiences?" or "How does eating affect symptoms?" are often elucidating questions.

Although food intake rapidly increases abdominal pain associated with gastroesophageal reflux disease (GERD), pain associated with pancreatitis and/or symptomatic gallstones increases 30 minutes after eating. The "hunger" discomfort associated with peptic ulcer disease is often relieved with food ingestion. The type of food consumed is important. For example, fatty meals more often stimulate gallbladder contraction, and therefore, exacerbate the pain in patients with symptomatic gallstones.

Not only is the time course of the episode leading to evaluation critical, but a careful history to determine whether the patient has experienced similar acute episodes or chronic symptoms previously is necessary. If there have been previous episodes and the current symptoms are similar, the cause is probably the same. If the symptoms are of a different nature, other diagnoses should be considered. For example, acute gastritis or chronic pancreatitis can be reactivated each time the patient drinks alcohol.

Consideration for the possibility of pregnancy is important not only because pregnancy can cause abdominal pain, but the evaluation of abdominal pain in a pregnant woman requires special attention. Organs displaced by the uterus may dramatically change position. By the late second trimester, the appendix may be in the right upper quadrant.

PHYSICAL EXAMINATION

General Appearance How comfortable the patient is when the history is obtained provides the

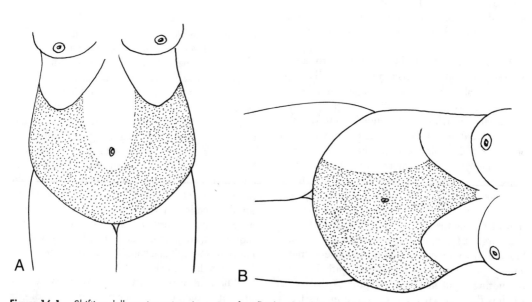

Figure 16.1. Shifting dullness in ascites. In ascites, free fluid in the abdomen will settle in the most dependent portion of the abdomen. Fluid in a supine patient will settle in the shaded area (**A**). Fluid in a patient lying on the left side will settle as in (**B**). Dullness to percussion localizes the fluid.

clinician with valuable information. Patients with acute gastrointestinal pain, a vascular aneurysm, or back pain radiating anteriorly may try to stay still to avoid increasing pain. In contrast, patients with renal calculi frequently writhe because of the nature of the pain. Patients with recurrent emesis or bleeding may appear weak and prefer to sit or lie down.

Vital Signs When there is a question of dehydration or bleeding, the clinician should personally determine the patient's pulse and blood pressure sitting or lying down, followed, at least, by checking the pulse standing. In young otherwise healthy patients, if there has been substantial volume loss while not taking medications that can suppress the sympathetic nervous system, the pulse will increase at least 20% with standing. This is followed by a decrease in systolic blood pressure as the amount of volume loss increases. The only exception is in a pregnant woman who without dehydration or bleeding may develop classical orthostatic changes during pregnancy. Elderly patients or patients receiving drugs that suppress the sympathetic nervous system may only decrease systolic blood pressure. The presence of orthostatic changes that do not respond rapidly to fluid intake is an indication for hospitalization.

The presence or absence of fever can be important in reviewing a patient with abdominal pain. Fever is common in infectious etiologies including pneumonia, peritonitis, cholecystitis, and pelvic inflammatory disease (PID). A low-grade fever can occur with pancreatitis, bowel perforation, or peptic ulcer disease. Fever may be low with sepsis of any cause including bowel perforation. The respiratory rate can increase with fever, acidosis, or acute pain. Pulmonary and cardiac causes of abdominal pain are often associated with increased respiratory rate.

Neck Examination Lymphadenopathy can indicate an active infectious process or malignancy, such as lymphoma. Advanced gastric carcinoma can be associated with very firm or matted nodes near the clavicle.

Cardiac Examination Decreased blood volume from bleeding or dehydration can cause tachycardia and a flow murmur along the left sternal border. Some infectious causes of abdominal pain can be associated with endocarditis. If the patient's history includes leaning forward for relief of upper abdominal pain, auscultation of the heart for signs of pericarditis, including a rub and/or distant heart sounds, is essential.

Pulmonary Examination A subdiaphragmatic abscess, which may occur with cholecystitis, can cause an elevated diaphragm and pulmonary atelectasis. Congestive heart failure or pneumonia at the pulmonary bases may be associated with abnormal breath sounds and an elevated diaphragm from pleural effusion. Abdominal ascites may be associated with pulmonary effusions.

Abdominal Examination The patient should initially be asked to graphically point to the areas of discomfort. The location may not be the same as indicated by the history. Focal areas of pain may provide an important clue as to etiology. In each area, the underlying structures may be the etiology of pain or the pain can be referred from another abdominal region or extra-abdominal process.

The examination begins with direct visualization of the contours of the skin on the abdomen. Tense bulging with fullness most prominent at the lateral flanks, which is common with massive ascites, appears different than obesity. Surgical scars can deform anatomical landmarks, such as the umbilicus. A pulsatile liver or aneurysm can sometimes be appreciated in lean patients. If there is acute abdominal pain, the patient should be requested to point to where the pain began and where it is most severe.

Before palpating, auscultation in several different areas should be completed. Silence or high-pitched rushes can be a clue of gastrointestinal obstruction. Vascular bruits can radiate from aneurysms. Percussion can be used to determine liver size and the presence of shifting dullness indicating ascites.

The amount of information available on palpation is determined by the degree of guarding and the skill of the examiner. A tense abdominal wall can limit the amount of information obtained about the abdominal cavity from palpation alone. Beginning palpation with a gentle touch often decreases abdominal guarding. Positioning the patient with flexed knees may discourage contraction of the abdominal wall.

Patients will allow a more comprehensive examination if palpation begins with a light touch that gradually and gently becomes deeper. Palpation should include liver, spleen, large intestine, and aorta. In selected patients, examination of genitalia, the spine, and a focused neurological examination are indicated. Rectal examinations are especially important if appendicitis is a consideration.

In acute abdominal pain, there is a spectrum of peritoneal inflammation. A rigid, boardlike abdomen can indicate a ruptured organ. Less severe peritoneal inflammation is tested by examining the patient for rebound tenderness. There are major ways to determine whether rebound is positive and therefore, occurring. During deep palpation of any abdominal area, the examiner rapidly lifts his or her hand and observes the patient for evidence of pain. Alternatively, rebound is present if, while pressing firmly and deeply in any area with a positive test, pain is elicited with coughing. Also, determine the area of greatest referred pain. If acute abdominal pain occurs, rebound is one sign of the possible need for emergency surgery. The absence of rebound does not exclude the need for surgery. For example, elderly patients with a perforated ulcer or acute mesenteric ischemia may not have rebound.

Areas of discomfort should receive special attention. At times, it can be difficult to determine if the pain is in the abdominal wall or in the abdominal cavity. If the etiology of the pain is deep to the abdominal wall, attempts at deep palpation with head flexion will be less painful, as the abdominal wall contracts and blocks palpation. With cholecystitis, the gallbladder is palpable in 25 to 50% of patients. A positive Murphy's sign is defined as the development of pain or hesitation in respiration while palpation of the gallbladder region is done during cough or deep inspiration.

The evaluation for the presence of ascites includes an examination for shifting dullness. This is most easily attempted after determining the liver span so that examination for fluid can be done inferior to the liver edge. With the patient still supine, the lateral flank is percussed slowly medially and anteriorly (Fig. 16.1). Because the small intestine usually contain gas, the central abdomen will be more resonant (more hollow sounding). After determining the location where percussion tone changes, the patient is rolled laterally. The maneuver is repeated. Because of gravity, free fluid in the abdominal cavity lies in the most dependent areas. In shifting dullness, the point of dullness moves in the opposite direction than the patient rotated from mid-line.

An aortic aneurysm is usually appreciated just left to the midline as a pulsatile, nonpainful mass. The diameter of upward pulsatile activity can be monitored over time for changes in size. Bruits may be appreciated over the pulsation or over the femoral arteries.

Back and Local Neurologic Examination Visualization, auscultation, and palpation of the back may provide important clues in determining the etiology of abdominal pain. Visualization should include looking for the erythema or subsequent skin vesicles from herpes zoster, hematoma

from ruptured aneurysm or trauma, or asymmetric bulging flanks from a malignancy. Palpation should include seeking spinal tenderness. Often dermatomes extending around the flanks to the anterior abdominal wall begin at the level of pain posteriorly.

Pelvic Examination The source of lower abdominal pain can be best determined by integration of information from abdominal, pelvic and rectal examinations. On pelvic examination, the lateral fornices provide an entry to examine intestine as well as ovaries. Examination of the right fornix is frequently painful in appendicitis. In sigmoid diverticulitis for example, the left ovary may be normal on palpation and the patient have a bulging fullness that is tender on examination. The pregnant patient should be assessed for the development of fibroids.

Rectal Examination If there is an acute abdominal pain, rectal examination with stool guaiac becomes essential. When acute appendicitis is considered, serial rectal examinations may be required to determine whether there is fullness and tenderness in the right lower quadrant of the abdomen. In addition, the presence of even microscopic evidence of bleeding is important when considering the diagnoses GERD, ulcer disease, gastritis or evaluating patients with gastrointestinal bleeding or anemia.

Laboratory Evaluation Any patient with abdominal pain who might be pregnant should have a blood beta human chorionic gonadotropin (HCG) determination. Not only can pregnancy present with many abdominal symptoms, but the management of many conditions would be affected by the presence of pregnancy.

For the evaluation of acute abdominal pain, a complete blood count, electrolytes, liver function tests, amylase or lipase are often adequate. An elevated WBC can occur in cholecystitis, pancreatitis, PID or gastroenteritis. A low WBC may be associated with chronic alcohol use or gastroenteritis. In patients with active bleeding, serial examinations are required. Usually 6 hours are required for blood loss to be reflected in the measured hemoglobin and hematocrit. Prior CBC reports used for comparison can establish the onset of anemia or the importance of an elevated WBC count.

In pancreatitis, the amylase level has been the historic laboratory test that has false positives and negatives. Problems include the many non-pancreatic causes of an increased amylase and the rapid fluctuations in amylase level. In comparison, a lipase level is more sensitive and specific and remains elevated longer after an acute episode. In pancreatitis associated with gallstones, liver function tests are also elevated.

Plain films of the abdomen are indicated if intestinal obstruction or perforation is a possibility. With vascular calcification, aortic aneurysms can be appreciated. Ultrasound and CAT scan are increasingly initially used for the evaluation of acute abdominal pain. Pancreatitis and cholelithiasis can best be initially diagnosed by ultrasound. If the examination is limited by technical problems including overlaying gas, a CAT scan can often provides more definitive information.

Differential Diagnosis

The possible causes of abdominal pain are multiple (Table 16.1). (Note that gender specific causes are listed at the end of each section.) Patients may have more than one precipitating cause of abdominal pain. For example, almost all women experience some abdominal pain during pregnancy. Common causes include increasing pressure from an enlarging uterus, heartburn, and constipation. Yet, a pregnant woman may also develop appendicitis.

The initial evaluation of the individual patient with abdominal pain requires attention to the clinical history and physical examination. Usually, a differential diagnosis can be developed that can be further refined as further tests and serial examinations are completed. The mid-epigastric area provides the largest challenge because of the number of possible diagnoses that begin with pain in this area. Mid-epigastric pain may be related to pancreatitis, cholecystitis, peptic ulcer disease, reflux or early appendicitis. Figure 16.2 reviews the etiologies of pain that can begin in the mid-epigastrium.

Initial evaluation of patients suspected to have active bleeding of any cause includes determination of who will require immediate hospitalization and transfusion because of ongoing blood loss. Orthostatic hypotension often occurs before a significant decrease in hemoglobin and hemocrit. After acute bleeding, it takes the body 5 or 6 hours to shift fluid to the circulation to replace the lost blood. This dilutes the blood, causing a decrease in hematocrit.

In this section the evaluations required to make common diagnoses for GERD, ulcer disease, gastritis, cholecystitis, pancreatitis, appendicitis, nonspecific abdominal pain, expanding aneurysm, and vascular ischemia are reviewed.

GASTROESOPHAGEAL REFLUX DISEASE

Gastroesophageal reflux disease (GERD) is caused by reflux of gastric acid secretions into the esopha-

Table 16.1.
Differential Diagnosis of Acute Abdominal Pain: Etiologies of Referred Abdominal Pain

Chest: pulmonary (pneumonia, pulmonary emboli) or cardiac (coronary ischemia, congestive heart failure, aortic aneurysm, pericarditis)

Back: renal (urinary tract infection, renal abscess or hematoma, renal calculi) or spinal cord (disc disease), growth (infectious or malignant))

Abdominal wall: muscle, skin (e.g., Herpes zoster)

Genitalia: pelvic inflammatory disease, venereal disease in men and women, prostatitis

Age-specific causes

Young
  Acute nonspecific abdominal pain
  Gastroenteritis
  Constipation
  Appendicitis
  Hepatitis
  Trauma causing contusion or bleeding
  Back or hip pain
  Diabetic ketoacidosis without abdominal pathology
  Sexually transmitted diseases including pelvic inflammatory disease in women
  Pregnancy
  Ruptured ovarian corpus luteum cyst
  Tuboovarian lesions such as torsion or ectopic pregnancy
  Endometriosis
  Prostatitis

Middle Years
  Diverticulitis
  Pancreatitis
  Peptic ulcer disease
  Cholecystitis
  Adhesions
  Renal calculi
  Vascular: aneurysm, ischemia
  Malignancies involving intestines, pancreas, gallbladder, liver, lymph glands, pelvic organs
  Fibroids
  All listed under "Young"

Geriatric
  Adhesions
  Hernias
  Growths (malignant and benign)
  Volvulus
  Bowel ischemia
  Abdominal aortic aneurysm
  All listed under "Young" and "Middle Years" except ovarian follicle, pregnancy

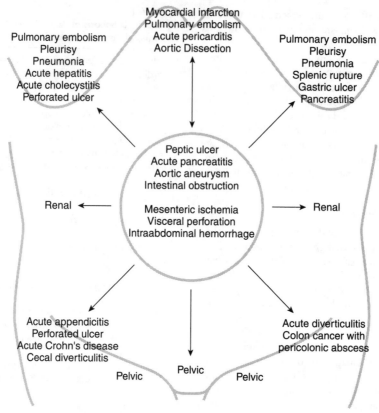

Figure 16.2. Central abdominal pain. Many causes of abdominal pain begin in the central abdomen, only to "migrate" subsequently into a more "localizing" position in the abdomen. When severe abdominal pain persists without localization to one specific quadrant, those entities listed in the periumbilical area of the figure must be especially considered. (Adapted from Reilly Practical Strategies in Outpatient Medicine, 2nd edition. 1991;13:761.)

gus resulting in esophageal mucosal injury including erosion and ulceration. This disease is often associated with abnormal esophageal pressures. Men have more physiologic reflux than women and produce more basal gastric acid. Severe blood loss can occur with advanced mucosal injury. Mechanical stimuli to reflux include eating a large meal; such body characteristics as central obesity, wearing a tight girdle, or pregnancy; and lying down after a meal. Decreased lower esophageal tone and increased symptoms occur with consumption of alcohol, caffeine, mint, chocolate, and tobacco. About 25% of individuals using nonsteroidal antiinflammatory drugs (NSAID) chronically have symptoms of GERD.

Reflux symptoms occur in about 40% of all pregnancies. The etiology is both hormonal and mechanical. Progesterone decreases lower esopha-

geal sphincter tone. Increasing uterine size is associated with increasing constipation and increasing reflux. The later decreases when the fetus lowers further into the pelvis.

Esophagitis and its complications are the pathologic complication of GERD. In about 10% of patients with esophagitis, strictures develop in the distal esophagus from fibrosis that involves at least the submucosal surfaces. Esophageal strictures can result in obstruction. Barrett's esophagus occurs when columnar epithelium replace squamous epithelium and is associated with an increased risk of adenocarcinoma.

GERD is suspected when a patient describes heartburn, symptoms of a central burning sensation especially behind the sternum, and the regurgitation of meals within 3 hours of eating. Fatty and large meals are frequent precipitants. Symptoms are aggravated by lying down or bending. Usually, antacids provide some relief. Patients with peptic stricture often experience dysphagia.

The symptom of heartburn is neither specific or sensitive for GERD. Although heartburn frequently occurs, extreme esophageal mucosal ulceration is less often found on investigation. The frequency of heartburn symptoms in the population has increased over the last two decades.

Because reflux symptoms are so ubiquitous, most clinicians believe selection of patients requiring further evaluation should be selective. Simple measures such as not eating before bed, especially in patients with mechanical factors such as pregnancy or obesity may provide adequate relief (Table 16.2). When simple measures fail, further investigation with upper endoscopy allows staging of GERD.

Dysphagia (difficulty swallowing) must be aggressively evaluated by upper endoscopy or barium swallow. The differential diagnosis of dysphagia includes not only peptic stricture, but esophageal cancer. Lesions external to the esophagus can cause dysphagia including severe osteoarthritis with large osteophytes. During endoscopy, peptic strictures can be managed with dilation.

Table 16.2.
Conservative Measures for Managing Gastroesophageal Reflux Disease

Mechanical
In obesity decreased weight
Avoid girdles and constricting clothes
Sit or stand after eating
Elevation of head of bed (cinder blocks)

Foods and exposures to avoid
Alcohol
Caffeine including chocolate
Mints
Tobacco smoke or chewing tobacco
Large meals
Fatty foods
Avoid medications that decrease lower esophageal
    tone (e.g., nitrates)

Medical therapy
Antacids
H_2 blockers from low to high doses
Prokinetic motility agents
Increase lower esophageal sphincter tone
Prevent gastric acid secretion

Surgical therapy
Antireflux surgery—fundoplication (gastric fundus
    wrapped around lower esophagus)

PEPTIC ULCER DISEASE (PUD)

Ulcer disease includes peptic ulcer disease (ulcers present in the duodenum) and gastric ulcers. The understanding of the pathogenesis of ulcer disease has radically altered over the past decade. The 1994 Consensus Development Conference affirmed that *Heliobacter pylori (H. pylori)* is an etiologic agent for almost all peptic ulcer disease and often gastritis and gastric ulcer disease. *H. Pylori,* a spiral gram negative bacillus, may colonize the mucous gel coating of the gastric cells and less often the cells themselves. The epidemiology of *H. pylori* and its mode of transmission is not well defined. Currently, diagnosis is dependent on results of endoscopic biopsy. Other less invasive means of diagnosis, such as a special breath test, are not yet in common use. The successful eradication of *H. pylori* infection usually prevents the recurrence of ulcer disease.

Another common etiology of ulcer disease is the use of nonsteroidal anti-inflammatory drugs (NSAID). Compared with non-users, individuals with NSAID use have at least three times the risk of gastrointestinal problems. Chronic use of aspirin, (even one tablet daily) or other NSAIDs may cause superficial erosions diagnosed by endoscopy. Gastric ulcers occur in 10–20% while peptic ulcer disease occurs in only 5-10% of chronic NSAID users. The adverse affects of NSAIDs are probably mediated by decreased gastrointestinal prostaglandins and perhaps local microvascular damage.

Peptic ulcer disease (PUD) is common and may occur at any age. Often PUD is a chronic, recurring problem with a genetic component. In peptic ulcer disease, basal acid secretion may be higher than in GERD and men have more basal acid secretion than women. Tobacco exposure increases the incidence of PUD and decreases the efficacy of treatment. The use of NSAIDs increases the risk of bleeding from PUD. Progressive increasing progesterone levels during pregnancy is thought to confer protection from PUD.

In comparison, the incidence of gastric ulcers increases with increasing age. They are less common than PUD. Etiologies include *H. pylori* and defective mucosal resistance (i.e., from NSAID or cancer). Because the prognosis with gastric cancer is related to the extent of disease at time of diagnosis, early diagnosis is important. Accurate diagnosis of benign stomach ulcer disease is especially important as gastric carcinoma often initially presents as a gastric ulcer.

Ulcer disease can cause significant blood loss due to chronic low level oozing or erosion through a blood vessel. In addition, blood loss from the stomach may be caused by gastritis and cancer. Other sites of gastrointestinal blood loss include the esophagus (i.e., Mallory-Weiss tear, esophagitis, varices), small intestine (i.e., polyp or cancer), colon (i.e., diverticulitis, vascular malformation, polyp, cancer). With significant blood loss and slow transit time, changes in the stool can be noted. Melena is black stool that occurs from the interaction of blood with hydrochloric acid from the stomach to produce hematin. Similar black stools can also occur after exposure to iron, bismuth (an active ingredient in pepto-bismol), or licorice.

Peptic ulcer disease (PUD) classically produces epigastric pain that increases at night and improves immediately after eating only to return one and a half to three hours after eating. The pain is characterized as being a hunger pain, aching, gnawing, or stabbing. However, patients may have significant blood loss from ulcer disease without abdominal pain. Antacids, as well as food, may decrease symptoms. Gastric ulcer pain may be similar, however, it may not improve with food and antacids. Tobacco exposure is a potent risk factor for ulcer disease. Some complications of PUD can be predicted from the patient's history. When eating attempts repeatedly result in emesis, the development of a gastric outlet obstruction should be considered. If hematemesis develops, treatment for acute hemorrhage should be initiated. When pain becomes relentless, radiates posteriorly, or is no longer improved with antacids, the possibility of perforation must be considered.

The most common life-threatening complication of ulcer disease is bleeding followed by perforation. If there has been significant blood loss (usually more than 500 ml), symptoms can include weakness, lightheadedness, wooziness, or even orthostatic dizziness (i.e., lightheaded upon standing). With this history, the patient should be immediately evaluated for orthostatic hypotension and fluid status. Patients with slow chronic blood loss usually present with fatigue and iron deficiency anemia. A less common, but more dangerous complication is intestinal perforation that is only occasionally associated with severe pain and more often diagnosed because of hypotension.

The diagnoses of ulcer disease should be considered when there is a typical history of pain or the development of iron deficiency anemia in a patient with risk factors for PUD. Symptomatic patients require evaluation before the diagnosis of ulcer disease is made since symptoms can occur with GERD or gastritis. It is especially important to determine a specific diagnosis in the elderly patient with associated weight loss.

Controversy persists in the initial evaluation of symptomatic patients. Many physicians suggest initial endoscopy because the detection of ulcers, esophagitis, gastritis, and duodenitis is more accurate than upper gastrointestinal radiograph using single or double contrast. In addition, endoscopic biopsy specimens can be examined for the presence of *H. pylori*.

Initial evaluation by upper gastrointestinal (UGI series) radiographs taken after swallowing barium are less invasive and expensive. Sedation of the patient is not required. PUD, reflux, severe esophagitis, and masses in the esophagus, stomach or duodenum can be diagnosed by the UGI series although endoscopy is more sensitive and specific. Gastritis, pancreatitis, and less severe esophagitis are rarely diagnosed by UGI series. Endoscopy is required only if the upper gastrointestinal radiograph is not diagnostic or reveals a potentially malignant gastric ulcer. The prognosis of gastric carcinoma is related to the stage at diagnosis. Careful follow-up of gastric ulcers until complete resolution is essential to avoid missing an early gastric carcinoma.

The specific presentation of blood provides important information when considering the source of acute bleeding. Hematemesis (vomiting of blood) indicates bleeding from the esophagus, stomach or duodenum. Melena (black, tarry stool) usually indicates bleeding from the esophagus, stomach, duodenum, and less often the jejunum, ileum, or ascending colon. Hematochezia (bright red blood per rectum) usually indicates blood loss from sites distal to the duodenum, although it can occur from rapid upper tract hemorrhage. The most common causes of upper and lower intestinal blood loss are reviewed in Table 16.3.

Table 16.3.
Etiology of Gastrointestinal Bleeding: Upper Versus Lower

Upper
Peptic ulcer disease
Gastritis
Varices and portal hypertension
Mallory-Weiss syndrome (esophagogastric mucosal tear)

Lower
Hemorrhoids/fissures
Diverticula
Colonic polyps
Colon cancer
Angiodysplasia

GASTRITIS

Gastritis is inflammation of the stomach that is classified as either erosive/hemorrhagic, nonerosive, chronic, or specific. Causes of nonerosive gastritis include *H. pylori,* viral infections, Crohn's disease or gastroenteritis. Erosive/hemorrhagic gastritis is diagnosed when subepithelial hemorrhages and erosions are visualized during endoscopy. Etiologies include NSAIDs, alcohol ingestion, or "stress" in critically ill patients. Only a small proportion of patients with erosive/hemorrhagic gastritis develop clinically significant bleeding. Nonerosive chronic gastritis is caused by *H. pylori* or pernicious anemia.

Gastritis may be asymptomatic or associated with heartburn and significant bleeding. New onset *H. pylori.* colonization can cause the acute onset of abdominal pain associated with nausea and vomiting lasting several days.

Gastritis is an endoscopic diagnosis. It is frequently associated with GERD or ulcer disease. Currently, the gold standard for the determination of *H. pylori* colonization requires endoscopy.

PANCREATITIS

The etiology of acute pancreatitis is most often alcoholism or gallstones. Less common causes include other causes of pancreatic duct obstruction (i.e., tumor, worm infestations such as ascariasis, drug reactions, and idiopathic pancreatitis). The mechanism by which pancreatic enzymes are released in acute pancreatitis is still not well defined. The resulting cascade of inflammation may be related to auto-digestion and local ischemia. Whether gallstone-induced pancreatitis is related to bile reflux or only obstruction of pancreatic drainage has not been determined despite many studies.

Pancreatitis is often associated with continual pain between the upper or central anterior abdomen and the back directly posterior. The pain may decrease sitting bent forward with flexed knees, and does not significantly improve after emesis. Eating may dramatically increase the pain. Patients often experience associated abdominal bloating, nausea, and vomiting. The severe abdominal pain radiating posteriorly can also occur with cholecystitis, peptic ulcer disease (especially perforation), dissecting aortic aneurysm, acute intestinal obstruction, pneumonia and diabetic ketoacidosis. All these diagnoses may also be associated with nausea and vomiting. Cholecystitis and biliary colic are located more laterally to the right and have a more gradual onset. Severe peptic ulcer disease is often associated with bleeding and sometimes a history of abdominal pain that is better with eating. A dissecting aneurysm is often associated with hypotension.

Most patients with acute pancreatitis have moderate abdominal pain that is best managed by limiting oral intake and providing intravenous hydration. Because mortality may be as high as 9% in the 25% of patients who have severe attacks, patients with active pancreatitis are usually admitted to the hospital for observation and treatment. A small number of patients with mild symptoms will adequately respond to an all-liquid diet. The prognosis of patients with acute pancreatitis depends on the etiology and severity and can be estimated utilizing the Ranson criteria.

CHOLECYTITIS

Gallstones are either composed of cholesterol or calcium bilirubinate (pigmented stones). The former are the more prevalent type of stone in the U.S., while the latter are more common in the Orient. The pathogenesis of cholesterol gallstones is multifactorial: high bile cholesterol levels; development of a crystal nucleus; stone growth; delayed gallbladder emptying and associated stasis of gallbladder contents. Symptoms develop from mechanical obstruction or local inflammation.

Gallbladder stones frequently form during pregnancy. In late pregnancy, high levels of progesterone further decrease gallbladder contracture. Acute cholecystitis is rare during early pregnancy and occurs more commonly after delivery when progesterone levels decrease and contraction of the gallbladder resumes.

Gallstones are more common with obesity and in women. Biliary colic is sharp abdominal pain often associated with nausea and vomiting that occurs in the middle or right upper quadrant. It usually lasts several hours followed by a residual aching that can last days. An episode of pain may be precipitated by a fatty meal, or eating after fasting. Symptoms may be less in the elderly.

Besides acute right upper quadrant tenderness, cholecystitis is characterized by fever and leukocytosis. Most patients report a prior similar episode. Hepatitis can cause discomfort in the same area, but usually the pain is not as severe. In contrast, most peptic ulcer disease improves with eating. Ultrasound confirms the presence of gallstones. Isotopic scans showing lack of gallbladder function aid in diagnosing cholecystitis.

APPENDICITIS

The history is critical in making an accurate diagnosis of appendicitis. Anorexia is frequently present.

Usually, it presents as a periumbilical or diffuse epigastric abdominal pain that is often associated with nausea and vomiting. The pain eventually shifts to the right lower quadrant.

Appendicitis is inflammation of the vestigial sac of the distal small intestine that begins as mucosal ulceration and without intervention may evolve to gangrene and perforation. Morbidity and mortality are adversely affected by perforation. Appendicitis can occur at any age, but is most common between the ages 20 and 40 years. Gender incidence is similar except for a higher incidence in males between puberty and age 25. Lack of insurance increases the risk of appendiceal rupture.

The differential diagnoses are broad and can include acute gastroenteritis, and in women: ruptured corpus luteum cyst; PID; ectopic pregnancy; and endometriosis. Careful serial examinations will at times allow differentiation. With appendicitis, there should be point tenderness on the abdominal, rectal, flank or pelvic examination. Even experienced clinicians can have difficulty making an accurate diagnosis. Collaboration across provider specialities may aid in care. Often surgical exploration is required to both confirm the diagnosis and provide treatment.

PREGNANCY

Even uncomplicated pregnancy is frequently associated with abdominal pain. The enlarging uterus presses on contiguous organs and causes the stretching of muscle and skin. Even before the uterus is large, women often experience discomfort with the stretching of the broad ligament or pain after emesis.

VASCULAR DISEASE

Abdominal aneurysms are pathologic dilation of an abdominal blood vessel wall often associated with atherosclerotic disease. As with other types of atherosclerotic disease, aneurysms are more common with tobacco smoke exposure. Vascular leakage can cause abdominal pain, although usually there is no warning prior to rupture.

Acute mesenteric ischemia occurs because of decreased intestinal vascular perfusion. Often the etiologies include hypovolemia due to bleeding or low cardiac output states as in congestive heart failure or myocardial infarction. Ischemia can also occur from emboli associated with cardiac arrhythmia.

Aneurysms are usually asymptomatic with gradual expansion. However, dissection or rupture may

cause both acute abdominal pain radiating to the back and severe hypotension. Acute mesenteric ischemia is associated with abdominal pain 75% of the time. Nausea and vomiting indicate disease progression. Sepsis and hypotension are late complications.

Patients presenting hypotensive with upper abdominal pain radiating to the back can be experiencing a massive myocardial infarction or aneurysm expansion or rupture. Once severe hypotension has occurred, the prognosis is grave even with aggressive management.

Acute mesenteric ischemia is a clinical diagnosis. Once nonspecific symptoms such as epigastric or left lower quadrant abdominal aching occur, there is about an 80% one year mortality. Laboratory tests are nonspecific and may include increased WBC, amylase and alkaline phosphatase. By the time plain films confirm the diagnosis, the patient has a high risk of death. Angiography is required to make a definitive diagnosis.

NONSPECIFIC ABDOMINAL PAIN

The pathophysiology of nonspecific abdominal pain is currently unknown. It is only recently that patients who present with acute right lower abdominal pain without appendicitis have been studied as a group. Only a small number of these patients have recurrent episodes. These patients are most likely to have a pathologic condition such as endometriosis.

About 40% of patients referred for evaluation of appendicitis do well with observation alone. The clinical course is initially similar to appendicitis with the development of right lower quadrant abdominal pain. But, patients gradually improve without another specific diagnosis being successfully proven. This is a diagnosis of exclusion, which is made retrospectively.

Management

Management of the patient with abdominal pain is usually straightforward if the diagnosis is correct. This section will review management of specific diseases. Also reviewed are drug therapies commonly used in the outpatient setting.

GERD

The spectrum of disease severity varies. Treatment modalities begin with simple measures and progress through the use of medications towards a definitive surgical procedure (Table 16.2). Many patients respond to dietary changes and avoid reclining after eating. Pharmacologic therapeutic options have increased in the last decade and provide adequate symptomatic control for most patients. Often, higher doses and longer treatment with (H2) histamine 2 blockers are required (Table 16.4). Fundoplication, anti-reflux surgery, should be considered for patients with severe symptoms not fully responsive to drug therapy and for young patients requiring long term pharmacologic treatment. Many asthmatics with GERD have improvement in their respiratory symptoms with successful GERD treatment.

ULCER DISEASE/GASTRITIS

The accurate diagnosis of *H. pylori* is currently under active investigation. Although the current gold standard is endoscopy with biopsy, less invasive diagnostic procedures are actively being developed. The treatment of *H. pylori* is discussed later in this chapter. Completion of an effective treatment regimen and resolution of symptoms may be accepted as indication of a cure. With treatment of *H. pylori,* fewer patients require long term H2 blocker maintenance therapy.

Tobacco cessation and avoidance of second-hand smoke exposure will improve the success of pharmacologic treatment and decrease the PUD recurrence rate. The diagnosis of PUD should be used as an opportunity to encourage patients to understand the connection between tobacco use and health. Longer pharmacologic treatment courses should be considered in individuals unable to decrease exposure to tobacco.

Surgical therapy of ulcer disease has decreased as medical management has improved. Current indications for surgery are limited to persistent bleed-ing that is not responding to medical therapy and patients who cannot tolerate medical therapy. Admissions for perforated ulcers are increasing especially in women over the age of 65.

CHOLECYSTITIS

Acute cholecystitis may require hospitalization for intravenous hydration and bowel rest. About 25% of patients do not improve in the first few days and require emergency cholecystectomy. Of the 75% of patients who initially improve, recurrence of cholecystitis will occur in 25% within one year and 60% within 6 years. Because of the high risk of recurrence, after an episode of acute cholecystitis patients may choose prophylactic cholecystectomy.

Laparoscopic cholecystectomy is a well tolerated and popular surgical procedure. Lithotripsy has short and long term problems. Initially, the passage of gallstone fragments after lithotripsy can cause biliary colic and less often pancreatitis. Long term, patients need to use medical therapy to prevent stone recurrence.

Medical therapies for symptomatic gallstones are less effective and will be discussed in the drug section. Chenodeoxycholic acid (CDCA) or urso-deoxycholic acid (UDCA) can result in partial or complete dissolution of radiolucent cholesterol gallstones in about half of carefully selected patients with a functioning gallbladder. Higher success rates occur if stones are also small and floating. Successful treatment may require two years of daily therapy. Potential drug side effects include diarrhea and increased transaminases. Once stones have dissolved, medication is continued to prevent recurrence. In summary, the use of medical therapy for gallstone dissolution is associated with a substantial

Table 16.4.
Dosage of H$_2$ Blockers

Drug	Active Ulcer Disease	Ulcer Relapse Prevention	GERD
Cimetidine (Tagamet)[a]	400 mg twice daily or 800 mg every night	400 mg every night	400 mg every night or 400 mg every 12 hr Maximum 400 mg every 6 hr
Ranitidine (Zantac)[a]	150 mg twice daily or 300 mg every night	150 mg every night	150 mg twice daily Maximum 150 mg every 6 hr
Famotidine (Pepcid)[a]	20 mg twice daily or 40 mg every night	20 mg every night	20 mg twice daily Maximum 40 mg twice daily
Nizatidine (Axid)[a]	150 mg twice daily or 300 mg every night	150 mg every night	150 mg twice daily

[a]Available without prescription.

failure rate and the necessity of long term treatment with an expensive medication.

APPENDICITIS

The definitive treatment is surgical removal of the appendix. Since the risk of perforation increases with time, delaying surgery is not without risk. By 48 hours, rupture may occur in 80% of acute appendicitis cases. Patients with a mass 3 to 5 days after symptoms may have substantial inflammation and require inpatient antibiotic treatment before surgery. To avoid missing the diagnosis, accept that some proportion of excised appendixes may be benign.

VASCULAR DISEASE

The management of an aneurysm depends on its size and rate of expansion. The risk of rupture increases with increasing size. Elective repair is recommended for most aneurysms greater than 5 cm because elective vascular surgery has a substantially lower morbidity and mortality than emergent surgery. The treatment of a rapidly expanding aneurysm requires hospitalization and preparation for surgical repair.

Acute mesenteric ischemia has a poor prognosis even with aggressive management. Acute mesenteric ischemia can be caused by thrombosis, low cardiac output or emboli. Surgical embolectomy will only aid some patients with a documented embolus after angiography locates the exact lesion. In patients with suspected thrombosis or low cardiac output surgery provides no benefit.

DRUGS

Drug therapy of abdominal pain is commonplace. Revenues from the sale of histamine blockers are consistently in the top five among all drugs. Drugs used in the treatment of upper gastrointestinal disorders are reviewed in this section.

Antacids Antacids have an acid neutralizing capacity. Antacids are alkaline and increase the pH of gastric contents, deactivate pepsin and may increase lower esophageal sphincter tone. Several different compounds are available. Magnesium-containing antacids may have a laxative effect and in renal failure, blood magnesium levels increase. Aluminum-containing antacids may bind with other drugs, can cause constipation and absorption of aluminum with decreased renal functioning, and can result in encephalopathy. Phosphorus-containing antacids bind with calcium-decreasing absorption. Calcium-containing antacids have the ad-

ditional benefit of increasing calcium absorption. The sodium content of different antacids varies widely (Table 16.5). Antacids are available in tablet and liquid form with the latter being more effective, but more difficult to carry.

Antacids are widely used for a variety of symptoms. Frequently, antacids are utilized as well as other medications for reflux, gastritis, or PUD. Other medications should not be taken at the same time. To treat PUD effectively with only antacids, dosing would be required seven times daily. Antacids do not affect the course of pancreatitis or gallstones.

Therapy for *H. pylori* The variety of current antibiotic regimens to treat *H. pylori* is growing rapidly (Table 16.6). The most studied regimens for cure still require multiple agents. As research

Table 16.5.
Antacids in Treatment of Duodenal Ulcer

Antacid (liquid)[a,b]	Dose to Neutralize 140 mEq Acid (ml)	Sodium per 30 ml (mg)
Maalox TC (aluminum hydroxide, magnesium hydroxide)	33	7.2
Delcid (aluminum hydroxide, magnesium hydroxide)	17–34	9
Mylanta-II (aluminum hydroxide, magnesium hydroxide, simethicone)	39	6.6
Gelusil-II (aluminum hydroxide, magnesium hydroxide, simethicone)	32–47	7.8
Maalox Plus (aluminum hydroxide, magnesium hydroxide, simethicone)	60	15
Gelusil (aluminum hydroxide, magnesium hydroxide, simethicone)	65	4.2
Riopan Plus (aluminum hydroxide, magnesium hydroxide, simethicone)	78	4.2
ALternaGEL (aluminum hydroxide)	63	4
Amphojel (aluminum hydroxide)	100	42

[a]Omitted from this table are the many antacids that contain either calcium or carbonate, each of which is at least theoretically contraindicated in the treatment of peptic ulcer disease.
[b]Magnesium-containing antacids often cause diarrhea. Antacids that contain only aluminum are more often constipating.
From Drake D, Hollander D: Neutralizing capacity and cost effectiveness of antacids. Ann Intern Med 94: 215–217, 1981. Dutro MP, Amerson AB: Comparison of liquid antacids (letter). N Engl J Med 302:1967, 1980.
Adapted from Reilly Practical strategies in outpatient medicine, 2nd ed. Philadelphia. Saunders, 1991; 13:771.

Table 16.6.
Treatment Regimens for Treatment of H. Pylori

Classic triple therapy

Two week course of bismuth 2 tablets four times daily; plus metronidazole 250 mg four times daily; plus tetracycline or amoxicillin 500 mg four times daily

Classic therapy with antisecretory agent

Above agents with ranitidine 300 mg at bedtime for up to 4 months

or

Above agents with omeprazole 20 mg twice daily for 4 weeks

Modified triple therapy

Amoxicillin 500 mg three times daily and metronidazole 250 mg four times daily for 14 days; plus ranitidine 300 mg at bedtime for 4–6 weeks

continues, the optimum regimen with the highest efficacy, least expense and fewest side effects continues to change. The specific drugs, doses and duration of treatment vary from regimen to regimen. Newer regimens include antibiotics and medications to decrease acid secretion.

When a regimen with a high success rate is successfully completed and the patient becomes asymptomatic, treatment is empirically considered successful. Patients who are still symptomatic may require a repeat endoscopy. As less invasive techniques to determine *H. pylori* colonization become available, tests of cure may be used rather than endoscopy for patients remaining symptomatic.

HISTAMINE-2 (H2) BLOCKERS

Since the introduction of H2 blockers, these agents have become the "gold standard" of treatment for ulcer disease. Indications for their use have expanded to include GERD, esophagitis and gastritis. There are currently four H2 blockers available in the United States: cimetidine; ranitidine; famotidine and nizatidine. These agents attach to the histamine receptors of the gastric parietal cell which usually produce gastric acid. This results in a decrease in intracellular cAMP levels and a significant decrease in gastric acid secretion during baseline conditions and after stimulation (including physiologic nighttime surges and food). Since cimetidine and ranitidine can increase prolocatin levels, rarely women may experience galactorrhea or breast swelling and men may experience gynecomastia.

Efficacy of treatment for GERD, esophagitis, gastritis, and ulcer disease improves with increasing dose and duration of treatment. Usually acute disease is treated for 6 to 8 weeks followed by maintenance therapy, which is given before bed (qhs) since physiologic acid levels are highest at night. The doses required for GERD are greater than for other indications (Table 16.4). With the introduction of these agents, elective and emergency surgery for ulcer disease has dramatically decreased. Cimetidine, the first agent to be released, has the least effect on gastric acid secretion and famotidine the greatest. Currently, only cimetidine is available in generic form and this preparation is the least expensive. Because these agents are excreted by the kidney, renal function and age can affect drug clearance and should affect dosing.

H2 blockers are not only effective, but well tolerated. The most common side effects from H2 blockers is interaction of cimetidine with other pharmacologic agents. Cimetidine is the only one of these agents to bind with P450 cytochromes in the liver and therefore decreases clearance of other medications degraded through P450 cytochromes. This results in higher blood levels of multiple medications including diazepam, warfarin, beta blockers, phenytoin and theophylline. All these agents occasionally cause headache, fatigue, muscular pains, or diarrhea. Patients who are old or have renal insufficiency are at greatest risk for confusion.

SUCRALFATE

Sucralfate is a sticky gel that includes aluminum hydroxide that especially adheres to the epithelial cells at the base of the ulcers and is generally not absorbed. Sucralfate is an effective and safe agent to treat and prevent active ulcer disease, if the patient can comply with the QID regimen using sucralfate before meals. It is as effective as cimetidine in healing ulcers and more effective while being used in preventing relapse. Simultaneous use of antacids or food does not affect gel adherence. However, an acid environment activates the drug so doses of sucralfate and antacids should be separated by at least 30 minutes. The mechanisms of action of sucralfate are multiple including resistance to degradation of the gel layer and stimulation of prostaglandin release. Sucralfate also absorbs bile acids, pepsin and trypsin and impairs absorption of coumadin, erythromycin, propranolol and diazepam. The dose prescribed for PUD is 1 gram QID with medication ideally taken 1 hour before each meal and at bedtime. The dose for prophylaxis is 1 gram twice a day. Constipation and dry mouth are rare side effects.

OMEPRAZOLE

Omeprazole totally inhibits the gastric parietal cell proton pump and causes gastric acid suppression. While it is very effective, omeprazole is only currently approved for short-term use in PUD, erosive esophagitis or poorly responsive GERD and is only gradually being utilized in longer treatment regimens. There are two major concerns about omeprazole. In patients with GERD, discontinuation of therapy often causes recurrence of symptoms. Also, gastrin levels rise in patients on omeprazole more than three months and return to normal after stopping treatment. In rats, high gastrin levels were associated with the development of gastric carcinoid tumors. In humans with elevated gastrin levels from Zollinger-Ellison syndrome or pernicious anemia, there is also increased risk of gastric carcinoid tumors. Monitoring of gastrin levels are recommended in patients using omepazole more than 3 months. The usual dose is 20 mg orally each morning.

MISOPROSTOL

Misoprostol is the first prostoglandin E. analogue available. It inhibits the secretion of gastric acid, inhibits gastric mucosal damage, and improves healing after an insult. Misoprostol protects mucosa from damage in the first weeks of therapy as well as long term. Diarrhea, a common side effect, less frequently occurs when misoprostol is taken after meals and lower doses are used. Unfortunately, the lower dose only protects the gastric mucosa, and higher doses are required to protect stomach and duodenum. Fortunately, the diarrhea often is mild and may spontaneously resolve even when misoprostol is continued. The usual dose is 100 mg QID with food followed by 200 mg QID. Gradually increasing dose decreases GI side effects.

PROMOTILITY AGENTS

Cholinergic medications increase bowel motility for some patients. These agents increase lower esophageal sphincter pressure and improve gastric emptying. These agents may decrease symptoms of reflux and constipation in some patients. The oldest agent is metoclopramide which has the most cholinergic side effects. Usually the dose is 10 mg about half an hour before meals and before bedtime. Side effects include drowsiness, irritability, and rarely urinary retention.

Newer agents include cisapride which decreases symptoms and improves endoscopic healing of esophagitis similar to H2 blockers (10 mg QID or 20 mg QID) and is beginning to be utilized at lower doses (10 g BID) as maintenance therapy. Because cisapride stimulates serotonin receptors to enhance release of acetycholine from the mesenteric plexus it is less frequently associated with the side effects noted with metoclopramide. Occasional side effects include headache, nausea, vomiting, diarrhea and rhinitis. Cisapride may increase the effect of anticoagulant drugs.

ILLUSTRATIVE CASES WITH SELF-ASSESSMENT QUESTIONS AND ANSWERS

Case 1

D.T. is a 42-year-old obese man with new-onset heartburn. He notes that over the last year he has gained an additional 10 pounds since learning his son's diagnosis of HIV disease. The pain is worse after eating, especially fatty foods. Use of antacids has caused diarrhea.

QUESTION: *What is your diagnosis?*

a. Gastritis
b. GERD
c. Ulcer disease
d. Gallbladder disease

ANSWER: b. *Although GERD is the most probable, any of these diagnoses are possible. All initial lab tests are normal.*

QUESTION: *What treatment would you recommend?*

a. Support group
b. Changing antacid from magnesuim containing to aluminuim containing
c. Endoscopy for definitive diagnosis
d. Anti-anxiety medications

ANSWER: c. *Definative diagnosis with upper*

endoscopy will guide therapy most effectively. Changing antacid type will alter drug side effects. Be sure to remind the patient that H2 blockers and antacid use should be separated to avoid decreased efficacy of H2 blockers. A support group could be helpful in adjusting to his son's new diagnosis. If his son is gay and that is an emotional issue, your patient may benefit from contacting Parents and Friends of Gays (See "The Spectrum of Patients" chapter). Anti-anxiety medications are not indicated in this situation.

Case 2

P.D. is a 25-year-old sexually active nulliparous woman whose last menses was on time 2 weeks ago. She developed left lower quadrant pain last night a few hours after eating a large meal of take-out Chinese food from a new restaurant. She had a normal bowel movement the morning before.

QUESTION: What is your preliminary diagnosis?

a. Viral gastroenteritis
b. Food poisoning
c. PID
d. Appendicitis
e. Mittelschmerz
f. Ectopic pregnancy

ANSWER: c, e, and **f** are the most likely choices. Localized left lower quadrant pain would be uncommon as the only symptom of gastroenteritis, food poisoning, and appendicitis.

QUESTION: What further questions would not aid in evaluation?

a. Did she have close contact with anyone ill?
b. Did she eat alone? If not, did anyone else become ill?
c. Could she be pregnant?
d. Did she have a recent respiratory infection?
e. Was her last menses typical?

ANSWER: d. The first two questions help define the possibility of viral gastroenteritis and food poisoning. The character of recent menses is helpful in the consideration of mittelschmerz. An ectopic pregnancy is only possible if the patient is pregnant. A history related to a recent respiratory infection does not aid differential diagnosis.

QUESTION: Immediate evaluation should not include which of the following?

a. Full neurologic examination
b. Abdominal examination
c. Pelvic examination
d. Rectal examination
e. Pregnancy test

ANSWER: a. Only the neurological examination is not essential initially. In this patient, examination is remarkable for diffuse left lower abdominal pain without rebound. Pelvic examination reveals tender left adenexa without cervical motion tenderness or vaginal discharge. The pregnancy test is positive.

QUESTION: What evaluation should be completed next?

a. Immediate laproscopy
b. Plain film of abdomen
c. Ultrasound
d. CAT scan

ANSWER: c. Xrays including CAT scan should be avoided in pregnancy since fetus radiation exposure increases the risk of childhood leukemia. An ultrasound can rapidly diagnosis intrauterine versus ectopic pregnancy. This patient had an ectopic pregnancy.

Case 3

M.L. is a 50 year-old-man with a long history of alcohol and tobacco use being seen for the first time at your community clinic. In the past, after heavy alcohol consumption, he has experienced pancreatitis requiring hospitalization. Although he is drinking less, over the last few weeks he's developed severe pain after eating that and is not responding to large doses of antacid. He denies alcohol withdrawal symptoms. This abdominal pain is different than prior episodes. He has been more tired than usual, but has not felt lightheaded.

QUESTION: Your differential diagnosis includes which of the following?

a. Pancreatitis
b. Gastritis
c. Gallbladder disease
d. Ulcer disease
e. All of the above

ANSWER: e. *All of the above, but the presumptive diagnosis would be gastritis or gastritis with associated ulcer disease that responded to antacids initially. Because symptoms are different than prior episodes, pancreatitis is less likely.*

QUESTION: *After obtaining a history and an examination that reveals upper mid-abdominal tenderness and guaiac negative stool, what tests would you order for completion the same day?*

a. CBC
b. Amylase
c. LFT
d. Ultrasound
e. Endoscopy

ANSWER: a, b, c. *Initial immediate assessment would include a CBC, amylase and LFT. The CBC will be scrutinized for evidence of anemia as well as pancytopenia as can occur from bone marrow supression by chronic alcohol use. The liver function tests and amylase are obtained to define his extent of chronic disease.*

Abnormalities are limited to Hb/Hct of 12/36 with an increased red cell distribution width and slightly elevated SGOT greater than SGPT. Given the patient's upper abdominal symptoms, the source of blood loss will most likely be upper abdominal.

QUESTION: *What diagnostic procedure is indicated?*

a. Ultrasound
b. UGI series
c. Endoscopy

ANSWER: c. *Endoscopy will provide accurate diagnosis and currently is the only test to define the presence of H. pylori infection.*

Upper endoscopy revealed gastritis without H. pylori infection.

QUESTION: *Your treatment and advice to the patient includes?*

a. Triple antibiotic regimen for *H. pylori* eradication
b. H2 blocker treatment
c. Sucralfate
d. Antacid use
e. Stopping alcohol consumption
f. Stopping tobacco consumption
g. Avoiding NSAID agents

ANSWER: b, f, g. *Treatment for H. pylori infection is only indicated with documented infection. H2 blocker use at appropriate treatment doses would be the preferred treatment of active gastritis compared to sucralfate which requires a QID regimen and antacids which require 7 x daily dosing. Before recommending acute termination of alcohol use, it is critical to review symptoms of alcohol withdrawal in detail with the patient. When there is previous history of acohol withdrawal seizures or potential for suicide, inpatient detoxification is indicated. Tobacco and NSAIDS should be avoided.*

Case 4

B.T. is a 72 year-old-woman with severe osteoarthritis and longstanding diabetes with associated peripheral neuropathy and peripheral vascular disease who reports solid foods get "stuck" going down over the last few months. She usually takes daily NSAIDs, but doesn't smoke or drink.

QUESTION: *Your initial differential diagnoses include which of the following?*

a. Cancer in the esophagus or stomach
b. Autonomic disease involving the esophagus
c. Ulcer in the pyloric channel causing obstruction
d. Esophageal stricture
e. Osteophytes compressing the posterior esophagus
f. All of the above

ANSWER: f. *All of the above.*

QUESTION: *On further questioning she notes her symptoms haven't changed since onset and she has found drinking large volumes of liquids helps. Does this alter the differential diagnosis?*

ANSWER: *Careful history often provides important clues. A progressive process often causes progressive symptoms (i.e., cancer or ulcer disease). The inflammation associated with a large pyloric ulcer can cause obstruction of the* *pyloric channel. Usually, patient presents with emesis of all food once obstruction occurs.*

QUESTION: *What diagnostic procedure would be indicated?*

a. Upper Gastrointestinal X-ray series (UGI series)
b. Endoscopy
c. No examination, re-assurance that "it will pass"

ANSWER: b. *While an UGI series will further define the problem, many of these diagnoses will also require endoscopy. If an esophageal mass is seen, direct visualization and biopsy is required. If an esophageal stricture is found, dilation is indicated. The patient underwent endoscopy and the only abnormality was an esophageal stricture that was dilated without complications. Her symptoms resolved.*

DIARRHEA AND CONSTIPATION

Diarrhea and constipation affect all individuals at some time or other. The incidence of diarrhea and constipation is probably under reported. Unless acute, these symptoms are often mentioned at the end of the clinical encounter because of the patient's embarrassment. About ten percent of adults in the United States are regular laxative users.

Pathophysiologic Correlation

The functions of the small intestine and colon are to reabsorb water and ions, absorb nutrients, secrete ions and dispose of waste. About 9L of fluid enter the small intestine daily (2L by ingestion, 7L by secretion in the upper GI tract). About 8L of fluid are absorbed by the small intestine and 800 cc by the colon, so that the usual water content in the feces is 200 cc daily. Water absorption follows absorption of protein, fat, sugars and vitamins and minerals occurring predominately in the small bowel and absorption of sodium occurring in the small bowel and colon. Transit through the gut depends in part on neural regulators. Defecation occurs when the rectum distends, the internal anal sphincter relaxes, and the external anal sphincter is voluntarily relaxed.

Processes which interfere with normal structure or function of the bowel cause constipation or diarrhea. A primary abnormality of motility is seen in irritable bowel syndrome and neurologic diseases

such as multiple sclerosis. Abnormal secretory function is seen in infectious diseases of the bowel and with some laxatives. Drugs and diet can affect bowel function by changing intraluminal osmotic factors leading to increased water in the gut lumen, or by interfering with neurologic function (b-blockers) or muscle tone (verapamil). Inflammation of the gut lumen, as seen in ulcerative colitis or Crohns disease can cause osmotic and/or secretory diarrhea. Painful defecation as seen with anal hemorrhoids or fissures can lead to constipation if the patient voluntarily withholds feces.

Clinical and Laboratory Evaluation

The history and physical examination often will permit accurate diagnosis of the cause of constipation or diarrhea. Because of the many etiologies of constipation and diarrhea, the work-up may be minimal or extensive. Commonly ordered diagnostic tests will be discussed.

HISTORY

Define exactly what the patient means by constipation or diarrhea. The description should include the volume, frequency and consistency of feces. Foul smelling, floating diarrhea indicates steatorrhea, as seen in pancreatic insufficiency. Massive diarrhea is seen in small bowel disorders. Small calibre, pencil-thin stools are seen in colon cancer.

Next, elicit the patient's normal bowel pattern. Some normal patients defecate every other day, some, three times a day. If the bowel pattern has changed from the patient's norm, it is significant.

Obtain other pertinent history, such as the onset of the constipation or diarrhea, aggravating or relieving factors, presence of symptoms before or after a meal or when asleep, associated symptoms, and bleeding. The clinician needs to learn the patient's family history, travel history, drug and medical history, and history of concomitant illness. It is helpful to have a knowledge of disease outbreaks in the community.

PHYSICAL EXAMINATION

The examination of the patient with diarrhea or constipation focuses on the abdomen and rectum. The abdominal examination has been thoroughly described in the abdominal pain chapter.

Rectal examination begins with inspection of the anus and perianal area for signs of inflammation or masses. Palpation with a gloved, lubricated finger, rotating 360° to feel the entire distal rectum can locate hemorrhoids, abscesses and firm masses. About 50% of colon cancers are palpable on digital rectal examination. A stool sample is saved for guaiac testing.

LABORATORY EVALUATION

Guaiac testing is done on every patient, the exceptions being constipation whose etiology is certain and situations where results of testing would not be helpful. If cancer is suspected, serial testing is indicated as outlined in Chapter 3. A CBC should be checked if the patient's stool is guaiac positive, or there is evidence of weight loss or palpable mass. Liver function tests, including a serum albumin assay are ordered if cancer is suspected.

Barium enema is less expensive than colonoscopy and is often used as an initial evaluating tool for patients with constipation. Barium enema is not a very sensitive test for rectal pathology or for polyps or tumors when there is other structural abnormality in the colon, like diverticuli.

Fiberoptic flexible sigmoidoscopy and colonoscopy are the two techniques that provide direct visualization of colonic and sometimes distal small bowel mucosa. These procedures have the advantage of allowing for biopsy of any unusual lesions and of being more sensitive than barium enema in regions of the gut where there is overlap or other anatomic abnormality that would obscure the x-ray view. In experienced hands, these procedures are done with mild to moderate discomfort to the patient.

Besides guaiac testing, other tests of the stool are helpful in evaluating diarrhea. A stool smear stained with Wrights stain or methylene blue can be inspected microscopically for leukocytes. Fecal leukocytes are found in diseases that disrupt the gut mucosa, such as Shigella infection or ulcerative colitis. Culture and sensitivity of stool specimens is sometimes ordered, particularly for immunosuppressed patients. Testing for ova and parasites can be useful in travelers or the immunosuppressed. Blood tests are usually not diagnostic.

Although plain films of the abdomen are not helpful, x-ray studies have special merit in the evaluation of diarrhea. If small bowel pathology is suspected, an upper GI x-ray and small bowel follow through or direct installation of barium into the small bowel by enteroclysis can be ordered to secure the diagnosis. The small bowel is difficult or impossible to directly visualize by current endoscopic techniques. Sigmoidoscopy and colonoscopy aid in diagnosing inflammatory bowel disease and in long-term surveillance.

Differential Diagnosis

This section discusses the common causes of constipation and diarrhea seen in an ambulatory practice. The diagnoses of constipation will be presented first, followed by the diagnoses of diarrhea.

CONSTIPATION

The question the clinician must consider when examining an adult with constipation is, "Is this a symptom of cancer?" Although cancer is not the most common cause of constipation, it is the most serious. For this reason, cancer will be discussed first.

Cancer   Colorectal adenocarcinomas begin as adenomatous polyps. Polyps may cause bloody stool, but most are asymptomatic and can be diagnosed by screening sigmoidoscopy. Adenomatous polyps are more likely to be malignant if they are >2.5 cm and sessile. Polyps smaller than 1.5 cm are rarely malignant. The risk factors for colorectal cancer are inflammatory bowel disease, hereditary bowel syndromes (such as familial polyposis of the colon) and perhaps dietary factors such as high cholesterol, low fiber diets. The dietary factors are not proven, but are supported by population studies.

As a polyp grows, it invades the colon wall and the lumen. Symptoms typically are related to the lumenal growth, either blood loss and anemia from right colon tumors or obstruction (cramping, pencil-thin feces) and hematochezia (red blood per rectum) from left colon tumors. Colon cancer is the second most common cause of cancer death. Because of its prevalence, any non-menstruating patient who has anemia, guaiac positive stool, or new unexplained constipation should have a colonoscopy or barium enema.

Drugs/Diet   Several commonly prescribed drugs cause constipation. Among the most common are opiates, beta blockers, verapamil, iron, and aluminum containing antacids. (Table 16.7). The clinician must review the patient's medications to

Table 16.7.
Medications That Cause Constipation

Narcotics
Aluminum or calcium containing antacids
Iron
Calcium channel blockers
Anticholigerics (many antidepressants and antipsychotics)
Beta-blockers

look for an iatrogenic cause of constipation. Dietary causes include changing to decaffeinated coffee, increasing milk intake, or eating low fiber diet. Most diet related constipation will resolve as the gut adapts to the change.

Irritable Bowel Syndrome The irritable bowel syndrome can present with crampy abdominal pain and constipation, alternating diarrhea and constipation, or intermittent diarrhea. Symptoms can be present off and on for years and are more common in young or middle aged women. The pathology of this bothersome disease relates to altered intestinal motility and increased response to distension of the gut. Stress may worsen symptoms. The diagnosis is based on chronic, intermittent symptoms that are precipitated or worsened by stress in a patient with a benign physical examination including guaiac negative stool. Lactase deficiency, which can present with similar symptoms, can be ruled out if a trial of avoidance of milk products does not improve symptoms.

Anal/Rectal Pain Hemorrhoids, varicose anal veins, can cause constipation if they are inflamed and tender. Anal fissures, (small tender skin excoriations), anal fistulae, and abscesses can also cause constipation for the same reason—it hurts to pass the feces through the inflamed area. These lesions are visible and/or palpable on digital rectal examination. Hemorrhoids look blue and are collapsible and distensible, unless thrombosed when they are firm and tender. Fistulae result from perirectal abscesses, which are tender and feel fluctuant on examination.

DIARRHEA

Infection causes most cases of acute diarrhea. Irritable bowel syndrome and inflammatory bowel disease are common causes of chronic diarrhea that are treated in the ambulatory setting. Drugs and dietary factors can cause acute or chronic diarrhea.

Infection The most common cause of acute diarrhea in the U.S. is non-invasive bacterial or viral infection. However, more serious causes are sometimes found, such as parasitic infection or invasive bacterial infection. Most diarrhea infections are spread by the fecal-oral route. A patient who presents with symptoms of diarrhea, but has an otherwise benign history and physical examination (no orthostatic hypotension) probably has a self-limited infection and needs no diagnostic evaluation. A patient who presents with bloody diarrhea, high fever, significant risks (immunosuppression or recent travel to a third world country), or whose symptoms don't improve, should be evaluated.

Wrights Stain or methylene blue stain of the stool should be done to look for leukocytes. Examine the stool for ova and parasites. Cultures for invasive enteric pathogens should be sent if salmonella, shigella, camplylobacter or yersinia are suspected based on the presence of fecal leukocytes, bloody diarrhea, or fever.

Traveler's diarrhea is caused by *E. coli*, and like the bacterial entities in the previous paragraph, is transmitted by the fecal-oral route. Although it is usually not life threatening, treatment is often instituted to decrease the duration of symptoms. The diagnosis is likely in any well-appearing patient who has recently travelled to an unsanitary area.

Irritable Bowel Syndrome As reviewed in the section on constipation, irritable bowel syndrome can present as intermittent diarrhea, or alternating diarrhea and constipation. The evaluation and differential diagnosis has been discussed in the constipation section. Because hyperthyroidism can cause diarrhea and both hyperthyroidism and irritable bowel syndrome are prevalent in young women, it is reasonable to check thyroid function tests in any young woman with chronic diarrhea.

Inflammatory Bowel Disease Patients with inflammatory bowel disease present with bloody diarrhea, abdominal pain, and sometimes with fever, weight loss, malaise. The course may be acute at presentation, but on history, the patient may recall previous, less severe exacerbations of the disease. The disease is diagnosed most often in the third decade. It is more prevalent in people of Caucasian and Jewish ancestry. The cause is unknown, although it may be infectious or immunologic. Other symptoms of inflammatory bowel disease include arthralgia or arthritis (seen in 25% of patients, usually in knees, wrists or ankles), skin abnormalities such as erythema nodsum (a tender, red, raised lump on the shin) or aphthous ulcers (painful, flat ulcers in the mouth), in 15% of patients. Abnormal liver function tests can be seen due to fatty liver or local inflammation. Inflammation in the portal areas will lead to elevations of alkaline phosphatase. Usually, these abnormalities of liver function are mild and do not require further diagnostic intervention in the patient who has no liver or biliary symptoms.

Inflammatory bowel disease describes two distinct conditions: ulcerative colitis and Crohn's disease. Ulcerative colitis diagnosed when an area of continuous ulcerated hemorrhagic colonic mucosa is seen endoscopically. The rectum is almost always involved and the diagnosis can be made by flexible sigmoidoscopy. Tenesmus is a common symptom of rectal involvement. Biopsy specimens show involvement of the mucosa that does not extend into the colonic wall.

Crohn's disease is characterized by discrete areas of thickening of the bowel wall separated by normal bowel. The mucosa may appear normal or hyperemic early in the course of the disease. In severe cases, there is nodularity of the mucosa. Inflammation extends through all the layers of the bowel wall, and may cause adjacent loops of bowel or mesentery to fibrose together. Small ulcerations may penetrate the bowel, forming abscesses. The disease can involve the large and/or small bowel, but is most common in the terminal ileum. Biopsy specimens may demonstrate granulomas.

Drugs/Diet A number of drugs can cause diarrhea (Table 16.8). Magnesium-containing antacids, levothyroxine, theophylline and laxatives are common offenders. Broad-spectrum antibiotics alter the normal colonic flora and can cause diarrhea. A common dietary cause of diarrhea in adults is lactase deficiency, which can be diagnosed clinically when symptoms improve on a milk-free diet.

Management

The management of constipation and diarrhea ranges from the simple "tincture of time" to the complex. The discussion of constipation and diarrhea and their treatment will be presented in the same order as in the Differential Diagnosis section.

CONSTIPATION

Cancer After colonoscopy gives biopsy-proof of cancer, the question of treatment comes to the forefront. Cancers diagnosed early, while still con-

fined to polyps, can often be completely excised, with follow-up colonoscopy every three years thereafter. Cancers that cannot be excised by colonoscopic means should be surgically removed. A search for metastatic disease , including assessment of liver function tests and chest x-ray should be done. A carcinoembryonic antigen (CEA) test is useful to check prior to surgery. Elevation of CEA level in the months after surgery correlates with metastatic disease. Patients who have colon cancer that has spread to regional lymph nodes have about a 50% five year survival. Most patients with metastasis to liver or lung die within 5 years. (Fig. 16.3). Discussion of what the future holds should be factual and supportive, but reserved until the patient is ready for it.

Drugs/Diet Once the diagnosis of drug induced constipation is made, the sensible response is to discontinue the offending drug. If the drug is necessary, the provider may offer dietary counseling and/or prescribe a laxative for a limited period. Dietary causes of constipation are usually treated with modification of diet. General recommendations include: increase fiber in diet (whole grains, bran, and green vegetables), increase water intake, and exercise regularly.

Stool softeners, such as docusate 200 mg daily will increase water and fat content of feces. Psyllium in dosages of 2 tsp in a cup of water twice daily will increase the water content of the feces and stimulate a reflex peristalsis. Cathartic agents are avoided for usual management of constipation because they are habit forming. However, agents such as bisacodyl 10 mg at bedtime or 2 tbsp. Milk of magnesia can be recommended to treat the occasional bout of constipation.

Irritable Bowel Syndrome The treatment of irritable bowel syndrome focuses on three goals. The patient must be reassured that the disease is not life threatening. The clinician should limit diagnostic tests. The constipation and/or diarrhea must be controlled.

The clinician must teach the patient that stress worsens the symptoms and must offer ways to handle the stress. Avoidance is the simplest method, but stress management in the form of distraction (reading, listening to music, walking) can be helpful, as can biofeedback. If the predominant symptom is constipation, high fiber diet is likely to be helpful. Psyllium can be helpful for constipation and diarrhea. Patients with diarrhea unresponsive to psyllium can sometimes control symptoms with Kaopectate 2 ounces q.i.d., but will often require an opoid agent such as diphenoxylate, 5 mg orally t.i.d.- q.i.d. as needed to control diarrhea. Diphe-

Table 16.8.
Medications That Cause Diarrhea

Laxatives/stool softeners
Magnesium containing antacids
Broad spectrum antibiotics
Angiotensin-converting enzyme inhibitors
Beta-blockers
Caffeine
Colchicine
Digoxin
Diuretics
L-dopa
Lipid lowering drugs
Lithium
Nonabsorbable sweetners
Nonsteroidal anti-inflammatory drugs
Theophylline
Thyroid preparations

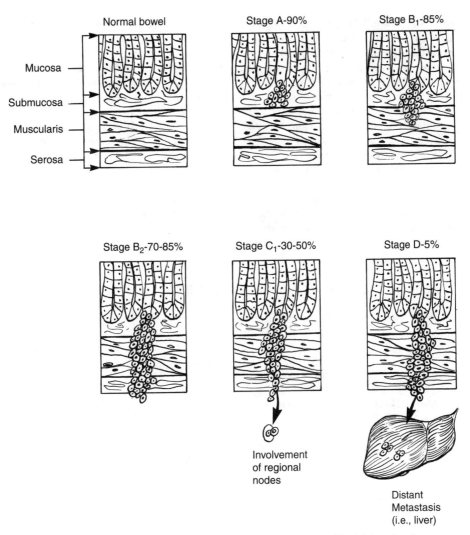

Figure 16.3. Estimated 5-year survival for colorectal cancer by modified dukes classification.

noxylate is a poor analgesic and has low potential for addiction.

Anal/Rectal Pain Hemorrhoids and fissures can usually be managed with local soaks, emollients, suppositories or creams and dietary changes to soften the stool and improve the ease of defecation. Hemorrhoids that do not respond can be treated by application of a band, laser, or surgery. Abscesses and fistulas require incision and drainage.

DIARRHEA

Infection Non-bloody diarrheas in an otherwise well patient are usually self-limited and can be treated by waiting a few days for the symptoms to abate. The patient should drink liquids as toler-ated. If dehydration is present, this should be corrected orally or parenterally. Even invasive pathogens causing dysentery can be treated in this fashion, if the patient is otherwise healthy. For the immunosuppressed or very ill patient, specific antibiotic therapies exist, and should be instituted depending on culture and sensitivity results. In general, antidiarrheals should be avoided.

Treatment of traveler's diarrhea does help if instituted early. Trimethoprim/sulfamethoxazole 160 mg/800 mg b.i.d. or ciprofloxacin 500 mg b.i.d. for 5 days is the antibiotic of choice. Parasitic infections can be treated with quinacrine 100 mg t.i.d. after meals for 5 days (giardiasis) or metronidazole 750 mg t.i.d. for 10 days followed by iodoquinol 650 mg t.i.d. for 20 days (amebiasis).

Inflammatory Bowel Disease For either ulcerative colitis or Crohn's disease a gastroenterologist will likely be involved in diagnosis and management of the patient. Anti-inflammatory drugs are the cornerstone of therapy. Sulfasalazine in doses up to 6 g daily is used during exacarbations. Sulfasalazine 2 g daily decreases relapse when ulcerative colitis is in remission. Steroids such as prednisone can be used, starting with doses of 60 mg daily and tapering as rapidly as symptoms permit.

Because of obstruction, fistula, or abscess most patients with Crohn's disease will require abdominal surgery sometime in the course of their disease. The clinician must be vigilant for signs of these complications (vomiting, pain, prolonged fever, malaise as diarrhea improves), especially in the patients treated with glucocorticoids. Patients who have inflammatory bowel disease are at increased risk for colon cancer. Surveillance colonoscopy every 1–3 years should be done for patients who have had inflammatory bowel disease for 10 or more years, regardless of their age.

Drugs/Diet If at all possible, the offending drug should be discontinued. If the drug is necessary, an antidiarrheal may be added, along with recommendations to decrease fiber in the diet. If lactase deficiency is diagnosed, avoidance of milk products will control symptoms. A folk remedy for diarrhea is to eat more white bread and white rice.

ILLUSTRATIVE CASES WITH SELF-ASSESSMENT QUESTIONS AND ANSWERS

Case 1

Karen Ayers is a 23-year-old college student who just returned from a 2 week tour of the archeological ruins of Mexico. She has had watery diarrhea, yellow in color, 5–6 times daily since she returned. She has had abdominal cramps and notes that her diarrhea worsens if she eats. She is otherwise healthy.

QUESTION: *What lab test is indicated?*

ANSWER: *None. A physical examination should be done.*

QUESTION: *What treatment is indicated?*

ANSWER: *This is probably traveler's diarrhea. She does not require treatment, but Trimethoprim/Sulfamethoxazole 160 mg/800 mg b.i.d. is inexpensive and will decrease the duration and severity of her symptoms.*

Case 2

Henry Allard is a 62-year-old painter who has had several months of difficulty passing his stool. He states he needs to strain. He has had a few bouts of constipation in the past that resolved in a short time. He feels well. He is hypertensive and has asthma. Both are controlled.

QUESTION: *What test is indicated?*

ANSWER: *Rectal examination and guaiac testing of the feces is indicated. Mr. Allard is at risk for colon cancer.*

QUESTION: *What is missing from his history?*

ANSWER: *Missing from his history are his medications, dietary practices, information about pain with defecation, and a description of the feces.*

QUESTION: *He started taking a new antihypertensive, verapamil, 3 months ago, about the time these symptoms started. Does this change your plans for diagnostic evaluation?*

ANSWER: *The verapamil may be the cause of the constipation. However, he is of the age to have screening tests for colon cancer. If serial stool guaiacs and/or sigmoidoscopy have not been done in the past year, they should be done now. If he is guaiac positive, he should be evaluated colonoscopically or by barium enema for colon cancer. If he is guaiac negative, he can be* *observed as another medication is substituted for verapamil. If his symptoms abate, no other workup is necessary.*

JAUNDICE AND/OR ABNORMAL LIVER ENZYMES

Because most medications are metabolized by the liver clinicians periodically check their patients' liver function tests. This leads to the not infrequent occurrence of the unanticipated abnormal laboratory value. The clinician faces the dilemma of whether to and how to work up the unexpected elevation of hepatobiliary enzymes. Decisions are more straight forward when dealing with a jaundiced patient. Whether or not a patient is symptomatic, the evaluation can be logical, systematic and even cost effective.

Pathophysiologic Correlation

A review of the commonly ordered liver function tests are presented in this section. This review discusses the significance of each individual test. A review of bilirubin metabolism and the pathophysiology of jaundice is included.

AMINOTRANSFERASES

These are hepatic enzymes which are a sensitive, but not a specific marker for hepatocellular injury. To fully comprehend the role of aminotransferases in the evaluation of the hepatobiliary system a review of their anatomic environment is necessary.

Elevated serum levels of hepatic enzymes are due to their release from injured or necrotic hepatocytes. The amount measurable in serum is rate dependent upon the extent of hepatocellular involvement and its extra vascular distribution. Because of their minimal presence in bile and urine these avenues do not have a major role in their removal. This is readily demonstrated by their relatively fast rate of clearance in the face of continued biliary obstruction.

Aspartate Amino Transferase (AST)/Serum Glutamate Oxaloacetate (SGOT) This is a catalytic enzyme found both in cytosol and mitochondria. As a measurable enzyme, it is also concentrated in cardiac muscle, kidney, brain, pancreas, lung, leukocytes and erythrocytes (from higher to lower concentrations). Its activity in the liver is 60–70% mitochondrial. Its level becomes elevated when there is injury to the hepatocytes, particularly the mitochondria. In alcohol abuse or insult by hypoxia, toxins etc. the centrolobular region of the

liver appears most vulnerable. Increased concentrations of mitochondrial AST leak into the serum in levels greater than ALT.

Alanine Aminotransferase (ALT)/Serum Glutamate Pyruvate Transaminase (SGPT) This is a cytosol enzyme and therefore high concentrations are localized to the liver, particularly the periportal area. This is a more specific marker of hepatocellular damage than AST. Its synthesis is dependent upon a coenzyme pyridoxyl 5' phosphate. When this is depleted in alcohol liver disease, the proportion of AST produced in the liver exceeds that of ALT. A serum ratio of AST:ALT greater than 2+ is highly suggestive of alcohol as the source of hepatocellular damage. This ratio is further exaggerated by the predilection of alcohol to injure the centrilobular area where AST is predominantly released.

ALKALINE PHOSPHATASE

This hydrolytic enzyme has its origin in multiple tissues. Towards the end of the third trimester of pregnancy the level of serum alkaline phosphatase can double and still be considered normal. In bone it is a measure of osteoblastic activity and can therefore be normally elevated in childhood and adolescence. To a lesser extent it is found in leukocytes, renal tissue and the small intestine. For the most part serum alkaline phosphatase is used to indicate hepatobiliary disease, particularly hepatic cholestasis. The phenomena of elevated alkaline phosphatase have been much studied. There appears to be more than one mechanism which leads to an altered serum level. Hepatic alkaline phosphatase is located on the hepatocyte membrane and the bile cannaliculi membrane. As cholestasis occurs, there appears to be an acceleration of alkaline phosphatase syntheses. This, combined with other theorized mechanisms, causes disruption of membranes and leads to the facilitation of alkaline phosphatase leakage into the serum. Its level cannot be used to determine whether the cholestasis is secondary to an extra or intra hepatic etiology.

Measurement of Alkaline Phosphatase Although isoenzymes of alkaline phosphatase can be measured, the process itself can be cumbersome and the results confusing. More commonly we look to other enzymes which have their origin in the liver to assist with the challenges of determining the cause of its elevation. Two frequently used enzyme markers are 5' nucleotidase and gamma glutamyl transferase (GGT).

5' Nucleotidase This is a hydrolytic nucleotide enzyme which is located on membranes throughout the entire hepatobiliary system. Although it is also found in tissues of the pancreatic, heart, brain and vascular system its pathologic elevation almost always indicates obstructive hepatobiliary disease. It lags behind the elevation of alkaline phosphatase in biliary tract obstruction. An elevated 5' nucleotidase is useful in determining that increased alkaline phosphatase is due to cholestasis.

GAMMA GLUTAMYL TRANSFERASE (GGT)

GGT is a transfer enzyme whose function is unclear. At present it serves as a useful tool in the correlation of hepatobiliary disease with the abnormal serum alkaline phosphatase. GGT is a sensitive indicator of hepatic disease as it is seen elevated in greater than 95% of all categories of disease involving the liver. GGT is, however, particularly sensitive to stimulation by drug and chemical. This allows it to be helpful in identifying ETOH liver disease where hepatocyte release of GGT is augmented in the face of ETOH. In the absence of cirrhosis, the GGT/AP ratio can be used to identify hepatic disease secondary to alcohol hepatitis in the face of mild to moderate elevations in alkaline phosphatase. The ratio of GGT/AP greater than 2.5 reinforces the possibility of alcohol involvement. Isolated elevation of GGT is a sensitive screening test for excess alcohol use.

BILIRUBIN

The term jaundice is used to describe the consequences of hyperbilirubinemia, conjugated or unconjugated, which in excess, is readily deposited in skin, mucous membranes and the sclerae. Humans produce approximately 4 mg per kg (body weight) of bilirubin per day. The majority of this production can be attributed to the breakdown of red blood cells. A small contribution comes from the degradation of heme containing proteins in the liver as well as the destruction of erythroid cells secondary to ineffective erythropoiesis. The normal range of total bilirubin in humans is 0.3 mg/dl-1.0 mg/dl. Jaundice usually becomes clinically evident at levels greater than 2.5 mg/dl. Total bilirubin levels reflect both direct as well as indirect bilirubin. To best understand the difference and importance one must simply examine the pathway of bilirubin metabolism. Almost eighty percent of bilirubin is derived from the breakdown of red blood cells in the reticuloendothelial system. It is transported to the liver for further metabolism

bound to albumin. Once in the liver there are three phases to metabolism: 1. Uptake-dissociation from albumin, 2. Conjugation-addition of one or two molecules of glucuronic acid, 3. Excretion-via bile, which overall is the rate limiting step. Bilirubin prior to conjugation with glucuronic acid is considered indirect bilirubin. Indirect bilirubin is insoluble in water; however, it is lipid soluble allowing for easy diffusion across membranes. Direct bilirubin is bilirubin conjugated to glucuronic acid, which is water soluble and allows for intestinal excretion in bile. Finally, the pathway does have a loophole at the end. Approximately 25% of the secreted conjugated bilirubin is changed by intestinal bacteria to urobilinogens. Most of the urobilinogen is reabsorbed and transported back to the liver. This loophole constitutes the enterohepatic circulation; a portion of the urobilinogen is diverted to the kidneys and excreted in the urine (Fig. 16.4). An excess unconjugated bilirubin implies a problem in bilirubin metabolism at the level of conjugation or any of the preceding steps. Specifically, this means overproduction of bilirubin (i.e., hemolytic syndromes); poor hepatic uptake (secondary to drugs, i.e., rifampin) or a defect in conjugation (i.e., Crigler-Najjar syndrome). Conjugated hyperbilirubinemia is often termed cholestatic jaundice. The term cholestasis refers to the failure of normal amounts of bile to reach the intestine. It is at the rate-limiting step of hepatic excretion that the defect is typically found. Impaired hepatic excretion can be divided further into intrahepatic vesus extrahepatic cholestasis. Intrahepatic refers to the transport from the hepatocyte to the intrahepatic ducts (defects can be seen with certain medications). Extrahepatic refers to problems occurring in the extrahepatic bile ducts (typically seen with mechanical obstruction). The evaluation of jaundice may not be clear because many etiologies affect multiple steps in the pathway of bilirubin metabolism.

Clinical and Laboratory Evaluation

When approaching the patient with abnormal liver functions, a thorough history and physical examination will guide the workup in a logical manner. Although laboratory tests are always necessary, the workup can be directed and cost effective.

HISTORY

Most commonly, without regard to etiology, the patient complains of fatigue and malaise. He/she may or may not experience anorexia and weight loss. In acute processes that are caused by inflam-

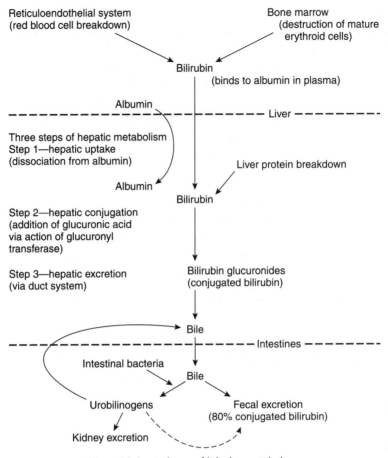

Figure 16.4. Pathway of bilirubin metabolism.

mation or infection (i.e., hepatic abscess, alcohol/ viral hepatitis), there may be fever. Pain is often isolated to the right upper quadrant. It may represent hepatic swelling (i.e., CHF), an infectious (hepatic abscess), obstructive (cholecystitis) or a combined etiology (hepatitis, cholangitis). A patient may experience episodes of agitation, flushing, and sweating from hypoglycemia. This often indicates severe liver disease in either hepatic failure or ETOH consumption without proper nutrition. It represents diminished gluconeogenesis and glycogen stores. Table 16.9 reviews the pertinent aspects of the history.

The jaundiced patient may complain of pruritis, increased abdominal girth, right upper quadrant pain, easy bruising, dark urine or pale stools. The symptoms may be as nonspecific as nausea, anorexia or weight loss. In a male patient there may be a complaint of increased breast size or decreased testicular size. The onset of symptoms can help delineate an acute versus chronic process.

Imperative to a good history is the social history, in particular use of alcohol or drugs, sexual history, possible exposure to hepatitis and recent travel. A well detailed medication list can often lead to the etiology of jaundice (Table 16.10). In the medical history, a history of gallstones, any previous abdominal surgery, or malignancy should be addressed.

PHYSICAL EXAMINATION

The physical examination should include a general assessment. Refer to Table 16.11 for details. Does the patient appear to have been healthy prior to this complaint or does the patient appear chronically ill with wasting of the extremities or general loss of muscle mass? Meticulous evaluation of the abdomen is necessary. One should note any abdominal tenderness, distention, or the presence of ascites.

Table 16.9.
Pertinent Aspects of Patient History

Historical Data	Important Relationship
Age	"Normal" elevation alkaline phosphatase in childhood, adolescence
Gender	"Normal" elevation alkaline phosphatase in pregnancy. W > M incidence of cholelithiasis. W > M incidence autoimmune hepatobiliary disease and primary biliary cirrhosis
Pertinent medical conditions	Congestive heart failure—hepatomegaly/passive congestion. COPD-alpha 1 antitrypsin deficiency. Diabetes-steatohepatitis. Inflammatory bowel disease-sclerosing cholangitis
Prescription and over-the-counter drug use	Cholestasis: estrogen, TMP-S, chlorpromazine, diabenese etc, chronic hepatitis: dilantin, INH, erythromycin, Oxacillin
Illicit drug use	Infectious hepatitis, HIV
Alcohol intake	Ethanol hepatitis masks another cause of hepatobiliary disease
Travel	Areas with endemic infectious hepatitis, hepatic liver flukes, amoeba
Sexual history	Infectious hepatitis, HIV
Transfusion history	Acute/chronic infectious hepatitis
Family history	Hemochromatosis, Wilson's disease

Hepatomegaly and splenomegaly should be noted along with the presence of any masses. The rectal exam must not be deferred. Presence of occult blood in the stool can be from an upper gastrointestinal source (varices) or from a lower source (i.e., neoplasm causing biliary obstruction). The character of stool should also be noted, as biliary obstruction can cause pale stools. Cutaneous changes include spider telangectasias, palmar erythema, xanthomas, and ecchymoses. In men, gynecomastia and testicular atrophy may be noted. Hepatic encephalopathy can present occultly as subtle mental status changes. It can also present more obviously with ataxia, asterixis and severe confusion, even coma. A good history and clinical evaluation coupled with routine laboratory tests has a sensitivity of eighty percent in correctly pinpointing the etiology of the jaundice. When interpreting laboratory tests, a general rule of thumb in biliary obstruction is the transaminases will be less than ten times normal and the alkaline phosphatase level is typically greater than 3 times normal.

Table 16.10.
Some Commonly Used Drugs That Cause Jaundice

Acetaminophen	Megace
Allopurinol	Methimazole
Augmentin	Methotrexate
Bactrim	Methyldopa
Benzodiazepines	Niacin
Calan	Nitrofurantoin
Captopril	Orinase
Carbamazepine	Phenothiazines
Cimetidine	Phenytoin
Clindamycin	Procardia
Colchicine	Quinidine
Contraceptive steroids	Salicylates
Coumadin	Sulfasalazine
Danazol	Tamoxifen
Diabenese	Tetracyclines
Erythromycin	Thiazides
Isoniazid	Tricyclics
Ketoconazole	

This is not an exhaustive list. If a medication is suspected as the cause of jaundice, consult the reference.

LABORATORY EVALUATION

Other than the tests discussed in the pathophysiologic correlation section, selected tests may be useful for confirming the final diagnosis of liver disease. If a conjugated hyperbilirubinemia is found, ultrasound is the first choice in non-invasive diagnostic imaging, chiefly because of its lower costs and the absence of any radiation exposure. Dilated bile ducts on ultrasound point to biliary obstruction. Limits to the use of ultrasound include patient obesity. Support for the use of CT scan comes from the fact that it is considered to be superior in the detection of pancreatic and other intraabdominal tumors. CT scannning and ultrasound are consid-

Table 16.11.
Pertinent Aspects of Physical Examination

Physical Findings	Pathophysiologic Causes
Scleral icterus	Decreased bilirubin excretion as seen in extrahepatic obstruction or hepatic necrosis
Fetid breath	Decreased liver clearance of sulfur byproducts in hepatic failure
Lymphadenopathy	Infiltration by infection (mononucleosis, HIV), lymphoma, or metastatic disease
Telangectasias/angiomata	Vascular effect of impaired metabolism of androgens and estrogen in cirrhosis
Gynecomastia/testicular atrophy	Impaired metabolism of androgens and estrogen in cirrhosis
Hepatomegaly	Enlargement caused by steatohepatis (diabetes, ethanol), infiltration (malignant, infectious), passive congestion (congestive heart failure)
Splenomegaly	Either secondary to increased portal hypertension or sequestration
Increased abdominal girth/ascites	Increased portal hypertension from all conditions leading to cirrhosis
Ecchymoses	Inability to produce clotting factors in liver failure
Xanthomas	Reflects elevated levels in serum lipids
Neurologic: asterexis, ataxia, confusion	End-stage liver disease with portosystemic shunting

ered equal with regards to sensitivity and specificity in finding a cause of jaundice. Ultrasound should be the initial diagnostic test of choice unless limits to its use are anticipated.

If suspicion of extrahepatic obstruction remains high despite a negative ultrasound and CT scan, one should pursue a more invasive means of testing. The two main options are percutaneous transhepatic cholangiography (PTC) and endoscopic retrograde cholangiopancreatography (ERCP). Both of these procedures have equivalent high sensitivity and specificity (99%) in diagnosing extrahepatic obstruction. The success of PTC depends on having duct dilatation, whereas greater skill and expertise is required to perform ERCP. ERCP is the procedure of choice because of a lower complication rate. A third invasive procedure that deserves mention is percutaneous needle biopsy of the liver. This procedure has a role when hepatocellular disease is considered as a possible cause of jaundice. Typically, ultrasound or CT scan is used to guide the biopsy, if there is a mass.

Confirmation of the etiology of hepatocellular disease can be achieved by obtaining viral studies, such as hepatitis serologies, or by ordering a liver biopsy to diagnose cirrhosis, infection, infiltration, metabolic disease or carcinoma. Table 16.12 lists commonly ordered tests for viral hepatitis and their significance.

Differential Diagnosis

The differential diagnoses of biliary disease are presented in Figure 16.5 and Figure 16.6. The algorithm for evaluation of elevated alkaline phosphatase is presented in Figure 16.7. The differential diagnoses of hyperbilirubinemia are presented in Table 16.13.

VIRAL HEPATITIS

DNA and RNA viruses are known causes of hepatic infection and inflammation. Hepatitis A is contracted through the fecal/oral route. It is a self-limited infection that does not lead to permanent hepatic damage. Hepatitis B and C both could have been contracted by blood transfusion before universal testing was implemented. They can also be contracted through parenteral exposure to an infected person's body fluid. Hepatitis B and C can lead to chronic infection and/or progressive hepatic disease. Diagnosis is confirmed by demonstrating antigen or antibody to hepatitis virus in the patient's blood. Common symptoms include malaise, nausea, and anorexia. The patient may become jaundiced, although not all people do. Symptoms usually last a few weeks and then resolve. Chronic hepatitis is common with hepatitis C, less so with B, and probably nonexistent with A. The serologic tests for viral hepatitis are listed in Table 16.12.

Table 16.12.
Serum Markers for Viral Hepatitis

Hepatitis A
  HₐIgM (antibody)   Acute infection disappears by 6 months
  HₐIgG (antibody)   Appears in acute infection; persists for life
Hepatitis B
  HBₛ Ag   Appears with acute infection; usually disappears by 6 months; persists in chronic
                                 hepatitis B
  HBₛ Ab (surface antibody)   Appears after acute infection; persists for life; absent in chronic hepatitis B
  HB_C IgM (core antibody)   Appears with acute infection; disappears by 1 year or persists at low level there-
                                 after
  HB_C IgG   Appears late in infection; persists for life
  HBₑ Ag (e antigen)   In chronic hepatitis B, suggests infectively
  Abₑ Ab (e antibody)   In chronic hepatitis B, suggests low infectivity
Hepatitis C
  HC Ab   Relatively new test to document hepatitis C infection
  RIBA (RNA test)   More specific than hepatitis C Ab

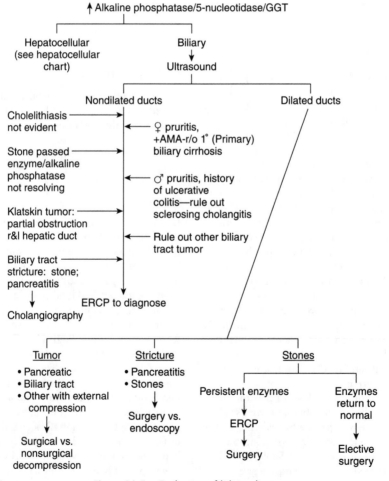

Figure 16.5. Evaluation of biliary disease.

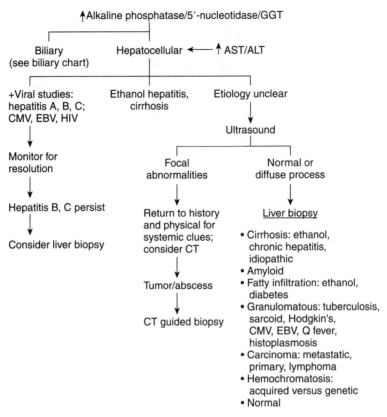

Figure 16.6. Evaluation of hepatocellular disease.

CIRRHOSIS

This is the pathophysiologic description of the endstage structural changes which occur within the liver. It represents an irreversible process characterized by hepatocellular necrosis, fibrosis and nodularity. Diagnosis is based on physical findings, and is confirmed by biopsy. Any condition which causes chronic hepatocellular necrosis can lead to cirrhosis. Common etiologies include hepatitis B and C, alcohol and other drugs/toxins. The liver is small and firm. The patient will likely have wasting, ascites, spider angiomata, and positive stool from variceal bleeding.

CARCINOMA

Malignancies of the hepatobiliary system include primary hepatocellular carcinoma, cholangiocarcinoma and much less commonly angiosarcoma. The liver is a common site for metastatic disease. They can be divided into those with portovenous drain-

age (colon, gastric, and pancreas); solid tumors (breast, lung, etc.); hematologic malignancies (lymphomas, etc).

CHOLELITHIASIS

This term denotes the presence of stones within the gallbladder. It is often asymptomatic. It is the symptomatic obstruction of these stones in the cystic or common bile duct (choledocholithiasis) which often brings the patient to the doctor's attention. Cholecystitis, acute or chronic, is the term which describes the inflammatory, edematous changes within the gallbladder. Diagnosis is confirmed by ultrasonography. Cholangitis signifies infection and is manifested by jaundice, colic, fever, and chills (Charcot's triad).

DRUG-INDUCED HEPATOBILIARY DISEASE

Drugs, even in therapeutic dosages, can cause acute and/or chronic liver damage. This can present as

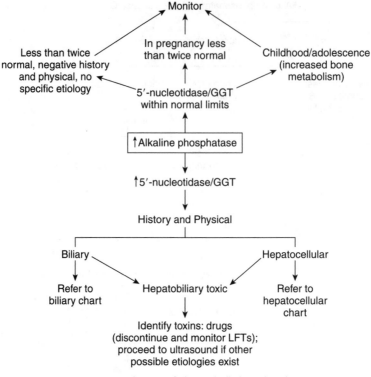

Figure 16.7. Evaluation of elevated alkaline phosphatase.

a hepatocellular and/or cholestatic picture. The list includes over the counter drugs, illicit drugs, as well as those routinely prescribed by physicians (See Table 16.10).

Management

Management is typically directed towards the underlying medical condition. When considering treatment options in a jaundiced patient, the most important determination to be made is extrahepatic obstruction versus intrahepatic nonobstructive cholestasis. Extrahepatic obstruction requires a surgical, radiologic or endoscopic intervention. Jaundice secondary to intrahepatic cholestasis or non obstructive jaundice requires treatment of the underlying cause.

VIRAL HEPATITIS

In the acute state of hepatitis management is directed towards supportive care (hydration and alimentation) and managing systemic symptoms such as nausea, vomiting and fever. Fulminant hepatitis care is supportive and directed towards preventing/treating complications (sepsis, etc). When hepatitis

B or C cause hepatocellular changes there may be a role for treatment with interferon. Prolonged prothrombin time (indicating the inability of the liver to synthesize clotting factors) is a poor prognostic finding.

CIRRHOSIS

There is no cure for cirrhosis as it is irreversible by definition. Management is directed towards preserving any remaining hepatic function and providing supportive care. This can mean removal of the causative agent (i.e., alcohol). Nutrition is important to maintain because patients often have anorexia. Because of malnutrition and loss of plasma proteins, fluid management is a mainstay of therapy. Limiting liquids orally and strictly avoiding sodium can control swelling and ascites.

CARCINOMA

The treatment is focused towards localization and pathologic diagnosis. In the case of metastatic carcinoma to the liver (breast, etc.) therapy is directed towards the primary malignancy. In primary hepatobiliary tumors often by the time of diagnosis the tumor is nonoperative. In this scenario, palliative therapy is directed towards the alleviation of bile obstruction by intra or transhepatic stent placement. This will decrease pruritis and the incidence of sepsis.

CHOLELITHIASIS

Treatment of this remains primarily surgical. In asymptomatic cholelithiasis surgical intervention remains controversial. Uncomplicated cholecystitis can be treated with laparoscopic cholecystectomy. Once complications arise such as an increase in liver enzymes or pancreatitis, common bile duct stones are suspected. The patient would likely undergo ERCP and traditional open cholecystectomy.

DRUG-INDUCED HEPATOBILIARY DISEASE

The mainstay of management of drug induced hepatobiliary disease is the withdrawal of the causative agent and supportive measures during the time of recovery. Corticosteroids have not proven to be effective. In the case of acetaminophen overdose, N-acetylcysteine is used to counteract hepatic toxicity.

Table 16.13.
Differential Diagnoses of Hyperbilirubinemia

Unconjugated hyperbilirubinemias	
Overproduction of bilirubin	Hemolytic syndromes
	Ineffective erythropoeisis
Impaired hepatic uptake	Drugs
	Gilbert's syndrome
	Sepsis
	Neonatal jaundice
Decreased Conjugation	Drugs (e.g., chloramphenicol)
	Gilbert's syndrome
	Crigler-Najjar syndrome
	Hepatocellular disease
	Neonatal jaundice
	Sepsis
Conjugated hyperbilirubinemias	
Impaired Hepatic Excretion	Drugs (e.g., oral contraceptives)
	Hepatocellular disease
	Sepsis
	Postoperative
	Pregnancy
	Dubin-Johnson syndrome
	Rotor syndrome
	Benign recurrent cholestasis
	Primary biliary cirrhosis
Extrahepatic Obstruction	Gallstones
	Tumor
	Strictures

ILLUSTRATIVE CASES WITH SELF-ASSESSMENT QUESTIONS AND ANSWERS

Case 1

This is the first visit for this patient who is a 48-year-old white man. He has never seen a physician in his adult life and feels it is time to get "checked out." The patient offers no physical complaints. He tells you he is recently divorced and became unemployed around the same time. Through the history he tells you that he typically has 2 to 3 scotch and water drinks in the evening. On the weekend he would have "a few more." During the physical examination you note scleral icterus, gynecomastia as well as testicular atrophy. The rest of the physical examination is unremarkable.

QUESTION: Given your findings of scleral icterus, what would you expect his total bilirubin levels to be?

a. >10
b. <1.5
c. >5.0
d. >2.5

ANSWER: d. *The finding of jaundice on physical exam typically occurs when serum bilirubin levels exceed 2.5 mg/dl.*

QUESTION: *What do you suspect to be the likely etiology for this patient's asymptomatic hyperbilirubinemia?*

a. Gilbert's Syndrome
b. Sepsis
c. Alcohol
d. Asymptomatic gallstones

ANSWER: c. *The patient's history raises a suspicion of alcohol abuse. Although Gilbert Syndrome is a distinct possibility given its 7% prevalence in the general population, it is the history and the supporting evidence on physical exam (gynecomastia and testicular atrophy) that make alcoholism a more likely etiology. Sepsis and gallstones are unlikely in this patient.*

QUESTION: *Assuming you suspect alcohol as the likely etiology of jaundice in this patient, which test results would be most supportive of your diagnosis?*

a. SGOT 40
   SGPT 40
   Alk Phos 150
   5'Nucleotidase wnl
   GGT wnl
b. SGOT 100
   SGPT 40
   Alk Phos 150
   5'Nucleotidase wnl
   GGT wnl
c. SGOT 100
   SGPT 100
   Alk Phos 300
   5'Nucleotidase inc
   GGT wnl
d. SGOT 100
   SGPT 40
   Alk Phos 300
   5'Nucleotidase inc
   GGT in (increased)

ANSWER: d. *Hepatocellular damage secondary to alcohol typically gives a ratio of SGOT/ SGPT greater than 2. Also an elevated GGT is a sensitive screen for excessive alcohol use. Further support for alcohol as the likely etiology would be a GGT/AlkPhos ratio greater than 2.5.*

Case 2

The patient is a 65-year-old obese Asian man who has noted a 20-pound weight loss over the past 6 months. He also states that his family has noted a change in his skin color. The patient himself complains of progressive body itching. He denies any abdominal pain. The physical ex-

amination reveals jaundice and a palpable nontender gallbladder. His laboratory tests show mildly elevated transaminases, a markedly elevated direct bilirubin, alkaline phosphatase and 5' nucleotidase.

QUESTION: *Given the above scenario, what is the most likely etiology for jaundice in this man?*

a. Viral hepatitis
b. Alcohol abuse
c. Tumor
d. Gilbert's Syndrome

ANSWER: c. *The lab data appear to be consistent with a conjugated hyperbilirubinemia/cholestasis picture. Gilbert's Syndrome typically presents as a mild unconjugated hyperbilirubinemia. Because he has a prominent palpable gallbladder the tumor is most likely distal to the entry of the cystic duct. The history as well as mild elevation of transaminases do not support alcohol or viral hepatitis as likely causes.*

QUESTION: *Which test would you order next as part of your diagnostic workup?*

a. Ultrasound
b. Cat scan of the abdomen

ANSWER: b. *Ultrasound is often the first test ordered in the face of a nonspecific exam and abnormal liver function studies. However, this patient presented with a palpable gallbladder and tumor is highly suspected. A CT scan would provide more information as to the exact location and any involvement of adjacent or distant structures. Ultrasound can also be limited by obesity.*

QUESTION: *Assuming that a mass lesion in the distal common bile duct with mild duct dilatation is demonstrated on CT scan, what would be the next step in the workup?*

a. Percutaneous transhepatic cholangiography (PTC)
b. Endoscopic retrograde cholangiopancreatography (ERCP)
c. Percutaneous needle biopsy

ANSWER: b. *In this situation, the ultimate goal is to obtain a tissue diagnosis as well as provide palliation if possible pending surgical evaluation.*

ERCP gives the opportunity to biopsy as well as place an internal shunt to facilitate bile drainage. Bile drainage is important to help reduce the incidence of biliary sepsis. If an internal stent cannot be placed during ERCP, an attempt to place a percutaneous shunt should be made. In the face of mild duct dilatation this becomes more difficult. Typically tumors of the bile duct are adenocarcinoma and they typically ocur in older men. The majority of these tumors are located in the common bile duct and are not resectable at the time of diagnosis. Tumors limited to the distal duct system with no extension can be treated with the Whipple procedure. Only approximately 10% of those with biliary tumors achieve a cure. The mainstay of therapy is palliation.

SUGGESTED READINGS

Abdominal Pain

Collen MJ, Abdulian JD, Chen YK. Age does not affect basal acid secretion in normal subjects or in patients with acid-peptic disease. Am J Gastroenterol 1994; 89: 712–716.

DeVault KR, Castell DO. Current diagnosis and treatment of gastroesophageal reflux disease. Mayo Clin Proc 1994; 69:867–876.

Epstein FB. Acute abdominal pain in pregnancy. Emerg Med Clin North Am February 1994; 12(1): 151–165.

Isselbacher KJ, Braunwald E, Wilson JD, Martin JB, Fauci AS, Kasper DL. Harrison's Principles of Internal Medicine, 13th Edition. McGraw-Hill, Inc. 1994.

Steinberg W, Tenner S. Acute pancreatitis. NEJM 1994; 330(17):1198–1210.

Weltman DI, Zeman RK. Acute diseases of the gallbladder and biliary ducts. Radiol Clin North Am 1994; 32(5):933–950.

Diarrhea and Constipation

Lipsky MS, Adelman M. Chronic diarrhea: evaluation and treatment. Am Fam Phys 1993; 48:1461–1466.

Shafik A. Constipation. Pathogenesis and management. Drugs 1993; 45:528–540.

Jaundice and/or Abnormal Liver Enzymes

Bass NM, VanDyke RW. Diseases of the liver and biliary system. In: Andreoli TE, Bennett JC, Carpenter CJC, et al. eds: Cecil Essentials of Medicine. 3rd ed. Philadelphia: WB Saunders Co, 1993; 320–349.

Gordon SC. Jaundice and cholestasis: some common and uncommon causes. Postgrad Med 1991; 90:65–71.

Herlong HF. Approach to the patient with abnormal liver enzymes. Hosp Pract 1994; 32–38.

Isselbacher KJ. Jaundice and hepatomegaly. In: Wilson JD, Braunwald E, Isselbacher KJ, et al. eds. Harrison's principles of internal medicine. 12th ed. New York: McGraw-Hill Inc., 1991; 264–269.

King PD. Abnormal liver enzyme levels. Postgrad Med 1991; 89:137–141.

McKnight JT, Jones JE. Jaundice. Am Fam Phys 1992; 45:1139-1148.

chapter 17

NEPHROLOGY
Lori A. Lemberg, Stella Pierre

URINARY TRACT INFECTION

Urinary tract infections (UTI) are the most common bacterial infections encountered in the adult female and the geriatric population. They are also the most frequent cause of bacteremia in the elderly patient residing at home or in a chronic care facility. Therefore, they are a major source of morbidity and financial cost to the medical profession. The signs and symptoms of UTI and the patient's individual risk factors should be recognized to institute an appropriate work-up and therapy, where warranted. For example, the approach to UTI differs between children and adult, male and female, and finally between the pregnant and nonpregnant female.

Pathophysiologic Correlation

The pathophysiology that underlies UTI varies greatly depending on the age and sex of the patient. Most of these differences are secondary to anatomic differences between males and females, and changes that occur with the pregnant state or with aging. Therefore, it is useful to discuss the pathophysiology of UTI in the context of the female patient versus the male patient.

FEMALES

Symptomatic urinary tract infections and asymptomatic bacteriuria are much more common in females than males starting with school-age children, with only a slight male preponderance in the neonatal period. In the neonatal period, most UTIs reach the urinary tract through hematogenous spread, whereas infections occurring after this period are mostly secondary to ascending infection. UTI in the pediatric patient needs further evaluation to rule out congenital anomalies in the newborn or anatomic defects such as vesicoureteral reflux in the prepubescent child.

Sexually active women are one of the populations at greatest risk for urinary tract infections. Hence, comes the expression "honeymoon cystitis." This is due to a combination of host factors and virulence factors of the bacteria. Bacteria that commonly cause UTI are found in the periurethral area in about 20% of adult women. The vaginal introitus is colonized by this bacteria, which can then easily ascend the short female urethra to the bladder and cause asymptomatic bacteriuria or clinically apparent UTI. The risk of UTI is further increased by sexual intercourse and the use of diaphragms with spermicidal jelly. Tampon use, oral contraceptives, and direction of wiping after a bowel movement are not risk factors for UTI. There are also important genetic factors that are known to predispose women to UTI. Women who are of P1 blood group have epithelial cell receptors that mediate attachment of bacteria and may have recurrent episodes of UTI as well as pyelonephritis, an infection of the renal parenchyma in which the bacteria ascend from the infected bladder up the ureter(s).

The establishment of a bladder infection also depends on the virulence of the present bacteria, the inoculation, and the presence or absence of normal host defense mechanisms. The urinary tract has a number of means to minimize attachment and growth of pathogenic bacteria to the mucosa of the urethra, vagina, and vaginal introitus. The normal commensal periurethral flora competes with pathogenic bacteria for sites of attachment. Various urinary immunoglobulins, proteins and mucopolysaccharides can offer protection by functioning as false receptors for bacteria, thus preventing the bacteria from attaching to the bladder mucosa. Urine itself has many chemical properties that render it an effective antibacterial agent. These include a high urea concentration, an acidic pH and high osmolality. The use of diaphragms with spermicidal jellies increases vaginal pH and allows proliferation of urogenital bacteria. The diaphragm in itself appears to decrease maximum flow rate of urine and to significantly increase urethral resistance. Normal voiding habits, especially after sexual intercourse, aid in elimination of some organisms.

There are two major physiological changes in pregnancy that predispose to upper urinary tract infection. First, the placenta secretes a high concentration of progesterone, which has an inhibitory effect on ureteral peristalsis. Second, the gravid uterus, as it enlarges and ascends out of the pelvis may extrinsically compress the ureters, leading to further stasis of urine. This stasis allows migration of bacteria from the bladder into the ureters and renal parenchyma. The sigmoid colon tends to cushion the left ureter, rendering it less compressible, thus most cases of pyelonephritis in pregnancy are right-sided. Patients who have left-sided or bilateral pyelonephritis are more likely to have structural anomalies of the urinary tract.

Urinary tract infections remain common in postmenopausal and elderly women. The ratio of women to men with UTI, however, is not as extreme in this population. Postmenopausal women become more readily colonized with Enterobacteriaceae, which increases the susceptibility to UTI in this age group. Other risk factors predispose to UTI in this population. These include patients who have had a cerebrovascular accident, or are functionally limited for other reasons, and are unable to empty their bladders at regular intervals, or have a neurological basis for urinary stasis. Other disease states that may promote urinary stasis secondary to neurological involvement include diabetes mellitus, multiple sclerosis, or spinal cord injuries. Instrumentation of the urinary tract or obstruction with ureteral or renal calculi also increase the risk of urinary tract infections.

MALES

As stated previously, UTI in males is a rare infection until men reach an older age group. Newborn and pediatric-aged males should always be evaluated after an episode of UTI for congenital anomalies or anatomic defects. These usually present fairly early in life. UTI in young males is usually due to a urethritis secondary to a sexually transmitted disease or instrumentation of the genitourinary tract. Homosexual men engaging in anal intercourse or heterosexual men having vaginal intercourse with a partner colonized with a uropathogenic strain of Escherichia coli (E. coli) may develop clinically relevant UTI. Other risk factors

include lack of circumcision and human immunodeficiency virus (HIV) infection with a CD4 lymphocyte count less than 200.

Middle-aged men may have an increased incidence of UTI secondary to an increase in the size of the prostate gland. This is a common occurrence in men older than 50 to 65 years. As the gland begins to enlarge, obstruction of the bladder outflow of urine may occur, leading to urinary stasis in the bladder and the possibility of a bacterial infection. Prostatic secretions appear to have decreased antibacterial activity in this age group, adding to the increased risk of infection. Infection of the prostate itself may also serve as a nidus for recurrent UTI.

Elderly men have similar risks to UTI as elderly women. In addition, continued prostatic enlargement may be a contributory cause to obstruction and urinary stasis. Urinary incontinence, condom or urethral indwelling urinary catheters, and a history of previous UTI are all risk factors. Studies have also demonstrated an increased adherence of bacteria to uroepithelial cells in elderly men as well as a decrease in a protective protein in the urine of elderly persons. Both these findings indicate a decrease in host mechanisms to protect oneself against infection.

Clinical and Laboratory Evaluation

The history and physical examination are essential in guiding the health care professional in the appropriate choices for laboratory evaluation. It is important to take into account the underlying medical conditions of the patient including previous history of UTI, the chronicity of the symptoms of UTI, as well as the age and sex of the patient to determine if a more aggressive and invasive work-up is indicated. One must recognize that a number of clinical syndromes exist with similar complaints, ranging from acute urethral syndrome (acute urethritis, symptomatic abacteriuria), lower urinary tract infection (or cystitis), and upper urinary tract infection (or acute pyelonephritis). The health care provider should effectively use the history and physical examination to choose the correct laboratory tests to help differentiate between these clinical syndromes and initiate appropriate therapy.

HISTORY

The classic complaints for UTI, especially in women, include dysuria or burning with urination, urinary frequency, hesitancy, and suprapubic pressure or pain. Many patients, however, will present with a minimal number of complaints or complaints of a much more vague nature. It is, therefore, essential that the health care provider ask specific questions to elucidate a coherent history. It is important to ask a sexual history in a female patient, because a significant temporal relationship exists between sexual intercourse and a UTI, especially if it is a new sexual partner. Urethritis or vaginitis may be more likely if the new partner had complaints of a penile discharge at the time of sexual intercourse. In young men presenting with symptoms of UTI it is also important to inquire about sexual behavior, including homosexuality, or any recent penile discharge to help differentiate between urethritis and UTI. Other important questions to ask a sexually active woman concern vaginal discharge or odor. Women with a vaginitis or urethritis may have symptoms of itching and "external" dysuria as opposed to "internal" dysuria of UTI. "External" dysuria suggests that burning occurs at the end of the urine stream, when urine is passing over the vaginal introitus or labia, whereas "internal" dysuria indicates burning with initiation of the urine stream as it leaves the bladder and enters the upper urethra, the source of infection and inflammation in a lower UTI.

Questions need to be asked to try and differentiate between cystitis and pyelonephritis since the evaluation of the patient and the therapy differ. Unfortunately, it is a very difficult differentiation to make on clinical grounds alone. If the patient complains of severe flank pain, fevers, and other systemic complaints such as nausea and vomiting, it makes the diagnosis of pyelonephritis fairly obvious. Again, the patient may only complain of one of the above symptoms, or the complaints may be more vague. Other helpful information may be the chronicity of the symptoms as well as a history of UTI in the past and if therapy was given. Recurrent infection may occur in some patients. Recurrence may be secondary to relapse (in which the original organism is suppressed by antimicrobial therapy) or to reinfection with a new organism. A majority of relapses may be secondary to renal parenchymal disease. It is important to ask about underlying medical conditions such as diabetes mellitus or other disease states, which may increase urinary stasis or impair host defense mechanisms. At the minimum, these are considered complicated urinary tract infections and treated differently. A history of an anatomic defect such as vesicoureteral reflux or obstructive uropathy secondary to known renal calculi or prostate enlargement may help the practitioner consider an upper urinary tract infection.

Elderly patients may present to the health care provider or hospital with no urinary complaints whatsoever. The family may have brought him or her in for more systemic complaints such as anorexia, nausea, vomiting or change in mental status. Fever is not a common symptom in the elderly population even in the event of sepsis secondary to a UTI. The practitioner must ask about functional status of the patient before the event and any recent history of genitourinary instrumentation or changes in urinary voiding habits, color, and smell of the urine. Again, it is essential to establish if the patient is suffering from any underlying medical conditions.

PHYSICAL EXAMINATION

As always, the first step in a thorough physical examination is evaluation of the vital signs. An increased temperature is indicative of a more systemic process. It is important to also document blood pressure and heart rate.

The elderly patient may not have a fever with an infection but only tachycardia or hypotension especially with overwhelming sepsis. In the female patient, one should palpate the suprapubic region for pain or distension and percuss the costovertebral angles (flanks) for any tenderness.

Extreme flank tenderness with minimal percussion may indicate pyelonephritis. Sexually active women should also have a pelvic examination to note any vaginal or cervical discharge, erosions or vesicles and a bimanual examination to search for cervical motion tenderness suggesting pelvic inflammatory disease (PID). Examination in men is similar in that the suprapubic region should be palpated for distention or discomfort and the flanks percussed for tenderness. In addition, the urethral meatus of the penis should be examined for the presence of any erythema or discharge and the testes and epididymides for any swelling or tenderness. A prostate examination should be performed to check for any enlargement, nodularity or pain on palpation. If acute prostatitis is suspected, a gentle examination should be performed to minimize the risk of causing bacteremia.

All these physical signs may be absent in the elderly patient with UTI or urosepsis unless the underlying etiology is obstruction, when a distended bladder may be palpable.

LABORATORY EVALUATION

Urinalysis All patients who present with reports of UTI, at a minimum, should have thorough urinalyses. Urine should be collected using a clean-voided technique to avoid possible contamination especially in the female patient. The urinalysis consists of a chemical evaluation, which includes urine color, pH, specific gravity, and concentration of glucose, protein, ketones, nitrites, leukocyte esterase, heme and bilirubin usually performed using a quick and easy "dipstick" method. A microscopic examination of the urine is essential to look for the presence or absence of white blood cells (WBC) and white blood cell casts, red blood cells (RBC) and bacteria. The most predictive indicator of infection is the presence of pyuria or white blood cells in the urine. Greater than 2–5 WBC per high-powered field on microscopy of unspun urine is indicative of UTI. The presence of WBC casts is more suggestive of a renal infection such as pyelonephritis. RBC alone without pyuria may be more suggestive of renal calculi and not infection, but hematuria often accompanies pyuria in UTI secondary to mucosal irritation of the bladder. Another important component to search for is the presence of bacteriuria. This is very difficult to identify without a Gram-stain evaluation of the urine. One organism per high-powered field of unspun urine examined with Gram-stain techniques represents clinically relevant bacteriuria (greater than 100,000 organisms per milliliter). The presence of pyuria without bacteriuria or hematuria is much more suggestive of acute urethral syndrome or urethritis secondary to *Chlamydia trachomatous* or *Neisseria gonorrhea*.

Urine Culture Traditionally, the urine culture has proven useful for two reasons. First, it allowed identification of the pathogenic bacteria, as well as quantification of colony count to identify true infection from contamination. Secondly, it allowed for antibiotic sensitivities to be performed in order to select the appropriate therapy. Currently, the use of urine culture to diagnose UTI in every potentially infected female and the colony count that is significant to diagnose UTI has been challenged in the outpatient setting.

The value of quantifying bacteriuria is questionable in the young woman with acute symptoms of UTI. The colony count on a urine culture that had been considered indicative of an infection was greater than or equal to 100,000 bacteria/ml. Current evidence suggests that this high bacteria count does not diagnose many women with bacterial infections of the lower urinary tract who would benefit from therapy. Colony counts of equal to or greater than 100 bacteria/ml are diagnostic of true coliform infection. Also, urine cultures are not helpful in identifying chlamydial, gonococcal, or other forms of urethritis or the presence of vaginal

infections. The majority of organisms that cause UTI in the young woman with symptoms of acute infection are sensitive to the commonly prescribed antimicrobial agents. Even when an organism is labeled as "resistant" to an antibiotic with disk-sensitivity testing, it is usually sensitive to the high concentration of antibiotic present in the urine and the patient is treated effectively. Therefore, urine cultures are not cost-effective in the young woman with an uncomplicated lower UTI. They are mandatory, however, in female patients with recurrent infection, symptoms or signs of upper urinary tract infection or pyelonephritis, urosepsis, complicated UTI secondary to underlying systemic diseases, or known anomalies of the genitourinary tract.

Unlike women, all men presenting with UTI need a urine culture performed as well as urinalysis and microscopic examination of the urine. This is secondary to the wider range of causative organisms responsible for infection as well as the greater variability of antibiotic sensitivities. A diagnosis of UTI is justified based on the isolation of 1000 bacteria per ml of urine of one type of organism. A culture with less than 1000 bacteria/ml of one type of organism or containing three or more organisms without one organism being predominant is considered contaminated and not indicative of true infection.

Other Tests Other more invasive urinary tract studies are often of low yield in helping to make a diagnosis in the initial UTI or recurrent infection in women. These include intravenous pyelography (IVP), excretory urography and cystoscopy. These radiographic and urological evaluations should be reserved for women with a history of UTI in childhood and suspected anatomic abnormality, when obstruction is likely or renal insufficiency is developing. In men, the widespread belief is that all UTI are secondary to anatomic or functional defects of the urinary tract. This has led to the routine use of IVPs when a UTI is observed in the male patient. There is little evidence to support utilizing this test in men unless the patient has recurrent infection, or suspected upper tract obstruction or pyelonephritis, as its use in lower urinary tract infection adds little information to aid in management. IVP will also give an estimate of the postvoid residual of urine. However, this can be accomplished dye-free by use of renal ultrasound, which is also helpful for evaluating possible obstruction. Another method to evaluate postvoid residual is straight catheterization of the bladder after the patient has voided. This is useful in the elderly or ill patient in which recurrent infection is felt to be secondary to neurogenic bladder and incontinence.

Other laboratory tests used depend on the clinical scenario. In the toxic appearing patient, measurement of serum white blood cell count and blood cultures to identify hematogenous spread of infection is indicated. If urethritis from sexually transmitted disease is suspected as causing the presenting symptoms, cervical cultures in the female or urethral cultures in the male are necessary to evaluate for chlamydia or gonorrhea.

Differential Diagnosis

FEMALES

Many different clinical syndromes can cause acute dysuria in women. It is important to use clinical and laboratory information to distinguish between them since management differs. The variability in these different syndromes is related to the presence or absence of infection and the anatomic location of the infection.

Acute Urethral Syndrome The first syndrome is commonly called acute urethral syndrome, acute urethritis or symptomatic abacteriuria. Women with this syndrome usually have a stuttering or prolonged course of dysuria, and may have findings on pelvic examination of discharge or cervicitis. The urinalysis is helpful in these women because classically they will have pyuria without bacteriuria. The most common cause is *Chlamydia trachomatous*, but also may be caused by *Neisseria gonorrhoeae* or *herpes simplex* virus. Occasionally, *Trichomonas vaginalis* or *Candida albicans* can cause urethritis without symptoms of vaginitis, but the diagnosis can be easily made on pelvic examination and microscopic examination of the vaginal discharge.

Cystitis and Pyelonephritis A much more difficult distinction to make at times is between lower urinary tract infection or cystitis and upper urinary tract infection or pyelonephritis. In acute pyelonephritis with a truly toxic-appearing patient and supporting laboratory evidence the diagnosis is made easily. However, there may be patients with subacute pyelonephritis with symptoms smoldering over a longer period or infection difficult to eradicate. These patients are difficult to identify based on history and physical examination alone, and may necessitate more laboratory studies. Certain clinical risk factors seem to increase the likelihood of pyelonephritis and need to be identified by the clinician so that the diagnosis is not missed. These include known underlying urinary tract disease, history of

urinary tract infections in childhood, diabetes mellitus or other conditions or therapies producing an immunocompromised state, a history of documented relapse with the same organism, or symptoms for 7 to 10 days before seeking medical attention. Other syndromes of dysuria may have minimal pyuria secondary to early infection, or absence of pyuria altogether. These are much more rare entities not commonly seen in practice and a detailed discussion of them is beyond the scope of this chapter. Their names for reference purposes are vestibular adenitis or burning vulva syndrome, painful bladder syndrome or interstitial cystitis, and urethral pain without obvious pathology (UPWOP).

MALES

In men, the differential diagnosis of dysuria is much more narrow. The main distinction needs to be made first between UTI and urethritis secondary to chlamydia or gonorrhea, much the same way it is done in the female patient. All UTI in men are treated as a complicated infection, such that subacute pyelonephritis is much less of a clinical problem. In patients not responding to therapy or with recurrent infection, one must be concerned of a prostatic source of infection and studies and therapy may need to be addressed to this possibility.

Management

There are many issues in management that have undergone changes in approach and therapeutic options based on recent research (Tables 17.1 and 17.2). The extent of evaluation and workup has changed as discussed in the section on laboratory evaluation, as have the length and choice of antibiotic therapy in young women.

ANTIBIOTIC THERAPY

There has been a trend towards shorter courses of antibiotic therapy for uncomplicated lower UTI in young healthy women. Many studies supported the notion that single-dose regimens could produce almost the same results as 7–10 day regimens with significantly fewer adverse effects. The benefits of single-dose regimens include less organism resistance to antibiotics, decreased incidence of vaginal candidiasis, diarrhea, rash, or adverse drug reaction, decreased cost of therapy and improved compliance. The patient needs to follow up with a health care provider to insure the infection was eradicated. A 3-day course of antibiotic therapy achieves a slightly higher cure rate, but still has most of the

Table 17.1.
Management of UTI: Females

Age	Presenting Symptoms/Signs	Laboratory/Clinical Evaluation	Antibiotic Therapy & Duration of Therapy
Young adult female Pregnant	Asymptomatic bacteriuria	UA, UCX	3 days Ampi 500 mg PO QID or Amox 500 mg PO TID or Oral cephalosporins For resistant organisms—Augmentin
	Mild-moderate lower UTI Dysuria, urgency, frequency Fevers/chills/flank pain	UA, UCX	3–7 days of above antibiotic regimen
	Subclinical (highly suspected) Pyelonephritis or acute pyelonephritis	UA, UCX BCX ×2, BUN/CR, Serum WBC. Follow-up UCX 2–3 days after therapy. If bilateral or 2 sided pyelonephritis, consider IVP after delivery. UA for leukocytes/nitrites every prenatal visit after treatment.	Inpatient treatment with IV antibiotics. After acute therapy, patients should receive *daily* prophylaxis with sulfisoxazole 1.0 gm or nitrofurantoin macrocrystals 100 mg because of 20–30% likelihood to develop recurrent UTI.
Nonpregnant	Asymptomatic bacteriuria	UA	No therapy unless underlying medical or anatomic problem, or patient with frequent recurrent UTI.
	Mild-moderate lower UTI	UA	1–3 days: GNRs TMS (DS) 1 dose 2 tablets or 1 tablet PO BID × 3 days. CIPRO 1 dose 1 gm or 500 mg PO BID × 3 days. GPCs Ampi 3 gm PO × 1 dose or 500 mg PO QID × 3 days. or Amox 3 gm PO × 1 dose or 500 mg PO TID × 3 days. If relapse occur-same antibiotic as previously used × 2 weeks.
	Subclinical pyelonephritis Prolonged symptoms, documented relapse, infection with same organism, >3 UTI/year, history of acute pyelonephritis during year.	UA, UCX Follow-up UCX 2–3 days after therapy completed.	12–14 days: TMS (DS) 1 tablet PO BID Cipro 500 mg PO BID
	Acute pyelonephritis	UA, UCX with follow-up UCX after therapy. BCX ×2 BUN/CR, WBC (serum).	Inpatient-IV antibiotics

Patient group	Condition	Workup	Treatment
Postmenopausal women with no medical problems	Asymptomatic bacteriuria	UA	No therapy, unless known structural anomaly or recurrent UTI
	Mild-moderate lower UTI	UA	3–7 days of above nonpregnant regimen
	Subclinical pyelonephritis	UA, UCX, follow-up UCX, BCX ×2, Bun/CR, serum WBC, follow-up UCX after therapy	14 days of above nonpregnancy regimen
	Acute pyelonephritis		Inpatient-IV antibiotics
With medical problems—diabetes, immunocompromised or known genitourinary abnormality	Asymptomatic bacteriuria	UA, UCX	Treat 3–7 days of above regimen
	Mild-moderate lower UTI	UA, UCX follow-up UCX 2–3 days after therapy	7–10 days of the above regimen
	Subclinical-acute pyelonephritis	UA, UCX, BCX × 2 BUN/CR, Serum WBC Follow-up UCX after treatment	Minimum 14–21 days of PO antibiotics; if very suspicious, inpatient with IV antibiotics
Elderly females	Asymptomatic bacteriuria	UA	No therapy unless underlying medical/anatomical problem or history of recent catheterization/instrumentation
	Mild-moderate lower UTI	UA, UCX, BUN/CR, WBC. Follow-up UCX after therapy	7–10 days of the above regimen
	Subclinical-acute pyelonephritis	UA, UCX, BCX × 2, BUN/CR, WBC Follow-up UCX after treatment	Inpatient therapy with IV antibiotics

UA: urinalysis with microscopic evaluation and Gram stain of unspun urine; UCX: urine culture; BCX: blood culture; US: ultrasound; IVP: intravenous pyelography; IV: intravenous; GNR: gram-negative rods; GPC: gram-positive cocci; WBC: white blood cells; UTI: urinary tract infection; Ampi: ampicillin; Amox: amoxicillin; TMS: trimethoprin-sulfamethoxazole; DS: double strength; CIPRO: ciprofloxacin; BUN: blood urea nitrogen; CR: creatinine.

Table 17.2.
Management of UTI: Males

Age	Presenting Symptoms/Signs	Laboratory/Clinical Evaluation	Antibiotic Therapy & Duration of Therapy
Young Males	Mild-Moderate UTI Dysuria, frequency, urgency ("uncomplicated")	UA, UCX, Bun/CR, serum WBC	7–10 day course of TMS (DS) 1 tablet PO BID for GNR's or Amox 500 mg PO TID for GPC's Can be changed after UCX organisms and sensitivities are available.
	"Complicated" UTI With known renal parenchymal disease, obstruction, recurrent infection or prostatic involvement	UA, UCX, Bun/CR, serum, UBC, Renal US and/or IVP Identification and correction of any treatable precipitants such as obstruction or dysfunction.	6–12 weeks with antibiotic coverage that penetrates the prostate and covers resistant organisms. Norfloxacin 400 mg PO BID or TMS (DS) 1 tablet PO BID More expensive, but more effective.
	Acute Pyelonephritis	Evaluation as above. BCX ×2	Inpatient management, IV antibiotics.
Middle Aged Males (50–65)	Mild-Moderate UTI	UA, UCX, BUN/CR, serum WBC	Treatment as above for mild-moderate UTI.
	"Complicated" UTI With known prostate hyperplasia and bladder outflow tract obstruction with post void residual +problems as listed above.	Work-up as for "complicated" UTI in a young male.	Treatment as above for "complicated" UTI.
Elderly males	Acute pyelonephritis	Evaluation as above for young males	Inpatient management, IV antibiotics
	Asymptomatic bacteriuria	UA	No therapy, unless underlying medical or anatomic problem, or history of recent catheterization/instrumentation
	Mild-moderate UTI	UA, UCX, BUN/CR, serum WBC	7–10 day course of antibiotics as above for young males and middle-aged males
	"Complicated" UTI versus suspected pyelonephritis. Patient may appear septic or with more vague symptoms such as change in mental status, failure to thrive.	UA, UCX, BCX ×2, BUN/CR, serum WBC Urologic evaluation-straight catheterization/or renal ultrasound US to rule out obstruction.	Inpatient management, IV antibiotics

UA: urinalysis with microscopic evaluation and Gram stain of unspun urine; UCX: urine culture; BCX: blood culture; US: ultrasound; IVP: intravenous pyelography; IV: intravenous; GNR: gram-negative rods; GPC: gram-positive cocci; WBC: white blood cells; UTI: urinary tract infection; Ampi: ampicillin; Amox: amoxicillin; TMS: trimethoprin-sulfamethoxazole; DS: double strength; CIPRO: ciprofloxacin; BUN: blood urea nitrogen; CR: creatinine.

advantages seen with the one-dose regimen. It requires a patient be more compliant as far as taking 3 days of antibiotic therapy, but follow-up evaluation is less essential. Patients that are not good candidates for short term therapy include patients with diabetes or immunosuppression from other medical or chemical causes, as well as patients with a history of relapses, recurrence, or more than three UTIs in 1 year. These patients should be treated with more conventional antibiotic courses. Because all UTI in males are considered in some sense "complicated" and no studies have been done using shorter therapeutic courses in men, there is no role for short course antibiotic therapy in male patients.

Choice of antibiotic agent should be based on the Gram stain identity of the organism found in the urine as well as some knowledge of the most common organisms known to cause outpatient UTI. In women, about 80% of uncomplicated lower UTI are caused by *E. coli* and about 11% are secondary to *Staphylococcus saprophyticus* (*S. saprophyticus*) a recently recognized pathogen that causes infections in patients usually between the ages of 16–25 and occurs most commonly in the warm months. *E. coli* is also the primary cause of acute pyelonephritis in community and hospital-based settings. Other responsible organisms for approximately 2–3% of outpatient infections include *Proteus mirabilis, Enterococcus faecalis, Klebsiella* species and mixed organisms. *Enterobacter* species become more common in postmenopausal women. Approximately 30% of outpatient acquired UTI with *E. coli* are now ampicillin-resistant, as are *S. saprophyticus* strains mostly producing B-lactamases. Trimethoprim/sulfamethoxazole (TMS) or the fluoroquinolones such as ciprofloxacin (cipro) or norfloxacin are very useful against gram-negative rods. Currently, there is a 15% resistance of *E. coli* to TMS in some areas, but its much lower cost compared with the fluoroquinolones makes it the drug of choice unless indications for another choice of antibiotic therapy exists. The use of Augmentin (amoxicillin-clavulanic acid) allows the health provider to overcome the B-lactamase issue when a penicillin is the preferred drug of choice, although again, the higher cost of this medication should be acknowledged. In men there exists a wider range of causative agents and more variability in antibiotic sensitivities. When infection is secondary to a single organism, about 25% of the cases are due to *E. coli,* and 50 % of infections are from other gram-negative rods including *Proteus mirabilis, Pseudomonas aeruginosa,* and *Providencia.* The remaining 25% are due to *coagulase-negative staphy-*

lococci and *enterococci.* In an initial infection antibiotic therapy can be started based on the Gram stain identity of the organism. TMS is a good choice for gram-negative rods and amoxicillin for gram-positive cocci pending urine culture results. When the patient has a more refractory or recurrent infection, Cipro or norfloxacin may be a better drug of choice.

ASYMPTOMATIC BACTERIURIA

Another important management issue centers around asymptomatic bacteriuria — who should be screened and who should be treated? Asymptomatic bacteriuria is a laboratory diagnosis based on the presence of bacteria in the urine of a woman with no UTI symptoms. A continuum exists because asymptomatic bacteriuria can become symptomatic or bacteriuria can persist after symptoms have resolved. Although both asymptomatic and symptomatic bacteriuria can spontaneously resolve, urine is more likely to become sterile after therapy. But, because there exists high rates of recurrence and resolution, long-term follow-up of asymptomatic bacteriuria after treatment will show no significant improvement after short-term therapy. Therefore, risk factors must be identified to make screening and treatment for asymptomatic bacteriuria necessary and beneficial. These high- risk populations include pregnant women, children, patients with diabetes mellitus, elderly males with urological abnormalities or prostatic enlargement, before and after instrumentation, all patients recently catheterized, and patients with known renal calculi or structural abnormalities of the urinary tract. Pregnant women with inadequately treated or undiagnosed asymptomatic bacteriuria have a 20–40% chance of subsequently developing acute pyelonephritis. These women have a 5–10% risk of preterm labor and delivering a premature infant, and therefore all pregnant women presenting for their first prenatal visit should have a screening urinalysis and urine culture. Children have an increased risk of renal scarring and should be screened and treated when appropriate. Diabetic patients have an increased risk of complicated UTI including papillary necrosis and perirenal or intrarenal abscess formation and should be at least closely observed and monitored, if not treated for asymptomatic bacteriuria. In the elderly population, previous studies had indicated a decreased survival duration in people with asymptomatic bacteriuria when compared with a population without this condition. More recent studies have not substantiated this claim and have not shown that elimination of bacteriuria with antibiotic therapy decreases mortality rates. Therefore, in the absence of obstructive uropathy, significant underlying medical disease or symptomatic UTI, asymptomatic bacteriuria should not be treated in the elderly patient.

CHRONIC SUPPRESSIVE ANTIBIOTIC THERAPY IN RECURRENT UTI

The last issue to discuss in management of UTI is if there is a role for chronic, suppressive antibiotic therapy in recurrent UTI. One study by Stamm et al. (1) suggested that the effectiveness of prophylaxis was limited to the 6 months that prophylaxis was given. Women with three or more infections during the year prior to prophylaxis were more likely to develop UTI after prophylaxis was discontinued. There seemed to be no increase in resistance to antibiotics by *E. coli*, but non-*E. coli* infections were more likely to occur after prophylaxis was stopped. Who then would benefit from antibiotic prophylaxis? Pregnant women after treatment for acute pyelonephritis have a 20–30% likelihood of developing recurrent UTI, and should receive daily prophylaxis for the duration of the pregnancy. Young, healthy sexually active women can use other methods to try and prevent recurrence if they have frequent UTI. Voiding after sexual relations helps decrease the bacterial load and urinary stasis in the bladder for a prolonged period. If the woman is using a diaphragm with spermicidal jelly and has a history of recurrent UTI, another form of birth control may be explored. There are some health care professionals who advocate prophylaxis with a single tablet of TMS or amoxicillin about 1 hour before anticipated sexual relations. This may at least decrease the frequency or severity of infection. In postmenopausal women there is some benefit to using topical vaginal hormone cream to prevent recurrent infection, presumably by changing the vaginal flora back to the premenopausal state and minimizing the Enterobacteriaceae. There may be some role for chronic suppression in frail, elderly patients with distended bladders and large postvoid residuals either secondary to large prostates in men or neurogenic bladder, although again, benefit is limited to the length of prophylaxis. In patients with chronic indwelling urinary catheters, bacterial colonization is the norm. Probably what is most useful for preventing recurrent infection in these patients is routine changing of the catheter, and prompt treatment of clinically apparent infection. Agents such as mandelamine or ascorbic acid (vitamin C) which acidify the urine and improve its bacteriostatic properties may have limited benefit in these patients.

ILLUSTRATIVE CASES WITH SELF-ASSESSMENT QUESTIONS AND ANSWERS

Case 1

A 22-year-old female has complaints of acute dysuria, frequency, urgency, and urinary hesitancy at the initial presentation.

QUESTION: *What other questions would you like to ask this woman to complete your history-taking?*

a. If she is sexually active with a new partner? Any vaginal discharge or vaginal or pelvic complaints?
b. Any history of previous UTI, or similar symptoms in the past?
c. Any history of childhood infections of the urinary tract? Or any significant medical conditions?

d. What form of birth control is being used, and when her last menstrual period was, to rule out possible pregnancy.
e. All of the above.

ANSWER: e. *All of the above. All the information above would help you to decide what to look for on physical examination and which laboratory evaluation would prove useful. She tells you that this is a new sexual partner, and she has been using a diaphragm with spermicidal jelly. She has no vaginal discharge or discomfort and has been treated in the past for UTI, her first infection being when she became sexually active at age 20 and her most recent infection was 3 months ago. She has no other medical problems. Her last menstrual period ended 2 days ago. She is afebrile on* physical examination, with no flank tenderness, only mild suprapubic tenderness and distention. Her pelvic examination is within normal limits with no vaginal discharge noted.

QUESTION: *What laboratory tests would you request in this patient?*

a. Intravenous pyelography
b. Renal ultrasound
c. Urine culture
d. Urinalysis and gram stain of the unspun urine
e. None of the above

ANSWER: d. *All clinical clues in this patient point to an uncomplicated UTI. A urinalysis and Gram stain would help document the presence of pyuria and bacteriuria, and help identify the responsible organism. The urinalysis and Gram stain show 10–15 white blood cells per high-powered field and many gram-negative rods are seen on microscopy. The patient has no known drug allergies.*

QUESTION: *What antibiotic therapy and for what duration would you prescribe for this patient?*

a. Ampicillin 250 mg po TID for 7 days
b. Trimethoprim-sulfamethoxazole double strength tablets, 2 tablets now
c. Ciprofloxacin 750 mg po BID for 14 days
d. Augmentin 250 mg po TID for 5 days
e. None of the above

ANSWER: b. *TMS would probably be the drug of choice in this female with mild symptoms and signs of lower UTI because of less organism resistance than with Ampicillin, and reasonable cost. Also, she would very likely have cure with a one-dose regimen given her mild complaints.*

QUESTION: *What advice can you give this woman to try and minimize recurrent infection?*

a. Empty the bladder after sexual relations
b. Consider alternate birth control methods other than the diaphragm and spermicidal jelly
c. Chronic suppressive antibiotic therapy daily
d. All of the above
e. A and B above

ANSWER: e. *Both the information in A and B may be helpful to the patient. She does not make criteria to even consider chronic suppressive therapy. What has been more useful in these women is taking one antibiotic tablet before sexual relations.*

Case 2

You are asked to consult on a 65-year-old male with persistent UTI with the same organism despite two weeks of antibiotic therapy. He has no significant known medical history.

QUESTION: *What findings would you look for on physical examination?*

a. Fever and/or tachycardia or other signs that the patient is toxic
b. Change in mental status, confusion, delirium
c. Flank tenderness, suprapubic tenderness or distention with palpable bladder, enlarged prostate, any prostatic tenderness or bogginess
d. All of the above
e. None of the above

ANSWER: d. *All the above findings would be useful in helping to differentiate a toxic, acutely ill patient with pyelonephritis or an intrarenal or perinephric abscess versus a patient with a prostatic nidus for infection and obstruction.*

QUESTION: *What laboratory evaluation would be useful in this patient?*

a. IVP
b. Renal ultrasound to evaluate kidneys and postvoid residual
c. Urinalysis and urine culture
d. Blood urea nitrogen and creatinine, serum white blood cell count
e. All of the above

ANSWER: e. *All of the above tests would help define the anatomy and any structural defects, as well as the presence of pyuria and bacteriuria, identification of the responsible organism, and evaluation of the man's renal function. The patient has normal kidneys by IVP and renal ultrasound but both show significant obstruction secondary to an enlarged prostate. His renal function is normal, but he has a slightly elevated serum* *white count. His urine culture grows E. coli, the same organism he has previously grown with the same antibiotic sensitivities as previously. He has a known allergy to sulfa drugs.*

QUESTION: *What antibiotic regimen and for what duration would you treat the patient?*

a. Augmentin 500 mg po TID for 3 weeks
b. TMS (DS) one tablet po BID for 6 weeks
c. Norfloxacin 400 mg po BID for 10 weeks
d. Ampicillin 500 mg po QID for 10 days.
e. None of the above

ANSWER: c. *There is a real need in this patient to select a drug with good prostatic penetration as well as a low incidence of organism resistance. Prolonged therapy is necessary because of the persistent infection despite 2 weeks of therapy already and the presence of a prostatitis. TMS would not be a choice in this patient with a documented sulfa allergy. Once the infection has resolved, the prostatic hypertrophy needs to be addressed to prevent recurrent UTI based on obstruction.*

RENAL INSUFFICIENCY

Renal insufficiency is a common diagnosis in adult medical patients especially the elderly. It is frequently discovered as a laboratory abnormality, i.e., a rising trend in the blood urea nitrogen and creatinine. It is usually asymptomatic in the early stages of the disease. The manifestations of renal insufficiency become evident as the disease progresses. These manifestations include disturbances of water balance and acid base function, underexcretion of toxic substances and abnormal production of various hormones such as erythropoietin, parathyroid hormone, 1–25 Dihydroxy vitamin D_3, renin and prostaglandins. This chapter will cover the pathophysiology, diagnosis and management of chronic renal insufficiency.

Renal failure is usually classified as acute or chronic. Because the causes of acute and chronic renal failure are not mutually exclusive, a review of chronic renal insufficiency should include an overview of acute renal failure. Acute renal failure is defined as a sudden compromise in renal function leading to accumulation of nitrogenous waste products and in some cases, retention of water. It can be classified in three categories: prerenal, renal, and postrenal. The prerenal state comprises all the disturbances leading to decreased perfusion of the kidney. It can result from severe volume depletion such as hemorrhage and dehydration, vasomotor changes such as vasodilation in sepsis or vasoconstriction in drugs and cardiovascular failure. The renal causes include intrinsic glomerular and tubulointerstitial processes. The postrenal causes involve obstructive processes (Table 17.3). These can be intrarenal or extrarenal. Many of these previously described processes if managed appropriately and in a timely fashion, can allow resolution to normal kidney function. However, there seems to be a critical mass of nephron destruction which will lead to chronic renal insufficiency and even end stage renal disease (l). It thus follows that acute renal insufficiency can lead to chronic renal insufficiency and even end stage renal disease. With endstage renal disease, the patient develops the manifestations known as the uremic syndrome.

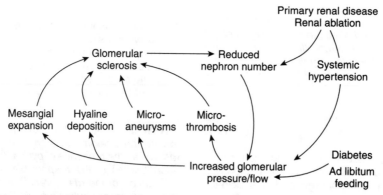

Figure 17.1. Hypothetical scheme detailing the progression of renal disease. Reductions in renal mass, systemic hypertension, whether primary or secondary to renal mass, diabetes mellitus, and ad libitum feeding all increase glomerular pressures and flows. (Modified from Meyer TW, Scholey JW, Brenner BM. Nephron adaptation to renal injury. In: Brenner BM & Rector, FC Jr eds. Brenner & Rector's The Kidney, 4th ed. WB Saunders, Philadelphia 1991: 1896.)

Table 17.3.
Causes of Acute Renal Failure

Disorder	Examples
Prerenal	
Hypovolemia	Skin, renal, gastrointestinal volume loss; hemorrhage; extracellular fluid sequestration (burns, peritonitis)
Peripheral vasculature	Vascular pooling (sepsis); vasodilatation or vasoconstriction (drugs); arterial or venous occlusion
Cardiovascular failure	Impaired cardiac output (infarction, arrhythmia, tamponade)
Postrenal	
Extrarenal obstruction	Urethral occlusion; bladder, pelvic, prostatic, retroperitoneal neoplasms; surgical accident; drugs; calculi; pus; blood clots; bladder rupture, trauma
Intrarenal obstruction	Crystals (uric and oxalic acids, drugs)
Parenchymal renal failure	
Acute tubular necrosis	
Ischemia	All conditions for prerenal failure
Toxins	Antibiotics; contrast material; anesthetics; heavy metals; organic solvents
Pigments	Hemoglobinuria, hemolysis (transfusion reaction, malaria); myoglobinuria, rhabdomyolysis (muscle trauma and disease, potassium or phosphate depletion)
Pregnancy	Septic abortion; uterine hemorrhage; eclampsia
Glomerulitis and vasculitis	Post streptococcus; immune complex (systemic lupus erythematosus), antiglomerular basement membrane (Goodpasture's); malignant hypertension; thrombotic thrombocytopenic purpura; scleroderma
Interstitial nephritis	Drugs; hypercalcemia; infections; radiation; idiopathic

(From Espinel CH. Diagnosis of acute and chronic renal failure In Preuss HG, ed. Clinics in laboratory medicine, Vol. 13, No. 1, WB Saunders, Philadelphia, 1993: 90.)

Pathophysiologic Correlation

A review of the pathophysiology of renal insufficiency involves an understanding of many interrelated events. These are the pathway leading to glomerular sclerosis, the nephron adaptation to renal injury and the pathophysiology of uremia. These processes operate in all forms of renal disease leading to progressive renal insufficiency and end stage renal disease.

PATHWAY TO GLOMERULAR SCLEROSIS

The basic functional unit of the kidney is the nephron. It consists of the glomerulus, the proximal tubule, the loop of Henle, the distal nephron and the collecting duct. Together they carry out the major renal functions namely glomerular ultrafiltration, tubular resorption and secretion. In renal failure any or all of these processes may be impaired. The pathophysiology of renal disease regardless of the underlying etiology, involves the progressive loss of nephrons resulting in functional and structural adaptations of remaining nephrons. To counteract the functional loss that would otherwise result from the decreased number of nephrons, the remaining nephrons undergo hyperfiltration.

These changes, which are compensatory initially, prove later to be maladaptive and are accompanied by morphological changes such as mesangial expansion, obliteration of glomerular capillaries. All of these morphologic changes result in the histological picture of glomerular sclerosis (Fig. 17.1). Several hormones such as growth and inflammatory factors have been implicated in the genesis of these morphological changes. Several other factors have been implicated in the acceleration of this process namely systemic hypertension, proteinuria, hyperlipidemia, dietary proteins, and phosphates.

ADAPTATION TO RENAL INJURY

In renal insufficiency, the glomerular filtration rate (GFR), a measure of kidney function begins to fall. With the decline in renal function, there must be a progressive increase in the rate of solute excretion to maintain balance. The following equation applies to any solute:

Solute excretion = glomerular filtration rate × plasma solute concentration − tubular solute reabsorption (S) + tubular secretion

The kidney is crucial in the maintenance of sodium and water balance. However, disorders of sodium and water balance do not become apparent until the later stages of the disease. This is because in mild to moderate renal insufficiency the percentage of filtered sodium that is excreted to maintain balance increases dramatically. For example, an individual with a normal GFR around 100ml/min filters about 25000 meq of sodium per day. If he ingests 100 meq, he will have to excrete 100 meq to maintain sodium balance approximately 0.4 percent of the filtered load. If his GFR drops to 50 ml/min and he ingests 100 meq of sodium, he still needs to excrete 100 meq to maintain balance, approximately 0.8 percent of the filtered load. Most patients with renal insufficiency are able to maintain potassium balance until their disease is advanced. The regulation of potassium balance is multifactorial involving the gastrointestinal tract, cellular uptake and renal excretion. In renal insufficiency and a tendency toward hyperkalemia, the colonic and tubular secretion increases.

PATHOPHYSIOLOGY OF UREMIA

There has been much debate as to why uremic syndrome develops in patients with renal failure. The most prominent hypothesis involves the presence of uremic toxins. This is partly validated by the fact that some of these symptoms disappear with dialytic therapy. Many substances have been proposed such as urea, trace metals, and inorganic ions. Various animal studies have shown that a progressive increase in urea causes a syndrome much like uremia with malaise, anorexia, bleeding diathesis, stupor, coma and even death. Although general correlations can be made between the concentrations of certain solutes and the presence of uremia, no single solute can account for all the symptoms. Many have postulated a significant endocrine contribution to the pathophysiology of uremia, i.e., secondary hyperparathyroidism and its complications, inadequate secretion of 1,25 dihydroxy vitamin D_3 and decreased metabolic clearance of certain hormones.

Clinical and Laboratory Evaluation

The history, physical examination, and laboratory evaluation will give invaluable information about the etiology of renal insufficiency and its prognosis.

HISTORY

Chronic renal insufficiency is usually asymptomatic in the early stages. The patient rarely presents to the clinician with a referrable complaint. Frequently, an abnormal blood urea nitrogen and creatinine is noted on routine laboratory examination, and this prompts the search for the underlying cause. The patient should be questioned at this point about polyuria, and nocturia, fatigue, disturbed sleep patterns, anorexia, nausea. With the exception of nocturia and polyuria reflecting a decrease in renal concentrating ability, most of the other symptoms are present only in advanced disease. The pattern of urine flow such as hesitancy or dribbling can suggest an obstructive etiology. The history should focus on the presence of concurrent medical problems known to be implicated in renal disease, such as hypertension, diabetes mellitus, gout, and immunodeficiency. A history of similarly affected family members can be the first clue to the presence of a congenitally acquired form of renal disease such as polycystic kidney disease or Alport syndrome. A history of drug use is mandatory including prescription, over the counter and illegal drugs.

PHYSICAL EXAMINATION

A complete physical examination is essential to correct diagnosis paying close attention to certain features. The patient's general appearance should be noted. General malaise and lethargy are suggestive of more advanced disease.

Vital Signs   An elevated blood pressure can be a contributor or a clue to the presence of renal disease. This is especially important in a patient with previously controlled blood pressure. The respiratory rate can be increased if there is concurrent metabolic acidosis.

Fundoscopic examination   The presence of retinopathy both hypertensive and diabetic should be investigated. Most patients with diabetic nephropathy will have evidence of retinopathy. The reverse, however, is not necessarily true.

Cardiovascular Examination   An S4 gallop or a ventricular lift suggest left ventricular hypertrophy, which is common in longstanding untreated hypertension. Hypertension, as mentioned previously, represents a significant cause of renal insufficiency. The presence of bruits in the carotid, renal, femoral area can be significant in establishing the cause of renal insufficiency.

Abdomen Examination   The presence of abdominal masses and bruits can be very significant. In polycystic kidney disease the kidneys are frequently palpable through the abdominal wall. The presence of an enlarged bladder can reveal a chronic obstructive process.

Genitourinary System Examination An enlarged prostate coupled with a history suggestive of prostatism can be a significant clue to the presence of obstruction. Extensive pelvic tumors with retroperitoneal involvement compromising the patency of the urinary tract can contribute to renal insufficiency.

Neurological Examination The presence of neurological deficits such as change in mental status or sensory motor neuropathy can be seen in advanced renal disease.

LABORATORY EVALUATION

Because of the relative paucity of signs and symptoms in early chronic renal insufficiency, the laboratory examination is helpful in establishing the diagnosis. A urinalysis is usually among the first tests ordered after a diagnosis of renal insufficiency has been made. It consists of a chemical analysis and a microscopic examination. The chemical analysis includes the specific gravity, pH, protein glucose, ketones, bilirubin and nitrite. A low specific gravity can be indicative of a renal concentrating defect. The patient's fluid status must, however, be kept in mind. It is perfectly normal for a patient who has just ingested a large amount of free water to pass urine with a low specific gravity. The finding of significant proteinuria is indicative of glomerular disease. In a patient in whom the clinician suspects amyloidosis or multiple myeloma and the urine is negative for proteins on routine urinalysis, a test for the presence of light chains in the urine using sulfasalicylic acid should be done. The microscopic evaluation of the urine consists of identifying cells, casts and crystals. Many kidney diseases leading to chronic renal insufficiency present with pyuria, hematuria and cellular casts. The finding of hematuria accompanied by red cell casts suggests glomerulonephritis. Abnormal shaped red blood cells in the urine; a condition termed dysmorphic hematuria, also suggests a glomerular process. A complete blood count should be obtained looking for the presence of anemia. The anemia of chronic renal insufficiency is usually normochromic and normocytic. A full biochemical profile should also be done looking for electrolyte abnormalities. More specialized tests such as serum complements, serum protein electrophoresis, hepatitis serologies, and even HIV antibodies should be obtained in cases where the history is suggestive.

Renal Ultrasound The renal ultrasound is done mostly to assess kidney size, cortical thickness, and echogenicity. It can detect the presence of hy-

dronephrosis or atrophic kidney. Hydronephrosis suggests an obstructive process, whereas, an atrophic kidney suggests renovascular disease. Increased renal echogenicity correlates well with the presence of intrinsic renal disease.

Assessment of Glomerular Filtration Rate When renal insufficiency has been diagnosed, it is useful to get an estimation of the patient's glomerular filtration rate. This will help to establish the level of renal insufficiency and lead to appropriate management. The glomerular filtration rate can be obtained in several ways. The most accurate method is the inulin clearance. Since inulin is freely filtered in the glomerulus and is neither reabsorbed, metabolized, nor secreted in the tubules, it is the ideal marker of glomerular filtration rate. It is, however, cumbersome and is not performed routinely. Traditionally, the creatinine clearance (Cr cl) is obtained. It is easy to perform because creatinine is an endogenous substance that is freely filtered and is not reabsorbed. It is, however, secreted in the tubule and this secretion increases in renal insufficiency. Because of this, it overestimates glomerular filtration rate. Although, less than an ideal marker, its clearance approximates glomerular filtration rate and is frequently used. A 24-hour urine collection of creatinine is obtained and a serum creatinine is obtained at the end of the collection. The creatinine clearance formula is as follows:

Creatinine clearance = urinary creatinine concentration $\times$ urine volume $\div$ plasma creatinine concentration $\times$ 1440 min

The creatinine clearance is expressed in ml/min. To check for the adequacy of the collection one can calculate the predicted creatinine level in the urine and see if it corresponds to the observed value. The formula in men is as follows:

expected creatinine = weight in kg $\times$ [28–0.2 (age)]

A 60-kg man who is 60 years old is expected to have 960 mg of creatinine. The formula in women is weight in kg $\times$ [(23.8–0.17 (age)]. If the observed value is much lower, one can conclude that this was an undercollection. Creatinine clearance can also be obtained using the Cockroft and Gault formula:

$$\text{creatinine clearance} = \frac{(140\text{-age}) \times \text{body wt kg}}{72 \times \text{serum Cr}}$$

Multiply the result by 0.85 for women.

Differential Diagnosis

The diagnosis of chronic renal insufficiency is straightforward. The challenge lies in establishing the etiology. Because of extensive monitoring and analysis of patients entering dialysis centers, there are reliable data about the causes leading to endstage renal disease (Table 17.4). As chronic renal insufficiency is part of that continuum, the same data are probably applicable. Diabetes mellitus represents the most common cause leading to end stage renal disease closely followed by hypertension. Together, they account for over half of the cases. Glomerulonephritis also contributes significantly to end stage renal disease. Analgesic abuse with nephropathy, secondary amyloidosis resulting from multiple myeloma, and hereditary problems like polycystic kidney disease and Alport's syndrome also contribute to the number of patients with end stage renal disease, but are substantially less prevalent. The history, physical examination, and laboratory tests will suggest the etiology in most cases and a renal biopsy is rarely needed to confirm the diagnosis.

Management

The clinician managing a patient with chronic renal insufficiency must keep in mind several important principles. The most important one is to establish a correct diagnosis and treat or attempt to arrest the process as soon as possible. The second is to identify risk factors contributing to the progression of renal disease. The third is to anticipate metabolic complications resulting from renal insufficiency. The fourth is to continually assess the progression of the disease. The last is to know when to refer for a higher level of care.

Table 17.4.
Incidence of Treated ESRD by Detailed Primary Disease; USRDS 1993 Annual Data Report—Combined Data 1987–1990

Diabetic nephropathy	34.2%
Hypertension	29.4%
Glomerulonephritis	14.2%
Cystic kidney disease	3.4%
Urologic disease	2.3%
Other	5.9%
Missing information	6.6%

Adapted from incidence and causes of treated ESRD. USRDS 1993.

RISK FACTORS CONTRIBUTING TO THE PROGRESSION OF RENAL DISEASE

Hypertension The traditional thinking is that hypertension accelerates the decline in glomerular filtration rate regardless of the underlying cause of the renal disease. The mechanism through which hypertension damages the kidney is unclear, but is thought to involve increased intraglomerular pressure and increased arteriolar wall thickness leading to ischemia. There is a growing body of evidence to suggest that treatment of hypertension retards the progression of renal disease (1–3). There has been recent attention to the use of angiotensin converting enzyme inhibitors and calcium channel blockers. The ACE inhibitors are believed to lower intraglomerular pressure in addition to systemic blood pressure. They also decrease proteinuria which is an additional risk factor for end stage renal disease. Their use, however, is not without complications especially the potential for hyperkalemia. Calcium-channel blockers are thought to decrease mesangial expansion, which is an important step in the pathway toward glomerular sclerosis. There is not an ideal drug for every patient, and many factors must be considered in the choice of an antihypertensive agent. The goal of therapy should be reduction of diastolic blood pressure to less than 90 mm of mercury.

Proteinuria Proteinuria is a sign of renal injury. It is increasingly being recognized as a risk factor for progression of renal disease. Several studies have shown a worse prognosis in patients with renal disease and significant proteinuria. There seems to be a correlation between treatment of proteinuria and the stabilization of renal disease.

A restricted protein intake in patients with progressive renal insufficiency is known to decrease the uremic symptoms such as nausea and acidosis. Many animal studies and a few human studies have suggested that dietary protein restriction retards the progression of renal insufficiency. The mechanism behind this observation is thought to be multifactorial, i.e., decreased growth factors, decreased lipids and a concomitant decrease in dietary phosphate which usually accompanies a protein restricted diet.

A recently published trial, the modification of diet in renal disease (MDRD) study, attempted to settle this question (4). The conclusions were that in patients with moderate renal insufficiency (Crcl between 25 and 55 ml /mIn) there was a small benefit to be derived from a restricted protein intake, whereas in patients with advanced renal insufficiency (Crcl between 13 and 24 ml/min) there was no significant benefit between a low protein diet and a very low protein diet with ketoacid-amino acid supplementation. However, because of the limitations of the study, i.e., the underlying diagnoses leading to renal insufficiency, and the short term of follow up, one cannot make general recommendations about every patient with renal insufficiency. Given the current evidence available, it appears safe to prescribe modest protein restriction (0.6 to 0.8 g/kg/day) to halt the progression and prevent some of the manifestations of progressive renal insufficiency. It is, however, essential to avoid a negative nitrogen balance.

Hyperlipidemia The treatment of hyperlipidemia may be beneficial in preventing progression of renal insufficiency. The use of lipid lowering agents may be helpful, although special attention to dosing must be considered (Table 17.5).

METABOLIC COMPLICATIONS OF RENAL INSUFFICIENCY

Metabolic complications of renal insufficiency affect every system of the body. Serious and/or treatable complications will be reviewed in this section.

Anemia The anemia of chronic renal failure is a major cause of disability and symptoms previously attributed to the uremic state such as lethargy, and dizziness are now thought to be related to anemia. The pathogenesis of anemia in renal failure is multifactorial and includes iron deficiency and low levels of erythropoeitin. The iron deficiency may come about through occult bleeding and shortened survival of red blood cells frequently observed in patients with renal failure. It can result from secondary hyperparathyroidism leading to osteitis fibrosa cystica and significant bone marrow fibrosis. The primary cause of anemia in renal failure, however, comes from erythropoeitin deficiency. Erythropoeitin is a hormone predominantly synthesized in the kidney which stimulates the bone marrow to produce red blood cells. It is secreted in the presence of anemia and hypoxemia. The abnormal kidney is unable to synthesize and secrete appropriate amounts of erythropoeitin for the level of anemia. When evaluating anemia in renal insufficiency, iron deficiency should be ruled out and corrected. In the early stages this might be all that is necessary. As erythropoeitin level starts to fall, replacement therapy is inevitable in order to maintain adequate hemoglobin level. The benefits of correcting the anemia are immeasurable including a greater sense of well being, increased energy, and increased sex-

ual function. The risks in adequate supervision are low, however, but still present including seizures, hypertension, and strokes. The cost of erythropoeitin can also be a limiting factor as it is very expensive.

Metabolic Acidosis With progressive renal insufficiency, the tubular secretion of hydrogen ions decreases, hence, their accumulation in the serum resulting in metabolic acidosis. The deleterious effects of acidosis include bone demineralization, renal osteodystrophy, protein catabolism, hyperkalemia and resistance to insulin. The therapy involves restriction of foods yielding increased hydrogen such as proteins and the addition of carbonate in the form of sodium or calcium carbonate. Calcium carbonate is the preferred mode of treatment because it addresses both the acidosis and the hypocalcemia frequently present in advanced renal insufficiency.

Calcium and Phosphorus Balance For many years secondary hyperparathyroidism was explained via the trade-off hypothesis. It was believed that after a meal the phosphorus level was transiently elevated, the available calcium would bind to phosphorus, thus reducing the level of calcium and this would trigger the secretion of parathyroid hormone. This long-held theory was disputed by studies in which hyperparathyroidism was present in hypercalcemia. It is currently believed that hyperparathyroidism results not from hypercalcemia, but from decreased endocrine feedback on the parathyroid gland by the calcium-regulating hormone 1,25 dihydroxy vitamin D_3. This hormone is thought to increase the calcium sensitivity of the parathyroid gland, decrease the level of calcium at which the gland is suppressed, inhibit parathyroid cell proliferation and hyperplasia, and increase the intestinal absorption of calcium and phosphorus. The metabolism of vitamin D_3 is ultimately regulated by the kidney. The pathway to the active form of vitamin D_3 is as follows: after ingestion or metabolism of cholesterol in the skin, cholecalciferol is 25-hydroxylated in the liver to produce 25 (OH) cholecalciferol. It is metabolized in the kidney by 1 alpha hydroxylase to its active form 1,25 dihydroxy vitamin D_3. In renal failure, there is a decrease in the activity of 1 alpha hydroxylase leading to decreased production of active vitamin D_3.

Bone Disease in Renal Failure Chronic renal failure may result in renal osteodystrophy, which includes three forms of bone disease: osteomalacia, osteosclerosis and osteitis fibrosa cystica. The sequence of events previously leading to in-

Table 17.5.
Therapeutic Interventions During the Course of Chronic Renal Failure

Stage of Chronic Renal Impairment (GFR)	Blood Pressure	Dietary Protein (g/kg per day)	Calcium Supplementation (mg/day)	Phosphorus Restriction (mg/day)	Hyperlipidaemia	Proteinuria
Early (50–80 ml/min)		0.1–1.2	500–1000	≤900		
Moderate (25–50 ml/min)	Requires treatment throughout course of disease	0.8–1.0	1000–1200	700–900 with mealtime calcium carbonate	Aim to reduce serum cholesterol by diet and drug therapy if ≥6.5 mmol/l	Aim to reduce if in excess of 3 g/24 h
Advanced (5–25 ml/min)		0.6 (high biological value protein)	1200–1500	≤700 with 1200 mg mealtime calcium carbonate		
Dialysis		1.2–1.4	1200–1800	As for advanced impairment although higher doses of phosphate binders may be required		

Protein restriction at GFR values below 25 ml/min is indicated to improve metabolic acidosis and to decrease phosphorus intake.
(From Klahr S. Chronic renal failure—management. Lancet 1991; 338:424.)

creased parathyroid hormone have been previously outlined. This increase in parathyroid hormone in conjunction with decreased vitamin D metabolism, metabolic acidosis, and increased levels of phosphorus all contribute to bone disease in renal failure. Bone disease is more common in children with renal failure, however, radiographic evidence is substantial in a large majority of adults with chronic renal insufficiency. In osteomalacia, x-rays reveal demineralization and pathologic fractures. This is thought to be due to hypocalcemia and low vitamin D levels. The clinical syndrome consists of bony deformity, bone pain and pathologic fractures. Osteosclerosis is recognized on x-rays by increased densities in the upper and lower parts of the vertebral bodies with an area of demineralization between them giving the so called rugger jersey spine appearance. Osteitis fibrosa cystica is characterized by bone resorption and subperiosteal erosions. The bone diseases are best prevented by altering the conditions which lead to secondary hyperparathyroidism and increased phosphorus level. This can be accomplished in some cases with administration of vitamin D and phosphate binders such as calcium carbonate. Of note, the use of aluminum phosphate binders in the past contributed to an aluminum-induced form of bone disease, which is rare now given the recognition of this entity.

PROGRESSION OF RENAL DISEASE/REFERRAL FOR HIGHER LEVEL CARE

Frequently, despite appropriate management of renal insufficiency the disease inexorably follows its course, albeit at a reduced rate, to endstage renal disease. The indications for initiation of dialysis are the presence of uremic symptoms, volume overload, hyperkalemia, refractory acidosis, pericarditis

and generalized failure to thrive. At this point, replacement therapy in the form of dialysis or renal transplantation has to be started to maintain life. Dialysis is divided into hemodialysis and peritoneal dialysis. To undergo hemodialysis the patient must have a surgically created arteriovenous fistula for access. The concept involves the diffusion of a high concentration of toxins across a semipermeable membrane into the dialysate (which is a fluid with a low concentration of solutes). Removal of water occurs by ultrafiltration. The patient usually receives three treatments at a dialysis center lasting 3 to 4 hours each. Peritoneal dialysis involves the similar process of diffusion of solutes and removal of water. The semipermeable membrane in this instance is the peritoneum. A surgically implanted catheter is placed in the abdominal wall extending into the peritoneal cavity. Dialysate is introduced in the peritoneal cavity and allowed to remain there for several hours. During that time, the diffusion of water and solutes occurs. At the end of the process, the patient empties the cavity and the fluid is discarded. This procedure is repeated four times over a 24-hour period. This form of dialysis offers the convenience of home dialysis and the freedom of not being tied down to a dialysis center. It is preferred by motivated and active patients. The patient, however, needs to be well trained in aseptic techniques and to be taught to recognize the signs of peritoneal inflammation which include local tenderness, nausea and general malaise. Renal transplantation is the best form of replacement because it basically restores all the functions of the healthy kidney including the endocrine functions. The patient will require immunosuppressive therapy for the rest of his or her life to prevent rejection. He or she will also need to be monitored by specialists trained in this type of care.

ILLUSTRATIVE CASES WITH SELF-ASSESSMENT QUESTIONS AND ANSWERS

Case 1

A 60-year-old black man comes to your office for an insurance physical examination. He is asymptomatic and says that he has not seen a doctor in a long time. He is concerned, however, because he was told that his insurance premiums were going to be much higher because his kidneys are not working well.

The pertinent lab tests are as follows:

Hg: 12.9   Hct: 39.2   Na: 138   K: 4.5   Chloride: 102
HCO_3: 24   BUN: 22   Creat: 2.3   Glucose: 110

QUESTION: *Which of the following questions should be asked?*

a. Any prior history of diabetes?

b. Any prior history of hypertension?
c. Any family history of kidney disease?
d. Does he smoke?
e. Does he use any drugs including over the counter?

ANSWER: *All of the questions are important as they help to narrow the diagnostic field.*

QUESTION: *What would you do next?*

a. Perform a complete physical exam and screening lab tests, i.e., urinalysis, repeat CBC SMA$_{20}$.
b. Refer to a nephrologist.

ANSWER: a. *Perform a complete physical and baseline laboratory exams. He may need a nephrologist at some point, but a thorough and careful history and physical examination should reveal the etiology in many cases. The physical examination is remarkable for elevated blood pressure I60/I00 narrowed arterioles on fundoscopic exam and the presence of femoral bruits. His urinalysis is significant for 1+ protein.*

QUESTION: *What is the most likely diagnosis?*

a. Diabetic nephropathy
b. Hypertensive nephropathy
c. Glomerulonephritis

ANSWER: b. *The most likely diagnosis is hypertensive nephropathy. He does not have diabetes nor significant proteinuria.*

QUESTION: *What would you do next?*

a. Control his blood pressure.
b. Evaluate his dietary habits and cholesterol status.
c. Stress that he should not abuse NSAIDS.

ANSWER: *All of the above. He will need close supervision to stabilize his renal disease and avoid further deterioration.*

HEMATURIA

Hematuria is defined as the presence of red blood cells in the urine. It is classified as microscopic or macroscopic depending on the amount of red blood cells present. The presence of persistent hematuria may be a sign of urologic disease and as such needs to be evaluated. A wide number of conditions may cause hematuria including urinary tract infections, glomerulonephritis, interstitial nephritis, kidney stones, renal infarction, papillary necrosis, endometriosis, trauma, vigorous exercise, renal tuberculosis and urologic neoplasm. This chapter will concentrate on kidney stones and the evaluation of persistent hematuria to detect urologic neoplasm.

Pathophysiologic Correlation

The urinary tract is made up of the kidneys, the ureters, the bladder, the urethra, and in the male the prostate which encircles the bladder neck discharging its secretions into the urethra. Any process causing luminal injury such as inflammation, crystalluria or disruption of the normal epithelium (as in tumors) will result in hematuria. The timing of hematuria to the urinary stream, i.e., initial versus terminal hematuria, may help localize the pathology to a specific region of the urinary tract. Initial hematuria suggests a lesion in the urethral meatus whereas terminal hematuria suggests a lesion in the bladder neck. Total hematuria suggests pathology at or above the level of the bladder.

Clinical Laboratory Evaluation

Hematuria, whether gross or microscopic, is a fairly common problem encountered by the clinician. The history, physical, and laboratory examination will help elucidate the etiology in most cases. In some setting the diagnosis may remain unclear.

HISTORY

The evaluation of hematuria begins with the history. The patient should be asked about symptoms of dysuria, urinary urgency and frequency as these point to the presence of an underlying infection. Sudden onset of flank pain radiating anteriorly and down the groin causing nausea and vomiting is pathognomonic of renal calculi. A history of vigorous exercise especially in the young can help to confirm a benign cause. The passage of large clots is suspicious for bladder cancer. The patient's demographics such as age and gender should be taken into account because the risk of urologic neoplasm is higher in the male and increases sharply after age 50. In addition, he or she should be asked about risk factors for urologic cancer such as tobacco use, occupational exposures to dyes, pelvic irradiation, analgesic abuse (phenacetin), *S. haematobium* infection (See Table 18.1). A thorough review of medications may be especially helpful when the cause of hematuria is particularly elusive. Hematuria in a patient taking anticoagulants should be considered significant because lesions can be discovered early in such patients. A family history of renal disease should always be sought.

PHYSICAL EXAMINATION

A complete physical examination is essential, paying special attention to the clues obtained in the history. The presence of fever usually suggests an infectious process. It can also suggest a systemic process such as glomerulonephritis. The presence of abdominal masses raises the suspicion of renal tumors or polycystic kidney disease. The presence of flank pain and costovertebral angle tenderness suggests kidney stones or infection. Frequently, the physical examination is unremarkable especially in the case where the hematuria was discovered incidentally.

LABORATORY EXAMINATION

A thorough history and physical examination will significantly narrow the differential diagnoses. The laboratory examination will help to confirm the clinical suspicion. The most appropriate initial test is the urinalysis. Figure 17.2 illustrates common urinary sediment findings. It will help to quantitate the level of hematuria, i.e., number of RBCs per high power field (HPF). The level of hematuria which constitutes an abnormality is unclear, but the finding of three or more RBCs/HPF on multiple specimens should be concerning. Several other findings may be obtained from the urinalysis, such as the shape of the red blood cells, the nature of the sediment and the presence of proteinuria. The finding of hematuria with pyuria suggests a urinary tract infection. This combination of findings can also be seen in the setting of kidney stones. The presence of red cell masts confirms glomerulonephritis. The finding of persistent hematuria on urinalysis in a patient with significant risks of urologic malignancy should lead to an aggressive search for malignancy. After excluding urinary tract infection with a urine culture, the patient should be evaluated with urine cytologies, intravenous pyelogram (IVP) or renal ultrasound and if warranted cystoscopy and abdominal CT scans.

Differential Diagnosis

In a compilation of studies examined by Sutton (1) in JAMA, he found that the cause of hematuria will fall into one of these categories: urologic malignancy, kidney stones, renal disease, urinary tract infection, prostate hyperplasia with a few unknown cases. Kidney stones and urologic malignancy will be discussed further in the following paragraphs. Urinary tract infection, renal disease and prostatic hyperplasia are covered elsewhere.

KIDNEY STONES

Kidney stones are of four types: calcium, uric acid, struvite, and cystine. Calcium stones are by far the most common and make up about 80% of all kidney stones. Calcium stones are usually small stones whereas struvite, uric acid and cystine stones can grow quite large and fill up the entire renal calyceal system creating staghorn calculi. The pathophysiology of kidney stones involves the interplay of three important factors: supersaturation, nucleation, and the lack of inhibitors of crystal aggregation. Normal urine contains many crystals of different salts such as calcium oxalate, and phosphate. These crystals may be at a concentration higher than their solubility, but not high enough to promote aggregation (2). Any factor such as decreased urinary volume, change in pH can create a condition where these crystals precipitate and start aggregating. The process of crystal aggregation is called nucleation. It can be homogeneous as described above or heterogeneous where a crystal anchors itself to the luminal epithelium or any debris thereby facilitating the process. Uric acid crystals can serve as a nidus for aggregation of calcium crystals. Usually, these aggregatory complexes are prevented from growing because of increased urine flow and intrinsic inhibitors of crystallization found in the urine such as citrate or other kidney proteins. A situation in which these inhibitors are deficient will enable the crystallization process to take place. The process of supersaturation, nucleation, and aggregation of crystals is common to all types of kidney stone formation. Certain factors, however, favor the formation of one type of stone versus another. Calcium oxalate stones may occur in the setting of idiopathic hypercalciuria, hyperuricosuria, primary hyperparathyroidism with increased urinary calcium excretion and hyperoxaluria. Uric

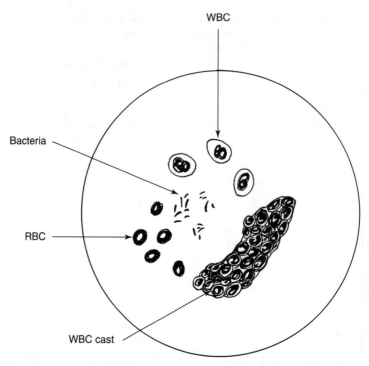

Figure 17.2. Sediment from a centrifuged urine sample. Note the presence and relative size of bacteria, red blood cells, white blood cells, and the white blood cell cast.

acid stones are much less prevalent in the United States accounting for about five percent of all stones. They are, however, prevalent in patients with gout or asymptomatic hyperuricemia. They may precede the articular disease in patients with gout. The three most important factors in patients with uric acid stones are hyperuricosuria, acidic urine, and low urinary volumes. Struvite stones occur in the setting of urinary infection with urea splitting bacteria. These are usually proteus species, but some strains of Klebsiella, Pseudomonas, and Enterococcus may also be responsible. *E. coli* never cause them. Because of their size and the tendency to fill up the renal calyceal system, these stones can deteriorate renal function. They can also cause life-threatening sepsis. Cystine stones are very rare accounting for less than one percent of kidney stones. They occur exclusively in patients with hereditary defects causing them to excrete excessive amounts of cystine in their urine. Figure 17.3 illustrates the appearance of crystals seen in nephrolithiasis.

UROLOGIC NEOPLASM

The primary reason for working up persistent asymptomatic hematuria is to detect a potentially life threatening disease such as a urologic neoplasm. Urologic neoplasm comprises a variety of tumors including prostate, kidney, bladder, and ureters. Bladder cancer may present as gross painless hematuria. It can also be associated with irritative symptoms such as dysuria, urgency, and frequency. It may be discovered during an episode of acute urinary retention. Renal cancer may present as a triad of abdominal mass, flank pain, and hematuria in a minority of cases. Despite these possible manifestations, these entities are more often asymptomatic in the early stages thus making an aggressive work up imperative.

Management

The clinician managing a patient with hematuria must keep in mind several principles. The most

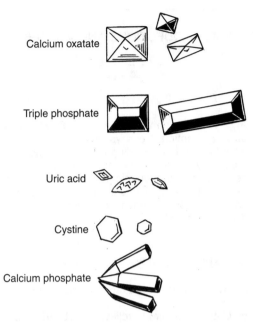

Calcium oxatate

Triple phosphate

Uric acid

Cystine

Calcium phosphate

Figure 17.3. Urinary crystals seen in nephrolithias. Note the pyramid shape of calcium oxalate crystals, the coffin lid shape of triple phosphate crystals, the rhomboidal shape of uric acid crystals, and the hexagonal shape of calcium phosphate crystals.

important one is to establish a correct diagnosis especially to rule out malignancy in the patient with a suggestive history and significant risk factors. Once a diagnosis has been established the management should proceed accordingly.

KIDNEY STONES

The patient with kidney stones will fit into one of several categories: acute renal colic, asymptomatic kidney stones noted on x-rays or recurrent kidney stones. The management of acute renal colic focuses on analgesia and generous hydration to facilitate the passage of the stone. During the acute episode the patient's urine should be collected and strained through a filter so that the stone can be analyzed if passed. An intravenous pyelogram or renal ultrasound should be done to localize the site of the obstruction. A urologic consultation should be obtained because if the stone becomes lodged in the urinary tree and is not progressing downward, the patient might need urologic intervention.

The patient who is incidentally found to have kidney stones on an abdominal x-ray and who has no evidence of active stone disease can be watched and any work up postponed unless the disease becomes active or there are metabolic abnormalities on routine blood tests precluding such an approach. The patient with active stone disease falls into a different category. This patient should be asked about prior history of stone analysis to determine which kind of stone he might have. A routine biochemical profile including renal function tests, uric acid, and calcium levels will be very helpful in ruling out some of the conditions previously outlined. A 24-hour urine for calcium, oxalate, uric acid, citrate, and phosphate, the urine pH, and a urine culture will be especially helpful. For example, in the case in which idiopathic hypercalciuria is found the treatment with thiazide diuretics may be very helpful. In a patient with uric acid stones found to have hyperuricosuria, acidic urine and low urinary volume the treatment involves alkalinizing the urine. This can be done with the administration of potassium citrate whose metabolism yields bicarbonate thereby raising the urinary pH. Allopurinol which blocks the oxidation of xanthine or hypoxanthine to uric acid will help decrease the uricosuria.

Persistent Hematuria/Rule Out Neoplasm

The finding of persistent hematuria should prompt an aggressive search for urologic neoplasm. The initial step should begin with a urinalysis. The presence of a positive sediment (i.e., pyuria, WBC and RBC masts) will point toward infection or glomerulonephritis. A negative sediment should lead to visualization studies either urography or ultrasound. These tests can be used interchangeably especially in the patient at risk for contrast nephropathy (3). They can also be complementary in the patient in whom a renal mass has been found on IVP to classify the mass as either cystic or solid. A cystic mass might have benign radiographic characteristics and could be followed by serial sonograms whereas a solid or mixed mass may be followed by abdominal CT and or selective arteriogram. A negative IVP or ultrasound should be followed by cystoscopy to completely visualize the bladder mucosa. Urine cytologies should also be obtained concurrently during that process. This work up will identify almost all urologic neoplasms. If negative and all medical causes of hematuria have been excluded, this patient can be evaluated at 6-month intervals with urine cytologies.

ILLUSTRATIVE CASES WITH SELF-ASSESSMENT QUESTIONS AND ANSWERS

Case 1

A 68-year-old man with new onset diabetes mellitus has moderate blood on routine office dipstick for the second time this month. He is completely asymptomatic. The history is significant for tobacco use, which was stopped 4 years ago. The physical examination is unremarkable.

QUESTION: *How would you proceed?*

a. Repeat a formal urinalysis.
b. Give the patient a 6-month appointment for evaluation.

ANSWER: a. *You opt to repeat the urinalysis to confirm and quantitate the level of hematuria and to examine the sediment. It is not appropriate to give him a 6-month appointment without an evaluation. The urinalysis is significant for nine red blood cells, no leukocytes, nitrite, protein and two white blood cells. You decide to obtain a urine culture to rule out occult infection. The urine culture is negative.*

QUESTION: *How would you proceed?*

a. Urine cytologies x 3
b. Renal ultrasound or intravenous urography
c. Referral to the urologist
d. All of the above

ANSWER: d. *All of the above. The urine cytology is important because it may demonstrate atypical cells that will further guide your diagnostic work up. It is best to collect the first voided specimen of the day because of the greater likelihood of detecting an abnormality. The imaging studies ie the renal ultrasound and the urography may visualize lesions along the urinary tract. The urine cytologies are negative as well as the renal ultrasound. The urologist decides to perform a cystoscopy, which is also negative. Your advice to the patient at this point is to continue routine follow up with you, which include periodic urinalysis and urine cytologies.*

Case 2

A 72-year-old man comes to the ER with acute urinary retention. He says that for the last few days he has been voiding clots, which got progressively larger. He became concerned when he developed suprapubic pain and difficulty urinating. The history reveals active tobacco use and the physical examination is significant for a distended bladder.

QUESTION: *What would you do next?*

a. Hydrate him in an attempt to induce him to urinate.
b. Catheterize him to relieve the obstruction.
c. Call the urologist.

ANSWER: b *and* **c.** *This man needs to be catheterized to relieve the urinary obstruction. In addition, he needs a urologic consultation because his passage of large clots is ominous. The urologist sees him and decides to fit him in an open slot for a cystoscopy. The patient has a large fungating lesion in the bladder.*

SUGGESTED READINGS

Urinary Tract Infection

Goroll AH, May LA, Mulley Jr, eds. Primary Care Medicine. 3rd ed. Philadelphia: JB Lippincott Company, 1995.

Kumin CM. Duration and treatment of urinary tract infections. Am J Med 1981; 71:849–854.

Neu HC. Urinary tract infections. Am J Med 1992; 92:4a-635–4a-5.

Richardson DA. Dysuria and urinary tract infections. Obstet Gynecol Clin North Am 1990;17:881–888.

Renal Insufficiency

Brenner, Barry M. Nephron adaptation to renal injury or ablation. Am J Physiol 1985;249 (Renal Fluid Electrolyte Physiol):F324-F337.

Giovanetti S, Cupisti A, Barsotti G. The metabolic acidosis of chronic renal failure: Pathophysiology and treatment. The kidney today: Selected topics in renal science. Contrib Nephrol (Basel, Karger) 1992;100:48–57.

Humphries JE. Anemia of renal failure use of erythropoietin. Med Clin North Am 1992;76: 2.

Jacobson HR. Chronic renal failure: Pathophysiology. Lancet 1991;338:419–423.

Klahr S. Chronic renal failure: Management. Lancet 1991;338:423–427.

Schaefer F, Mehls O, Ritz E. New insights into endocrine disturbances of chronic renal failure. Miner Electrolyte Metab 1992;18:169–173.

Hematuria

Aslaksen A, Gadehoh G, Gothlin JH. Ultrasonography in the evaluation of patient with microscopic hematuria. Br J Urol 1990;66:144–147.

Brenner BM. Brenner and Rector's the Kidney. 5th ed. Philadelphia: WB Saunders, 1996.

Coe FL, Parks JH, Asplin JR. The pathogenesis and treatment of kidney stones. NEJM 1992;327:1141–1152.

Sutton JL. Evaluation of hematuria in adults. JAMA 1990;263:2475–2481.

REFERENCES

Urinary Tract Infection

1. Stamm WE, Counts GW, Wagner KF, et al. Antimicrobial prophylaxis of recurrent urinary tract infections. Ann Intern Med 1980;92:770–775.

Renal Insufficiency

1. Beckie M, Burke JF Jr. Chronic renal disease: New therapy to delay kidney replacement. Geriatrics 1994;49:33–38.
2. Parving HH. Clinical experience in the treatment of diabetic renal disease (type 1 and 2); Summary and concluding remarks. Kidney Intl 1994;45:S165-S166.
3. Oldrizzi, Rugiu C, Biase V, et al. The place of hypertension among the risk factors for renal function in chronic renal failure. Am J Kidney Dis 1993; 21:119–123.
4. Klahr S, Levey AS, Beck GJ. The effects of dietary protein restriction and blood pressure control on the progression of chronic renal disease. N Engl J Med 1994;330:no.13.

Hematuria

1. Sutton JL. Evaluation of hematuria in adults. JAMA 1990; 263:2475–2481.
2. Coe FL, Parks JH, Asplin JR. The pathogenesis and treatment of kidney stones. NEJM 1992;327:1141–1152.
3. Aslaksen A, Gadehoh G, Gothlin JH. Ultrasonography in the evaluation of patient with microscopic hematuria. Br J Urol 1990;66:144–147.

chapter 18

ENDOCRINOLOGY AND METABOLIC DISORDERS

Robert L. Braham, Lori A. Lemberg, Perry Pong,
Lisa M. Rucker and James K. Stulman

DIABETES MELLITUS

Diabetes mellitus is an extremely common disease—affecting about 6% of Americans older than 40 years of age. Because of the multiplicity of serious complications, it is a disease that causes a very high number of visits to clinicians. It is the second most common diagnosis prompting a visit to an internist, the fifth most common diagnosis prompting a visit to general and family practitioners and an extremely common predisposing illness prompting visits to ophthalmologists, general surgeons, and many other specialists (1).

There are two major types of diabetes. The first is marked by absolute deficiency of insulin secretion and a tendency toward ketosis. The second is marked by a resistance of the liver and muscle tissues to the effect of insulin. In 1979, the National Diabetes Data Group set clearer definitions for these syndromes and also changed the criteria for the diagnosis of diabetes mellitus (Table 18.1). The first major type was called Type 1 or insulin-dependent diabetes mellitus (IDDM). The second group was called Type 2 or noninsulin dependent diabetes mellitus (NIDDM). These terms superseded older terms like adult-onset diabetes, juvenile diabetes, and a host of others. Because many Type 2 diabetics are treated with insulin, many health care providers feel that the terms Type 1 and Type 2 are less confusing than IDDM and NIDDM, and these terms will be used in the remainder of this chapter.

Type 1 diabetes mellitus is more common in Caucasians whereas Type 2 diabetes is more common in Native Americans, Hispanics, and Blacks. Irrespective of ethnicity, Type 2 diabetes is much more common in obese individuals and becomes increasingly prevalent in countries that have adopted a lifestyle of increased caloric intake and decreased exercise.

The criteria for the diagnosis of diabetes mellitus of either type were set by the Diabetes Data Group to require fasting blood sugars of over 140 mg/dl and/or random blood sugars in excess of 200 mg/dl. In addition to clarification of the terminology of the two major types of diabetes mellitus, the Diabetes Data Group eliminated the terminology "prediabetes" and substituted "impaired glucose tolerance" for patients whose fasting blood sugar is between the values of 115 and 140 mg/dl and/or whose 2-hour post prandial blood sugar is between 140 and 200 mg/dl (the range between normal and overt diabetes). This was done because many patients with this level of glucose intolerance do not eventually go on to develop overt diabetes, and the adverse psychological effects of "labeling" these patients as diabetics and/or the dangers of treating them with pharmacological agents outweighed any benefit from identifying them as diabetics.

Because of the benefits on fetal outcome of identifying and treating hyperglycemia during pregnancy and the alterations of glucose metabolism in the pregnant state, the criteria for diagnosis of gestational diabetes have been set somewhat differently (See Table 18.1).

Pathophysiologic Correlation

A discussion of the pathophysiology of diabetes mellitus involves a review of the normal physiology

341

Table 18.1.
National Diabetes Data Group Classification of Diabetes Mellitus

Class	Clinical Characteristics	Diagnostic Criteria
Insulin-dependent diabetes mellitus (IDDM, type I)	Ketosis prone; dependent on insulin for survival; usual onset in youth; absolute insulin deficiency; anti-islet cell antibodies often present at diagnosis	Unequivocal elevation of blood glucose with polyuria, polydipsia, weight loss, weakness
Non-insulin-dependent diabetes mellitus (NIDDM, type II)	Ketosis resistant; usual onset after age 40; majority obese; insulin resistance often present with inadequate insulin secretion	Same criteria as for IDDM; fasting plasma glucose (PG)[a] $\geq$ 140 mg/dl on more than one occasion, or 75 g oral glucose tolerance test (OGTT) yields 0.5, 1.0, or 1.5 hr PG and 2 hr PG values $\geq$ 200 mg/dl
Secondary diabetes	Diabetes in association with other conditions, including pancreatic disease (e.g., chronic pancreatitis), endocrine diseases (e.g., acromegaly or Cushing's syndrome), and certain medications (e.g., thiazides, glucocorticoids)	Same criteria as for IDDM and NIDDM
Impaired glucose tolerance	Asymptomatic; may represent normal variation of glucose in the population; however, one third eventually develop NIDDM; not at risk for long-term diabetic complications but at risk for cardiovascular complications	OGTT yields fasting PG < 140 mg/dl; 0.5, 1.0, or 1.5 hr PG $\geq$ 200 mg/dl; and 2 hr PG of 140–200 mg/dl
Gestational diabetes mellitus	Glucose intolerance with onset during pregnancy (usually at 24–30 weeks' gestation); associated with increased perinatal complications; glucose intolerance corrects after delivery, but NIDDM occurs in 30%–50% within 10 years; occurs in 2%–3% of all pregnancies	100 g OGTT[b] yields at least two of the following values: fasting PG $\geq$ 105 mg/dl, 1 hr PG $\geq$ 190 mg/dl, 2 hr PG $\geq$ 165 mg/dl, 3 hr PG $\geq$ 145 mg/dl

[a]Venous and capillary whole blood glucose levels are 10%–15% lower than plasma values.
[b]A 50 g one-hour screening test is now recommended for all pregnant women at 24–28 weeks. If the 1 hr PG is $\geq$ 140 mg/dl, a 100 g OGTT should be administered.

and pathophysiology of the hormonal control of glucose metabolism, a presentation of the differences between Type 1 and Type 2 diabetes mellitus and a discussion of the complications of diabetes. For these complications, emphasis will be placed on pathophysiologic mechanisms and the evidence for benefit of interventions that improve blood glucose metabolism and/or lipid metabolism.

PHYSIOLOGY OF HORMONAL CONTROL OF GLUCOSE METABOLISM

In normal individuals, the level of plasma glucose remains in a relatively narrow range (60-140 mg/dl) in both the fasting and postprandial states and

increases in a similar pattern following meals that are vastly different in relative composition of carbohydrates, protein, and fat. After a meal, the pancreatic secretion of insulin is stimulated and the combination of hyperglycemia and hyperinsulinemia increase the uptake of glucose into the liver, gut and muscle tissues. The hyperinsulinemia suppresses hepatic glucose output by promoting glycogen storage and inhibiting gluconeogenesis. Insulin also promotes lipogenesis by increasing very low density lipoprotein (VLDL) and triglyceride production by the liver and by stimulating the lipoprotein lipase in capillaries, which in turn promotes adipose tissue deposition.

In the fasting state, the concentration of insulin decreases and the concentration of other "counter-regulatory" hormones increases. Glucose is taken up and metabolized principally by insulin-independent tissues like brain and splanchnic organs and this disposal rate is precisely matched by the output of glucose by the liver. The major physiologic counterregulatory hormone is glucagon, which is secreted by the alpha cells of the pancreatic islet in response to a decrease in blood glucose and insulin levels. Glucagon increases blood sugar by promoting gluconeogenesis and glycogenolysis and also promotes lipolysis and the production of ketones from the free fatty acids produced by this lipolysis. The other counterregulatory hormones have a less important role in the normal fasting state but may be important in glucose regulation in periods of stress or specific pathologic states (e.g., Cushing syndrome). Cortisol, growth hormone, and catecholamines all increase hepatic glucose output and lipolysis and decrease the rate of glucose utilization by muscle. Beta endorphins increase the secretion of glucagon.

PATHOPHYSIOLOGY OF HORMONAL CONTROL OF GLUCOSE METABOLISM

From this description, it follows that diabetes mellitus can develop from defects in β-cell secretion of insulin, in the overproduction or abnormal regulation of counterregulatory hormones, and in resistance to the effects of insulin in the major target organs of liver and muscle.

Insulin is produced by the pancreatic β cell first as a 109 amino acid peptide (preproinsulin) and after several steps is secreted into the circulation as a 51 amino acid peptide (insulin) and another fragment (C peptide) in equimolar amounts. In normal individuals, plasma insulin begins to increase within the first 10 minutes of an increase in blood sugar (first phase) and continues to be elevated as long as there is hyperglycemia. This is most easily demonstrated in an intravenous glucose tolerance test. In Type 1 diabetes, the production of insulin is greatly diminished or absent. In the earliest stages of Type 2 diabetes, the first phase of insulin secretion is blunted but the total amount of insulin secreted is usually normal or high. As time passes, in the usual course of Type 2 diabetes, the amount of insulin secreted falls to normal or subnormal levels. The exact etiology of this progressive fall in insulin secretion in Type 2 diabetes is still under investigation, but the preponderance of the evidence suggests that it is due to "glucose toxicity," a diminution in the ability of the β cell

to respond to a hyperglycemic challenge. This concept is bolstered by the clinical and experimental observation that any mechanism that improves metabolic control of blood sugar (diet, exogenous insulin therapy, sulfonylureas) will increase endogenous insulin secretion in Type 2 diabetics in whom the levels have decreased.

In both Type 1 and Type 2 diabetes, the decrease in insulin levels prompts the increased secretion of glucagon despite the presence of hyperglycemia. This increased glucagon to insulin ratio promotes glycogenolysis and gluconeogenesis—increasing hepatic glucose output.

In periods of severe physiologic stress, like infections, trauma, or myocardial infarction, the levels of epinephrine, norepinephrine, cortisol, growth hormone, and β-endorphins are elevated. As described, above this tends to increase hepatic glucose output and promote ketogenesis. This can be further exacerbated in otherwise well-compensated Type 2 diabetics by the suppressive effects of catecholamines on endogenous insulin secretion. Stimulation of alpha adrenergic receptors in the islets suppresses insulin secretion; beta adrenergic receptor stimulation has the opposite effect. In physiologic stress, the suppressive effect of the adrenergic receptors predominates.

Lastly, major deficiencies in the control of blood glucose can be engendered by resistance of peripheral target tissues to the action of insulin. This can occur because of the opposition of counterregulatory hormones but occurs more commonly as a primary defect in Type 2 diabetes mellitus. Insulin is a peptide hormone that acts on target cells by attaching to a membrane receptor and then effecting numerous "post receptor" chemical events. The details of these events and the experimental basis of the conclusions are beyond the scope of this chapter. In brief, the elevation of blood sugar seen in both types of diabetes is due to a decrease in the insulin-mediated uptake of glucose in muscle and an increase in hepatic glucose output unrestrained by insulin action. In Type 1 diabetes, this is due to a deficiency of endogenous insulin production. In Type 2 diabetes, a resistance to the effect of insulin appears to predate the deterioration in glucose metabolic control and to be the major factor in its pathogenesis. Most of this resistance in both muscle and hepatic tissues appears to be at the post-receptor level, although Type 2 diabetics (particularly if obese) seem to have fewer insulin receptors per target cell. As fasting and post prandial hyperglycemia develop in Type 2 diabetics, stimulation of the β-cell causes more hyperinsulinemia and a down regulation of both receptor number and post-receptor events, thereby exacerbating the insulin resistance.

TYPE 1 AND TYPE 2 DIABETES

The two major types of diabetes are principally differentiated by the absence or near absence of endogenous insulin secretion in Type 1 and by peripheral insulin resistance with variable insulin secretion in Type 2.

The pathogenesis of Type 1 diabetes is thought to involve an autoimmune etiology with 70-80% of patients having anti islet cell antibodies. The trigger to this autoimmune response is under investigation, with some evidence that it may be due to viral infection in genetically predisposed individuals. There is a higher prevalence of HLA types DR-3 and DR-4 in Type 1 diabetics; these HLA types are associated with other autoimmune diseases. However, the inheritance of Type 1 diabetes is not as strong as that of Type 2 diabetes; the concordance in monozygotic twins is only about 40%. Islet cell antibodies have been detected years before the onset of diabetes in first degree relatives of Type 1 diabetics. If these relatives have both antibodies and the same HLA type, the likelihood of developing Type 1 diabetes is 50% in the next 7 years. At present, studies are underway to determine a safe way to prevent full blown Type 1 diabetes in predisposed patients like these.

Type 2 diabetes is much more common than Type 1 diabetes, accounting for about 92% of the total cases in the US, with the prevalence increasing with age and adiposity. The inheritance is strong with a concordance of almost 100% in monozygotic twins. There is a very strong association between Type 2 diabetes and obesity, atherosclerosis, hyperlipidemia, and hypertension. Several investigators have believed that all of these defects are linked via the mechanism of insulin resistance and hyperinsulinemia and have dubbed this constellation "Syndrome X." Hyperinsulinemia may act as a growth factor to induce proliferation of components of arterial walls to initiate or aggravate macrovascular disease and, via similar effects on arterioles,to promote hypertension. This tendency to hypertension is aggravated by the effect of hyperinsulinemia to promote renal tubular absorption of sodium. As previously described, hyperinsulinism promotes lipogenesis and the hepatic production of VLDL and triglycerides.

From a clinical standpoint, Type 1 diabetes generally occurs in younger people, rarely presenting

after age 40, and usually presents as polydipsia, polyuria, polyphagia, weight loss, and fatigue of abrupt onset. Type 2 diabetes occurs principally in older obese individuals who may have nonspecific symptoms and usually cannot precisely date the onset of the disease.

In addition to the two major types, there are several "secondary" forms of diabetes. The first is due to destruction of pancreatic islets as a result of chronic pancreatitis—usually from alcoholism, but occasionally from other diseases like hemochromatosis. It is necessary to lose about 90% of islets before clinical diabetes is manifest, and patients with chronic pancreatitis usually manifest exocrine insufficiency (diarrhea) before endocrine insufficiency. When manifest, the diabetes is more like Type 1, except that there is usually less glucagon secretion. As discussed below, diabetes in alcoholics is a dangerous disease requiring skilled management. Diabetes, or at least glucose intolerance, can be caused by the overproduction of the main counterregulatory hormones—cortisol in Cushing syndrome, catecholamines in pheochromocytoma, and growth hormone in acromegaly. However, the vast majority of the cases of diabetes secondary to "counterregulatory" hormone excess is due to the iatrogenic Cushing syndrome seen in the estimated 5 million Americans each year who are given corticosteroid hormones for the treatment of inflammatory diseases. Lastly, several commonly used medications, including thiazide diuretics, β adrenergic blockers, and phenytoin cause a deterioration in glycemic control by blunting the secretion of insulin in response to a hyperglycemic challenge.

PATHOPHYSIOLOGY OF COMPLICATIONS OF DIABETES

The pathophysiology of many of the complications of diabetes mellitus has been extensively scrutinized in recent years from the standpoint of both general pathophysiologic mechanisms and the likelihood that complications can be prevented by specific therapeutic interventions – usually "tight control" of blood glucose and attention to blood pressure and blood lipid levels. Although controversies about tight control persist, in the past few years evidence has accumulated favoring tight control as a factor in preventing complications in Type 1 diabetics, and trials in progress should help settle the remaining questions in Type 2 diabetics.

Thus far, efforts to find a single pathogenic mechanism to explain all of the complications of diabetes have been unsuccessful. Numerous abnormalities have been noted. The first group is clearly associated with hyperglycemia and is manifest by abnormalities in polyol (especially sorbitol) metabolism and in the excessive glycation of circulating and membrane bound proteins. The second group is associated with vascular abnormalities including accelerated atherosclerosis, changes in the endothelium, and changes in supporting cells like mesangial cells in the glomerulus and pericytes in the retina. The third group of abnormalities are found in platelet and granulocyte function and several growth factors.

Retinopathy. Retinopathy occurs in both Type 1 and Type 2 diabetics and, like all complications of diabetes, is likely to be more severe the longer the patient has had the disease. There are two stages of retinopathy—non proliferative (or "background") and proliferative. The latter is much more likely to cause impairment in vision. The first changes in the retina usually occur about 3-5 years after the onset of the disease and begin with microaneurysms (<100 μm) that arise from the terminal capillaries of the retina. As these microaneurysms begin to leak, erythrocytes cause dot and blot hemorrhages and serous fluid causes "hard" exudates. Unless there is leakage near the macula, there is generally no loss of vision from these nonproliferative changes. As time passes and the vessels become occluded, infarctions occur in the nerve layer of the retina and are seen as "cotton wool" exudates. In response to ischemia, new vessels develop (neovascularization). The fragile new vessels proliferate out of the retina into the vitreous (proliferative retinopathy) and usually leak and bleed. These vitreous hemorrhages will sometimes acutely impede vision but are usually absorbed in a few months. Unfortunately, as they are absorbed, fibroproliferative changes occur that exert traction on the retina and cause subsequent retinal detachment and loss of vision. The course of progression of retinopathy with conventional therapy is somewhat variable, but about 50% of patients will develop non proliferative retinopathy within seven years, and 90% will develop nonproliferative retinopathy in 20 years. The ability to detect mild non proliferative retinopathy by ophthalmoscopy is much less sensitive than by other techniques, such as seven field stereoscopic fundus photography and fluorescein angiography. This last technique is the most sensitive in detecting rare isolated microaneurysms in early non proliferative retinopathy.

The pathogenesis of retinopathy has not been completely clarified but seems to be at least partially due to the effects of hyperglycemia on the glycation of proteins in the retina and to an effect on the pericytes of the retina.

Cataracts and Other Changes in the Lens. During periods of hyperglycemia, changes in osmotic forces cause changes in refraction of the lens, hence patients often experience a blurring of vision. These visual symptoms generally resolve with better glycemic control, and patients should not seek new eyeglasses until two months after metabolic control is established. In addition, hyperglycemia causes excess production of sorbitol in the lens over a longer period of time. It is thought that these chronic changes in osmolality cause the development of cataracts—an irreversible process.

Nephropathy. Nephropathy is a less common complication of diabetes than retinopathy, occurring in about 40% of patients with Type 1 and less than 20% of patients with Type 2 diabetes. The earliest detectable abnormality in diabetic nephropathy is the development of microalbuminuria (30 to 300 mg of albumin in 24 hours), which may occur as early as 5 years after the onset of diabetes. If the disease progresses, in another 5-10 years overt proteinuria (> 300 mg/day of albuminuria) and hypertension develop, and the glomerular filtration rate begins to decrease. Endstage renal disease does not usually develop before 20 years of diabetes, unless other conditions coexist (e.g., poorly controlled hypertension). Unlike retinopathy, whose prevalence continuously increases with the duration of diabetes, nephropathy is unlikely to develop in patients who do not develop overt proteinuria after 25-30 years.

The histopathologic changes in diabetic nephropathy follow a progression beginning with an increase in size of the glomeruli (principally mesangium and basement membrane) and a consequent increase in total renal size. As the disease progresses, arteriosclerosis of afferent and efferent arterioles begins, some glomeruli close, and others hypertrophy. The pathognomonic lesions of Kimmelstiel – Wilson nodular glomerulosclerosis occur in a minority of patients with diabetic nephropathy, but all patients with endstage diabetic nephropathy eventually develop small, atrophic kidneys with diffuse glomerulosclerosis.

Much like diabetic retinopathy, the pathogenesis of nephropathy is still incompletely understood. Nephropathy may result from an interplay of genetic, metabolic, and hemodynamic alterations (3). In terms of the question of correlation with glycemic control, there is a large body of evidence demonstrating that an increase in nonenzymatic glycosylation of glomerular basement membrane and collagen in blood vessel walls occurs in the setting of hyperglycemia and that this may be important in the pathogenesis of diabetic nephropathy.

Neuropathy. There are three distinct types of neuropathy in patients with diabetes mellitus. The most common is a distal symmetrical sensorimotor neuropathy. Patients with this disorder have primarily sensory disturbances in a proximal to distal gradient that is worst in a distribution that would be covered by stockings and gloves—prompting the name "stocking glove neuropathy." The sensory symptoms are often unnoticed by patients and can include loss of proprioception, vibratory sense, pain, temperature perception, and light touch. As the process progresses, patients may notice that they have lost sensation in their feet and that their shoes feel "softer" (or more ominously, they do not notice pebbles or other irritating bodies that have gotten into their shoes). They may also notice unsteadiness of gait associated with the loss of proprioception. Less commonly, this symmetrical polyneuropathy causes hyperesthesia in the affected areas, ranging from mild tingling to excruciating lancinating pain exacerbated by light touch (e.g., bed clothes). It is common for patients with hypesthesia associated with poor glycemic control to go through a brief period of mild hyperesthesia as they achieve better glycemic control. The clinician should warn them about this and emphasize that it is a sign of improvement in nerve function that almost never lasts or progresses to truly painful neuropathy. Motor abnormalities are less clinically significant than sensory abnormalities but can be manifest by a diminished ability to move and separate the toes. This may be important in creating different pressure points on the toes and in subsequent callus and ulcer formation. Loss of strength in the interosseous muscles of the hand may be perceived as weakness of grip and inability to open jars.

In a process similar to that thought to be important in the pathogenesis of cataracts, hyperglycemia is associated with an accumulation of sorbitol in Schwann cells in nerve tissue. This causes an increase in intracellular osmolality and subsequent swelling, anoxia, and demyelination. In addition, the concentration of myoinositol in peripheral nerves is decreased in hyperglycemia − a factor thought to be associated with dysfunction. There is a strong correlation between glycemic control and the symptoms of this polyneuropathy.

The second type of neuropathy in diabetics is asymmetric and associated with one nerve trunk (mononeuritis) or more than one trunk (mononeuritis multiplex). Commonly affected nerves are cranial, particularly the third cranial nerve, and nerves that are subject to external pressure or entrapment (e.g., carpal tunnel). Onset of dysfunction is usually sudden and there is partial or complete recovery in a period of months. Because these neuropathies are more common in older Type 2 diabetics and have characteristics suggesting acute ischemic events, it is generally thought that there is a vascular contribution to their pathogenesis.

The third type of neuropathy in diabetics is autonomic dysfunction. Although the most common presenting symptom of autonomic neuropathy is impotence in men, further questioning and specific testing will usually reveal that more than one autonomic function is abnormal. Many patients will have bladder abnormalities that may be manifested early by an increase in the intervals between voidings and progress to other symptoms of poor emptying and bladder distention. Patients will frequently have resting tachycardia and orthostatic blood pressure changes. The cardioregulatory dysfunction can be quantitated by measuring the beat to beat (R-R interval on EKG) variation in response to a Valsalva maneuver. These cardiovascular abnormalities have been found to have an adverse effect on overall life expectancy and on perioperative mortality. Symptoms of gastrointestinal autonomic dysfunction include gastric atony (manifested as early satiety), occasional nausea and vomiting, and diarrhea, which is usually due to small bowel dysfunction. The diarrhea is usually episodic and worse at night. Impaired sensation of fecal distention may lead to incontinence.

Infections. Infections are commonly seen in diabetics due to several different factors. Hyperglycemia inhibits the phagocytic activity of granulocytes. Candidal infections of the skin and mucous membranes, furuncles of the skin, and external otitis are all more common in diabetics. Infections are more likely to occur in the static conditions of bladders and small intestines of patients with autonomic neuropathy. Infections in the feet occur because of patients' inability to feel irritants in their shoes and because vascular disease and a diminished ability to adjust the muscles and bones of the foot to fit shoes lead to ulceration. Once ulceration has occurred, the likelihood of osteomyelitis dramatically increases, and the compromised blood supply makes antibiotic treatment less efficacious.

Cardiovascular Disease. Cardiovascular disease is the most frequent cause of death in diabetics and occurs at double the rate of nondiabetics in patients stratified for other risks of cardiovascular disease. Its onset is earlier and the pattern of atherosclerosis is often more diffuse than in non diabetics. Arterial insufficiency of the lower legs is particularly more prevalent in diabetics than in other patients with atherosclerosis. Diabetics with coronary artery disease sometimes have ischemia or infarction without pain, presumably owing to abnormalities in afferent nerve fibers.

The pathogenesis of this macrovascular disease is thought to be somewhat different from the microvascular disease of the retina and glomerulus. As described earlier, the hyperinsulinism of Type 2 diabetics is associated with an increase in the hepatic synthesis of VLDL, and diabetics generally have lower levels of HDL than nondiabetics. In patients with chronic hyperglycemia, circulating lipoproteins become glycosylated, which seems to decrease their turnover and increase their deposition in arterial walls.

Clinical and Laboratory Evaluation

The history and physical examination can give information about the consequences and severity of the diabetes mellitus and the length of time glucose intolerance is likely to have been present. In addition, certain findings can alert the clinician to a differentiation of Type 1 and Type 2 diabetes or to one of the rarer secondary causes of diabetes. Laboratory evaluation is principally used to assess the nature of the consequences of diabetes on the specific target organs and to make decisions about initial therapy.

HISTORY

The diagnosis of Type 1 diabetes is made relatively easily in a patient who was previously well and describes the subacute onset of polyuria, polydipsia, polyphagia (the "polys") and a general loss of strength and feeling of good health. If the patient presents with ketoacidosis, he or she is often too ill to accurately describe the onset of the symptoms but should be able to do so after treatment. The diagnosis of Type 2 diabetes is more difficult to make from historical data, as the patients may not notice the more gradual and less severe onset of the "polys" and may be asymptomatic or only complain of vague symptoms of malaise. Because of the chronicity of the disease and its multiple consequences, it is more common that the initial visit to a specific clinician occurs after the diagnosis has been made and treatment has been instituted. In either case, once the diagnosis of diabetes mellitus

is made, the history should review any prior treatment; help evaluate the adequacy of glycemic control; determine the presence or absence of the chronic complications of diabetes; and help to formulate an overall management plan.

When inquiring about prior treatment, not only the type of pharmacologic or nonpharmacologic treatment that was used should be elicited, but also as much detail as possible about its success or reasons for failure (e.g., diet therapy that failed because of poor compliance or the use of other medications that may affect blood glucose concentrations). In this light, prior educational interventions with regard to diet, exercise, and, if applicable, home glucose monitoring should be sought. Any history of episodes of ketoacidosis or severe hypoglycemia should be recorded, as well as prior episodes of infections—particularly of the skin, foot, oral cavity, and genitourinary systems. Specific attention is paid to eliciting symptoms or prior laboratory tests that would be helpful in determining the extent of the consequences of diabetes on the eye, heart, kidney, central and peripheral nervous systems, lower extremities and cerebral circulation and on sexual function. Lastly, as other risk factors for atherosclerosis greatly add to the likelihood of development of vascular disease, data concerning smoking habits, hypertension, obesity, and hyperlipidemia must be obtained.

PHYSICAL EXAMINATION

The examination should focus on the consequences of diabetes in the major target organs and, at least briefly on the signs of the rare diseases that can cause secondary diabetes. In children, attention must be paid to the possibility of delayed growth and maturation. In all patients, the clinician should measure weight and assess adiposity, and blood pressure should be determined (with orthostatic measurement). A funduscopic examination, preferably with dilatation, and examination of the heart and peripheral pulses are necessary to assess vascular status. Examination of the feet should be done carefully to assess for sensory function (touch and vibration), Achilles tendon reflex, skin and nail changes, and for evidence of prior infection or ulcer. The patient's shoes should be examined for irregularities as part of an educational process to prevent future ulceration. Sites of frequent infection like the skin, oral cavity, and female genital tract should be examined for evidence of past or current infection. In addition to being checked for the signs of autonomic nervous system dysfunction elicited by orthostatic changes in blood pressure, and being tested for diabetic polyneuropathy in the feet, patients should have neurologic examinations to assess for the possibility of prior cerebrovascular accidents. The majority of authors recommend that all patients with diabetes be referred to an ophthalmologist for a comprehensive eye exam at the time of initial diagnosis, and certainly all patients with visual abnormalities should be referred.

LABORATORY EVALUATION

All patients should have an initial laboratory evaluation to establish the diagnosis of diabetes, determine the degree of glycemic control, and define associated complications and risk factors. This should include a single fasting blood glucose (or random glucose if the patient is symptomatic); a glycosylated hemoglobin determination; a fasting lipid profile with cholesterol fractionation; a serum creatinine and urinalysis; and an EKG in adults. In addition, urine culture, electrolyte measurement, testing for microalbuminuria and sophisticated neurologic testing should be done in selected patients.

The utility of the measurement of glycosylated hemoglobin (Hgb A_{1c}) as an index of chronic glucose levels is well established. Hgb A_{1c} is the nonenzymatic product of glucose and hemoglobin and reveals the mean blood glucose concentration during the half life of the protein. As the average life span of an erythrocyte is 120 days, a measurement of Hgb A_{1c} reflects the mean glucose level over the previous 60 days. The range of normal for the level of this protein varies slightly depending on the laboratory methods but is less than 6.4% in normal adults. The frequency of measurement of this protein as a guide to the adequacy of metabolic control depends on the expectations of the tightness of glucose control in individual patients. For Type 1 diabetics in whom very tight control is a goal, measurements need to be done at least four times yearly, and the target range is a level less than 7.5%. In Type 1 diabetics in whom the rigors of a regimen of tight control are impractical or unacceptable, a measurement of glycosylated hemoglobin should be done four times a year, but the target range is 7.5-9.5%. In Type 2 diabetics, the frequency and target range of glycosylated hemoglobin measurements is still somewhat controversial awaiting better data on the effects of tight control on the complications of Type 2 diabetes, but many clinicians use periodic glycosylated hemoglobin measurements in a manner similar to that used in Type 1 diabetics.

Differential Diagnosis

Once it has been determined that the patient has hyperglycemia, consideration of the history, physical examination, and laboratory tests can establish whether the patient has simply impaired glucose tolerance; either Type 1 or Type 2 diabetes; generalized pancreatic insufficiency from another cause; gestational carbohydrate intolerance; or hyperglycemia secondary to an excess of counterregulatory hormones. As mentioned previously, fasting blood sugars between 115 and 140 mg/dl and/or 2-hour post prandial blood sugars between 140 and 200 mg/dl are characteristic of impaired glucose tolerance, a condition that may progress to true diabetes mellitus. The diagnosis of Type 1 diabetes is rarely difficult once considered. The patients almost always present with polyuria, polydipsia, polyphagia, weight loss, and generalized fatigue (or stupor in cases in which the patient delayed seeking medical attention) developing in an abrupt way—the patient may be able to give the exact date of the onset of symptoms. The diagnosis can usually be confirmed by the presence of ketosis and, in severe cases, acidosis. The differentiation between Type 1 and Type 2 diabetes is rarely difficult, but in some cases of Type 2 diabetes in which endogenous insulin secretion is low, the clinical pictures are similar. There is almost never a clinical reason to differentiate between Type 1 and this stage of Type 2 if the patient requires exogenous insulin for treatment, but the presence and level of endogenous insulin secretion can be determined by measurement of levels of C peptide in the blood. Generalized pancreatic insufficiency is most commonly seen as a late stage of alcoholic pancreatitis and features of both exocrine insufficiency (diarrhea) and endocrine insufficiency (diabetes) are seen. Rarer causes include cystic fibrosis, amyloidosis, and hemochromatosis.

Diabetes is also more commonly seen in some muscular dystrophies, Friedrich's ataxia, and Turner's syndrome. A rare syndrome with extreme insulin resistance and acanthosis nigricans has been described. Diabetes mellitus can be a feature of the rare multiple endocrine failure syndrome (Hashimoto's thyroiditis, diabetes mellitus, hypophysitis, premature gonadal failure, Addison's disease, hypoparathyroidism) thought to be due to autoimmune causes.

Gestational diabetes mellitus and drug-induced glucose intolerance associated with thiazide diuretics, corticosteroids, or phenytoin are conditions that often remit when delivery occurs or the offending drug is discontinued. Diabetes mellitus associated with Cushing syndrome, pheochromocytoma, and acromegaly can usually be diagnosed because of specific symptoms of these diseases. Because of the low prevalence of these diseases and the high prevalence of obesity and hypertension in routine Type 2 diabetics, there is a high probability of false positive tests in patients undergoing work-up for nonspecific symptoms like obesity or hypertension. Therefore, extensive work-up should be reserved for more specific signs and symptoms or for patients who do not respond to treatment.

Management

All patients with diabetes need education to deal with a chronic serious disease for which changes in lifestyle, often major ones, are necessary. This can be challenging to the clinician and patient as the life style changes are usually more onerous than those in the other extremely common, minimally symptomatic disease—hypertension. The challenges of changing behavior in a middle-aged asymptomatic patient with Type 2 diabetes are different from those encountered in an adolescent patient with Type 1 diabetes who is in the midst of dealing with issues of autonomy and relationship to authority figures. In addition to changes in eating patterns and the use of medications, instruct patients in exercise regimens and to work toward a plan so that they can participate as much as possible in achieving metabolic control. Cessation of smoking is extremely important to decrease the likelihood of development of vascular disease. As it is unlikely that any health care provider will have the time to deal with these issues in the desirable detail, numerous booklets intended for patient use have been created and made available by the American Diabetes Association (1660 Duke Street, PO Box 25757, Alexandria, VA 22313; 1-800-232-3472), the US Public Health Service National Diabetes Information Clearinghouse (Box NDIC, Bethesda, MD 20892; 301-468-2612), and several pharmaceutical manufacturers.

RELATIONSHIP BETWEEN HYPERGLYCEMIA AND COMPLICATIONS

As described earlier in this chapter, although there are good pathophysiologic reasons to suggest that many of the complications of both Type 1 and Type 2 diabetes are due to the effects of hyperglycemia, until recently there was no well-controlled prospective trial to demonstrate that treatment of diabetics to achieve near normoglycemia ("tight control") actually prevented complications.

In the early 1980s, a large NIH-sponsored multicenter study was begun to determine whether intensive treatment with the goal of maintaining blood glucose concentrations close to the normal range could decrease the frequency and severity of these complications in Type 1 diabetics – the Diabetes Control and Complications Trial (DCCT) (4). Because this is a very important and frequently quoted study, some of the detail of the study design will be described so the reader can understand the applicability of the findings to the general population of Type 1 and Type 2 diabetics. Between the years 1983 and 1989, 1441 patients with Type 1 diabetes were recruited at 29 medical centers (average of 8 patients per center per year) and randomized into a regimen of intensive therapy or conventional therapy and followed for a mean of 6.5 years. Approximately half of these patients were without retinopathy at baseline (primary prevention cohort), and the other half had mild retinopathy (the secondary intervention cohort).

The patients assigned to intensive therapy self-administered insulin three or more times daily by injection or an external pump. The dosage was adjusted according to the results of self monitoring of blood glucose performed at least four times a day (including a weekly 3 AM measurement), dietary intake, and anticipated exercise. The goals of this intensive therapy included preprandial blood glucose concentrations between 70 and 120 mg/dl; postprandial concentrations of less than 180 mg/dl; 3 AM blood sugars greater than 65 mg/dl, and glycosylated hemoglobin determinations in the normal range (less than 6.05%). Patients in this group visited the study center at least once monthly and were contacted frequently by telephone to review and adjust their regimens.

Patients assigned to conventional therapy self administered one or two daily injections of insulin (including mixed intermediate and rapid acting insulins), self-monitored urine or blood glucose daily, and were educated about diet and exercise. These patients were not encouraged to make daily adjustments to their insulin regimen. Goals of therapy included the absence of symptoms attributable to glycosuria or hyperglycemia; the absence of ketonuria; the maintenance of normal growth, development, and ideal body weight; and freedom from severe or frequent hypoglycemia. Patients in this group were examined every 3 months. At the end of the study, the mean glycosylated hemoglobin concentration for the intensive therapy group was 7.0% and the level for the conventionally treated group was 9.1%.

Patients assigned to the intensive treatment group had less severe retinopathy, less albuminuria and less neuropathy at the end of the study. As the patients were young, the number of events attributable to macrovascular disease was small, and the reduction in the number of macrovascular complications in the intensively treated group was not statistically significant. There was no difference in death rates between the groups, and the major adverse effect of intensive treatment was a three fold increase in the incidence of severe hypoglycemia in the intensively treated group.

As a result of this study, the predominant opinion is that for most patients with Type 1 diabetes, intensive therapy with insulin is the preferred treatment but that large logistical barriers exist in trying to motivate patients to adhere to such a regimen and to provide the support necessary to make this therapy available. For the much larger group of Type 2 diabetics, the predominant opinion is that improvement in glycemic control probably decreases the incidence and progression of microvascular complications, but that data are not yet sufficient to decide whether treatments other than diet therapy are effective in decreasing the likelihood of complications. Intuitively, the greatest benefit should accrue to younger Type 2 diabetics who have enough life expectancy to benefit from interventions that should retard complications years in the future. As described earlier in this chapter, hyperinsulinism and insulin resistance are associated with weight gain, a worsening of lipid profiles, hypertension, and macrovascular complications. There is a theoretical concern that intensive insulin or oral hypoglycemic therapy may exacerbate macrovascular complications, the leading cause of morbidity and mortality in this disease. At the time of this writing, a trial is underway in the United Kingdom to determine the best way to avoid complications in Type 2 diabetics. Until the results of this trial are available, patients with Type 2 diabetes should be encouraged to adopt appropriate diet and exercise routines and only if these fail (by the criteria of "conventional therapy" in the DCCT trial), to begin oral hypoglycemic therapy or insulin therapy.

SELF MONITORING OF METABOLIC CONTROL

There are at least two reasons for patients to learn to monitor metabolic control themselves. Firstly, it is an excellent method for them to learn how changes in diet, exercise, and pharmacological therapy affect metabolic control and to involve them actively in the process of controlling their blood sugar. Secondly, it gives them a much better "early warning" system for acute or subacute changes in control due to intercurrent illness or other factors. This permits them to seek medical attention or self adjust therapy before the situation deteriorates further.

Historically, urine glucose and ketone measurements have been used by both Type 1 and Type 2 diabetics to monitor glycemic control. Although painless, relatively easy, and inexpensive, this technique suffers from several disadvantages. Firstly, there is an inability to distinguish moderate hyperglycemia from normoglycemia and hypoglycemia because of a renal threshold that prevents excretion of glucose until the blood level is 180 mg/dl or higher. Additionally, urine glucose determinations are affected by fluid intake (dilution of urine) and reflect an average level of blood glucose since the last voiding, not the level of blood glucose at the time of the test.

In recent years, technology has developed to permit patients to determine their own blood sugar levels with small samples of blood obtained via a fingerstick. This self monitoring of blood glucose (SMBG) is becoming more and more widespread, and it is estimated that over one million diabetics now use this technique. The number will continue to rise as the criteria for its use are broadened from only selected patients with difficult to control Type 1 diabetes to all patients in whom achievement of a goal of near normoglycemia is attempted. Clinicians should choose patients for whom achievement of this goal is advisable and who appear to be able to learn the technique (or who have significant others who will help them with it). The actual teaching is usually done by nurses, dietitians, pharmacists, manufacturers' representatives, and clinicians. Students should observe at least one such session, even if they do not plan to do such teaching, as it will be helpful to them in choosing patients who can comply with the instructions. In studies done on appropriate patients, 50-70% of patients who receive formal instruction can obtain results within 20% of the reference standard(5). In addition to the discomfort associated with a fingerstick, the other major factor inhibiting widespread use is the cost. Patients checking fingerstick blood glucoses four times daily will incur costs of 50-100 dollars a month for reagent strips.

The objectives of this technique are several. The first is the development of a data base concerning the patient's blood glucose profile under a variety of circumstances (e.g., changing meal and exercise patterns). This profile should be reviewed by the patient and health care provider to make adjustments in therapy and to enhance the patient's understanding of diabetes. In selected patients this technique permits increased flexibility in their lifestyle—permitting them to vary meal schedules and to engage in vigorous physical activity without undue concern about unappreciated major variations in glycemic levels. Lastly, it permits patients to recognize and respond to urgent or emergent situations like hypoglycemia, hyperglycemia associated with intercurrent illness, or ketoacidosis. In that light, specific instructions for the frequency of SMBG vary depending on the clinical situation. In patients in whom intensive therapy for Type 1 diabetes is prescribed, a regimen similar to that used in the DCCT is necessary. For patients with Type 1 diabetes in whom intensive therapy is unacceptable or impractical, once daily SMBG may suffice. For Type 2 diabetics, SMBG may not be necessary if goals of near normoglycemia are not attempted, but many patients report considerable satisfaction from more active participation in their own treatment program. As the goals for the "tightness" of control for Type 2 diabetics must vary according to individual patient's needs and abilities, the frequency of SMBG will vary. For many patients, a regimen of SMBG performed "twice a day, twice a week"—a fasting and a pre dinner check on one weekday and one weekend day—is sufficient to serve as a maintenance technique. Even if SMBG is not practiced on a regular basis by patients who are taught to do so, providers should instruct them that they should self monitor blood sugar at any time that they notice a specific or vague change in their health. An instruction that patients (or significant others) should perform SMBG "whenever you feel sick in any way" can often alert the patient and clinician to symptoms of hypoglycemia or severe hyperglycemia secondary to intercurrent illness.

DIET THERAPY

The approach to educating the patient about diet depends on the clinical situation. In some obese, Type 2 diabetics, diet is chosen as the first and only treatment for the glucose intolerance. In other diabetics, in whom insulin or oral hypoglycemic agents are selected for therapy, dietary habits may need to be tailored to the pharmacological time action of these drugs. In all diabetics, the underlying predisposition to accelerated atherosclerosis increases the importance of avoiding atherogenic foods.

Firstly, all diabetics should eat a diet similar to that recommended by the American Heart Association and the American Cancer Society in terms of fats, fiber, and other nutrients. Specifically, total fat should comprise <30% of total calories, saturated fat <10% of total calories, and cholesterol intake should be less than 300 mg/day. Protein intake should be about 0.8 g/kg of body weight; consideration of protein restriction should be made in patients with incipient renal disease. There is no evidence that diabetics need different amounts of vitamins and minerals than patients who do not have the disease.

In recent years, recommendations concerning carbohydrate intake have been modified so that a higher percentage of total calories (55-60%) should come from carbohydrates. Foods containing unrefined and complex carbohydrates with fiber should be substituted for highly refined carbohydrates, which are low in fiber. The former complete prohibition of sucrose and other refined sugars has been made more flexible so that some individuals may be allowed to consume modest quantities contingent on weight and metabolic control. All diabetics may be permitted an occasional "lapse" (e.g., birthday cake). As in most issues of self care in chronic disease, giving the patient some latitude and an understanding of the consequences of different actions may improve overall compliance.

In Type 2 diabetics, weight loss and exercise may be sufficient to normalize glycemia without need for pharmacological intervention. As opposed to the controversies regarding therapy with insulin and oral hypoglycemics in Type 2 diabetics, this therapeutic maneuver is universally recommended as the primary and best approach to most Type 2 diabetics. The metabolic improvements achieved with weight reduction include reduction in hyperglycemia, hyperinsulinemia, hyperlipidemia, hypertension, and proteinuria. Weight reduction also leads to improvement in pulmonary function, reduced perioperative risks, and reduced musculoskeletal problems. The problem with the diet and exercise therapy is not in its efficacy (Will it work under ideal circumstances?), but with its effectiveness (Will it work in patients who have the average level of compliance with the intervention?). Unfortunately, the success of health care providers is quite low in convincing patients to initiate and maintain weight loss over a long follow up period. Some patients will comply better with a regimen of caloric restriction and exercise if they are asked to perform self monitoring of blood glucose at home. The goal of this strategy is for patients to determine themselves that eating less and exercising more will improve glycemic control and to determine what kinds of meals or snacks raise blood sugar significantly. When used in this way, a month's trial of twice daily (fasting and pre dinner) self monitoring of blood glucose may help patients in complying with dietary therapy.

The timing and composition of meals and snacks must be tailored to the time of administration of insulin or oral hypoglycemic agents and to levels of exercise during the course of the day. This is particularly true in Type 1 diabetics, who have large swings in the level of blood glucose because of a complete absence of endogenous insulin secretion, and in Type 2 diabetics who are attempting to achieve near normoglycemia with the use of pharmacological treatments. A large percentage of patients eat the majority of their daily caloric intake after 6 PM—small breakfast, small lunch, large dinner and an evening of snacking while watching television. Ideally, it is preferable for these patients to spread out their calories over the day and efforts should be made to help them to do this. If this does not work out, at least patients should be instructed to keep their meal schedules consistent (don't skip meals); to understand something about the effect of unusual exercise in lowering blood sugar; and to understand the time action of the insulin or oral hypoglycemic agent they are taking in terms of specific times of the day at which they might be at greatest risk for large changes in blood sugar. The process of tailoring food intake and scheduling of pharmacological therapy is one that requires ongoing dialogue between the patient and clinician.

INSULIN THERAPY

Insulin therapy is absolutely necessary in the treatment of all patients with Type 1 diabetes and is used by many clinicians in the treatment of Type 2 diabetics. Almost all clinicians will use insulin or oral hypoglycemic agents in Type 2 diabetics if diet therapy fails to relieve symptoms of hyperglycemia (polyuria and polydipsia). Some clinicians choose insulin as the first therapy in this group of patients, while others choose oral hypoglycemic agents first and reserve insulin for patients in whom oral hypoglycemic agents do not achieve the desired effect. Still others use insulin in diabetics in whom diet therapy only improves glycemic control to a moderate extent (e.g., glycosylated hemoglobin in 7.5-9.5% range) to achieve tight metabolic control. The differences in approach and lack of firm guidelines reflect the lack of good evidence concerning the role of tight control using these agents in the initiation and progression of the complications of Type 2 diabetes.

Insulin Preparations. There are numerous preparations of insulin available in the United States. They vary in terms of species of origin, purity, concentration, and onset and duration of action. Standard grades of insulin are derived from the pancreases of pigs and beef cattle and are "purified" to contain less than 50 ppm of proinsulin. "Highly purified" preparations contain less than 10 ppm of proinsulin. Commercially available insulins are available in concentrations of 40, 100, and 500 units/mL (labeled U-40, U-100, and U-500, respectively). U-40 insulin is used infrequently, and U-500 insulin is used only in instances of extreme insulin resistance. The usual syringes available for insulin injection are calibrated for U-100 insulin. Pork and beef insulin differ from human insulin by one and three amino acids, respectively. Human insulin for commercial use is made with recombinant technology using yeasts or Escherichia coli. Despite the differences in amino acid composition between animal and human insulins, there is a very low incidence of antibody mediated insulin resistance or of local or systemic allergy to the animal preparations. There are very few diabetics who have an absolute indication for human insulin, but the only disadvantage of human insulin is the somewhat higher price (about 20%).

As is shown in Table 18.2, there are three general groups of insulin preparations in terms of their time of onset and duration of action—short, intermediate, and long acting. Different pharmaceutical companies have adopted different names for similar formulations, and human insulins usually have the most rapid onset and shortest duration of action followed by pork and then beef insulin. Regular and NPH insulins can be mixed in a syringe or bottle without loss of pharmacological properties and several preparations of a predetermined mixture of 70% NPH and 30% regular insulins are available. Similarly, different preparations from the lente series are able to be premixed without adverse effects but mixing of regular and lente insulins is not advised. In the United States, the most commonly used insulin preparations are regular and NPH insulin. Insulin bottles should be refrigerated when possible and carry expiration dates stamped on their labels. However, it is unusual for even unrefrigerated bottles to lose appreciable potency in less than 30 days. This is important for diabetics who must take multiple daily doses of insulin and

Table 18.2.
Insulin Preparations

Insulin Type	Specific Examples	Onset (hr)[a]	Peak Action (hr)[a]	Duration (hr)
Short acting	Regular, crystalline zinc insulin (CZI)	0.5–1.0	2–4	6–8
	Semilente	0.5–1.5	2–6	10–12
Intermediate acting	Neutral protamine Hagedorn (NPH)	2–4	4–12	10–24
	Lente	Same	Same	Same
Long acting	Protamine zinc (PZI)	8–14	14–24	24–36
	Ultralente	Same	18–24	Same

[a]The wide range in time action of these preparations relates to the fact that human insulins have a shorter time action than pork which is in turn shorter than beef. In addition, there is biologic variability between patients.

find it impossible to refrigerate the bottle during the day.

Insulin Injection. Insulin should be injected into the subcutaneous tissue of the upper arm, the anterior and lateral thigh, and the abdomen (except for a 2-inch radius around the navel). The injection site should be rotated to avoid local lipoatrophy or lipohypertrophy, and scar tissue or other poorly vascularized tissue should be avoided because of the unreliability of absorption. Insulin is absorbed more quickly from the anterior abdominal wall in a sedentary individual, but absorbed most quickly from an exercising limb (e.g., thigh in a jogger).

Timing and Dosing. The details of the timing and dosing of an insulin regimen depend on whether the patient has Type 1 or Type 2 diabetes and the level of tightness of control desired (Table 18.3). The most stringent schedule is necessary for Type 1 diabetics to achieve near normoglycemia and has been described above in the section concerning the DCCT trial. It requires at least four daily self monitorings of blood glucose (SMBG) and subcutaneous insulin injection by syringe or external pump at least three times daily. Each dose of insulin is adjusted by the patient in response to the SMBG result, dietary intake, and anticipated exercise. At the other end is so-called minimal therapy, in which the goal is avoidance of symptomatic hyperglycemia or hypoglycemia. In Type 2 diabetics, this can often be achieved with a single morning dose of a mixture of short and intermediate acting insulins. A middle course of average or conventional therapy sets a goal of near normal fasting blood sugars and glycosylated hemoglobin measurements in the 7.5-9.5% range. In some cases, insulin can be used in combination with an oral hypoglycemic agent. In one recent study, the addition of NPH insulin injected at 9 PM to a regimen

of oral agents given to Type 2 diabetics improved glycemic control without significant weight gain (6).

The most common initiation of insulin therapy in an ambulatory setting occurs in Type 2 diabetics who are not acutely ill and who have not achieved glycemic control after at least several weeks of diet therapy. The level of glycemic control desired and the length of a trial of diet therapy should be individualized. The initiation of insulin therapy is almost always done in these patients with an intermediate acting preparation. A safe initial dose for an individual who has never received insulin therapy is 15 units of NPH insulin before breakfast in a thin individual and 25 units in an obese one. During the initial phase of determining the correct total dose and the details of the dosing and timing of the regimen, it is necessary that the patient check metabolic control several times daily—either by urine glucose determinations or preferably with SMBG before each meal and at bedtime. Patients can usually increase the dose of insulin by 5 units every three days by keeping in telephone contact with a clinician. Specific additions of short acting insulin to the morning dose or additional daily injections are made using the results of SMBG or urine measurements (coupled with some blood measurements to establish the renal threshold). During this time, it is critical to remind the patient of the importance of keeping diet relatively constant in timing and composition and to note and record any reasons for major changes in metabolic control, like dietary indiscretions, unusual exercise, or intercurrent illness. This will give patients an understanding of factors that affect metabolic control for the future. It is also important to use this time to work with patients to achieve greater autonomy in controlling their disease and to assure them

Table 18.3.
Specific Insulin Regimens

Level of Therapy	Goal of Therapy	Sample Regimens	Monitoring Needed
Minimal therapy	Avoidance of symptomatic hyperglycemia or hypoglycemia in Type 1 and Type 2 diabetics Hgb A_{1c} 9.5–12%	Single early morning insulin injection: Most frequently mixture of intermediate and short acting insulins—e.g. 25 NPH and 10 regular.	Check urine or SMBG[a] if symptomatic of hyper or hypoglycemia or if "sick in any way"
Conventional therapy	Near normal fasting blood glucose in Type 1 and Type 2 diabetics—70–140 mg% Hgb A_{1c} 7.5–9.5%	Two insulin injections daily: *Example 1* Prebreakfast dose of 2/3 TDD[b] ~70% intermediate ~30% short acting Predinner dose of 1/3 TDD[b] ~70% intermediate ~30% short acting *Example 2* Prebreakfast dose of 3/4 TDD[b] ~70% intermediate ~30% short acting 9 PM dose of 1/4 TDD[b] All intermediate Combination insulin and oral agent: Oral hypoglycemic agent given in AM ~20 U intermediate insulin at 9 PM	Check urine or preferably SMBG[a] several times a week when stable. Example 1 Early AM and predinner twice weekly—one weekday and one weekend day Example 2 Early AM every day Patients should self monitor more frequently when sick or if regimen is being adjusted.
Intensive therapy	Near normal blood glucose throughout the day in Type 1 diabetics: Preprandial 70–120 mg% Postprandial <180 mg% Hgb A_{1c} <7.5%	Three or more insulin injections daily: Dosage adjusted individually for each insulin injection according to results of SMBG, dietary intake and anticipated exercise. *Example 1* *Prebreakfast* dose of combination of intermediate and short acting insulin *Predinner* dose of short acting insulin *9 PM* dose of intermediate acting insulin *Example 2* Short acting insulin given before breakfast lunch and dinner 9 PM dose of intermediate acting insulin *Example 3* Basal insulin rate supplied by insulin pump or ultralente insulin injection Short acting insulin given before breakfast lunch and dinner	SMBG at least four times daily including a weekly 3 AM measurement

[a]SMBG = Self monitoring of blood glucose.
[b]TDD = Total daily dose.
Premeal insulin should be administered 30–45 minutes before eating.

that the close dependence on the clinician will not be permanent. Reasonable control should be achievable within a few weeks.

If the pattern of SMBG or urine determinations is irregular and follows no pattern after months of treatment, the problem most commonly is poor compliance with diet or insulin administration. However, over the course of time, some patients will need more or less insulin to achieve glycemic control goals. Type 2 diabetics already have insulin resistance and may require more insulin if they gain weight. Intercurrent illness or trauma may increase insulin requirements but this should be apparent on clinical evaluation. A slow increase in insulin requirement may be due to the development of IgG antibodies to insulin that inhibit its attachment to membrane receptors. If patients are getting animal insulin, a switch to human insulin or a more purified product is warranted. If this doesn't work, a course of prednisone (40-60 mg/day) for 2 weeks will often dramatically decrease the immune insulin resistance. Discontinuation of the prednisone rarely causes the immune insulin resistance to recur.

Decreases in insulin requirements over time will occur in Type 2 diabetics who lose weight, in all diabetics who increase exercise, and frequently in diabetics who develop renal insufficiency. During pregnancy in established diabetics, insulin requirements decrease during the first trimester. If the patient is continuing to check urine or SMBG measurements, the emerging pattern of decreasing insulin requirements should be noted before severe hypoglycemia occurs.

Hypoglycemia. In patients who are unable or unwilling to self monitor metabolic control, those who have very irregular diet and exercise patterns, and patients who attempt very close metabolic control, hypoglycemia may be a problem. If the patient is awake, he/she will have symptoms of epinephrine release (tachycardia, diaphoresis, tremor, and anxiety) and be able to recognize the symptoms and eat. The oral treatment should include about 10 g of carbohydrate. This can consist of six ounces of soda or sweetened juice or the content of four "glucose tablets" sold in most pharmacies and easier for the patient to carry.

There are two circumstances where patients may be unable to recognize oncoming hypoglycemia—inadequate or blocked sympathetic response and sleep. Patients who have autonomic neuropathy associated with their diabetes will often lack the symptoms that warn them of impending hypoglycemia. Similarly, patients receiving adrenergic blockers for hypertension may lose these premonitory symptoms. Nighttime hypoglycemia is a problem because sleeping patients are unaware of premonitory symptoms and their stuporous state will not be noted by others. Sometimes patients with nighttime hypoglycemia will report nightmares, night sweats, or headaches when arising. Because of the surge of counterregulatory hormones stimulated by the hypoglycemia in the early morning hours, the fasting blood glucose may be high—the Somogyi phenomenon.

Treatment of severe hypoglycemia, at times when the patient is too stuporous to ingest carbohydrate, must be done either with intravenous administration of concentrated glucose solutions, or more easily with 1 mg subcutaneous injection of glucagon. Single dose prefilled syringes with 1 mg of glucagon are commercially available. Friends, relatives, and coworkers of patients prone to serious hypoglycemia can be instructed in the technique of administration.

ORAL HYPOGLYCEMIC AGENTS

Many clinicians administer oral hypoglycemic agents to Type 2 diabetics who continue to have symptoms of hyperglycemia after a trial of diet therapy (Table 18.4). The benefit of oral hypoglycemics or insulin in Type 2 diabetes in slowing the progression of complications is still unresolved awaiting results of clinical trials similar to the Diabetes Control and Complication Trial in Type 1 diabetics. A large trial of oral hypoglycemics performed in the 1960s, the University Group Diabetes Program (UGDP), was halted because of a statistically and clinically significant excess rate of cardiovascular deaths in the patients randomized to sulfonylureas (Tolbutamide). However, many questions relating to the applicability of the data have caused most clinicians to continue using these agents.

Sulfonylureas act principally by increasing beta cell responsiveness to secretagogues. A second category of oral hypoglycemic agents is the biguanides. This class of drugs appears to exert its major effect by inhibiting hepatic gluconeogenesis. One agent in this class, phenformin, was associated with the development of lactic acidosis and was withdrawn from sale in the U. S. in 1977. In December 1994, the FDA approved the U. S. sale of another biguanide, metformin.

The choice of a specific oral hypoglycemic agent depends on several factors, most importantly the duration of action, side effect profile and price. In patients with liver or renal disease, the mechanism

Table 18.4.
Oral Hypoglycemic Drugs

Generic Name	Daily Dose Range (mg)	Duration of Action (hr)	Approximate Cost (100 tablets)[a]	Comments
First-generation Sulfonylureas				
Tolbutamide	500–3,000	6–12	500 mg = $3.81	100% inactivated by liver
Acetohexamide	250–1,500	12–18	250 mg = $17.97 500 mg = $28.58	100% inactivated by kidney excretion
Tolazamide	100–1,000	12–24	100 mg = $4.21 500 mg = $12.58	Inactivated by both liver and kidney
Chlorpropamide	100–500	>36	100 mg = $2.11 250 mg = $3.61	100% inactivated by kidney excretion; has disulfiram like effects; can be associated with hyponatremia and prolonged hypoglycemia.
Second-generation Sulfonylureas				
Glyburide	2.5–20	16–24	2.5 mg = $17.63 5 mg = $21.43	Metabolized by liver; 50% excreted in bile 50% excreted in urine can be associated with hypoglycemia
Glipizide	5–40	12–24	5 mg = $14.73 10 mg = $27.95	100% inactivated by liver
Biguanides				
Metformin	1000–3000	12–24	500 mg = $46.27 850 mg = $78.66	Principally inactivated by kidney; contraindicated in renal or hepatic insufficiency because of possibility of lactic acidosis

[a]Except for metformin, all costs are average wholesale prices for generic equivalents—1995.

of inactivation is also important. Chlorpropamide is the longest acting of the sulfonylureas and can cumulate to toxic levels in patients with renal insufficiency, producing hypoglycemia. In elderly patients, chlorpropamide has been associated with water retention, hyponatremia, and a syndrome similar to inappropriate secretion of antidiuretic hormone (SIADH). It has also been associated with disulfiram like effects in patients who drink alcohol. The second generation sulfonylureas are more potent on a milligram per milligram basis because they are less firmly bound to plasma proteins. This sometimes decreases the likelihood of drug – drug interactions (see below). Glyburide, like chlorpropamide, is associated more frequently with prolonged hypoglycemia because of its prolonged duration of action. The second generation sulfonylureas are much more expensive than first generation drugs.

In a recent series (7), 63% of the episodes of severe hypoglycemia were associated with the use of oral hypoglycemics—principally chlorpropamide and glyburide. It is extremely important to recognize that patients who are made hypoglycemic

by long-acting oral hypoglycemic agents require more prolonged therapy than patients who are made hypoglycemic by short-acting insulins or oral agents. The latter can sometimes be treated with an injection of glucagon or 50% glucose solution and be returned home. The patients taking long acting agents must be treated with a constant infusion of 10% glucose solution for at least 24 hours and then monitored carefully to be sure that the effect of the long-acting agent has dissipated.

If the decision is made to initiate oral hypoglycemic therapy, patients should be warned that the initiation of the drug is an addition to, not a substitution for, the more onerous diet therapy that should continue. Patients are started on a relatively low dose of oral hypoglycemic medication. The dose is increased gradually over several weeks or months, depending on the compliance of the patient in urine or blood glucose monitoring, diet, and other factors. Optimally, the determination of dosing should be done in a manner similar to that for initiating and adjusting "conventional" insulin therapy. If a patient is unwilling or unable to comply with such a regimen, monitoring goals similar to "minimal" insulin therapy are appropriate. In the absence of further data concerning the efficacy of extremely tight control in Type 2 diabetes, oral hypoglycemics have not been used to achieve glycemic goals similar to those in "intensive" insulin therapy.

About 70% of patients will achieve glycemic goals in the "conventional" therapy range after a correct dose is established. In the remainder, even maximal doses of an oral hypoglycemic will not achieve these goals because of non compliance or inadequate β cell response. These patients are called primary failures. An additional 10% per year will become secondary failures because of the above reasons and/or weight gain. It is important to discontinue oral hypoglycemic therapy if glycemic goals are not achieved, to determine if they are partially contributing to glycemic control or are completely ineffective, as is often the case. There is no reason to continue oral hypoglycemics if they are completely ineffective. For patients who are primary or secondary failures, the choices are initiation of insulin therapy or the tolerance of hyperglycemia.

Sometimes the effectiveness of oral hypoglycemic therapy is altered by drug-drug interactions. Salicylates, some sulfonamides, phenylbutazone, and coumarin compounds all increase the hypoglycemic action of sulfonylureas by displacing them from plasma proteins or interfering with their metabolism. Thiazide diuretics, especially with concomitant hypokalemia, will diminish endogenous insulin release and so negate the effect of sulfonylureas. Similar blunting of sulfonylurea induced insulin release occurs with β sympathetic blocking agents used for hypertension and with phenytoin.

DIABETIC KETOACIDOSIS AND HYPEROSMOLAR NONKETOTIC STATE

Diabetic ketoacidosis and nonketotic hyperosmolar state are relatively infrequent complications of diabetes. With good patient education and SMBG daily, or at least at the time the patient "feels sick in any way," these complications should be avoidable. The patient should be able to avert acidosis or severe hyperglycemia with adjustment of medications under a clinician's guidance.

The pathophysiology and treatment of severe ketoacidosis or hyperosmolarity is beyond the scope of this chapter on ambulatory medicine, as it must be done in a hospital. However, the evaluation may be done in an ambulatory setting, and the clinician should be alert to consider these complications in any diabetic who has an intercurrent illness or who appears to be generally decompensating.

Ketoacidosis is much more common in Type 1 diabetics but is occasionally seen in insulupenic Type 2 diabetics. Hyperosmolar non ketotic state is more common in elderly Type 2 diabetics with renal insufficiency and/or dehydration. Recent recommendations from the American Diabetes Association are that patients with diabetic ketoacidosis should be hospitalized if their arterial pH is <7.35, their venous pH is <7.30, or their serum bicarbonate level is <15 meq/L. All patients with blood glucose >700 mg/dl should be hospitalized, as should patients with a combination of blood glucose >350 mg/dl, serum osmolarity >295 mosm and impaired mental status.

SPECIAL CONSIDERATIONS

Treatment and educational strategies in certain subgroups of patients may require special considerations. These include pregnant women, ethanol abusers, hypertensives, and patients who are treated with therapeutic corticosteroids.

Diabetes in Pregnancy. As mentioned earlier, the criteria for the diagnosis of gestational diabetes are somewhat different from that of non pregnant patients (Table 18.1). Gestational diabetes is defined as carbohydrate intolerance of variable severity with onset or first recognition during pregnancy. The offspring of mothers who experience hyperglycemia are at risk for intrauterine death or neonatal mortality, and surveillance and treatment of the hyperglycemia reduces the risk. Therefore, a screening test for gestational diabetes is recommended for all pregnant women at 24-28 weeks. This test consists of a single plasma glucose performed 1 hour after ingestion of 50 g of oral glucose. If the plasma glucose is equal to or greater than 140 mg%, a full oral glucose tolerance test is recommended.

In either gestational diabetics or in patients with known diabetes before pregnancy, close surveillance of blood glucose (preferably with SMBG) and close monitoring of fetal development are strongly recommended. Fetal and neonatal mortality can be reduced to that in the general population if glucose control is normalized and obstetrical care is optimal. Goals for glucose control are fasting plasma glucose 105 mg/dl or less and postprandial plasma glucose of 120 mg/dl or less. If this cannot be achieved through diet therapy, insulin therapy should be initiated. Oral hypoglycemic agents are not recommended at this time for pregnant women.

Diabetes and Patients Who Drink Alcohol. Although alcohol consumed in moderation is not contraindicated in diabetics, larger amounts of alcohol can cause two serious complications—hypoglycemia and ketoacidosis. These disorders, like diabetic ketoacidosis, are rarely encountered in office or clinic settings (the patients are too ill and present to emergency services), but the syndromes are important to understand in terms of education of patients and significant others to avoid these serious complications.

Hypoglycemia is a major concern in patients who drink alcohol to excess while continuing to take insulin or oral hypoglycemic medications. Alcohol is metabolized by alcohol dehydrogenase, and this metabolism raises the level of NADH, the reduced form of nicotinamide adenine dinucleotide (NAD). This increased NADH/NAD ratio decreases hepatic gluconeogenesis. In patients who have exhausted liver glycogen due to poor nutrition or chronic liver disease, this decrease in gluconeogenesis can be associated with severe hypoglycemia. The patients most at risk are poorly nourished binge drinkers with little liver glycogen who take their morning oral hypoglycemic agent or insulin, start drinking, and avoid eating—either as an oversight or due to alcoholic gastritis. As blood sugar falls in response to exogenous insulin or oral agents, there is no mechanism for them to prevent catastrophic hypoglycemia without gluconeogenesis, glycogenolysis, or direct absorption of oral carbohydrate. These patients are at additional risk because if observed to be stuporous (and smelling of alcohol), friends, family and passers-by may assume the problem to be simply due to alcohol. Because of the importance of the high NADH/NAD ratio in depressing gluconeogenesis, the hypoglycemia will eventually resolve (after possible neurologic damage) after complete metabolism of alcohol and the completion of the pharmacological time action of the oral hypoglycemic agent or insulin.

A second problem seen in ethanol abusers is so called alcoholic ketoacidosis. This disorder occurs most frequently in binge drinkers who are not true diabetics and who develop ketoacidosis in the setting of vomiting and dehydration. The pathogenesis of this syndrome appears to be related to a decrease in insulin levels and an increase in glucagon levels. Even in non diabetic ethanol abusers, there is a decrease in blood sugar during a binge that is caused by the same factors of decreased gluconeogenesis, diminished availability of glycogen, and absent food intake. This will cause a decrease in insulin levels in normal patients and a more serious deficiency in patients with chronic pancreatitis, impaired carbohydrate tolerance, or otherwise stable Type 2 diabetes. Vomiting, dehy-

dration, and metabolic or circulatory stress cause an increase in glucagon secretion. The increased glucagon/insulin ratio fosters lipolysis and ketogenesis. In the majority of cases, patients present to medical attention with this syndrome after the ethanol of a binge has been metabolized. They thus have absent or only mildly elevated ethanol levels. In the absence of overt diabetes, blood glucose is generally normal. The patients have a metabolic acidosis (ketones and sometimes lactate). Their blood pH depends on the severity of the coexisting metabolic alkalosis (secondary to vomiting) and respiratory alkalosis (secondary to delirium tremens or pain). Treatment is not done in the ambulatory setting and involves rehydration, glucose infusion, and electrolyte and thiamine replacement.

Patients with Hypertension. Hypertension is approximately twice as common in persons with diabetes than in non diabetics. Hypertension contributes to the progression of cardiovascular disease and nephropathy in diabetics and should be carefully monitored and treated. Control of hypertension has been shown to retard the progression of cardiovascular complications and nephropathy. As described above, some authors have felt that the association of hypertension and Type 2 diabetes is partially due to insulin resistance and hyperinsulinism and have dubbed the condition "Syndrome X" or CHAOS (**C**oronary heart disease, **H**ypertension and **H**yperlipidemia, **A**dult **O**nset Diabetes, **S**troke). The presence of both diabetes and hypertension requires an initial evaluation that includes the measurement of microalbuminuria, a determination of orthostatic blood pressure measurements, a careful examination of the eyes by a specialist, and an electrocardiogram—tests that may not be done in all diabetics. The goal of antihypertensive therapy is to achieve a blood pressure of ≤130/85 mm Hg, but this may not be possible in all patients (Fig. 18.1).

The choice of antihypertensive treatment should be individualized, but most authorities feel that an angiotensin converting enzyme inhibitor should be used in the majority of patients, as these agents have been shown to retard the progression of nephropathy in hypertensive and even normotensive diabetics. Low dose diuretics rarely worsen glycemic control, but β sympathetic blocking agents have several disadvantages and are thus less frequently recommended than in the non diabetic population. They may worsen glucose control by their effect on decreasing β cell secretion of insulin, prolong hypoglycemia by inhibiting the β sympathetic mediated glycogenolysis needed to recover

TREATMENT GOAL <130/85 mmHg

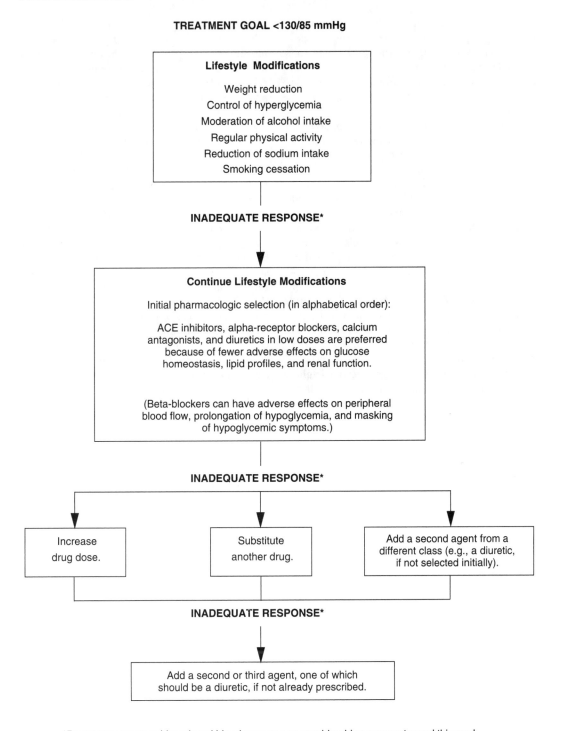

Lifestyle Modifications

Weight reduction
Control of hyperglycemia
Moderation of alcohol intake
Regular physical activity
Reduction of sodium intake
Smoking cessation

INADEQUATE RESPONSE*

Continue Lifestyle Modifications

Initial pharmacologic selection (in alphabetical order):

ACE inhibitors, alpha-receptor blockers, calcium antagonists, and diuretics in low doses are preferred because of fewer adverse effects on glucose homeostasis, lipid profiles, and renal function.

(Beta-blockers can have adverse effects on peripheral blood flow, prolongation of hypoglycemia, and masking of hypoglycemic symptoms.)

INADEQUATE RESPONSE*

| Increase drug dose. | Substitute another drug. | Add a second agent from a different class (e.g., a diuretic, if not selected initially). |

INADEQUATE RESPONSE*

Add a second or third agent, one of which should be a diuretic, if not already prescribed.

*Response means achieved goal blood pressure or considerable progress toward this goal.

Figure 18.1. Hypertension treatment algorithm for diabetic patients. (From the National High Blood Pressure Education Program Working Group Report on Hypertension in Diabetes. US Dept. of Health & Human Services. NIH publ. no. 94-3530, April 1994; 13.)

from hypoglycemia; and mask the symptoms of impending hypoglycemia that are due to β sympathetic overactivity (tremor, diaphoresis, tachycardia, and general premonitory anxiety). In addition, in patients with atherosclerosis, β sympathetic blocking agents can diminish an already compromised blood flow.

Patients Receiving Therapeutic Corticosteroids. More than 5 million Americans receive a course of corticosteroids each year for treatment of an inflammatory or allergic disease. The majority of these patients develop some abnormalities in carbohydrate tolerance. The corticosteroids used therapeutically for inflammatory diseases (e.g., prednisone and dexamethasone) are also known as glucocorticoids because of their stimulation of hepatic glucose production. This is accomplished in several ways. The first is via an increase in gluconeogenesis that is mediated by the catabolic effect of glucocorticoids on muscle and connective tissue, which releases alanine and other amino acids into the circulation. The increase in the plasma concentration of alanine stimulates glucagon release, and the combination of increased amino acid substrate and glucagon stimulation causes an increase in gluconeogenesis. The second is via an inhibitory effect on the uptake of glucose into peripheral tissues. Glucocorticoids are also necessary for normal accumulation of glycogen stores. The effects on gluconeogenesis and peripheral glucose uptake are dose related, and so patients who are treated with supraphysiologic doses of glucocorticoids must either increase insulin secretion appreciably or develop Type 2 diabetes.

From a clinical standpoint, this means that patients who are not known to be diabetic should have at least a random blood glucose or urinalysis performed soon after initiation of glucocorticoid therapy. For patients who exhibit only impaired glucose tolerance or mild Type 2 diabetes (glycemia in the "conventional therapy" range), no specific therapy should be instituted. However, the exacerbation of their inflammatory disease can be the stress that increases the secretion of counterregulatory hormones and worsens glycemic control, so the clinician should be alert to deterioration in glycemic control. For patients whose glycemia exceeds acceptable levels and for whom extended courses of glucocorticoids are planned, treatment for this "secondary" Type 2 diabetes should be similar to that of usual Type 2 diabetes.

ILLUSTRATIVE CASES WITH SELF-ASSESSMENT QUESTIONS AND ANSWERS

Case 1

A 46-year-old obese woman comes to see you because of vaginal pruritis for a few days and vague symptoms of fatigue and lightheadedness over the past few months. You diagnose and treat candidal vaginitis and note glycosuria but no proteinuria or pyuria on a urinalysis you routinely perform in patients with perineal pruritis or burning. To further evaluate this patient, you obtain a fasting blood sugar, of 235 mg% and a glycosylated hemoglobin of 11.5%. During her periodic health evaluation last year, she was normotensive, had a normal eye examination including ophthalmoscopy, and had a completely normal "routine" physical examination. As per the USPHS guidelines for asymptomatic adults, you did not check for diabetes or renal disease, but measured her total cholesterol as 210 mg%. She smokes cigarettes, has gradually gained 50 lb.

over the past 20 years, and is taking no medications.

QUESTION: *Which of the following diagnostic evaluations are important to do at this time?*

a. A careful foot and shoe exam that is not part of your "routine" physical exam: This includes careful evaluation of reflexes, sensory function (touch, vibration, position sense), examination of the skin and nails, and examination of her shoes to look for irregularities in the lining.
b. Orthostatic blood pressure measurements
c. A referral to an eye doctor for a more careful ophthalmologic examination
d. A serum creatinine
e. Tests for microalbuminuria

f. Fasting lipid profile including cholesterol fractionation
g. Electrocardiogram
h. Liver function tests

ANSWER: *According to the most recent recommendations of the American Diabetes Association, the correct answers are* **a, b, d, e, f,** *and* **g.** *Evaluation for microalbuminuria was recently added to their list of recommendations and has not yet been endorsed by all clinicians and authors. Measurement of orthostatic blood pressure changes and referral for more careful ophthalmologic examination should be individualized, and therefore* **b** *is correct because of her lightheadedness. Liver function tests are not recommended in the absence of specific indications.*

QUESTION: *What therapeutic interventions are necessary at this time?*

a. General educational sessions with clinician and other appropriate personnel to explain the nature of the chronic disease and its complications, and to help with necessary alterations in lifestyle, with special emphasis on smoking cessation and dietary modification
b. Education of patient with printed material on self care in diabetes mellitus
c. Initiation of therapy with oral hypoglycemic agents
d. Initiation of insulin therapy

ANSWER: **a** *and in most cases,* **b.** *Although some facilities have trained personnel who can initiate and follow through on the extensive educational interventions necessary, most clinicians supplement this with printed materials. Drug therapy for relatively asymptomatic Type 2 diabetics is initiated only after diet therapy has been determined to be ineffective in achieving glycemic goals.*

QUESTION: *How frequently should the patient come to see the clinician or a member of her staff over the next 3 months?*

a. Three times to see the clinician and four times to see other staff members
b. Once to see the clinician at the end of three months and four times to see other staff members
c. Once to see clinician at the end of three

months and once to see other staff members
d. It depends on factors relating to the patient's compliance, glycemic response, and adequacy of telephone contact to deal with problems

ANSWER: **d.** *There is no specific amount of time or frequency of visits necessary to educate the patient and to achieve glycemic goals. In general, all Type 2 diabetics should initially be encouraged to pursue the goals of "conventional" therapy with diet. This will take several hours of instruction via direct contact with clinicians and staff, printed materials, and telephone contact to monitor progress.*

Case 2

A 57-year-old obese man comes to see you for the first time after moving from a distant city. He has been taking glyburide 20 mg/day for the past 3 years. He was diagnosed as having Type 2 diabetes 10 years previously and has been placed on several different oral hypoglycemics over the years as his job has caused him to move. He was obese at the time of diagnosis, never adhered to a weight reducing diet and has continued to gain weight at about 2 lb/yr. He admits to overeating and although taught SMBG by a previous clinician, never did it regularly and has not done it for at least a year. However, he religiously takes his glyburide each day. He has no symptoms of hyperglycemia, cardiovascular disease, autonomic or other neuropathy or visual change and takes no other medications. As part of his initial evaluation, you obtain a fasting blood sugar of 275 mg% and a glycosylated hemoglobin of 13.5%.

QUESTION: *What changes would you recommend in his therapeutic regimen?*

a. Change of oral medication to glipizide at a dose of 30 mg/day and revisit in 3 months with no other intervention
b. Continuation of glyburide at the present dose with initiation of weight loss through diet therapy and exercise. Reinitiation of SMBG twice daily with a revisit to see you in 2 weeks to reassess the clinical situation and the SMBG record

ANSWER: **b.** *It is extremely unlikely that this secondary failure with one sulfonylurea can be* *ameliorated with the substitution of another sulfonylurea. In the absence of a drug-drug interaction that would decrease the effectiveness of the sulfonylurea (e.g., thiazide diuretics, phenytoin, or β sympathetic blocker) or noncompliance by the patient, the only intervention likely to restore drug effectiveness is weight loss. In the absence of symptoms, there is no immediate need to begin insulin therapy.*

QUESTION: *When you see him in 2 weeks, he has lost 2 pounds. His fasting blood sugars have been falling slightly over the past few days to the 250 mg% range, and his predinner readings are also falling to the mid 200s. You recommend:*

a. Continuation of glyburide at the present dose with continuation of weight loss through diet therapy and exercise and continuation of SMBG twice daily. You ask him to call you in 2 weeks to review the SMBG record and schedule a revisit to see you in 4 weeks to reassess the clinical situation.
b. You begin 20 U of NPH insulin at 9 PM in addition to his sulfonylurea therapy.
c. You discontinue his sulfonylurea therapy and initiate insulin therapy alone with a regimen eventually intended to achieve "conventional" therapy goals.

ANSWER: a *is the preferred answer because it appears that diet therapy may be having some effect. A 2-week course and 2-pound weight loss is not sufficient to determine if diet therapy will be effective.* **b** *and* **c** *would be options once it was determined that diet therapy had failed.*

QUESTION: *Another 3 months have passed, he has lost 12 pounds, his fasting and evening blood sugars are in the 125 to 175 mg% range, and his glycosylated hemoglobin is 9.0%. You decide to:*

a. Discontinue his sulfonylurea and have him call you about his SMBG record in one week
b. Continue his sulfonylurea at the present dose
c. Begin 20 U of NPH insulin at 9 PM in addition to his sulfonylurea therapy
d. Discontinue his sulfonylurea therapy and initiate insulin therapy alone with a regimen eventually intended to achieve "conventional" therapy goals

ANSWER: a. *Most clinicians would discontinue the sulfonylurea in this situation rather than continue it, decrease the dose, or begin the initiation of insulin therapy. In the absence of data to support "intensive" therapy goals in Type 2 diabetics, most clinicians would not add insulin. In patients such as this one, it is unlikely that the sulfonylurea is contributing to glycemic control, and there is no danger to abruptly discontinuing it if the patient is reliable, performs SMBG, and can call the clinician if glycemic control deteriorates markedly. The abrupt discontinuation of the sulfonylurea allows a quicker determination of its effectiveness than a slow taper of dose. If glycemic control deteriorates, the sulfonylurea can be restarted.*

THYROID DISORDERS

Thyroid abnormalities are the most common endocrine disorders, other than diabetes, that are seen in the out-patient setting. Thyroid disease is seen in all age groups and can range in severity from asymptomatic to life-threatening. This chapter will review the biochemistry and anatomy of the thyroid gland, and the diagnosis and treatment of thyroid diseases.

Pathophysiologic Correlation

The thyroid is a 5 × 5 cm butterfly-shaped gland. The thyroid is located below the thyroid cartilage and above the sternal notch. There are 2 lobes (right and left), a central isthmus, and sometimes a cephalad extension of the isthmus called the pyramidal lobe (Fig. 18.2). Thyroid hormones control the body's metabolism, influence growth and maturation of the tissues, and govern cellular respiration.

Histologically, the gland is composed of follicular cells, which synthesize the thyroid hormone and follicles, where thyroid hormone and its precursors are stored. Synthesis of thyroid hormone is accomplished in several steps. Plasma and iodide is "trapped" by the follicular cell, and then organification occurs, with loss of the negative charge (i.e., oxidation). Tyrosine molecules, which are part of the large thyroglobulin molecule, are iodinated. When one iodine atom is bound to tyrosine, the product is monoiodotyrosine or MIT. When two iodine atoms are bound, the product is diiodotyrosine or DIT. These precursors are then coupled to form triiodothyronine (T_3) or tetraiodothyronine (T_4), and the resulting hormone − thyroglobulin mass is stored in the follicle colloid space (Fig. 18.3). When needed, the T_4 and T_3 are cleaved from the thyroglobulin and released into the circulation as active hormone (Fig. 18.4).

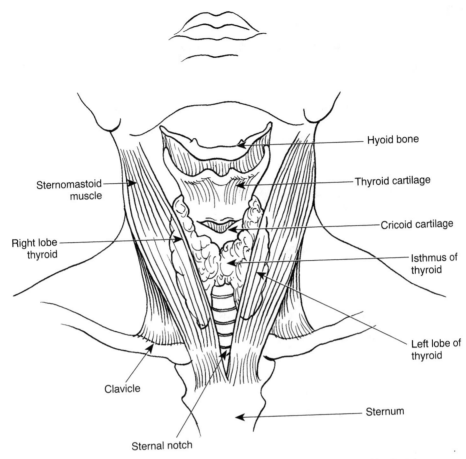

Figure 18.2. Location of the normal thyroid. Each lobe is 5 cm in length by 2 cm in width. The lobes are connected by the isthmus. (From Willms JL, et al. Physical diagnosis: bedside evaluation of diagnosis and function. Baltimore: Williams & Wilkins, 1994;189.)

Thyroid binding globulin (TBG) is the major carrier of T_4 and T_3 in the blood, although thyroid binding pre-albumin and albumin are also carriers. T_4 is 99.98% bound, T_3 is slightly less firmly bound (99.7%). The hormone that is "free" or not bound, is what exerts the metabolic effects. T_3 is approximately ten times more active than T_4 and is the more important of the thyroid hormones. Principally because of differences in plasma binding the half-life of T_4 in the blood is 7 days and the half-life of T_3 is 1.5 days.

T_4 is deiodinated predominately in the liver and kidney cells. Control of thyroid hormone production and release depends on hypothalamic release of thyrotropin releasing hormone (TRH), which in turn causes thyroid stimulating hormone (TSH) to be released by the pituitary gland. TSH, in its turn, stimulates the thyroid uptake of iodine and the formation and release of T_3 and T_4. T_3 and T_4 both complete the feedback loop by causing inhibition of TSH release by the pituitary gland (Fig. 18.5).

Clinical and Laboratory Evaluation

The clinician can make the diagnosis of thyroid disease in a healthy, young patient by doing a careful history and physical examination. Laboratory tests are confirmatory. The diagnosis is much more difficult to make in patients who are sick, very young or old.

HISTORY

Patients with thyroid disease can have a wide variety of symptoms because thyroid hormone affects vir-

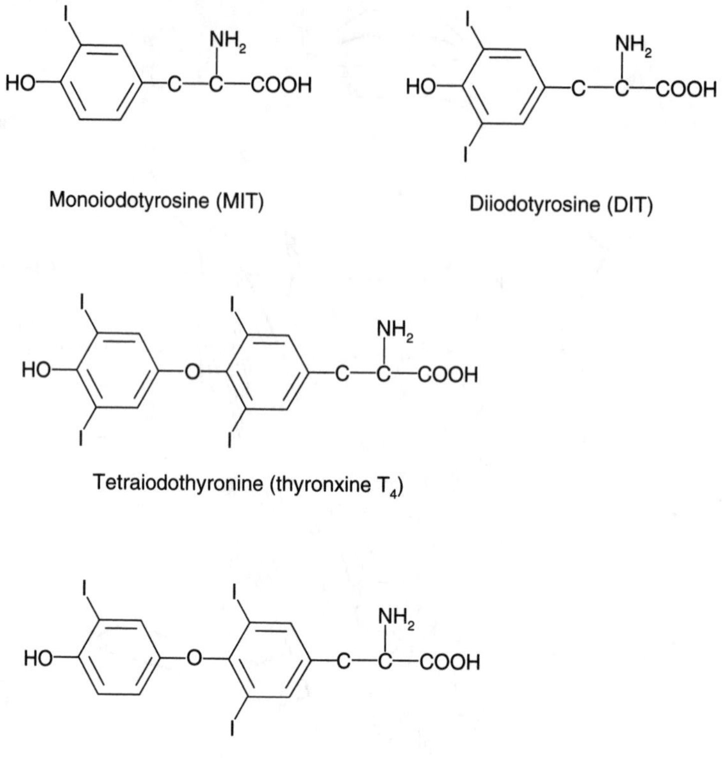

Monoiodotyrosine (MIT)

Diiodotyrosine (DIT)

Tetraiodothyronine (thyronxine T$_4$)

Triiodothyronine (T$_3$)

Figure 18.3. Thyroid hormones and precursors.

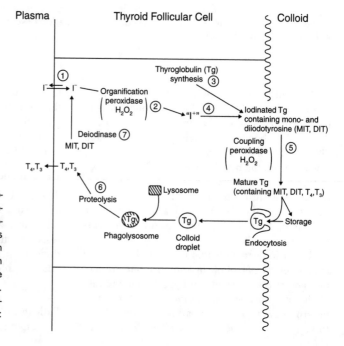

Figure 18.4. Intrahyroidal iodine metabolism. Principle steps in the synthesis and secretion of thyroid hormones. MIT = monoiodotyrosine; DIT = diiodotyrosine. The steps denoted by the numbers are those in which defects have been identified in patients with inherited abnormalities in thyroid hormone biosynthesis. (From Larson P. The Thyroid. In: Wyngaarden JB, et al. eds. Cecil Textbook of Medicine. 17th ed. Philadelphia: WB Saunders Co., 1985.)

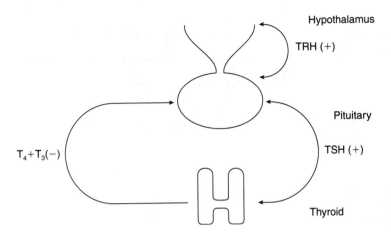

Figure 18.5. Current concepts of hypothalamic-pituitary-thyroid interrelationships.

tually every organ system in the body. Signs and symptoms of hyperthyroidism and hypothyroidism are listed in Table 18.5. The list of possible symptoms is long, therefore, high yield questions should be asked. In suspected hyperthyroidism, questions regarding thyroid enlargement, weight loss, eye signs, irritability, insomnia, muscle weakness, skin and hair changes, tremor, and family history of hyperthyroidism should be the most helpful. In suspected hypothyroidism, ask questions regarding use of lithium or iodine (which interfere with T_4 synthesis), thyroid enlargement, cold intolerance, sleepiness, constipation, dry skin and, in younger women, menorrhagia. A patient with a thyroid nod-

Table 18.5.
Signs and Symptoms of Hyperthyroidism and Hypothyroidism

Hyperthyroidism	System	Hypothyroidism
Anxiety, irritability, psychosis, insomnia, heat intolerance, tremor, tachycardia, hyperflexia	Neurologic or adrenergic	Confusion, slowed thinking, memory loss, slowed movement, delayed relaxation phase of reflexes
Decreased PTH secretion, increased cortisol turnover, decreased sensitivity to injected insulin	Endocrine	Increased prolactin, decreased cortisol turnover
Tachycardia, arrhythmia, congestive heart failure, pericardial effusion	Cardiovascular	Bradycardia, cardiomegaly paricardial effusion
Diarrhea, vomitting, frequent defecation, abdominal pain	Gastrointestinal	Constipation, elevated serum lipids
Pretibial myxedema, oncholysis, warm skin	Integumental	Dry skin and hair, myxedema, cool skin
Exopthalmos, periorbital edema, ophthalmoplegia, papilledema, decreased ability to converge	Ophthalmologic	Periorbital puffiness
Weakness, proximal myopathy, clubbing of digits, osteoporosis, hypercalcemia	Musculoskeletal	Muscle aches, stiffness
Infertility, ogliomenorrhea, testicular atrophy, gynecomastia, decreased libido	Reproductive	Infertility, menorrhagia, decreased libido, impotence
Increased appetite, weight loss	General	Decreased appetite, weight gain
	Renal	Decreased glomerular filtration rate, increase in body water
Normocytic anemia	Hematologic	Normocytic, B_{12}, folate, iron deficiency anemia
Decreased vital capacity	Pulmonary	Hypoventilation

ule should be asked about family history of thyroid disease, prior radiation, dysphagia, and hoarseness. Nodules in young males are more likely to be malignant than those in young females.

PHYSICAL EXAMINATION

The physical examination of the thyroid gland begins with inspection of the neck. The examiner should look for an enlargement below the thyroid cartilage. The patient should hyperextend his neck and swallow which will cause an enlarged thyroid to visibly move. Auscultation for bruits should be attempted with the bell of the stethoscope. A systolic bruit may be heard in hyperthyroidism.

Palpation of the gland is accomplished most easily when the examiner is standing behind the seated, relaxed patient. The examiner identifies the thyroid cartilage and places his fingertips 1-3 cm below its caudal border, on each side of the trachea. The patient then swallows a mouthful of water, causing the thyroid gland to move. The examiner can then estimate the size and configuration of the gland. Some thyroid glands are not palpable, particularly in patients with fleshy necks. To more completely examine the right lateral lobe, the examiner can instruct the patient to bend his neck to the right, while displacing the trachea laterally to the right and palpating anterior and then posterior to the sternocleidomastoid muscle during swallowing. This can then be repeated in the opposite direction for the left lobe.

The gland is not visible in most patients, nor should it be tender. If enlargement is noted, the examiner should note if it is diffusely enlarged, (as in Graves disease), if there are multiple nodules, or if there is a single nodule.

LABORATORY EVALUATION

Thyroid function tests (TFTs) can be difficult to interpret, at least by the novice. Part of the difficulty occurs because there are many non-thyroidal factors (Table 18.6) that affect the test results, especially a variety of acute and chronic illnesses that affect the serum binding protein levels and hence the levels of serum total T_4 and T_3. Some of the available tests include serum T_4 level; T_3 level; TSH level; and a "thyroid profile" consisting of T_4, T_3 resin uptake, and free T_4 index. Costs vary widely, but at an estimated cost of $20 for T_4, $50 for T_3, $60 for TSH, and $40 for thyroid profile, testing can be expensive. The initial testing depends on the patient's condition and the clinician's index of suspicion of the likelihood of thyroid disease. If the

Table 18.6.
"Non-thyroidal Factors" Affecting Thyroid Function Tests

Peripheral conversion of T_4 to >T3:
  Acute and chronic illness,
  Prophylthiouracil, propranolol
  Glucorticoids
  Iodinated radiographic dyes, amiodarone

Decreased Binding of T_4
  Acute illness
  Chronic illnesses—hypoproteinemia
  Renal failure
  Drugs—Heparin, ASA

Increased Binding of T_4
  Estrogens
  Familial High TBG

Secretion of TSH:
  Dopamine, Glucocorticoids,
Acute and chronic illness—medical and psychiatric

Radioactive iodine uptake:
  Iodinated radiographic dyes, amiodarone
  Bread
  Vitamin preparations (Kelp)

patient does not have confounding non-thyroidal factors listed in Table 18.6 and the clinician does not have a high index of suspicion, a T_4 level is a good initial screening test. If the patient has non-thyroidal factors and/or the clinician has a high index of suspicion, a TSH is the most reasonable initial test followed by a T_4 level. Laboratory confirmation of the diagnosis of hyperthyrodism requires finding a high T_4 (above 12 mg/100 ml) and a suppressed TSH (usually less than 0.5 micro IU/ml). T_3 levels are also likely to be elevated. Confirmation of hypothyroidism requires finding a low T_4 (usually less than 5 mg/100 ml) and an elevated TSH (usually above 10, and often above 20 micro IU/ml) (Table 18.7). Since the overwhelming majority of thyroid diseases are not secondary to pitu-

Table 18.7.
Thyroid Function Tests in Thyroid Disease

Test	Hypothyroidism	Hyperthyroidism
T4	↓	↑
T3	↓	↑
T3 resin uptake	↓	↑
T4 index	↓	↑
TSH	↑	↓

itary or hypothalamic disease, these testing regimens are reasonable. In secondary hypothyroidism, one would not expect the serum TSH level to be elevated.

Other commonly used diagnostic tests include thyroid ultrasound, radioactive iodine uptake, and needle biopsy. Radioactive iodine uptake (a radionuclide scan) measures the uptake and retention of iodine by the gland and hence its activity. The uptake is elevated in Graves disease. Uptake is decreased diffusely in thyroiditis and hypothyroidism and locally in most neoplasms. Iodine uptake of a normal thyroid gland will be low when there is excess iodine in the body from iodinated contrast media from x-ray procedures, vitamins containing iodine (such as kelp from health food stores), and bread (to which iodine is added as a surfactant).

Differential Diagnosis

Numerous diseases affect the thyroid gland. In the ambulatory setting, most thyroid disease will fall into one of five categories. The diagnostic strategies for hyperthyroidism, hypothyroidism, thyroiditis, goiter, and thyroid neoplasms are described in the following paragraphs.

HYPERTHYROIDISM

The most common cause of hyperthyroidism is Graves Disease. Secondary causes account for a minority of the cases. Anxiety disorder and primary cardiac dysrhythmias can present in a fashion similar to hyperthyroidism, but hyperthyroidism will have many more systemic signs and symptoms. In hyperthyroidism, laboratory tests will reveal elevated serum T_4 (and T_3) and suppressed TSH levels.

Graves Disease. Graves Disease tends to be a disease of young women. Graves patients produce a thyroid stimulating immunoglobulin (TSI) which activates TSH receptors and thus promotes increased T_3 and T_4 production by the thyroid gland. Physical examination findings peculiar to Graves disease are:

- *Thyroidopathy*—diffusely enlarged, symmetrical, homogeneous thyroid gland with a systolic bruit.
- *Ophthalmopathy*—exophthalmos and occasionally ophthalmoplegia caused by inflammatory infiltrates and by fat, mucopolysaccharide distribution and edema in the orbital structures surrounding the globe (Fig. 18.6).

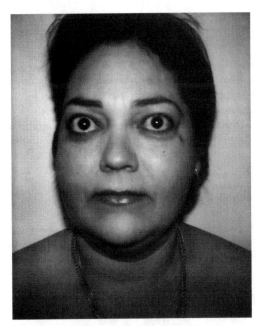

Figure 18.6. Ophthalmology.

- *Dermopathy*—fine skin and pretibial myxedema—a raised, thickened, demarcated area of skin on the shin, which is infiltrated with the same material as the orbit with ophthalmopathy, and whose cause is unknown.

If the clinician is unsure about the diagnoses of Graves disease versus toxic adenoma, a radioactive iodine uptake scan of the thyroid gland can be ordered. In Graves disease, the radioiodine scan will show a diffuse increase in uptake, while in toxic adenoma only the hyperfunctioning nodule(s) will show an increase in uptake.

Hyperfunctioning Adenoma. There are two classic physical examination presentations in the case of hyperfunctioning adenoma; a single palpable nodule in an otherwise normal sized gland or several nodules in a chronically enlarged gland. Thyroid scan can differentiate the two if the diagnosis is unclear. It is not known what causes thyroid adenomas to form and hyperfunction. They are virtually never malignant.

Thyroid Storm. Rarely, in extreme hyperthyroidism the patient becomes febrile, then delirious, and may suffer circulatory collapse and die. The clinician must determine if the patient's illness is caused by infection, hyperthyroidism or both, and treat agressively. When this diagnosis is entertained, hospitalization is required.

HYPOTHYROIDISM

The prevalence of hypothyroidism is 0.35% in the general population and is higher in the elderly. Most instances of idiopathic hypothyroidism are believed due to Hashimoto's thyroiditis (an autoimmune disease that may be an end result of Graves disease) or may be due to previous radioactive iodine ablation or surgical removal of an overactive thyroid gland. Hypothyroidism can be confused with depression and dementia. The diagnosis is made by finding a decreased T_4 (less than 5 mg/100 ml), and an elevated TSH (above 10 micro IU/ml, and usually higher) in a patient with a compatible picture. High levels of anti-thyroid antibodies are found in patients with Hashimoto's disease.

In untreated hypothyroidism or myxedema, the patient may present with stupor, coma, respiratory depression and hypothermia. Myxedema refers to the clinical constellation of puffy face, hands and feet, dry skin, coarse thinned hair, hoarse voice and slowed mentation owing to hypothyroidism. Inpatient evaluation and treatment are indicated.

THYROID MALFUNCTION IN THE ELDERLY

The elderly may not display the expected signs of hyper- or hypothyroidism. Older patients with hyperthyroidism may present with apathy, myopathy, or arrhythmia. Elderly patients with new atrial fibrillation deserve testing for hyperthyroidism. An elderly patient who appears to have dementia or depression should have her thyroid function tested because she may be hypothyroid.

THYROIDITIS

There are several types of thyroiditis—the two most common are Hashimoto's and subacute thyroiditis. Patients with so called sub-acute thyroditis, which is usually an acute illness, present with a history of a sore throat and/or ears a few days after an upper respiratory illness. The pain then localizes to the thyroid and may become severe. Some patients have fever and malaise as well. This disease is sometimes misdiagnosed as pharyngitis, earache or musculoskeletal neck pain. Inflammation of the gland may result in less thyroid hormone than usual being formed, but the hormone may leak out of the colloid. The gland is very tender on examination. TFTs may be consistent with hyper- hypo-, or euthyroidism, depending on the amount of leak. Diagnostic tests include elevation of the erythrocyte sedimentation rate and suppression of radioactive iodine uptake on scan.

GOITER

Enlargement of the thyroid gland is termed goiter. It is most often associated with euthyroidism, but patients may be hyper- or hypothyroid. Simple goiter in the US is thought to be caused by familial or idiopathic defects in the synthesis of thyroid hormone, but this is unproven. In third world countries, goiter is often caused by iodine deficiency and some of the affected children are hypothyroid. The gland hypertrophies in attempt to compensate for defects in T_3 and T_4 production. Patients with simple goiter may develop multiple nodules in the gland, but TFTs are usually normal.

THYROID NEOPLASM

Neoplasms, benign and malignant, occur in about 4% of adults, and are present at autopsy in 50% of adult cases. Most of these nodules are benign. Women tend to have nodules more often than men. Thyroid cancer has a clinical prevalence of 0.0025% and an autopsy prevalence of 2%. However, only about 1,000 persons a year die from thyroid cancer—mainly from the incurable and aggressive anaplastic type. Papillary carcinomas are the most benign type of cancer, followed by medullary carcinomas.

For the patient with a single, small nodule, a dominant nodule among many, or few cancer risk factors found by history, two algorithms for diagnosis are presented in Figure 18.7. The best approach varies depending on cost and expertise at each hospital. If the patient is likely to have a malignancy, based on physical examination abnormalities or multiple risk factors, needle aspiration should be the initial test (Fig. 18.7A).

Management

The management of thyroid disease is usually simple. Therapies are well tolerated and easy to comply with. It is gratifying to witness the response some patients have to therapy.

HYPERTHYROIDISM

There are three choices for treatment of hyperthyroidism. Each treatment has its advantages. The choice of method depends on the patient's condition, her preference, and the clinician's bias.

Graves Disease. Graves Disease can be treated with radioactive iodine (RAI), antithyroid drugs, or surgery. Radioactive iodine is the most commonly recommended treatment in the US. The RAI therapy has been used in more than half a

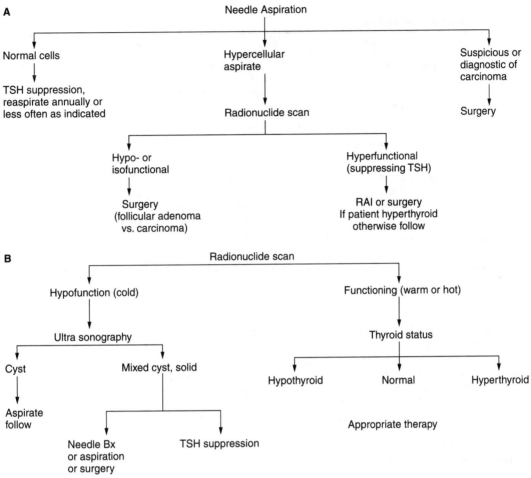

Figure 18.7. Schema for the diagnosis of a patient with solitary thyroid nodule. Panel A shows a schema for the diagnostic evaluation of a patient with solitary thyroid nodule based on aspiration biopsy cytology. Panel B presents an alternative solution to the same problem with a thyroid scintiscan. (Adapted from Larson P. The Thyroid. In: Wyngaarden JB, et al. Cecil Textbook of Medicine. 17th ed. Philadelphia: WB Saunders Co., 1985.)

million patients during the past 50 years, and has not been associated with subsequent cancers or genetic abnormalities. The dosage of radiation the gonads receive in RAI therapy is similar to that of a barium enema.

After RAI therapy, patients improve symptomatically in a month or so; TFTs improve in several months and normalize in 3-6 months. Beta blockers such as propranolol 10-60 mg every six hours are often given initially to control the hyperadrenergic symptoms, and are then tapered and discontinued after 2-3 months.

The advantage of RAI treatment is that usually only one dose is needed, although a second dose may be given if the hyperthyroidism doesn't respond within 3 to 6 months of the first dose. The disadvantages are that patients may remain symptomatic for a month or more after treatment, (although this can be minimized with drug therapy) and up to 80% will ultimately become hypothyroid.

Antithyroid drugs (Table 18.8), such as propylthiouracil and methimazole inhibit thyroid hormone synthesis. Propylthiouracil also inhibits peripheral conversion of T_4 to T_3. Propylthiouracil is preferred for use in pregnancy because it does not readily cross the placenta and is found in breast milk only in very small concentrations. Methimazole can be given once daily, as opposed to three

Table 18.8.
Comparison of the Antithyroid Drugs

	Propylthiouracil	Methimazole
Pharmacology	Serum half-life 75 minutes Highly protein-bound Inhibits T_4 to T_3 conversion	Serum half-life 4–6 hours Duration of action 40 hours
Pregnancy	Only small amounts cross placenta	Crosses placenta
Lactation	Minimal concentration in breast milk	Concentrates in breast milk
Toxicity	Rash, fever, athralgias, nausea 5%, agranulocytosis 0.5%, hepatocellular necrosis	Rash, fever, athralgias, nausea 5%, agranulocytosis less common if dose <30 mg daily Cholestatic jaundice Congenital scalp defect (possibly)
Advantage	Use in pregnancy and lactation	Once-a-day dosing
Initial dosage	100–150 mg every 6–8 hours	10 mg every 8 hours or 15–30 mg once daily

times daily for propylthiouracil. Either drug produces an improvement in TFTs in about a week, and TFTs normalize in 2-3 months. Clinical responses occur within weeks. The drugs are inexpensive and have few side effects. The only serious adverse effects are leukopenia, agranulocytosis and rash. These effects are rare and reversible. The starting dose of propylthiouracil is 100 mg three times daily, and of methimazole, 20 mg once daily. Beta blockers may be added to control adrenergic symptoms. TFTs should be monitored every 2-4 weeks, and the dosage should be adjusted as needed. Treatment is continued for 6-18 months. Up to 30% of patients will not require further therapy for hyperthyroidism after this period of time. Antithyroid drugs do not cause permanent hypothyroidism; however, a significant percentage of patients with Graves disease will ultimately develop hypothyroidism, which appears to be the natural course of the disease. Patients must be monitored for the onset of hypothyroidism during and long after treatment with any of these modalities.

Surgery is no longer used as a treatment for Graves disease. It is an option for patients who refuse or have failed other treatment modalities. If used, every attempt must be made to delay surgery until hyperthyroidism is controlled with antithyroid and/or beta-blocking drug therapy.

Hyperfunctioning Adenoma. Hyperfunctioning adenoma(s) can be treated with radioactive iodine or surgery. The RAI is concentrated in the adenoma and does little damage to the rest of the suppressed thyroid gland, resulting in a low incidence of permanent hypothyroidism. Beta blockers may be given for symptomatic control.

HYPOTHYROIDISM

The treatment of hypothyroidism is relatively simple, cheap, and well tolerated. Levothyroxine, given in doses of 0.1–0.15 mg daily is usually sufficient replacement therapy. TFTs should be checked a month after starting therapy, and adjustments in the dosage made accordingly. Hypothyroidism in young patients who are otherwise well can be treated with nearly full replacement doses of levothyroxine. The dosage should be monitored by measuring serum TSH values, which should not become supressed to subnormal levels.

THYROID MALFUNCTION IN THE ELDERLY

Most clinicians recommend RAI treatment for elderly patients with hyperthyroidism. It is well tolerated and effective. Elderly patients with hypothyroidism have risks for cardiovascular disease. Therefore, replacement therapy with levothyroxine is initiated in a dose of 0.0125 mg daily. The dosage is increased not more frequently than every 3-4 weeks, with close monitoring for signs and symptoms of angina, of congestive failure or other circulatory problems.

THYROIDITIS

Symptomatic subacute thyroiditis tends to be a self-limited disease but patients may require therapy with NSAIDS or low-dose glucocorticoids if there is severe pain and/or constitutional distress. In general, no treatment is necessary for hyper- or hypothyroidism because they are self limited. If symptoms of hyper- or hypothyroidism are severe or prolonged, treatment with antithyroid drugs, beta blockers, or levothyroxine can be instituted. TFTs should be monitored monthly, and treatments adjusted as the patient reverts to euthyroidism.

GOITER

Goiter often does not require treatment. Levothyroxine suppression (0.1–0.15 mg daily) may be useful, especially early in the course of goiter to control its size. Surgery may be done for cosmetic reasons or, rarely, obstructive symptoms.

THYROID NEOPLASM

Cysts and benign nodules may be observed clinically or treated by suppression with levothyroxine.

Ultrasonography or scan are helpful for following the dimensions of a cyst or neoplasm. Figure 18.7 outlines an apporach to the follow-up of cysts and nodules.

Thyroid cancers are of three main types. Papillary cancer accounts for 70% of thyroid cancer and tends to be slow growing and unlikely to metastasize to distant sites. It has a bimodal incidence—the 3rd and 7th decade. The treatment of choice is total thyroidectomy.

Follicular cancer accounts for 15% of thyroid cancer and tends to grow faster than does papillary and to metastasize sooner. Follicular cancer occurs in older patients. Here too, total thryroidectomy is the treatment of choice.

Anaplastic cancer is the most deadly thyroid cancer. It is seen in the elderly, is rarely curable, and accounts for 5% of thyroid cancers.

ILLUSTRATIVE CASES WITH SELF-ASSESSMENT QUESTIONS AND ANSWERS

Case 1

MG is a 33-year-old woman who presents with nervousness and neck swelling. Her symptoms began insidiously 2 months ago. Physical examination reveals a diffusely enlarged, non-tender thyroid gland, a heart rate of 112, and a fine hand tremor. She has protuberant eyes.

QUESTION: *Which of the following is the most likely diagnosis?*

a. Graves disease
b. Toxic multinodular goiter
c. Benign goiter
d. Thyroiditis

ANSWER: a. *Graves disease causes painless diffuse enlargement of the thyroid gland and hyperthyroidism. It is the only thyroid cause of exophthalmos.*

QUESTION: *What diagnostic test(s) would you order?*

a. T_3 resin uptake, T_4, TSH

b. TSH
c. T_4
d. T_3

ANSWER: b *and* **c.** *As an initial test for a patient who is likely to be hyperthyroid, TSH is the most reliable indicator. TSH should be suppressed. A T_4 level would be confirmatory. T_3 would be expected to be elevated, but is more expensive than T_4 as would be the combination T_3 resin uptake, T_4 and TSH. The T_4 level will be used to guide therapy.*

Case 2

HL is a 72-year-old male with congestive heart failure. He had atrial fibrillation at his previous clinic visit 2 weeks ago.

QUESTION: *What diagnosis should be suspected?*

a. Coronary arterial disease
b. Hyperthyroidism
c. Both A and B

ANSWER: c. *Although coronary arterial disease is much more prevalent, hyperthyroidism is treatable and curable. It would be essential to test for it.*

Case 3

JF is a 65-year-old woman who has sluggishness and weight gain. She has stable angina that requires no regular medication. On physical examination her voice is hoarse, her hair is coarse, she has a heart rate of 56, and a slightly enlarged thyroid gland. Her TSH is elevated and her T_4 is low.

QUESTION: *What is your diagnosis?*

a. Hyperfunctioning adenoma
b. Goiter
c. Pituitary neoplasm
d. Primary hypothyroidism

ANSWER: d. *Her complaints, physical examination, and laboratory tests are consistent with primary hypothyroidism. She is not euthyroid as in benign goiter, or hyperthyroid as in hyperfunctioning adenoma. In the case of pituitary tumor causing hypothyroidism, TSH levels should be low.*

QUESTION: *What treatment do you recommend?*

a. Levothyroxine 0.0125 mg daily, increasing by 0.0125 monthly if her angina does not worsen.
b. Levothyroxine 0.15 mg daily
c. Levothyroxine 0.025 mg daily, increasing daily to a dose of 0.1 mg
d. Levothyroxine 0.1 mg. daily

ANSWER: a. *Because her cardiac symptoms may have been "masked" by hypothyroidism, she is at risk of developing severe angina long before she reaches euthyroidism − maybe after just a week or two of therapy. Replacement doses should start low and be increased slowly, with regular clinical evaluation.*

HYPERLIPIDEMIA

Hyperlipidemia is not a pathologic condition; it is a risk factor for other diseases, principally coronary atherosclerosis. Clinicians are mainly concerned with cholesterol because it is high levels of cholesterol that are correlated with increased coronary death and myocardial infarction rates. Because heart disease is the leading cause of death in the United States, any change in its risk factors can have a great impact on the population.

This section reviews lipid metabolism, the measurement of lipids, and the diagnosis and general management of hyperlipidemia. It looks at the evidence that an elevated level of cholesterol is deleterious and that treating an elevated cholesterol is beneficial. Finally, it surveys current dietary and pharmacologic treatment.

Pathophysiologic Correlation

This section highlights lipid metabolism and the data that higher levels of cholesterol are related to higher levels of heart disease. There are many influences on the level of plasma cholesterol; greatest are the patient's genetic background and intake of saturated fat and cholesterol. The genetics of hypercholesterolemia are not all known, but most cases are polygenic. Knowledge is incomplete on cholesterol metabolism and the effects different variants of lipoproteins, enzymes, or receptors can have.

REVIEW OF LIPID METABOLISM

Cholesterol is a necessary constituent of cell membranes. It is also a precursor molecule for the synthesis of steroid hormones and bile acids. Besides dietary sources, cholesterol is synthesized in the liver and other tissues and is transported throughout the body and back to the liver. Cholesterol is also secreted into bile and reabsorbed in the small intestine. Triglycerides (TG) or fat, are made of fatty acids and a glycerol backbone. Fatty acids are essential fuel sources and are stored in fat cells in the triglyceride form.

Lipoprotein Transport and Function. Cholesterol and triglycerides cannot be transported in an aqueous solution, like plasma, without a hydrophilic coating. This coating is provided by apolipoproteins and phospholipids, which have hydrophobic and hydrophilic ends. Some apolipoproteins act as recognition signals for cellular receptors or enzymes. The hydrophobic core of fat and cholesterol esters surrounded by apolipoproteins, phospholipid, and small amounts of free cholesterol are called lipoproteins (Fig. 18.8).

The lipoproteins are best understood by their function. They are also classified by their buoyancy or density after centrifugation (Table 18.9). From

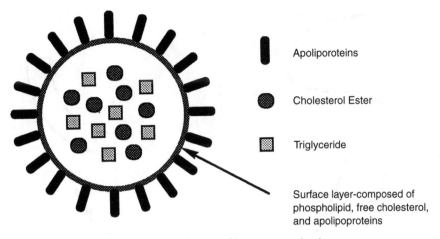

Figure 18.8. Schematic of lipoprotein molecule.

largest and least dense to smallest and most dense, they are: chylomicrons, very low density lipoprotein (VLDL), intermediate density lipoprotein (IDL), low density lipoprotein (LDL), and high density lipoprotein (HDL).

Intestinal Uptake: Chylomicrons. Chylomicrons bring ingested triglycerides and cholesterol to tissues (Fig. 18.9). Intestinal cells surround esterified cholesterol and triglycerides with phospholipid and apolipoproteins and secrete the newly formed chylomicrons into lymphatics. As they circulate, capillary lipoprotein lipase breaks down triglycerides into fatty acids for removal by tissues for energy and fat storage. Chylomicron remnants are taken up by the liver via receptors which recognize apolipoprotein B.

Hepatic Synthesis: Very Low Density, Intermediate Density, and Low Density Lipoproteins. The liver also manufactures and circulates cholesterol and triglycerides (Fig. 18.10). Very low density lipoprotein (VLDL), the largest lipoprotein synthesized, performs in a similar capacity as the chylomicrons. VLDL contains apolipoproteins, phospholipid, and has a high ratio of triglyceride to cholesterol. Triglycerides are again split into fatty acids for release to tissues. VLDL also interacts with high density lipoprotein to accept more cholesterol while releasing apolipoproteins and phospholipid. Of the remaining VLDL remnants, two-thirds are catabolized by the liver and one-third become intermediate density lipoprotein (IDL). Further removal of triglycerides, phospho-

Table 18.9.
Lipoprotein Characteristics

Lipoprotein	Density (g/ml)	Cholesterol % of Total Mass	Triglycerides % of Total Mass	Apolipoproteins
Chylomicrons	0.95	2–7	80–90	A-I, A-II, A-IV, B-48, C-I, C-II, C-III, E
Very low density (VLDL)	<1.006	10–22	50–70	B-100, C-I, C-II, C-III, E
Intermediate density (IDL)	1.006–1.019	30–40	40	B, E
Low density (LDL)	1.019–1.063	45–50	5–10	B-100
High density (HDL)	1.063–1.21	15–25	3–5	A, C, E

Adapted from Blackman M, Kern D, Clinical implications of abnormal lipoprotein metabolism in Barker L, Burton J, Zieve P. eds. Principles of Ambulatory Medicine. Baltimore: Williams & Wilkins, 1992.

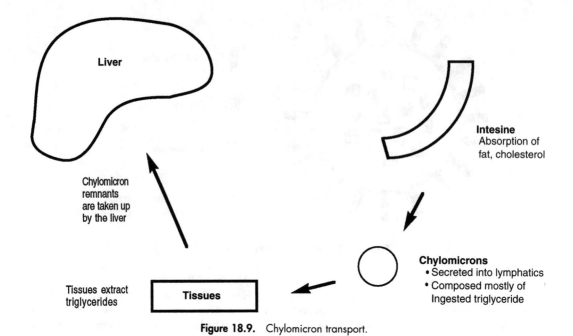

Figure 18.9. Chylomicron transport.

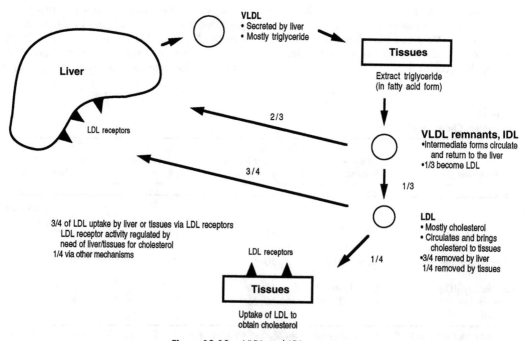

Figure 18.10. VLDL and LDL transport.

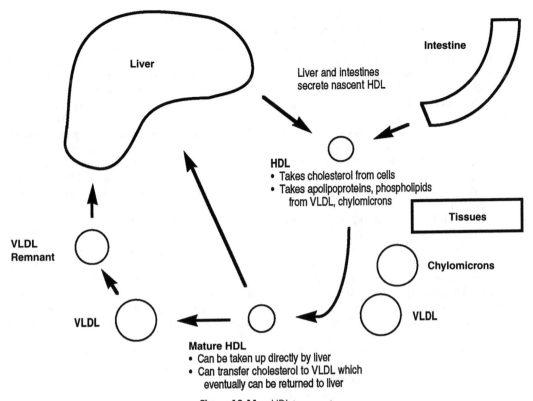

Figure 18.11. HDL transport.

lipid, and apolipoproteins from IDL results in the formation of low density lipoprotein (LDL), which is now cholesterol rich. The only apolipoprotein left on LDL is B-100.

LDL circulates and brings cholesterol to tissues. Of circulating LDL, the liver removes approximately ¾ and tissues ¼. Mechanisms utilizing specific cellular receptors that recognize apolipoprotein B-100 are responsible for ⅔ to ¾ of LDL uptake, both in the liver and in tissues. Poorly understood mechanisms not involving receptors account for the balance.

LDL can deposit in arterial walls, where it is engulfed by foam cells. These cells, thought to be derived from macrophages, accumulate LDL and oxidized LDL. Atherosclerosis can result, with the build-up of cholesterol, smooth muscle cells, connective tissue, and debris.

Return of Cholesterol to the Liver: High Density Lipoprotein. High density lipoprotein (HDL) is the main instrument of cholesterol reuptake for return to the liver. HDL is synthesized in the liver and in intestinal cells (Fig. 18.11). It begins as a hollow disk, composed of phospholipid and

apolipoproteins, and becomes filled with cholesterol esters. HDL also acquires apolipoproteins from chylomicrons and VLDL during its circulation.

The "reverse transport" of cholesterol has not been fully characterized, nor has the function of different HDL subclasses. The direct pathway consists of HDL uptake of cholesterol from cell membranes. The indirect pathway is thought to use transfer of cholesterol from HDL to VLDL. VLDL becomes VLDL remnants with subsequent hepatic catabolism.

LINKS BETWEEN ATHEROSCLEROSIS AND HYPERCHOLESTEROLEMIA

Is a high cholesterol level necessarily harmful? The clinician can examine several lines of evidence linking high cholesterol levels to coronary heart disease. Several types of studies have been done, including cross-sectional population, family, and cohort studies.

Cross-Sectional Population Studies. One method would be to look at different populations in different locales or countries, and plot cholesterol levels versus the incidence of heart disease. There is a positive relation between the level of cholesterol in a country's population and the number of deaths from heart disease (the higher the cholesterol, the higher the death rate from heart disease). The relation is strongest for middle-aged men. Using the total cholesterol to HDL ratio results in a stronger correlation. Lower levels of cholesterol are found in less developed countries, but also in some industrialized nations like Japan, where less meat is eaten. Migration studies of ethnic Japanese men from Japan, Hawaii and the continental United States also show that as cholesterol increases, heart disease increases (1,2).

Genetic Insights from Family Studies. Brown and Goldstein studied families with extremely elevated levels of cholesterol and early occurrence of myocardial infarction. They found patients who had defective LDL receptor activity and impaired LDL reabsorption (3). The patients produced great amounts of cholesterol because their livers received little negative feedback to control cholesterol production. Homozygous patients with two defective genes and without any working LDL receptors have cholesterol levels approaching 1000 mg/dl and suffer myocardial infarction as young adults. Heterozygous patients (1 of 500 in the general population) have cholesterol levels near 400 mg/dl and also have high rates of heart disease.

Epidemiologic Evidence: Cohort Studies.

More evidence for the role of cholesterol in coronary artery disease arises from examining populations over time. The Framingham Study followed 5209 men and women (Fig. 18.12). After 14 years, high cholesterol levels, hypertension, smoking, diabetes, and obesity were found in increase the risk for coronary artery disease. Men aged 30-49 who had levels of cholesterol between 265-294 mg/dl had 2.4 times the risk of developing coronary disease as men with cholesterol between 205-234 mg/dl (4). The level of HDL was inversely related to coronary disease (the lower the HDL, the higher the risk). This relation was true for women as well as men (5).

The Multiple Risk Factor Intervention Trial (MRFIT), screened 361,662 men, aged 35-57, for hypertension, smoking, and hypercholesterolemia. Six years later, records were searched to determine who had died of heart disease. Of the men without a prior history of coronary artery disease, there was a 17% increased risk of death from heart disease with each increase of 20 mg/dl of cholesterol (Fig. 18.13) (6). There was no cutoff level or "safe" cholesterol, so that there was a risk of heart disease at every level of cholesterol.

Clinical and Laboratory Evaluation

The clinician uses the history, physical examination, and laboratory results to properly diagnose

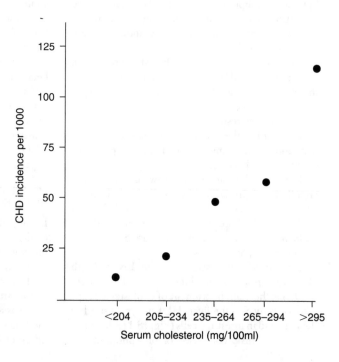

Figure 18.12. Risk of coronary heart disease over 6 years in men aged 30-49 according to serum cholesterol level in the Framingham Study. (From Castelli W. Epidemiology of coronary artery disease: the Framingham Study. Am J Med 1984;76:4.)

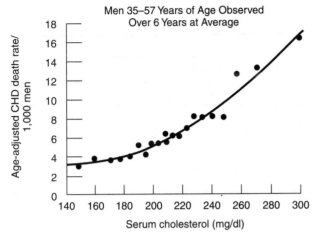

Figure 18.13. Relationship of cholesterol to coronary heart disease mortality in men aged 35-57 years over an average 6 years from MRFIT screening. (From the Johns Hopkins physician's lipid education program, a practical approach to the patient with a lipid disorder, 2nd ed. Baltimore: Johns Hopkins University, 1988.)

and treat the hyperlipidemic patient. Each can add important information. This section will review pertinent features of each category of data.

HISTORY

The clinician should inquire about symptoms of coronary artery disease. Exercise tolerance and normal activity level are helpful to check for limitation by ischemia or other diseases. The clinician should inquire about other vascular diseases such as stroke or claudication. Symptoms of hypothyroidism can be elicited. The clinician should also ask about a family history of elevated cholesterol, heart disease, or early cardiac death. Other risk factors for coronary disease should be sought, such as diabetes, smoking, hypertension, and obesity. A gynecologic history is necessary to determine menstrual status. The clinician should obtain a diet history, especially the intake of meats, dairy products, processed foods, fats and oils, snacks, and restaurant meals.

PHYSICAL EXAMINATION

High cholesterol levels result in few physical signs. Xanthelasmas are small yellowish plaques usually found around the eyelids. Xanthomas can be small nodules on tendon surfaces or diffuse cutaneous plaques and papules. Tendon xanthomas are hard and suggest familial hypercholesterolemia. The clinician evaluates for obesity by measuring height and weight.

LABORATORY EVALUATION

The laboratory evaluation begins with a determination of the total serum cholesterol. The patient

need not fast for the test. The National Cholesterol Education Program (NCEP) divides blood cholesterol into three classifications: "desirable" for cholesterol < 200 mg/dl; "borderline" for 200-239 mg/dl; and "elevated" for levels > 240 mg/dl (Table 18.10). If the cholesterol is greater than 240 mg/dl, or greater than 200 mg/dl and the patient has two or more cardiac risk factors, the NCEP recommends fractionation of the cholesterol.

Total cholesterol and HDL are measurable. The equation

Total cholesterol = VLDL + LDL + HDL

allows an estimate of LDL cholesterol. VLDL is approximated by dividing the triglyceride level by five. This method is inaccurate if the TG level is greater than 400 mg/dl. Some experts advocate obtaining HDL measurements on all patients, since it is also an independent risk factor for heart disease.

Considerations About Cholesterol Measurement. The most accurate and reproducible measurement is total cholesterol. Since LDL is calculated, there is a greater chance of error. It is not recommended to take action, especially prescribing medication, unless the cholesterol measurement has been repeated (7). It is sufficient to average the two results unless the results are widely disparate, when a third determination may be needed. The reliability and accuracy of HDL values are less well standardized than for total cholesterol. Cholesterol should also not be measured during acute illness or myocardial infarction, as the result will be lower than usual.

In the future, it may be possible to more easily order other lipoprotein measurements. There is

Table 18.10.
NCEP Classification of Cholesterol

Cholesterol	Category	Action
≥240 mg/dl	High	Determine HDL and calculate LDL
200–239 mg/dl	Borderline-high	If two or more risk factors,[a] determine HDL and calculate LDL
<199 mg/dl	Desirable	Counsel on diet, general health measures

[a]Risk factors

Positive Risk Factors
Age
   Male ≥ 45 years old
   Female ≥ 55 years old or premature menopause without estrogen replacement therapy
Family history of premature CAD
   Definite MI or sudden death before 55 years of age in father or other male first-degree relative, or before 65 years of age in mother
      or other female first-degree relative
Current cigarette smoking
Hypertension (blood pressure ≥ 140/90 or taking antihypertensive medication)
Low HDL cholesterol (<35 mg/dl)
Diabetes mellitus
Negative Risk Factors (subtract one positive risk factor for each negative risk factor)
High HDL Cholesterol (≥60 mg/dl)
Adapted from Expert Panel on Detection, Evaluation, and Treatment of High Blood Cholesterol in Adults (Adult Treatment Panel II).
   Second report of the National Cholesterol Education Program (NCEP) expert panel on detection, evaluation, and treatment of high
   blood cholesterol in adults (Adult Treatment Panel II). Circulation 1994; 89: 1334–1445.

great interest in which lipoprotein and apolipoprotein phenotypes and which subfractions of LDL and VLDL are most atherogenic. It may also be possible to quantitate HDL subtypes to better gauge the risk of a low HDL value.

Differential Diagnosis

When high levels of cholesterol are found, the clinician should rule out secondary causes of hyperlipidemia. This includes hypothyroidism, nephrotic syndrome, poorly controlled diabetes mellitus, obstructive liver disease, and medications such as progestins and anabolic steroids. This is easily done with a thorough history, physical examination, thyroid stimulating hormone (TSH) level, urinalysis, and glycosylated hemoglobin.

Certain patterns or phenotypes of familial hyperlipidemias are not uncommon. Depending on which lipoprotein fraction is elevated, serum triglyceride and/or cholesterol may be raised. For example, if the liver cannot remove chylomicrons normally, triglycerides would be very elevated. However, most syndromes are managed based on the cholesterol and triglycerides levels alone.

Management

The decision whether to treat an elevated cholesterol level depends on the individual's risk of coronary artery disease. The following table shows the

recommendations of the NCEP based on LDL cholesterol levels (Table 18.11). The clinician should also address other modifiable coronary heart disease risk factors such as smoking, obesity, and lack of physical activity to try to lower risk.

DIET

Dietary treatment is the cornerstone of treatment for hyperlipidemia. Reducing dietary saturated fat is more important than reducing dietary cholesterol. By replacing saturated fat calories with calories from unsaturated or monosaturated fat or carbohydrate, cholesterol will be lowered. The magnitude of the reduction depends on a person's prior diet. In the Lipid Research Clinics (LRC) and Helsinki Heart Trials, dietary counseling and education were able to reduce participants' cholesterol an average of 5%. The American Heart Association (AHA) Step One diet limits the amount of cholesterol to 300 mg/day, the proportion of calories derived from fat to 30%, and the proportion of calories from saturated fat to 10%.

If the patient's cholesterol level remains high after 2 to 3 months, intensified dietary modification is tried. The AHA Step Two diet limits cholesterol intake to 200 mg/dl and saturated fat to no more than 7% of total calories. A minimum of 6 months of dietary treatment is recommended as well as counseling by a nutritionist or dietician.

Table 18.11.
NCEP Recommendations Based on LDL Cholesterol

Patient Category	Initiation of Therapy	Goal of Therapy
Dietary therapy		
Without CHD and with fewer than two risk factors	≥ 160 mg/dl	< 160 mg/dl
Without CHD and with two or more risk factors	≥ 130 mg/dl	< 130 mg/dl
With CHD	> 100 mg/dl	≤ 100 mg/dl
Drug therapy		
Without CHD and with fewer than two risk factors	≥ 190 mg/dl	< 160 mg/dl
Without CHD and with two or more risk factors	≥ 160 mg/dl	< 130 mg/dl
With CHD	≥ 130 mg/dl	≤100 mg/dl

Adapted from Expert Panel on Detection, Evaluation, and Treatment of High Blood Cholesterol in Adults (Adult Treatment Panel II). Second report of the National Cholesterol Education Program (NCEP) expert panel on detection, evaluation, and treatment of high blood cholesterol in adults (Adult Treatment Panel II). Circulation 1994; 89: 1334–1445.

Greater reductions are possible; Dean Ornish (author of the popular book Eat More, Weigh Less) has shown that a program of a vegetarian diet, combined with regular exercise and stress management, can decrease total cholesterol up to 30% (8). A concern about low fat diets is that HDL cholesterol may be lowered along with LDL and total cholesterol. Some support replacing saturated fat calories with monounsaturated fats like olive oil rather than with carbohydrate.

PHARMACOLOGIC TREATMENT

First the clinician must decide to whom to offer pharmacologic treatment. The patient must also agree to drug therapy, as it is destined to fail without the patient's understanding of the nature and treatment of hyperlipidemia. One possible strategy would be for the clinician to discuss what is known about cholesterol modification and allow patients to choose the treatment they are comfortable with. In that manner, the patient is a participant and more likely to adhere to medical or diet therapy. Table 18.12 summarizes pharmacologic treatments currently available.

There are many approaches to pharmacologic treatment, depending on the provider's analysis of the literature. Does lowering cholesterol actually decrease morbidity or mortality? If it does, by what amounts? This section will review the two main primary prevention (patients without heart disease) trials published and one recent landmark study, the Scandinavian Simvastatin Survival Study (4S).

The Lipid Research Clinics Coronary Primary Prevention Trial (LRC) divided 3,806 middle aged men into two groups. One group received six packets of cholestyramine daily and the other placebo. Follow-up for signs of cardiovascular disease, including death, myocardial infarction, a positive stress test, stroke, or transient ischemic attack, continued for an average of 7 years. In the cholestyramine group, 8.1% of the participants suffered a heart attack or coronary death versus 9.8% of the placebo group. This 1.7% decrease was a 19% reduction in relative risk. It required 2 years before there was any difference in events. The treatment group's average decrease in total cholesterol was 8% and in LDL 11%. Total or all-cause mortality for the two groups was not significantly different (9,10).

The Helsinki Heart Trial studied 4,081 middle-aged, hypercholesterolemic, Finnish men for approximately 5 years. One group received gemfibrozil (600 mg twice a day) and the other placebo. With the drug, total cholesterol decreased 11%, LDL 10%, and HDL rose 10%. Of the treated group, 2.7% compared to 4.1% of the placebo group suffered a heart attack or definite coronary death. This absolute difference of 1.4% was a 34% reduction in risk (11). As in the LRC trial, it took 2 years before the groups diverged and there was no change in total death rate.

Both the Helsinki Heart and LRC trials led to similar conclusions: it was possible to decrease cardiovascular events by lowering cholesterol with drugs, but it did not save lives. This may be because the trials did not lower cholesterol enough, a fluke in the statistical data, or that drug treatment affects patients in ways we do not yet realize. Other limitations were that the trials only included middle-aged

Table 18.12.
Major Cholesterol Lowering Agents

Drug	Average Dosage	Mechanism of Action	Estimated Effect	Advantages	Disadvantages	Average Wholesale Cost
CHOLESTYRAMINE Questran, Questran Light **COLESTIPOL** Colestid	4g–12g BID-TID 5g–10g BID	Bile Acid Sequestrant • Increases LDL receptor activity • Increases excretion of bile acids	Lowers LDL 15–30%	Safe, Non-toxic Cholestyramine-lowered Coronary Heart Disease deaths in LRC Trial	Constipation Bloating Can increase triglycerides Can interfere with absorption of fat-soluble vitamins	Cholestyramine 4g TID = $3.64 a day Colestipol 10g BID = 2.98 a day
GEMFIBROZIL Lopid	600 mg BID	Increases Lipoprotein Lipase activity • Decreases incorporation of free fatty acids into triglycerides	Lowers LDL 5–15% Raises HDL 20% Lowers TG 20–50%	Lowered MI's in Helsinki Heart Trial Easy to take	GI upset Myositis possible with HMG-CoA Reductase Inhibitors Potentiation of warfarin Can increase gallstones	600 mg BID = $2.19 a day
LOVASTATIN Mevacor **PRAVASTATIN** Pravachol **SIMVASTATIN** Zocor **FLUVASTATIN** Lescol	20 mg qD up to 80 mg qD 5 mg qD up to 40 mg qD 20 mg qd up to 40 mg qD 20 mg qd up to 40–80 mg qD	HMG-CoA Reductase Inhibitor • Interferes with enzymatic step in cholesterol production • Increases LDL receptor activity	Lowers LDL 25–45% Raises HDL 10%	Lowered mortality and coronary mortality in Scandinavian Simvastatin Survival Study Easy to take Highly effective	Can increase LFT's in 1–2% of patients Myositis in 0.15% of patients Should not use with gemfibrozil, niacin or cyclosporine In dogs—cataracts; no evidence in humans.	Lovastatin 20 mg qD = $2.00 a day Pravastatin 20 mg qD = $1.80 a day Simvastatin 20 mg qD = $1.63 a day Fluvastatin 40 mg qd = $1.14 a day
NIACIN (NICOTINIC ACID)	500 mg–1 g tid start at 100 mg TID	Decrease synthesis of VLDL Inhibits lipolysis in fat	Lowers LDL 15–30% Raises HDL 20–30% Lowers TG 20–50%	Decreased subsequent MI's in Coronary Drug Project	Flushing Pruritis GI Upset } Can take with meals or with ASA to lessen Can increase LFT's glucose, uric acid	1 g TID = $0.18 a day
PROBUCOL Loreko	500 mg BID	Increases LDL catabolism	Lowers LDL 10–15% Lowers HDL 20–30%	Easy to take	Decreases HDL Can prolong QT Interval Recent MI, arrhythmias are contraindication GI upset	500 mg BID = $2.32 a day

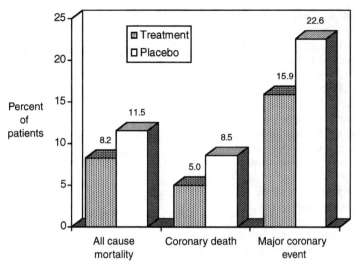

Figure 18.14. Scandinavian Simvastatin Survival Study. Comparison of mortality, coronary death, and major coronary events between treatment and placebo groups with a median 5.4 years of follow-up. (Adapted from Scandinavian Simavastatin Survival Study Group. Randomized trial of cholesterol lowering in 4444 patients with coronary heart disease: the Scandinavian Simavastatin Survival Study (4S). Lancet 1994;344:1386.)

men; it is not known if their results are applicable to women, elderly, or minority patients.

The Scandinavian Simvastatin Survival Study (4S), published in 1994, was the first study to show a lower mortality in patients treated pharmacologically to lower an elevated cholesterol. Patients (4,444) with a history of myocardial infarction or angina and total cholesterol levels between 213 and 310 mg/dl were divided into placebo and treatment groups. The treatment group took 20 to 40 mg of simvastatin daily to lower cholesterol to less than 213 mg/dl. Total cholesterol decreased an average of 25%, LDL 35%, and HDL rose an average of 8% on treatment. After a median follow-up period of 5.4 years, 8.2% of treated patients versus 11.5% of placebo patients had died (Fig. 18.14). This absolute reduction of 3.3% in mortality equals a 30% reduction in risk. A similar decline was found for coronary death rates, 5.0% vs. 8.5%, and major coronary events 15.9% vs. 22.6%. It took 1 year of treatment before the groups began to diverge. Upon subgroup analysis, treated women had 35% fewer major coronary events but did not show any difference in mortality compared to women taking placebo. In contrast, patients over 60 years of age did show decreases in mortality and major coronary events (12).

Resins or Bile Acid Sequestrants. Cholestyramine and colestipol are ion-exchange resins. They bind bile acid salts in the small intestine.

The liver manufactures more bile acids, and LDL receptor activity increases to enhance uptake of LDL. These two actions decrease plasma cholesterol. The resins are taken two to three times daily and can lower LDL 15–30%. Common side effects are constipation and bloating. They can interfere with the absorption of fat soluble vitamins and can raise triglyceride levels. An advantage is that they are not systemically absorbed.

Fibric Acids. Gemfibrozil is the only agent used in this class. It increases lipoprotein lipase activity and decreases the incorporation of free fatty acids into triglycerides, but how it lowers LDL and raises HDL is unknown. It can decrease LDL 5–15%, increase HDL 20%, and decrease TGs 20–50% in its usual dose of 600mg twice a day. It is convenient to take. Adverse effects include gastrointestinal upset, possible myositis if given with hydroxy-methylglutaryl coenzyme A reductase inhibitors, the potentiation of warfarin, and an increased incidence of gallstones. It is most useful for those patients with mildly increased LDL, low HDL, and/or high triglyceride levels.

Hydroxy-Methylglutaryl Coenzyme A (HMG Co A) Reductase Inhibitors. HMG Co A reductase inhibitors interfere with the last reversible enzymatic step in cholesterol production. They are the most potent agents to lower LDL, achieving reductions of 25–45%. They also increase HDL approximately 10%. The HMG Co A reductase inhibitors are simple to take and cost less than resins or fibric acids to obtain an equivalent reduction in cholesterol. There is an approximate 0.15% risk of myositis; this is increased with concomitant use of gemfibrozil, niacin, or cyclosporine. Thus, use of those agents with a HMG Co A reductase inhibitor is contraindicated. HMG Co A reductase inhibitors raise liver transaminases in approximately 1-2% of patients. It is prudent to monitor liver transaminases and creatinine kinase levels periodically. HMG Co A reductase inhibitors are most useful to treat elevated total cholesterol and LDL levels. Currently available formulations include lovastatin, pravastatin, simvastatin, and fluvastatin.

Niacin. Niacin or nicotinic acid, decreases synthesis of VLDL, and inhibits lipolysis of fat. It can lower LDL 15–30%, raise HDL 20–30%, and lower TG 20–50%. In the Coronary Drug Project, a secondary prevention trial, three grams of niacin daily decreased the occurrence of second non-fatal myocardial infarctions by 27% (8.9% in the treatment group vs. 12.2% in the control group) over an average of 5 years (13,14). Ten years after the trial ended, there was a slight survival difference when the patients were re-examined. The major adverse effects of niacin are flushing, pruritis, gastrointestinal upset, and elevations in liver transaminases. Aspirin can be given 30 minutes before to decrease the flushing. These symptoms usually abate with continued treatment. The sustained release form may lower the occurrence of flushing, but may increase gastrointestinal upset and hepatic toxicity. Niacin is most useful in patients with moderate hypercholesterolemia, low HDL, and/or elevated triglycerides.

Probucol. Probucol increases LDL catabolism. It can decrease LDL 10–15%, but also decreases HDL 20–30%. It is easy to take, but can cause a prolonged QT interval and gastrointestinal upset. Its unknown clinical effects of lowering both LDL and HDL levels make it problematic to use.

OTHER TREATMENTS

Other possible therapies include exercise, moderate alcohol consumption, and soluble fiber. Exercise can raise HDL levels and assist in weight reduction efforts. Alcohol in modest amounts, one to two drinks per day, may increase HDL levels. Soluble fiber (psyllium) has been studied as an adjunct to dietary treatment. In limited trials, it has been able to reduce total cholesterol by 5–8%.

SPECIAL CONSIDERATIONS IN TREATMENT

All of the major pharmacologic primary prevention trials were done in middle-aged men. There has been a paucity of studies on cholesterol levels and heart disease for the elderly and women. In addition, studies on the effect of treatment in minority groups is lacking. The benefits of lowering cholesterol in women or the elderly, and in minority groups needs to be studied further.

Women. Women get coronary artery disease later in life than men, yet as many women as men die each year of coronary disease. Women are much less likely to get coronary artery disease until after menopause. It is unknown how the menstrual cycle "protects" women from coronary disease. Estrogen replacement after menopause seems to lower LDL and raise HDL, but it is not known if there are other effects. In the future, women should be included in any major prevention trial. Women's cholesterol metabolism and the effects of drug therapy may be different.

Elderly. The elderly are the group with the highest rates of coronary heart disease, yet there have been few studies on whether pharmacologically lowering cholesterol is beneficial in this age group. Since coronary artery disease is common in the elderly, a small benefit may translate into an effect on a large number of people. High cholesterol levels in older adults contribute less to the relative risk for a heart attack than in younger adults with high cholesterols. Since it is a more common event, there is a wide range of cholesterol values in the elderly who develop coronary disease. In fact, the majority of myocardial infarctions in the elderly occur in people with "normal" cholesterol levels. It is not clear what policy should be for elderly patients without pre-existing heart disease.

Patients With Coronary Artery Disease. Treating these patients may lower the risk for a second heart attack. Niacin and simvastatin have been shown to reduce the actual incidence of subsequent non-fatal myocardial infarctions. In addition, the 4S trial was able to show that lowering cholesterol reduced mortality in patients with a prior myocardial infarction or angina (12). Several trials have used repeated coronary angiography to try to show that lowering of cholesterol may reduce the risk of progression of disease. This may not be true in patients with normal values of cholesterol however.

ILLUSTRATIVE CASES WITH SELF-ASSESSMENT QUESTIONS AND ANSWERS

Case 1

A 54 year-old male, without other coronary heart disease risk factors, has a cholesterol of 255 mg/dl.

QUESTION: *How should you intervene?*

a. Start him on a HMG Co A reductase inhibitor, since they are our most potent lipid lowering agents.
b. Start him on a Step One diet, since all patients should be given a trial of diet therapy.
c. Repeat his cholesterol and obtain HDL and a calculated LDL cholesterol.
d. Do nothing, since he has no coronary heart disease risk factors other than being male.

ANSWER: c. *Repeat his cholesterol and obtain HDL and a calculated LDL cholesterol. Before deciding on any treatment, it is necessary to confirm the total cholesterol. HDL and LDL information will help the clinician stratify his risk and make a more informed decision. His risk factor by NCEP criteria is being a male >45 years of age.*

Case 2

A 73 year-old female smoker, with diabetes mellitus and hypertension, is found on repeated measurements to have a total cholesterol of 285 mg/dl, a HDL of 40 mg/dl and a LDL of 200 mg/dl.

QUESTION: *What should you do?*

a. Start her on a HMG coenzyme A reductase inhibitor, since they are our most potent lipid lowering agents.
b. Start her on a Step One diet, since all patients should be given a trial of diet therapy.
c. Tell her that stopping smoking will have the greatest effect on her chances of having a heart attack.
d. Do nothing because she is already 73 years old.

ANSWER: c. *Tell her that stopping smoking will have the greatest effect on her chances of having a heart attack. Quitting smoking also has few adverse consequences. Answer B is also reasonable, since dietary modification, especially a Step One diet is a modest action. Though she has many risk factors for coronary artery disease, it remains to be proven whether lowering a 73-year-old female's cholesterol without coronary disease will decrease her chance of a cardiovascular event.*

Case 3

A 57-year-old male with single vessel coronary artery disease is found to have a cholesterol of 318 mg/dl with an LDL of 193 mg/dl and a HDL of 34 mg/dl. After 6 months of intensive diet modification, his cholesterol is now 288 mg/dl, with an LDL of 167 mg/dl.

QUESTION: *What do you advise him?*

a. Start him on a HMG coenzyme A reductase inhibitor, since they are our most potent lipid lowering agents.
b. Start him on a bile acid sequestrant, since it has been shown to lower the risk of a first heart attack.
c. Start him on gemfibrozil, since it has been shown to lower the risk of a first heart attack.
d. Do nothing, since he has nearly achieved a moderate level of LDL.

ANSWER: a. *Start him on a HMG coenzyme A reductase inhibitor, since they are our most potent lipid lowering agents. On the basis of the 4S trial, simvastatin decreases both cardiovascular event rates and mortality in men with past myocardial infarction or angina. Answers B (start him on a bile acid sequestrant) because it has decreased the risk of a first heart attack or C (start him on gemfibrozil) because it has decreased the risk of a first heart attack are both also reasonable. If he is started on medicines, they will have a greater effect if he remains on his diet. The NCEP guidelines recommend lowering LDL to <100 mg/dl for patients with known coronary ar-*

tery disease. However, this recommendation has not been studied in clinical trials.

Case 4

A 36-year-old female is referred because of a family history of early myocardial infarction. Her total cholesterol is 410 mg/dl, LDL 245 mg/dl, and HDL 75 mg/dl. You suspect a familial form of hypercholesterolemia.

QUESTION: *What do you advise her?*

a. Tell her you will start her on medicine anyway, so she can eat whatever she wants.
b. Tell her that her total cholesterol to HDL ratio is above average for a heart attack.
c. Tell her that she will require a comprehensive genetic evaluation.
d. Start her on a cholesterol-lowering diet.

ANSWER: d. *Start her on a cholesterol-lowering diet. Though it is very likely that she has a familial cause of her hypercholesterolemia, dietary therapy still has a role. Pharmacologic therapy is more effective if a diet is followed. Answer b is also correct, but LDL and HDL are independent risk factors for coronary disease. She is still at risk, because of her high LDL, though for women, it is not as strongly predictive as with men. If resources allow, a phenotype of her cholesterol elevation may be done, which is different than a comprehensive genetic evaluation.*

ABNORMAL WEIGHT AND NUTRITION

Large population studies conducted by life insurance agencies have demonstrated an association between increased body weight and mortality. Approximately 26% or 34 million adults in America are overweight. A significantly overweight individual is at increased risk for developing hypertension, diabetes, coronary artery disease, cerebrovascular disease as well as several other conditions.

Less often patients are concerned about being underweight. The clinician must, however, remain extremely vigilant when encountering involuntary weight loss, as it may be an indication of serious systemic disease. Additionally, the markedly underweight patient is at risk during periods of prolonged food deprivation or periods of high metabolic stress. Patients undergoing extensive pre-operative evaluation and those battling cancer are two groups of underweight patients likely to experience complications such as sepsis, poor wound healing and slower recovery in general.

The first problem encountered in any discussion of abnormal weight is to define what is normal weight. Ideal weights are difficult to derive because of the diversity of body types (i.e., frame sizes). The Metropolitan Life Insurance tables are the most widely used tables of desirable body weight (Table 18.13). Constructed in both 1959 and 1983, these tables reflect pooled data on nearly 5 million insured individuals, but have been frequently criticized for the inherent selection bias that people who seek life insurance are healthier and thinner than the general population.

Pathophysiologic Correlation

Two individuals with the same weight and height can have varying proportions of bone, muscle, and fat mass. Obesity is defined as an excess amount of body fat. An estimated 25% of Americans over age 20 are considered obese. The health risks of being overweight are directly associated with an increased percent of body fat. Moreover, the specific pattern of body fat distribution is also of great importance in predicting morbidity and mortality. There is no simple or reliable method to directly measure a persons total body fat. The most widely used measure of body composition is the body mass index (BMI).

$$BMI = weight\ (kg)/height\ (m)^2$$

BMI values help correct for changes in weight due to height and are thus useful in assessing the degree of obesity. BMI can also be determined by using a nomogram. The National Center for Health Statistics defines overweight as a BMI greater than the 85th percentile. This corresponds to a BMI of more than 27.8 kg/m^2 for men and above 27.3 kg/m^2 for women. It is felt that while most degrees of obesity (BMI<40) result from an increase in fat cell size (hypertrophy), extreme obesity (BMI>40) may involve an increase in total number of fat cells (hyperplasia).

Body composition can be estimated by measuring fatfolds. Two commonly used measures of total body fat are the fatfold thickness over the triceps muscle and in the subscapular area. Using skin calipers total body fat composition can be initially estimated and subsequently followed by remeasuring of fatfold thicknesses.

Table 18.13.
1983 Metropolitan Height and Weight Tables

Weights at ages 25 to 29 based on lowest mortality. Weights in pounds according to frame (in indoor clothing weighing 5 pounds for men or 3 pounds for women), shoes with 1-inch heels.

Men					Women				
Height		Small Frame	Medium Frame	Large Frame	Height		Small Frame	Medium Frame	Large Frame
(ft)	(inches)				(ft)	(inches)			
5	2	128–134	131–141	138–150	4	10	102–111	109–121	118–131
5	3	130–136	133–143	140–153	4	11	103–113	111–123	120–134
5	4	132–138	135–145	142–156	5	0	104–115	113–126	122–137
5	5	134–140	137–148	144–160	5	1	106–118	115–129	125–140
5	6	136–142	139–151	146–164	5	2	108–121	118–132	128–143
5	7	138–145	142–154	149–168	5	3	111–124	121–135	131–147
5	8	140–148	145–157	152–172	5	4	114–127	124–138	134–151
5	9	142–151	148–160	155–176	5	5	117–130	127–141	137–155
5	10	144–154	151–163	158–180	5	6	120–133	130–144	140–159
5	11	146–157	154–166	161–184	5	7	123–136	133–147	143–163
5	0	149–160	157–170	164–188	5	8	126–139	136–150	146–167
6	1	152–164	160–174	168–192	5	9	129–142	139–153	149–170
6	2	155–168	164–178	172–197	5	10	132–145	142–156	152–173
6	3	158–162	167–182	176–202	5	11	135–148	145–159	155–176
6	4	162–176	171–187	181–207	6	0	138–151	148–162	158–179

Reproduced with permission of Metropolitan Life Insurance Company. 1979 Build Study. Society of Actuaries and Association of Life Insurance Medical Directors of America, 1983.

The specific pattern of fat distribution is important in determining health risk. It is well established that central obesity, that is obesity occurring primarily at and above the waist, is associated with an increased incidence of diabetes, stroke, coronary artery disease and death, independent of total body fat. One simple measure of fat distribution is the waist to hip size ratio. As this ratio increases and approaches 1.0 in women and 0.8 in men, the risk for obesity related morbidity increases.

ENERGY BALANCE

Obesity is a result of an imbalance between energy intake and energy utilization. When energy intake exceeds requirements, this excess energy is stored as fat. Multiple other factors, many poorly understood, are involved in the complex physiology of obesity including mechanisms of fat storage, genetic influences on fat metabolism and psychological factors. In general, however, a basic approach to obesity starts with the following equation:

change in energy stores = energy intake
− energy output

Any attempt to decrease body fat must begin with influencing the above equation so that energy stored is negative. This goal is usually achieved by decreasing the quantity of energy intake while simultaneously increasing the energy output.

Energy Intake. Energy intake represents solely the amount of calories an individual consumes. Repeated studies have confirmed the association between increased caloric intake and weight gain. Conversely, reduced-calorie diets lead to a reduction in weight and fat stored in both obese and non-obese people. Previously obese people at near normal weights, however, appeared to require fewer calories to maintain their weight than people who were never obese. These findings have given rise to the set-point theory of obesity. Simply stated, this theory holds that the body chooses a specific weight it wants to be and regulates metabolic activity and eating behavior to maintain this weight. Alteration of energy intake is the chief means of reducing body weight.

Energy Output. The body expends energy in primarily two ways; basal metabolism is the sum of the energy required by the body to maintain constant functioning. The work of inhaling and exhaling, maintaining a beating heart, and keeping a steady body temperature are a few of the constant energy-consuming processes that make up one's basal metabolism. On average, the basal metabolic rate (BMR) is an extremely active process usually accounting for approximately 60% of the body's daily energy expenditure.

WEIGHT LOSS

Weight loss can result from one of three processes: l) decreased caloric intake; 2) increased nutritional losses; or 3) an increase in nutritional requirements. Major causes of decreased oral intake include anorexia, nausea, dysphagia, abdominal pain, substance abuse, poverty, senility or depression. Increased nutritional losses may result from malabsorption, diarrhea, diabetes mellitus, and nephrosis. Nutritional requirements are increased in the presence of fever, infection, neoplasm, burns, and trauma.

Insufficient caloric and protein intake results in protein-energy malnutrition (PEM). Total body protein depletion and weight loss are the hallmarks of significant malnutrition. Among developing nations, PEM is usually due to inadequate intake. In industrialized societies, PEM is most frequently seen in patients with underlying psychiatric or medical conditions.

PEM adversely affects virtually every organ system. Cardiac function is compromised with diminution of cardiac stroke volume and stroke index. Hepatic synthesis of vital proteins is reduced. Stores of glycogen in the liver are depleted triggering gluconeogenesis with consequent breakdown of muscle tissue. Endocrine changes are diverse including abnormal thyroid functioning and in women, amenorrhea. Wound healing is severely impaired as a result of protein depletion. Perhaps, most significant is the severely compromised immune system found in patients with PEM. Reduction in both total lymphocyte number and function predisposes the malnourished patient to infection.

Clinical and Laboratory Evaluation

The vast majority of cases of obesity are not due to medical conditions. In addition to advising the patient on means of weight loss, the clinician's attention should be focused on diagnosing and treating the complications associated with being overweight (Fig. 18.15). In contrast, unexplained weight loss must alert the physician to a prompt search for an underlying cause.

HISTORY

Obtaining an accurate history is the initial step in evaluation of the obese patient. Most patients will report gaining weight progressively through ado-

lescence and early adulthood. A careful family history may be useful in identifying individuals with a predisposition towards obesity; 80% of children with two obese parents will be obese and 40% with one obese parent, compared with 14% of children with normal-weight parents. Common precipitants of weight gain include a new sedentary lifestyle, increased dietary intake, and pregnancy. The clinician should review the patient's current diet and activities. Additionally, details regarding previous attempts at weight loss should be ascertained.

A history, which includes a more recent or rapid increase in body fat, should alert the clinician to an endocrine disorder. If endocrine causes such as disease of the pituitary, adrenal or thyroid glands, ovaries or hypothalamus have been excluded, then the remainder of the history should focus on the complications arising from obesity. Polyuria, polydypsia, polyphagia, blurred vision, and recurrent vaginal yeast infections are some of the classic symptoms of diabetes mellitus. Cardiac symptoms may include hypertension or signs of coronary artery disease with exertional chest pain, palpitations or generalized fatigue. Congestive heart failure may manifest as orthopnea, paroxysmal nocturnal dyspnea, peripheral edema or dyspnea on exertion. The patient should also be asked about other cardiac risk factors such as cigarette smoking and family history of coronary disease.

Obese patients should be asked about joint pains as they are at risk for developing osteoarthritis. Recurrent abdominal pain may suggest either cholelithiasis or gastroesophageal reflux disease. In addition, due to excessive weight on the chest wall with concomitant increased work of breathing, the obese patient is at risk for restrictive lung disease. A history of restless sleep, loud snoring and daytime somnolence may necessitate evaluation for sleep apnea.

A thorough history regarding weight loss should include information regarding dietary intake with an eye towards determining if weight loss has been volitional through dieting or use of appetite suppressants. A complete review of gastrointestinal symptoms is essential with a focus on bowel function and the presence of pain within the GI tract. An assessment of the patient's functional status as well as a review of psychiatric symptoms is often critical in disclosing the cause of weight loss.

PHYSICAL EXAMINATION

Careful documentation of height and weight is the initial step in examining the overweight patient.

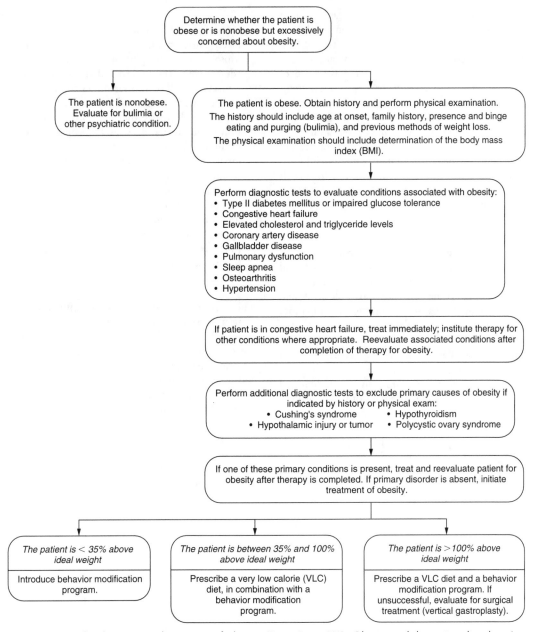

Figure 18.15. The diagnosis and treatment of obesity. (From Agras WS. Obesity and the eating disorders. In: Scientific American Medicine. New York: Scientific American, Inc. 1995; 9:(III):5.)

From this data, the BMI can be calculated. Waist and hip circumference ratio should also be determined. Blood pressure should be accurately measured using an appropriately sized cuff. Physical signs of endocrine-related obesity should be searched for. Corticosteroid excess may manifest with hypertension, buffalo hump, striae formation, hirsutism, acne, edema and hyperpigmentation.

The hypothyroid patient may have bradycardia, dry, coarse skin, hair thinning and swelling of the hands, face and extremities.

Weight loss should be carefully documented and expressed as a percent of original body weight. By most standards, a 10% weight loss due to illness is considered significant. The physical examination should be directed to searching for evidence of any acute or chronic disease that could cause weight loss. Loss of subcutaneous fat and bitemporal muscle wasting are hallmarks of significant weight loss. Pale conjunctivae suggest anemia of any origin. Lymphadenopathy may indicate the presence of malignancy or an infectious process. Organomegaly or a palpable mass on abdominal examination hint at neoplastic disease or a host of other systemic illnesses. Peripheral edema may mask underlying weight loss, but may also suggest severe protein deficiency. In the setting of unexplained weight loss the rectal examination with a stool test for occult blood is an important screen for gastrointestinal malignancies.

LABORATORY EVALUATION

All overweight patients should have routine screening for the presence of glucose intolerance and hyperlipidemia. Further studies investigating cardiac, pulmonary or orthopedic pathology should be guided by the history and physical examination. If endocrine causes of obesity are suspected, then the appropriate endocrinologic tests (i.e., thyroid function tests, serum cortisol measurement) should be performed.

Protein − energy malnutrition is best identified and quantitated by measurement of serum protein levels. The laboratory tests most commonly employed are the serum albumin and transferrin. Low total lymphocyte counts and anergy to skin test allergens are also evidence of malnutrition.

Further laboratory studies in the patient with weight loss should be guided by the history and physical examination. A complete blood count, liver function tests, blood urea nitrogen, creatinine, glucose, and thyroid functions may be helpful when no obvious cause of weight loss is found.

Differential Diagnosis

Most obesity is the result of overeating. The clinician should consider the possibility that an endocrine disorder could be responsible for weight gain. The major endocrine disorders which may manifest with **obesity** include:

1. Pituitary and adrenal dysfunction: Cushing's disease is characterized by an excess production of ACTH by the pituitary leading to increased cortisol secretion by the adrenal glands. Cushing's syndrome can be caused by primary hyperfunction of the adrenals, exogenous glucocorticoids or paraneoplastic secretion of ACTH. Cortisol excess leads to fat cell hypertrophy and central obesity along with hypertension and glucose intolerance.

2. Thyroid disease: Hypofunction of the thyroid gland can lead to modest weight gain, but rarely causes significant increase in fat tissues. Most increased weight can be attributed to edema which resolves with thyroid hormone replacement. (For further discussion of signs and symptoms associated with hypothyroidism, see the thyroid chapter).

3. Polycystic ovarian disease: The constellation of obesity, menstrual disturbances, and hirsutism suggests PCO. An overproduction of androgens by the ovaries is thought to underlie this condition.

4. Hypothalamic disease: Tumors or injury involving the hypothalamus may stimulate hyperphagia (the ventromedial syndrome) and thus lead to obesity. The most common tumors seen in this syndrome are craniopharyngiomas.

The diagnostic possibilities for **unexplained weight loss** are numerous. Unexplained weight loss can be associated with many diseases. Among the more commonly encountered are neoplasms, infection, diabetes, renal disease, hyperthyroidism, and psychiatric illness.

Cancer can lead to weight loss through several means. Lesions of the oropharynx, esophagus, stomach or colon may cause dysphagia, nausea, early satiety, abdominal pain or bloating which, in turn, often leads to decreased oral intake. Malignancies also produce weight loss by inducing a hypermetabolic state thus increasing nutritional requirements. Occasionally, certain neoplasms produce diarrhea, malabsorption and bleeding which result in increased nutritional losses.

Infection with concomitant fever represents another state of increased nutritional requirements. Prolonged febrile illnesses such as tuberculosis are frequently accompanied by significant weight loss.

Diabetes mellitus and nephrotic renal disease represent examples of two conditions associated with increased nutrient losses. Hyperglycemia with hyperglycosuria leads to weight loss through the urinary loss of body water. In addition, lack of insulin will stimulate gluconeogenesis and the utilization of primary energy stores with loss of lean body mass. Nephrotic renal disease has numerous causes, but all are associated with increased glomerular permeability and, by definition, at least 3.5 g of protein being lost in the urine. Severe hypoalbuminemia may result from this protein losing process.

The patient with hyperthyroidism frequently presents with unexplained weight loss despite normal dietary intake. Clinical presentation may include several of the classic signs and symptoms of increased thyroid hormone or, as frequently seen in the elderly, may be "masked" and have only a single manifestation.

Major depression is a common psychiatric illness often presenting with significant weight loss. These patients display a complete lack of interest in eating as part of their vegetative symptomology. Bulimia nervosa is a disorder characterized by alternating episodes of binge eating and severe dieting motivated by abnormal degrees of concern for body shape and weight. Anorexia nervosa is characterized by marked restriction of dietary intake and profound weight loss. The etiology of these last two disorders is unknown. They are most prevalent among women.

Poverty is a disturbing and often overlooked cause of weight loss especially among the elderly and others on fixed incomes. Patients are often reluctant to admit to financial hardship, therefore, it is incumbent upon the clinician to ask if a lack of funds is a cause of poor dietary intake. Social isolation or dementia may contribute to inadequate food intake as well.

Management

If a primary endocrine disorder is present, then treatment is directed towards that disease. Pituitary and adrenal tumors are usually treated surgically. Hypothyroidism is managed with thyroid replacement. Polycystic ovarian disease is frequently managed with hormone cycling.

The treatment of obesity is difficult, primarily because success is largely based on patient behavior modification. The role of the clinician is to establish a supportive environment for achieving reasonable weight loss goals. The major modalities for treating obesity are diet, exercise, and drugs.

DIET

For a diet to be successful the patient must be able to adhere to it for a long time. As is usually the case with crash diets, the satisfaction of quick weight loss is unsustainable as weight is invariably regained. Balanced reduced calorie diets are the safest and most likely to succeed as they insure nutritional balance and are more palatable. In patients who are severely overweight, very low calorie diets (300–700 calories) have been employed. Weight loss is initially very rapid, but side effects such as orthostatic hypotension, fatigue, and menstrual irregularities may occur.

For any diet to be successful in the long run, the patient must adopt a new attitude or relationship with food. Behavior modification attempts to make the patient more aware of the environment and stimuli which surround eating behavior. Careful documentation of intake, limiting oneself to three meals a day, concentrating while eating and eating slowly are some commonly used tactics.

EXERCISE

Exercise should be part of any weight reduction program. Obese people tend to be sedentary. Although energy expenditure by most activities is modest, exercise will assist in utilizing extra calories as well as improve cardiac and orthopedic conditioning.

PHARMACOLOGICAL TREATMENT

Pharmacological treatments for obesity have been disappointing. Some amphetamine derivatives may initially produce weight loss through appetite suppression. Over time, however, their addictive potential and disturbing side effects (i.e., insomnia, agitation, and psychosis) make them unsafe for chronic use. Fenfluramine is not addictive and does not cause psychomotor agitation, but can produce depression, sedation, and diarrhea. This, and similar drugs as well as the newer serotonergic antidepressants, may have short-term roles in the management of weight loss, but have not been proven efficacious in maintaining weight loss.

The management of weight loss is always directed towards the underlying cause whether it be medical, psychological, or social. For the severely malnourished patient nutritional support can be provided through a variety of means. Enteral feeding can be via the oral cavity or forced through a gastrostomy tube. Parenteral nutrition is administered through a peripheral or central vein. Both enteral and parenteral routes can provide either partial or total nutritional support. Similarly, feeding preparations can be adjusted to eliminate or supplement specific nutrients to fit the needs of the patient (e.g., low potassium diet in a patient with renal disease or increased water delivery in a volume depleted patient). Parenteral feeding, however, is not without its complications. Catheter-related complications include infection, pneumothorax and air embolus, while metabolic complications include electrolyte disturbances, hyperosmolarity and fatty liver.

NORMAL NUTRITION

The prudent diet which meets the body's needs must fulfill several criteria. First, the diet must provide adequate amounts of energy sources, minerals, vitamins and water. Second, the diet must be balanced as not to overemphasize a single food group. Third, calorie intake should be sufficient to maintain an appropriate weight, not produce weight gain or loss. Equally important, few diets are realistic if they do not offer a variety of palatable foods.

Nutrient Requirements. Nutrients are considered essential if a deficiency disease results from their absence in a diet. Scientific panels have established guidelines for Recommended Dietary Allowances (RDA's) of most essential nutrients (Table 18.14). RDA's are based on average heights and weights and will vary with sex, age, and whether the person is pregnant or lactating.

Daily water consumption must be adequate to replace losses. Insensible losses (exhalation and evaporation) account for about 500–1000 ml with approximately another 100 ml of water lost in feces and the remainder in the urine. Survival requires consuming about 700–1000 ml of water per day with 2000 ml representing a safe amount for maintaining basal activities.

Energy sources include protein, carbohydrate and fat. For the healthy adult energy requirements will vary with body size, age, sex, and level of activity. Protein is needed to maintain vital body functions and structure. An adequate diet includes proteins containing the nine essential amino acids. Protein should account for 10–15% of caloric intake.

Most carbohydrates derive from vegetable sources including sugars (simple carbohydrates)

Table 18.14.
Recommended Dietary Allowances (RDA), 1989[a]

Age (years)	Weight (kg)	Weight (lb)	Height (cm)	Height (inches)	Protein (g)	(RE) Vitamin A	(μg) Vitamin D	(mg) Vitamin E	(μg) Vitamin K	(mg) Vitamin C	(mg) Thiamin	(mg) Riboflavin	(mg equiv.) Niacin	(mg) Vitamin B$_6$	(μg) Folate	(μg) Vitamin B$_{12}$	(mg) Calcium	(mg) Phosphorus	(mg) Magnesium	(mg) Iron	(mg) Zinc	(μg) Iodine	(μg) Selenium
Infants																							
0.0–0.5	6	13	60	24	13	375	7.5	3	5	30	0.3	0.4	5	0.3	25	0.3	400	300	40	6	5	40	10
0.5–1.0	9	20	71	28	14	375	10	4	10	35	0.4	0.5	6	0.6	35	0.5	600	500	60	10	5	50	15
Children																							
1–3	13	29	90	35	16	400	10	6	15	40	0.7	0.8	9	1.0	50	0.7	800	800	80	10	10	70	20
4–6	20	44	112	44	24	500	10	7	20	45	0.9	1.1	12	1.1	75	1.0	800	800	120	10	10	90	20
7–10	28	62	132	52	28	700	10	7	30	45	1.0	1.2	13	1.4	100	1.4	800	800	170	10	10	120	30
Males																							
11–14	45	99	157	62	45	1000	10	10	45	50	1.3	1.5	17	1.7	150	2.0	1200	1200	270	12	15	150	40
15–18	66	145	176	69	59	1000	10	10	65	60	1.5	1.8	20	2.0	200	2.0	1200	1200	400	12	15	150	50
19–24	72	160	177	70	58	1000	10	10	70	60	1.5	1.7	19	2.0	200	2.0	1200	1200	350	10	15	150	70
25–50	79	174	176	70	63	1000	5	10	80	60	1.5	1.7	19	2.0	200	2.0	800	800	350	10	15	150	70
51+	77	170	173	68	63	1000	5	10	80	60	1.2	1.4	15	2.0	200	2.0	800	800	350	10	15	150	70
Females																							
11–14	46	101	157	62	46	800	10	8	45	50	1.1	1.3	15	1.4	150	2.0	1200	1200	280	15	12	150	45
15–18	55	120	163	64	44	800	10	8	55	60	1.1	1.3	15	1.5	180	2.0	1200	1200	300	15	12	150	50
19–24	58	128	164	65	46	800	10	8	60	60	1.1	1.3	15	1.6	180	2.0	1200	1200	280	15	12	150	55
25–50	63	138	163	64	50	800	5	8	65	60	1.1	1.3	15	1.6	180	2.0	800	800	280	15	12	150	55
51+	65	143	160	63	50	800	5	8	65	60	1.0	1.2	13	1.6	180	2.0	800	800	280	10	12	150	55
Pregnant					60	800	10	10	65	70	1.5	1.6	17	2.2	400	2.2	1200	1200	320	30	15	175	65
Lactating																							
1st 6 mo					65	1300	10	12	65	95	1.6	1.8	20	2.1	280	2.6	1200	1200	355	15	19	200	75
2nd 6 mo					62	1200	10	11	65	90	1.6	1.7	20	2.1	260	2.6	1200	1200	340	15	16	200	75

[a]The allowances are intended to provide for individual variations among most normal, healthy people in the United States under usual environmental stresses. Diets should be based on a variety of common foods in order to provide other nutrients for which human requirements have been less well defined. See the text for a more detailed discussion of the RDA and of nutrients not tabulated.
From: Recommended Dietary Allowance, © 1989 by the National Academy of Sciences, National Academy Press, Washington, D.C.

and starches and fibers (complex carbohydrates). Although a diet rich in fiber has been associated with a decreased incidence in colon cancer and diverticular disease, currently there is no official recommendation for carbohydrate ingestion. Americans lack fiber intake, therefore, increasing dietary fiber to 20–35 g. is considered advisable.

Fats are needed as carriers for many vitamins and provide a concentrated source of energy. A diet rich in fatty foods can promote hyperlipidemia and atherosclerosis. High intake of saturated animal fats raises LDL levels and promotes premature coronary artery disease. Dietary intake of fat should contain a balance of polyunsaturated and monounsaturated fats which are contained in foods such as corn oil and olive oil.

Nutritional Recommendations. A number of organizations including the Surgeon General's Office, the American Heart Association (AHA) and the National Cancer Institute have proposed dietary goals. Much of the emphasis is placed on limiting fat intake to less than 30% of calories ingested. In addition, protein should constitute 12% of total calories and carbohydrates about 60% with half of that being complex carbohydrates. In general, 1 g of either carbohydrate or protein contains 4 calories, 1 g of fat contains 9 calories, and 1 g of alcohol contains 7 calories. To reduce cardiovascular disease, the AHA recommends restricting dietary cholesterol to 300 mg and sodium to less than 3 g/day.

ILLUSTRATIVE CASES WITH SELF-ASSESSMENT QUESTIONS AND ANSWERS

Case 1

A 37-year-old man with no previous medical history presents with a 25-lb weight gain in the last 3 months. He takes no medications. He was recently laid off from his job and has been very sedentary. On physical examination the patient's blood pressure is 180/100. Central obesity is noted. Laboratory studies are significant for a blood glucose of 210.

QUESTION: *What is the most likely etiology for this patient's weight gain?*

a. Diabetes
b. Lack of exercise
c. Hypothyroidism
d. Cushings disease
e. Depression

ANSWER: d. *Although b and c are common reasons for weight gain and may be contributing factors, this degree of rapid weight gain in association with the onset of hypertension and diabetes suggest adrenal dysfunction. Serum cortisol and ACTH levels should be measured.*

Case 2

A 19-year-old woman presents with a 20-lb weight loss over 2 months. She reports extreme fatigue which she claims is due to insomnia. She is constantly thirsty and reports blurred vision and abdominal pains. On physical exam she is thin and ill appearing with a pulse of 110 and blood pressure of 90/60.

QUESTION: *What is the most likely cause of her weight loss?*

a. Depression
b. Cancer
c. Anorexia nervosa
d. Hyperthyroidism
e. Diabetes mellitus

ANSWER: e. *The patient suffers from the classic symptoms of diabetes. Hyperglycemia produces a hyperosmotic diuresis and increased thirst with signs of volume depletion. The patient's inability to sleep is at least partly due to sleep interruption by frequent nocturia.*

Case 3

An obese patient is placed on a 1800 calorie diet with 30% fat and 10% protein.

QUESTION: *How many grams of fat and protein per day may he consume?*

a. 50, 45
b. 60, 45
c. 70, 50
d. 80, 50
e. 90, 60

ANSWER: b. *To calculate fat restrictions, 30% of 1800 calories means 540 calories of fat. At 9 calories per gram, 540 calories is equal to 60 grams of fat. Similarly for protein, 10% of 1800 equals l80 calories of protein. At 4 calories per gram of protein, l80 calories equals 45 grams of protein that may be consumed.*

FEVER

Fever has proven to be a frustration to the health professional and a sign of illness and cause for concern to the patient throughout the ages. The patient interprets the fever as an indication of infection and need for therapy. The health provider is then placed in a position of finding the underlying cause for the fever, instituting appropriate treatment, and limiting the use of antibiotic therapy to when it is warranted.

Before a discussion of fever can be entertained, one must define the term "normal body temperature." Contrary to popular belief normal body temperature is not one reading of 98.6°F (37°C), but displays a circadian rhythm. In healthy individuals, mean rectal temperatures range from about 97°F (36.1°C) in the early morning to 99.3°F (37.4°C) in the late afternoon. Physiological factors such as exercise or the menstrual cycle can introduce even more fluctuation into the normal circadian rhythm. Clinically, it is important to recognize this variation may also exist in the disease state, with fever lowest in the morning and climbing in the evening. Therefore, frequent temperature readings may need to be made on the febrile patient to document the presence of fever.

Pathophysiologic Correlation

Fever is the result of physiologic processes that rely on intact homeostatic responses. Hyperthermia, on the other hand, occurs from thermoregulatory failure. Body temperature is based on a balance of heat produced as a byproduct of metabolic processes and heat lost from various body surfaces, especially skin and the lungs. The center of thermal control is located in the preoptic nucleus of the anterior hypothalamus. If the hypothalamus senses an increase in core temperature, efferent fibers of the autonomic nervous system produce vasodilation at the level of the skin and increase the rate of sweating. Conversely, heat is conserved by vasoconstriction and decreased sweating if a decrease in core temperature or skin surface temperature is sensed by the hypothalamus. Heat can only be generated by an increase in skeletal muscle activity, and may be manifested by an overt shiver. The febrile patient may experience myalgias as a result of this increased muscle tone. Fever occurs when circulating pyrogenic cytokines act to increase the hypothalamic set-point causing peripheral mechanisms to conserve and generate heat until the new, higher set-point is reached.

Clinically, this sudden increase in hypothalamic set-point for body temperature can present as a shaking chill or rigor due to the increased muscle activity responsible for raising body temperature. Even as the patient's temperature is rising, he or she will cover with blankets because of subjectively feeling cold. This is due to a decrease in surface temperature as a means to conserve heat and raise core temperature to the new set-point. The opposite occurs when a fever "breaks." Cutaneous vasodilation serves as a conduit for heat to be lost and allow a decrease in core body temperature. Clinically, the patient will be bathed in sweat as he or she defervesces.

Clinical and Laboratory Evaluation

The history and physical examination can contribute significant clues to the underlying cause of fever and help guide the health professional in a diagnostic path. In many cases, history and physical examination alone are sufficient to make a conclusive diagnosis. When laboratory studies are necessary, they can be very helpful in providing the health professional with useful information.

HISTORY

As discussed previously, when a patient comes to the health provider with a complaint of fever one must first ascertain that in fact a fever does exist. It is important to ask if the temperature was measured, and if so, what was the numerical value. Ask what time of day was the fever and elevated temperature noted and if this occurred only on one occasion or with several measurements. It is also useful to establish the duration of the "febrile illness." Once the health professional feels certain that the patient has been experiencing fevers, a systematic approach to the history may prove very useful.

Localizing Symptoms. Questions concerning localizing symptoms can be very helpful in directing the remainder of the workup and formulating a diagnosis. Complaints of sore throat, earache, and swelling in the neck accompanied by fever can be indicative of pharyngitis or an upper respiratory tract infection. These symptoms combined with a productive or nonproductive cough and pleuritic chest pain may point to a diagnosis of bronchitis or pneumonia. Questions concerning dysuria, urinary frequency and hesitancy should be asked. An affirmative answer to any of these questions may lead to the diagnosis of urinary tract infection. If the patient is a sexually active woman with a vaginal discharge one must consider pelvic inflammatory disease. Complaints of abdominal pain should be further investigated with questions concerning change in bowel habits such as diarrhea or constipation. It is also important to ask about accompanying nausea, vomiting and anorexia, or if the pain is related to meals. If diarrhea and abdominal cramping are the main symptoms, one needs to ask further about the type of diarrhea-mucus or watery of short duration points more towards a viral gastroenteritis. Bloody diarrhea associated with high fever may be more indicative of bacterial or amebic dysentery. If nausea and vomiting are the main complaints associated with abdominal pain, one needs to consider pancreatitis or acute cholecystitis.

Skin Rashes. Skin rashes are another important question to raise. An allergic reaction may present with fever and a hive-like pruritic rash. This may be associated with difficulty breathing or swallowing if the reaction is severe. Localized rash or erythema may represent an infection of the skin such as cellulitis, or inflammation over a deep vein thrombosis, and questions concerning calf pain or tenderness need to be raised. Diffuse rash may represent a viral exanthema with associated prodromal symptoms or a rickettsial infection such as Rocky Mountain spotted fever. Rash may accompany a spectrum of headache and neck stiffness to a change of mental status as seen with meningitis or encephalitis, viral or bacterial. Cranial tenderness in an elderly patient may suggest temporal arteritis and sinus pain may indicate acute sinusitis. Joint pain or tenderness from collagen-vascular disease or acute arthritis from other causes may also be seen with a rash and fever.

Host Factors. Host factors are another important part of the history to establish. Is the individual a basically healthy person or does he or she have underlying medical conditions and greater risk for certain infections or illnesses? Patients at the very extremes of life, that is very young or elderly may present with subtle findings of disease and be mildly febrile, afebrile or hypothermic, and in fact be overwhelmingly septic and near death. Patients

in an immunocompromised state such as those infected with the HIV virus, hematological malignancies, receiving chemotherapy, or on chronic steroid therapy are more likely to become ill from opportunistic pathogens or have more severe illnesses from common infectious agents. Other disease processes that may lead to a more adverse outcome and the need for earlier treatment intervention are those patients with diabetes mellitus or sickle cell anemia. Another consideration in a febrile patient is if there is a prosthetic heart valve, or hip prosthesis, which are more prone to be the site of infection. Does the patient exhibit high-risk behavior for an infectious etiology such as active intravenous drug use? Has the patient had a history of recurrent infections in the past? Urinary tract infections and pyelonephritis tend to relapse or recur.

Epidemiological Factors. One should inquire about epidemiological factors concerning the patient. Is anyone else sick in the household with similar symptoms? If the symptoms include gastrointestinal complaints, were any new foods ingested? Did anyone else eat these foods and also feel ill? What is occurring in the community may be helpful, as *Legionella* infection, viral hepatitis (ie. Hepatitis A), and viral syndromes in general tend to be clustered. Any recent travel history and to where is useful in screening for exposure to typhoid fever or malaria. Household pets may be the source of illness. Cats may cause cat-scratch fever from a scratch or bite, or toxoplasmosis from fecal contamination. Birds have been known to cause psittacosis and turtles can be carriers of salmonella. A history of an animal bite may be suggestive of rabies infection or a cellulitis of the area bitten. Is there any high risk sexual behavior or drug use activity that puts the person at increased risk for HIV disease? What is the person's occupation? Although not very common in the United States, leather workers are at increased risk of exposure to anthrax.

Medications. A careful review of all medications is essential in the history-taking from a febrile patient. Is there any previous history of allergies to any medications? Drug allergies, especially antibiotics are commonly associated with rash as well as fever. Is there any illicit drug use? Cocaine may cause pyrexia in certain individuals.

PHYSICAL EXAMINATION

The most important aspect of the physical examination begins with the measurements of the vital signs, then patients should be approached in a systematic fashion from top to bottom so no physical clues towards diagnosis are missed. After the vital signs are measured and known to be stable, the appearance of the patients should be noted. Do they look sick or toxic? Do they appear wasted and chronically ill? Do they appear well and basically healthy? This is important for obvious reasons. It will provide the health provider with crucial information concerning the overall health status and duration of the illness.

Vital Signs. Besides the documentation of the temperature, which may be normal at this time despite a report of fever at home, it is critical to note the heart rate, blood pressure and respiratory rate.

Most febrile illnesses are accompanied by tachycardia, especially if secondary to an infectious etiology. The exception to this "rule" is seen with typhoid fever which can present with a prolonged fever and relative bradycardia. Respiratory rate may be rapid if the fever is related to a pulmonary etiology, and hypotension in combination with fever may signify septic shock.

Head and Neck Examination. The head and neck is the first place to start the physical examination. The eyes should be examined for injected conjunctiva or exudate suggestive of a viral syndrome. The fundi should be viewed with an opthalmoscope for the presence of retinopathy, which may occur with collagen-vascular disease, or Roth spots secondary to septic emboli from bacterial endocarditis. The frontal and maxillary sinuses should be percussed for any signs of tenderness, as well as transilluminated with a pen light looking for evidence of sinusitis. The mouth should be viewed from the outside as well as inside. The lips should be examined for the presence of "fever blisters" or labial *Herpes simplex* which more often recur with infections secondary to pneumococcal pneumonia or meningococcal meningitis. The buccal mucosa can be visualized for any signs of ulcers or exudates. White thick plaques can be representative of oral thrush caused by *Candida* and seen commonly in patients suffering with AIDS or immunocompromised for other reasons. Vesicular eruptions on the hard and soft palate may accompany a viral syndrome. The dentition should be observed for any obvious signs of a tooth abscess. The back of the throat needs to be fully examined for the presence of erythema and exudates. If tonsils are present it needs to be noted if they are enlarged or if one is surrounded by exudate suggestive of a peritonsillar abscess. Exudative pharyngitis accompanied by sore throat and cervical adenopathy may be caused by Group A streptococcus and should be treated with antibiotics to prevent untoward consequences. The ears should be examined with an otoscope to see

both the external ear canal as well as the tympanic membrane. Signs of an acute otitis media which may be associated with ear pain and fever are erythema and bulging of the tympanic membrane. The neck should be palpated for the presence of any enlargement of the thyroid gland or any tenderness to touch. Also, the various lymph node chains should be palpated for any enlargement of a lymph node. If an enlarged node is palpated, it should be noted whether it is tender and freely mobile, or fixed in place. The former description is more likely associated with acute infection, the latter with infiltration of the node possibly by a malignancy. The neck should also be moved back and forth to see if any signs of nuchal rigidity are present suggesting meningeal irritation. Other signs to check for meningeal involvement are the Kernig signs and Brudzinski signs, both of which employ methods to stretch the spinal cord and meninges looking for reactions of pain to these movements.

Chest and Back Examination. The chest and back should first be visualized for any signs of skin rash. The patient's chest movements with respiration should be viewed for any paroxysmal motion, any shallowness to the respirations or any splinting on inspiration, which may suggest a musculoskeletal etiology versus a pulmonic process. The heart should be ascultated for the presence of any murmurs which may suggest endocarditis if the murmur is new or changed in quality. A pericardial friction rub should also be listened for, suggestive of pericarditis. The lungs should be percussed for any dullness to percussion or hyperresonance. Ascultation should be performed listening for any wheezing, or decrease in breath sounds that may accompany consolidation. The breasts in a female should be examined for any redness, tenderness or masses suggestive of a cellulitis of the skin or an abscess.

Abdomen Examination. It should first be noted if the abdomen is obese or thin. It is more difficult for obvious reasons to effectively palpate an obese abdomen. Before a hand is laid on the abdomen the four quadrants should be ascultated with a stethoscope for the presence of bowel sounds and the quality of the sounds. The absence of bowel sounds should alert the examiner to the possibility of a total bowel obstruction or acute peritonitis and an underlying surgical emergency. Palpation of the abdomen in all four quadrants is very useful and necessary. One needs to be aware of any tenderness on light touch or deep palpation as well as rebound or involuntary guarding. These again can be signs of an underlying surgical pathology. Palpation is also essential to search for any organomegaly or masses. The liver span should be approximated by percussion over the right upper quadrant and if enlarged and palpable, the edges should be felt for nodules. If the abdomen is large on physical examination, one should attempt to rule out ascites on clinical grounds by testing for a fluid wave or shifting dullness. Ascitic fluid can be the site of infection and peritonitis with concomitant fever and abdominal tenderness. The flanks and costo-vertebral angles should be percussed for tenderness suggestive of acute pyelonephritis.

Genitourinary Examination. Genitourinary examination is essential in a patient with an unknown source of fever. In the female a pelvic examination is necessary to search for signs of cervicitis and vaginal discharge on speculum examination. A bimanual examination is also necessary to search for cervical motion tenderness suggestive of pelvic inflammatory disease (PID) or adnexal masses which may represent a tuboovarian abscess. In males it is important to examine the penis for any ulceration or chancre and penile discharge suggestive of a sexually transmitted disease (STD). The testicles should be palpated for any enlargement or tenderness which may be from orchitis or epididymitis and the inguinal area palpated for any lymphadenopathy. The rectal examination is important in both sexes. Initially the health provider should visualize and palpate the perineum and anus for perirectal fissures or fistulas or a perirectal abscess. A digital examination should be carried out feeling for any rectal masses and stool obtained for the peroxidase reaction looking for occult blood. In the male patient, the prostate should be palpated for tenderness or "bogginess" suggestive of a prostatitis.

Extremities Examination. The extremities and joints are a necessary part of the physical examination in a febrile patient. The fingernails should be looked at for splinter hemorrhages and the hands for Osler nodes secondary to endocarditis. These are rare findings in this day and age of early detection and intervention of febrile illnesses. The skin should be examined for the presence of a diffuse rash, vesicles or bullae. One can also search for a localized rash such as erythema chronicum migrans seen at times with Lyme disease. Areas of erythema on the skin should be further examined for any signs of pus, edema or skin breakdown and may represent an early cellulitis. Especially in the lower extremities the calf area should be palpated for any tenderness or underlying "cord" in the vein signifying deep vein thrombosis (DVT). A phlebitis or thrombosis can also involve superficial veins. Joints should be palpated for tenderness, warmth and effusions and it should be noted if one joint is involved, (a monoarthritis) versus multiple joints. If it is a polyarthritis one should look for symmetry and which joints are involved (i.e., small, medium, or large joints) which may give clues to various collagen-vascular diseases. A monoarthritis is more likely secondary to an infectious etiology, gout or pseudogout.

Neurological Examination. Finally, a thorough neurological examination is essential. First, the health professional needs to note if the patient is alert and aware. Simple questions can be asked to ascertain orientation to time, place, and person. This initial information will already tell the examiner if any significant central nervous system (CNS) pathology is occurring. If the patient has a clear sensorium, is oriented and answering appropriately to the questions asked, a severe CNS infection is unlikely. As discussed previously, it is important to search for signs of meningeal irritation. A full neurological examination checking cranial nerves, motor strength and sensation is essential to rule out focal deficits. It is also important to observe gait and gross motor movements to rule out cerebellar disease.

LABORATORY EVALUATION

If a thorough history and physical examination in an acutely febrile patient points to an upper respiratory tract infection or viral syndrome, no laboratory data may be required for diagnosis. Otherwise, one needs to select wisely based on the history and physical examination which laboratory tests will be most useful in contributing to a diagnostic end. If an uncomplicated urinary tract infection in a woman is suspected, a urine specimen should be obtained for microscopic examination and gram stain looking for the presence of white cells (pyuria) and bacteria. A urine culture may be sent to the bacteriology lab as well for identification of the bacteria and antibiotic sensitivities. If the patient is presenting with a productive cough and fever and the physical examination suggests an infiltrate, then the next step for evaluation would be a chest radiograph to document a pneumonia. If the patient is able to produce sputum upon demand, a microscopic examination and sputum culture may be useful to identify the etiologic agent and antibiotic sensitivities. In the patient with diffuse rash felt to be secondary to a new medication or allergy one may make the diagnosis alone based on clinical grounds. If laboratory testing is performed, an elevated serum white count with an increase in eosinophils may be confirmatory.

In the event that the diagnosis is not so clearcut based on history and physical examination alone, more extensive laboratory evaluation can be undertaken. One should try to use the information gathered from the history and physical examination to guide the choice of tests and attempt to minimize the cost of the workup in monetary means as well as emotional and physical toll on the patient.

Blood Tests. Initial screening blood tests are relatively inexpensive and may be very useful in leading subsequent evaluations. A complete blood count (CBC) can provide a multitude of information. First, one should look at the total white count to see if it is normal, decreased or elevated. The ratio of neutrophils, lymphocytes, monocytes and eosinophils to each other is equally important. An elevated white count with a "left shift" (i.e., an increase in the relative number of neutrophils and precursors on a peripheral blood smear) is highly suggestive of a bacterial infection as is toxic granulation of the neutrophils. In contrast, a decrease in the relative or absolute number of neutrophils is commonly seen in patients that are immunocompromised from HIV disease or secondary to chemotherapeutic agents. An increase in lymphocytes or monocytes of one clonal colony may represent chronic leukemia. Immature cells in abundance on a peripheral smear suggest acute leukemia or lymphoma and need to be further investigated. The hemoglobin should be noted as well. Although very nonspecific, a normochromic, normocytic anemia may be secondary to chronic disease or inflammation. The platelet count may be useful as an indicator of the overall status of the patient, too. A mild reactive thrombocytosis may be seen in relation to an acute infection, as platelets can be an acute phase reactant. An increase in platelet count may also be seen in rheumatoid arthritis. This is in contrast to other collagen-vascular disease such as systemic lupus erythematosus (SLE) where thrombocytopenia is the norm.

The erythrocyte sedimentation rate (ESR) lacks specificity or sensitivity to serve as an adequate marker for the presence of infection, collagen-vascular disease or an occult malignancy. If the ESR is very elevated, however, especially in the elderly patient with headache or shoulder-girdle pain, one may suspect temporal arteritis and further studies may be indicated. Remember, the ESR is elevated in renal disease, and is not at all reliable.

Measurement of blood chemistries may be very helpful. A low sodium may be noted in a patient with an ongoing pulmonic process or CNS pathol-

ogy. A low bicarbonate may signify acidosis secondary to bacterial sepsis among other possible etiologies. Hyperglycemia in a diabetic patient previously in good control may suggest an occult infection. Profound hypoglycemia may accompany overwhelming sepsis. Liver function tests can be very useful. Elevations in the transaminases suggest hepatitis. Viral hepatitis can be screened for with serology tests for hepatitis A, B, and C. An isolated increase in the alkaline phosphatase alone may signify infiltration of the liver. Specific blood tests can be ordered if a diagnostic possibility exists. The evaluation for collagen-vascular disease includes serum for anti-nuclear antibody (ANA), rheumatoid factor (RF), and complement levels.

Cultures. Blood cultures may prove very useful if a hematogenous source is suspected. This is especially true in the patient with a prosthetic heart valve or hip prosthesis. It is essential to culture urine, stool and sputum as well where applicable. If other body fluid sources are obtainable, they should be cultured as well. For example, if the patient presents with a fever, headache and nuchal rigidity, a lumbar puncture should be performed and the cerebrospinal fluid (CSF) sent for culture. If the patient presents with a warm, swollen knee with a palpable effusion, this fluid can be obtained under sterile technique for culture. Mycobacterial, viral and fungal cultures should be collected as well if the suspicion arises. Anerobic cultures are also necessary with suspected gastrointestinal, pulmonary and pelvic infections. All fluids collected for culture should be examined by the gram-stain technique as well to look for the presence of white cells and bacteria. An India ink preparation can be done as well on CSF if cryptococcal meningitis is suspected in an AIDS patient. The presence of bacteria in a body fluid considered sterile such as CSF or ascitic fluid makes the presumptive diagnosis. Body fluids should also be sent to the laboratory for cell count and chemistry evaluation. As a generalization, bacterial, mycobacterial and fungal infections produce a low glucose and high protein in infected body fluids.

Radiographic Studies. Radiographic studies may prove helpful in selected cases. Chest x-rays may reveal an infiltrate, effusion, mass, or nodule even in the absence of physical findings. A plain film of the abdomen may help to elucidate ascites, air-fluid levels in the bowel or free air under the diaphragm in the upright view. Radiographic studies of a suspicious bony area correlated with a nuclear bone scan may reveal an osteomyelitis. When indicated, ultrasound or CT scan can be of great use. In the patient with an undiagnosed source of fever, a gallium scan may be helpful. White blood cells are labelled with a radioactive tag, and then the radioisotope emits gamma rays, which are captured by a gamma camera and a picture evolves. This may help elucidate the source of a fever if the cause is secondary to an infectious etiology or a malignancy (leukemia or lymphoma) with a preponderance of white cells.

Immunological Studies. Immunological studies may be helpful. In the patient with suspected HIV disease this should be confirmed providing the patient consents. Antistreptolysin O (ASLO) titers may be useful for acute rheumatic fever and other streptococcal infections. Heterophile testing can help make the diagnosis of infectious mononucleosis. Skin testing for tuberculosis (TB) can help confirm the diagnosis of active TB in the patient with consistent symptoms, radiographic findings and a positive skin reaction.

Biopsies. Lastly, biopsies may be a means to make a diagnosis based on pathological criteria. Bone marrow biopsy may be very useful not only in clarifying the histological nature of the marrow in a patient with an abnormal peripheral smear, but in diagnosing a disease entity as well, such as infection (histoplasmosis or tuberculosis), metastatic carcinomas, or primary hematological malignancies. A bone marrow biopsy can be useful as a "blind" study, that is when all previous laboratory examinations have proven fruitless. Lymph node biopsy may also prove useful if there is lymphadenopathy. Liver biopsy or tissue biopsy are usually of low diagnostic yield as a "blind" study, unless some abnormality is noted on radiographic studies and can guide the biopsy.

Differential Diagnosis

Most cases of febrile illnesses will present with localizing symptoms or temporally related events so that the diagnosis will be clear. The major categories to consider when attempting to make a diagnosis are infection, neoplasm, drug-related, and collagen-vascular disease. Most common causes will be those of infectious etiology, either viral or bacterial, and localized or systemic. It is important to make a diagnosis in these cases, especially when a bacterial infection is suspected so therapy can be initiated. The majority of cases will be diagnosed based on history and physical examination and the use of appropriate laboratory testing.

There is an entity that exists called "fever of unknown origin (FUO)." This label is attached to cases which meet certain criteria. The patient must have the illness of at least 3 weeks duration, with

Table 18.15.
Fever of Unknown Origin Etiology

Infections
  Systemic
    Tuberculosis
    Endocarditis
    AIDS-related, ie. Toxoplasmosis, cytomegalovirus
      (CMV), mycobacterum avium intracellulare
      (MAI), pneumocystis carinii, cryptoccus, etc.
    Salmonella
    Epstein Barr virus
  Abdominal
    Anicteric viral hepatitis
    Bacterial hepatitis
    Hepatic abscess
    Suppurative cholangitis
    Cholecystic or pericholecystic abscess
    Appendicial abscess
    Sub hepatic abscess
    Other abscesses
  Pelvic
    Tubo ovarian abscess
    Endometritis
    Pelvic abscess
    Prostatic abscess
  Retroperitoneal
    Pyelonephritis
    Perinephric abscess
Neoplasms
  Systemic
    Hematologic, i.e., leukemias and lymphomas
    Metastatic cancers especially to liver and bone
  Localized
    Atrial myxomas
    Renal cell carcinoma
Collagen-vascular disease
  Vasculitis allergic or polyarteritis
  Systemic lupus erythematosis
  Juvenile rheumatoid arthritis
Other Causes
  Inflammatory bowel disease
  Drug fever
  Pulmonary embolism
  Metabolic, i.e., Hyperthyroidism, post-ovulation,
    post-exercise
  Factitious fever
  Noninfectious granulomatous disease
  Hepatocellular necrosis with cirrhosis
  Idiopathic

Adapted from Jacoby GA, Swartz MN. Fever of undermined origin. N Engl J Med 1973; 289:1408.

temperature exceeding 38.3°C on several occasions, and no established diagnosis after one week of hospitalization. Hospitalization does not always have to be instituted, but it does allow for objective, repeated temperature measurements to document the presence of fever. It also may be useful to quicken the pace of the work-up, as a multitude of tests can be done sequentially as needed. The establishment of criteria are important to save the patient and health provider unnecessary emotional, physical and financial expense prematurely. The most common diagnoses made of an FUO are very similar category-wise to an acute illness, but perhaps a bit more occult (Table 18.15).

Management

The first question that arises is whether fever in itself dangerous to the patient. Most healthy individuals can tolerate temperatures up to 40.5°C (105°F) without adverse effects; however, many people will be symptomatic with this high temperature, necessitating therapy. High fevers should be treated in small children because of the concern that febrile convulsions may occur. Patients with cardiac disease should also receive antipyretic therapy. For each 1°F elevation in temperature, basal metabolic rate increases by 7 percent. This puts increased demands on the heart, which may precipitate cardiac ischemia or heart failure. Temperatures greater than 108°F may cause direct cellular damage and the mortality rate is appreciable.

The best initial therapy is to treat the underlying cause whenever possible. In the meantime, however, if patients are symptomatic from an increased temperature antipyretic therapy can be instituted with aspirin or acetaminophen dosed every four to six hours. Both of these agents appear to act on the hypothalamus to lower the thermal set point. More aggressive forms of lowering body temperature ex-

ist and should be used when necessary. These consist of physical cooling and range from undressing the patient and exposing the skin to cool ambient temperature which allows cooling or sponging the patient with cool water or alcohol which allows cooling by evaporation. In extreme cases, the patient can be immersed in an ice water bath. All methods of physical cooling run the risk of hypothermia and, therefore, should be discontinued once the patient's body temperature has fallen below the critical level. Methods of physical cooling can be very uncomfortable to the patient and, therefore, should be instituted only when the fever itself presents a medical problem.

Blind therapeutic trials in unidentified febrile illnesses are not a good practice. Many times these do more harm than good and complicate the situation with superinfection due to resistant pathogens, drug fever or toxicity, and negative cultures due to antimicrobial agents. The use of broad-spectrum antibiotics as empiric therapy should be reserved for the acutely toxic patient or a patient in a compromised state secondary to an underlying medical condition. This includes patients with HIV disease, diabetes or a malignancy, especially those patients receiving chemotherapy with depressed immune systems. If therapeutic trials are initiated, they should be done with a specific diagnosis in mind whenever possible. If an extensive work-up of a patient for an FUO proves fruitless in producing a diagnosis, the best approach is to start the work-up again. Never underestimate the importance of the history and physical examination in aiding the health professional in making the correct diagnosis.

ILLUSTRATIVE CASES WITH SELF-ASSESSMENT QUESTIONS AND ANSWERS

Case 1

A 45-year-old healthy male presents to your office with 1 week of "fevers" especially in the evening, never documented with temperature measurements. He also complains of sore throat, runny nose, and dry cough, and tells you both of his children had the same symptoms 1 week ago. Physical examination reveals a well nourished, well developed male who appears healthy. Vital signs are stable, temperature measured at 99.3°F orally. His throat is mildly erythematous, with no

exudates or tonsillar enlargement. There is no cervical lymphadenopathy, his tympanic membranes are clear and his lungs are clear on ascultation.

QUESTION: *What following tests would you perform of this patient?*

a. Chest radiograph
b. Complete blood count
c. CT scan-total body

d. No further tests
e. All of the above

ANSWER: d. *The diagnosis can be made without any further tests on this patient based on the history and physical examination.*

QUESTION: *What is his most likely diagnosis?*

a. Upper respiratory tract infection of viral etiology
b. Bacterial pneumonia
c. Acute allergic reaction
d. Rocky Mountain spotted fever
e. Secondary syphilis

ANSWER: a. *The history and physical examination all point to a viral syndrome, especially with other people in the home with similar symptoms, and a healthy appearing patient.*

Case 2

A 23-year-old white female comes into the clinic where you work with complaints of a diffuse, itchy rash and low grade fevers for 2 days.

QUESTION: *What other questions would be important to ask her?*

a. Any recent travel history?
b. Anyone else sick at home with similar symptoms?
c. Any other associated symptoms such as sore throat, runny nose or cough?
d. Any new medications?
e. All of the above

ANSWER: e. *All of the above are very important questions to ask to help guide you towards a diagnosis, even before a physical examination is carried out. On further questioning you find out that she was treated with penicillin by her dentist for a tooth abscess 1 week ago. She had never taken this antibiotic before so knows of no previous adverse reactions. She denies any other acute symptoms, and states the tooth pain has resolved 3 days after starting the antibiotic.*

QUESTION: *What is her most likely diagnosis given this history?*

a. Lyme disease
b. Infectious mononucleosis
c. Drug fever
d. Secondary syphilis
e. None of the above

ANSWER: c. *The diffuse, pruritic rash and low grade fever is most likely secondary to an allergic reaction to the penicillin. The most common cause of drug fever is due to a hypersensitivity reaction and antibiotics are a very common causal agent. The reaction usually occurs within the first week of exposure.*

QUESTION: *What is the therapy for drug fever in this patient?*

a. Systemic steroids
b. Stoppage of the offending agent
c. Supportive care with topical steroids for the rash and anti-histamines as well for the pruritis
d. Intubation to protect the airways and monitoring in an intensive care setting
e. B and C

ANSWER: e. *The penicillin should be stopped immediately and the patient told to avoid penicillin and penicillin-related antibiotics in the future. If her symptoms are severe enough and bothersome, the inflammatory reaction can be minimized with topical steroids and the pruritis diminished with an anti-histamine agent. The other answers are more appropriate for an anaphylactic reaction to an agent, and could happen if this patient was re-exposed to penicillin. If she still needs antibiotic therapy for the tooth abscess, an agent from another antibiotic family would need to be used.*

Case 3

A 55-year-old man comes to see you in your office with the complaint of fevers only at night, accompanied with some chills. This has been occurring almost nightly for at least the past two weeks. He also is complaining of generalized malaise and anorexia and has lost 5 pounds over the past month. On further questioning, he has a history of rheumatic heart disease and subsequent significant mitral stenosis. He was in his usual state of health until approximately 2 months ago when he had some dental work done.

QUESTION: *What findings would you look for on physical examination?*

a. Heart murmur or change in the quality of his murmur
b. Roth spots on opthalmoscopic examination
c. Splinter hemorrhages and Osler nodes of the fingernails and fingers
d. Hepatosplenomegaly
e. All of the above

ANSWER: e. *All of the above physical findings are important to look for when the history leads one to suspect bacterial endocarditis.*

QUESTION: *What diagnostic tests are important to perform on this patient?*

a. Serial blood cultures especially during fever spikes.
b. Transesophageal echocardiogram (ECHO)
c. A complete blood count, blood chemistries and liver function tests
d. A urinalysis
e. All of the above

ANSWER: e. *All of the above tests are important to establish the diagnosis of bacterial endocarditis and the extent of infection. Blood cultures will help identify the causative bacterial pathogen and antibiotic sensitivities. Drawing cultures during a fever spike usually helps to "catch" the organism at a period of hematogenous spread. Once the blood cultures are collected, antibiotic therapy can be initiated. The patient's history points to the seeding of the stenotic valve following a dental procedure and antibiotic coverage needs to cover for viridans streptococcal groups. Transesophageal ECHO will allow one to visualize the valve and the presence of any vegetations. The other laboratory tests will help to clarify if there is any other systemic involvement. Often with a large vegetation on a left-sided heart valve, septic emboli can be thrown to other organs such as the liver, spleen or kidneys.*

REFERENCES

Diabetes

1. Dept. of Health and Human Services, Centers for Disease Control. National ambulatory care survey. Vital Health Stat 1994;[13]116:1–110.
2. DeFronzo RA, Bonadonna RC, Ferrannini E. Pathogenesis of NIDDM. Diabetes Care 1992;15:318–361.
3. Reddi AS, Camerini-Davalos RA. Diabetic nephropathy. Arch Int Med 1990;150:31–43.
4. The Diabetes Control and Complications Trial Research Group. The effect of intensive treatment of diabetes on the development and progression of long-term complications in Insulin-Dependent Diabetes Mellitus. N Engl J Med 1993;329:977–986.
5. American Diabetes Association. Consensus statement on self monitoring of blood glucose. Diabetes Care 1994;17:81–86.
6. Yki Jarvinen H et al. Comparison of insulin regimens in patients with Non-Insulin Dependent Diabetes Mellitus. N Engl J Med 1992;327:1426–1433.
7. Seltzer HS. Drug induced hypoglycemia. A review of 1418 cases. Endocrinol Metab Clin North Am 1989;18(1):163–83.

Cholesterol

1. Simons L. Interrelations of lipids and lipoproteins with coronary artery disease mortality in 19 countries. Am J Cardiol 1986;57:5G–10G.
2. Kagan A, Harris BR, Winkelstein et al. Epidemiologic studies of coronary heart disease and stroke in Japanese men living in Japan, Hawaii, and California: demographic, physical, dietary and biochemical characteristics. J Chronic Dis 1974;27:345–64.
3. Brown M, Goldstein J. How LDL receptors influence cholesterol and atherosclerosis. Scientific American 1984;251:58–66.
4. Castelli W. Epidemiology of coronary artery disease: the Framingham Study. Am J Med 1984;76:4–12.
5. Castelli W, Garrison R, Wilson P, Abbott R, Kalousian S, Kannel W. Evidence of coronary heart disease and lipoprotein cholesterol levels; the Framingham Study. JAMA 1986;256:2935–2838.
6. Stamler J, Wentworth D, Neaton J. Is relationship between serum cholesterol and risk of premature death from coronary heart disease continuous and graded? Findings in 356,222 primary screenees of the Multiple Risk Factor Intervention Trial (MRFIT). JAMA 1986;256:2823–2828.
7. Expert Panel on Detection, Evaluation, and Treatment of High Blood Cholesterol in Adults (Adult Treatment Panel II). Second report of the National Cholesterol Education Program (NCEP) expert panel on detection, evaluation, and treatment of high blood cholesterol in adults (Adult Treatment Panel II). Circulation 1994;89:1334–1445.
8. Ornish D, Brown S, Scherwitz L et al. Can lifestyle changes reverse coronary heart disease? The Lifestyle Heart Trial. Lancet 1990;336: 129–33.

9. Lipid Research Clinics Program. The Lipid Research Clinics Coronary Primary Prevention Trial results. I. Reduction in the incidence of coronary heart disease. JAMA 1984;251:351–364.

10. Lipid Research Clinics Program. The Lipid Research Clinics Coronary Primary Prevention Trial results. III. The relation of reduction in incidence of coronary heart disease to cholesterol lowering. JAMA 1984; 251:365–374.

11. Frick M, Elo O, Haapa K et al. Helsinki Heart Study: primary prevention trial with gemfibrozil in middle-aged men with dyslipidemia. Safety of treatment, changes in risk factors, and incidence of coronary heart disease. NEJM 1987;317:1237–1245.

12. Scandinavian Simavastatin Survival Study Group. Randomised trial of cholesterol lowering in 4444 patients with coronary heart disease: the Scandinavian Simavastatin Survival Study (4S). Lancet 1994;344:1383–1389.

13. Coronary Drug Project Research Group. Clofibrate and niacin in coronary heart disease. JAMA 1975;231:360–381.

14. Canner P, Berge K, Wenger N, Stamler J, Friedman L, Prineas R, Friedewald W, for the Coronary Drug Project Research Group. Fifteen year mortality in coronary drug project patients: long-term benefit with niacin. J Am Coll Cardiol 1986;8:1245–1255.

SUGGESTED READINGS

Diabetes

American Diabetes Association. Clinical practice recommendations. Diabetes Care 1993;16 (Suppl 2):1–118.

American Diabetes Association. Standards of medical care for patients with diabetes mellitus. Diabetes Care 1994; 17:616–623.

Dept. of Health and Human Services, Centers for Disease Control. The prevention and treatment of complications of diabetes mellitus. A guide for primary care practitioners. Atlanta: National Center for Chronic Disease Prevention and Health Promotion, 1991:1–85.

Cholesterol

Expert Panel on Detection, Evaluation, and Treatment of High Blood Cholesterol in Adults (Adult Treatment Panel II). Second report of the National Cholesterol Education Program (NCEP) expert panel on detection, evaluation, and treatment of high blood cholesterol in adults (Adult Treatment Panel II). Circulation 1994;89:1334–1445.

Grundy S. Cholesterol and Atherosclerosis: Diagnosis and Treatment. NY: Gower Press, 1990.

Screening for high blood cholesterol. In: US Preventive Services Task Force. Guide to Clinical Preventive Services, An Assessment of the Effectiveness of 169 Interventions, Report of the U.S. Preventive Services Task Force. Baltimore: Williams & Wilkins, 1989.

Hyperlipidemia

Havel R, Rapaport E. Management of primary hyperlipidemia. N Engl J Med 1995;332:1491–8.

National Cholesterol Education Program. Second report of the Expert panel on detection, evaluation, and treatment of high blood cholesterol in adults (Adult Treatment Panel II). Bethesda: National Heart, Lung, and Blood Institute, National Institutes of Health, 1993.

Scandinavian Simvastatin Study Group. Randomized trial of cholesterol lowering in 4444 patients with coronary heart disease: the Scandinavian Simvastatin Survival Study (4S). Lancet 1994;344:1383–1389.

Screening for high blood cholesterol. In: US Preventive Services Task Force. Guide to Clinical Preventive Services, 2nd ed. Baltimore: Williams & Wilkins, 1996.

Sheperd J, Cobbe S, Ford I, et al. Prevention of coronary heart disease with pravastatin in men with hypercholesterolemia. N Engl J Med 1995;333:1301–7.

Abnormal Weight and Nutrition

Agras WS. Obesity, Bulimia nervosa and Anorexia Nervosa. In Rubenstein E, Federman DD, ed. Scientific American Medicine. New York: Scientific American, Inc. 1989.

Hamilton EMN, Whitney EN, Sizer FS. Nutrition: concepts and controversies. 5th ed. St. Paul: West Publishing Co., 1991.

Wyngaarden JB, Smith LH, Bennett JC, eds. Cecil Textbook of Medicine 19th ed. Philadelphia: W.B. Saunders Co. 1992.

chapter 19

UROLOGY
Linda McLaughlin, Thomas McGinn, and Sharon Parish

FEMALE VOIDING PROBLEMS

Incontinence of urine is defined as a condition in which urine is involuntarily lost. Incontinence of urine affects up to 30% of older women (1); and 38–83% of patients in long-term care (2–4), where females outnumber males by more than 2 to 1. The costs of incontinence are medical (cystitis, urosepsis, urinary tract infections, decubiti, perineal rashes, falls, fractures), psychosocial (dependency, embarrassment, disruption of social life, undermining of self confidence, physical discomfort, isolation, depression, and predisposition to institutionalization), and economic. In 1983 the U.S. Surgeon General estimated that the cost of additional care for the 15% of incontinent elderly who were institutionalized was $8 billion (5).

Pathophysiologic Correlation

The lower urinary tract functionally consists of a bladder and a sphincter. Anatomically, the bladder includes two parts, the bladder musculature (detrusor) and the trigone. The sphincter (or bladder outlet) is composed of the bladder neck and the proximal urethra. The detrusor is innervated chiefly by the pelvic nerves via the parasympathetic (cholinergic) nervous system. The bladder neck and the proximal urethra are innervated by the hypogastric nerves via the sympathetic (alpha-adrenergic) nervous system. The distal urethra is enclosed in striated muscle and is innervated by the pudendal nerves via the somatic nervous system (Fig. 19.1).

The two major tasks of the bladder are storage and expulsion of urine. A correctly functioning and coordinated bladder and sphincter mechanism are necessary for continence. The bladder is in charge of accommodating increasing volumes of urine while maintaining low pressures. Storage of urine is mediated by detrusor relaxation and closing of the sphincter. Detrusor relaxation is achieved by inhibition of parasympathetic tone by central nervous system centers in the brain; sphincter closing is mediated by a reflex increase in sympathetic and somatic neural activity. Normally, the bladder neck and urethra remain shut during bladder filling and at times of increased intra-abdominal pressure. Continence is thus preserved as long as bladder neck and urethral pressure is greater than intravesical pressure. Micturition transpires when detrusor contraction is coordinated with sphincter relaxation. Contraction is mediated by the parasympathetic nervous system, and relaxation by inhibition of somatic and sympathetic nerve impulses to the bladder outlet. The reciprocal relationship between the detrusor and the outlet is coordinated by a voiding center, probably located in the pons. Voluntary micturition transpires when intravesical pressure exceeds bladder neck and urethral pressure under cognizant and coordinated control.

Clinical and Laboratory Evaluation

In the majority of cases, a thorough history and focused physical examination can accurately predict which type of incontinence is extant, as well as whether a cause of transient incontinence is present. Laboratory studies may be necessary to delineate the kind(s) of incontinence in more complicated cases and may also be needed to confirm a reason for transient incontinence.

HISTORY

A precise micturition history is vital for the accurate classification of urinary incontinence in females. The first step should be to assess the features of the incontinence, such as the body position in which it transpires (e.g., supine, upright, sitting), intensifying conditions (e.g., coughing, sneezing, running); pattern of occurrence (episodic or continu-

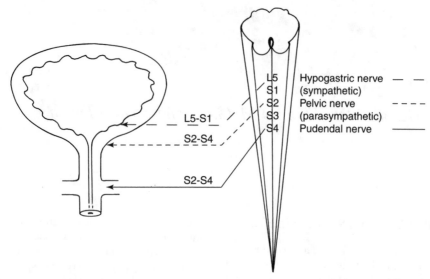

Figure 19.1. Neuroanatomy of lower urinary tract. (Adapted from Sloane B, Baum N. Urinary incontinence in women. Postgraduate Medicine 1988;84:252.)

ous); associated urologic characteristics (urgency, frequency, nocturia); amount or severity of leakage (a few drops, entire bladder contents); and the patient's cognizance of the incontinence (sensible or insensible fluid loss). Toileting abilities should also be assessed. (Table 19.1).

The existence of other medical disorders that may produce incontinence (e.g., Parkinson's disease, diabetes mellitus, multiple sclerosis, pernicious anemia, cerebrovascular accidents, seizure disorders) should be determined. Chronic pulmonary disease and upper respiratory tract infection often aggravate urinary incontinence because of the increased coughing that these disorders generate.

Symptoms or history of urinary tract infection should be sought, because the frequency and urgency such infection generates may increase incontinence. The existence of gross hematuria, particularly if no urinary tract infection is discovered, implies a pathologic disorder of the urinary tract (e.g., bladder carcinoma) and requires a more exhaustive urologic investigation.

The patient's gynecologic history is significant in evaluating her estrogen status. Estrogen-deficient conditions can result from ingestion of medicine (e.g., clomiphene) or, more frequently, menopause. Estrogen deprivation may cause atrophic vaginitis or atrophic urethritis, which predisposes to urinary frequency and/or urgency and can aggravate incontinence. A history of spinal, gynecologic, abdominal, or bladder surgery is significant because

such surgery could affect the anatomy and innervation of the lower urinary tract.

Ultimately, the history should include use of any medicines that could result in dysfunction of the lower urinary tract (Table 19.2). Medicines warrant particular attention, since drugs with effects on the urinary tract are so often prescribed for other purposes. Many urologically active drugs are attainable without prescription.

PHYSICAL EXAMINATION

In addition to executing the customary physical examination, the health care provider should do meticulous abdominal, pelvic, neurologic and rectal examinations. The abdomen should be observed for a distended bladder, which implies overflow incontinence. The pelvic examination evaluates the estrogen status of the vaginal mucosa. Atrophic vaginitis is commonly associated with atrophic urethritis. A urethral caruncle is also an indication of hypoestrogenism (a caruncle is a small, red, papillary growth, highly vascular, sometimes found in the urinary meatus in females). A search should be made for vaginal infection, which can frequently result in urinary incontinence.

A neurologic examination is executed to evaluate the fifth lumbar and the first, second, third, and fourth sacral nerves' sensory and motor supply to the pelvis and perineum. This includes the perineal response to light touch and pinprick. Evaluation

Table 19.1.
Clinical Evaluation of the Incontinent Patient

History
 Type (urge, reflex, stress, overflow, or mixed)
 Frequency, severity, duration
 Pattern (diurnal, nocturnal, or both; also, e.g., after
  taking medications)
 Associated symptoms (straining to void, incomplete
  emptying, dysuria)
 Alteration in bowel habit/sexual function
 Other relevant factors (e.g., cancer, diabetes, acute
  illness, neurologic disease, pelvic or lower urinary
  tract surgery.)
 Medications, including nonprescription agents
 Functional assessment
 Incontinence chart

Physical examination
 General medical examination
 Test for stress-induced leakage when bladder is full
 Observe/listen to voiding
 Palpate for bladder distension after voiding
 Pelvic examination (atrophic vaginitis/urethritis; pel-
  vic muscle laxity; pelvic mass)
 Rectal examination (resting tone and voluntary con-
  trol of anal sphincter; prostate nodules; fecal im-
  paction)
 Neurologic examination (mental status and elemen-
  tal examination, including sacral reflexes and peri-
  neal sensation)

Initial investigation
 Metabolic survey (measurement of electrolytes, cal-
  cium, glucose, and urea nitrogen)
 Measurement of postvoid residual volume
 Urine analysis and culture
 Renal ultrasound[a]
 Urine cytology[a]
 Uroflowmetry[a]
 Cystoscopy?[a]

[a]See text
Adapted from Resnick NM. Initial evaluation of the incontinent
patient. J Am Geriatr Soc 1990;38:314.

Table 19.2.
Common Causes of Transient Incontinence

Delirium or confusional state
Infection, urinary (symptomatic)
Atrophic urethritis or vaginitis
Pharmaceuticals
 Sedatives or hypnotics, especially long-acting agents
 Loop diuretics
 Anticholinergic agents (antipsychotic agents, antide-
  pressants, antihistamines, antiparkinsonian
  agents, antiarrhythmics (disopyramide), antispas-
  modics, opiates, and antidiarrheal agents)
 Alpha-adrenoceptor agonists and antagonists
 Beta-adrenergics and blockers
 Calcium-channel-entry blockers
 Analgesics
Psychological disorder, especially depression
Endocrine disorder (hypercalcemia or hyperglycemia)
Restricted mobility
Stool impaction

Adapted from Resnick NM. Initial evaluation of the incontinent
patient. J Am Geriatr Soc 1990;38:312.

are also mandatory. To evaluate metabolic conditions such as diabetes mellitus and hypercalcemia
accompanied by incontinence serum glucose and
calcium levels should be ordered.

In a female with a considerably increased post
void residual (i.e., over 200 ml), hydronephrosis
should be ruled out by renal sonography or, if the
results of renal sonography are indeterminate, by
intravenous pyelogram (IVP). If sterile hematuria
is extant, IVP and cystoscopy are indicated, as well
as a urine cytology. When the risk of carcinoma is
elevated (e.g., incontinence of new onset, or in a
patient who smokes and/or has been exposed to
aniline dyes), a urine cytology may be warranted
even with a lack of hematuria, as the sensitivity of
the urinalysis by itself is insufficient to rule out
bladder carcinoma. Although the merit of a urinary
flow rate in an elderly person remains questionable,
and although flow rates tend to decrease with age,
the flow rate remains a sensitive test. If the rate is
normal, it can be used to rule out clinically meaningful obstruction.

Several simple office procedures may be executed to delineate the type of the incontinence. To
begin appropriate treatment, the clinician needs
to distinguish between incontinence secondary to
abnormal bladder contraction (detrusor instability)
and that secondary to an anatomic defect. To quantify the amount of voided urine, the patient should
drink liquids to fill her bladder and then the health

of rectal sphincter tone and the existence or absence
of rectal masses or fecal impaction concludes the
physical examination. (See Table 19.1)

LABORATORY EVALUATION

Urinalysis should always be executed when assessing a patient for incontinence. The existence
of hematuria, pyuria, bacteriuria, or glycosuria requires further investigation. Urine should be sent
for culture if greater than five white blood cells per
high power field are present. Serum levels of urea
nitrogen and creatinine to establish renal function

care provider should watch her urinating into a measuring container. The amount of urine and mean flow rate (amount divided by the number of seconds taken to empty the bladder) should be documented. A low volume may indicate a small bladder capacity produced by bladder instability, neurologic impairment, or anatomic aberrations in the bladder. A diminished flow rate (<20 ml/sec) implies urethral obstruction or poor bladder contractility.

The volume of residual urine should be quantified by inserting a 14French or 16French catheter into the bladder while the patient is supine. An amount of 50 to 100 cc may indicate a disturbance in bladder emptying. Trouble in inserting the catheter may imply a large urethral diverticulum or urethral obstruction (quite uncommon in women).

With the catheter left in place, a bladder filling test is executed. The catheter is connected to the open barrel of a 50-ml irrigation syringe, which acts as a funnel. The syringe is held about 15 cm above the pubic symphysis and is filled with room temperature sterile water or saline solution. The patient's bladder is gradually filled to the volume she can tolerate, but not to more than 600 ml. Observe for trouble in filling the bladder, leakage around the catheter, and involuntary bladder contractions (indicated by upward movement of the fluid column). The patient relates the first feeling of a full bladder (bladder capacity). When she urinates, the fluid column within the syringe should increase, indicating a bladder contraction. The clinician should also observe whether the patient can sense the bladder contraction and intentionally prevent it (i.e., the fluid in the syringe would decrease).

Bladder instability classically results in urgency, with a bladder contraction that cannot be prevented. If 250 ml of water or saline solution is instilled and no bladder contraction transpires, bladder instability in the supine position is improbable. It is not uncommon for a normal person to be unable to initiate a contraction under these conditions.

The Marshall-Marchetti Test. The Marshall-Marchetti test is useful in discerning stress incontinence. To execute this procedure, the bladder is again filled through the catheter. Withdraw the catheter and request that the patient not urinate any fluid for 15 to 30 seconds. Observe and document whether there is any loss. As the patient coughs or performs the Valsalva maneuver, the health care provider watches the external meatus of the urethra for fluid leakage. If possible, have the patient stand. Again, request that the patient inhibit any flow for 30 seconds. If no loss transpires, request that the patient cough or perform the Valsalva maneuver. Again, observe for loss. If this test does not evoke incontinence, the patient is requested to run in place and is watched for urinary loss. Occasionally, these maneuvers cause uninhibited detrusor contractions, which produce a large amount of fluid leakage instead of the spurt that is observed in stress incontinence.

The urine volume ranges and signs and symptoms observed during simple cystometry should suggest what kind of incontinence the patient is experiencing (Table 19.3). Among the findings suggestive or indicative of urge incontinence are urgency at a bladder capacity of less than 300 ml, loss around the catheter; and loss after cough connotes urge incontinence with detrusor contraction provoked by exertion. Stress incontinence is manifested by loss during cough. A large residual volume (i.e., >100 ml) suggests overflow incontinence either from urethral obstruction or decreased bladder contractility. If 600 ml is instilled without a feeling

Table 19.3.
Typical Findings of Simple Cystometry in the Three Main Types of Incontinence

Findings	Urge (ml)	Stress (ml)	Overflow (ml)
Voided volume	<200	300–500	<200 or >600
Post-void residual	<100	<100	>100
Spontaneous contractions	<300	300–500	>600
Discomfort	<300	400–600	>600
Leakage			
Supine	<300		>600
Upright	<300		>600
Cough	Delayed	<600	

From Douglas KC. A bedside test for evaluating incontinence. Senior Patient 1990:41.

of fullness, incontinence may be associated with decreased feeling resulting in overflow. Reflex incontinence is suggested by spontaneous contractions without a concomitant feeling of the desire to void. While this kind of incontinence may be discernable with simple cystometrics, it is problematic.

The Bonney Test. Many clinicians use the Bonney test to foretell the success of surgery for incontinence. In this procedure, the health care provider lifts the bladder neck on each side of the urethra with the fingers. However, this test may yield a false-positive outcome because the urethra is squeezed (and may be obstructed) against the pubis. A false positive outcome can be averted by putting a slightly opened ring forceps in the vagina at the level of the bladder neck. The bladder neck is lifted with the ring forceps, and the patient is requested to strain or do the Valsalva maneuver. If the patient is continent during this test, the probability of success from a bladder-suspension surgery is high.

The Cotton-swab Test. Another procedure used to evaluate the loss of support of the urethra and bladder neck is the cotton-swab test. A lubricated cotton swab is introduced into the urethra to the level of the bladder neck. The patient is requested to cough or do the Valsalva maneuver. Excursion of the cotton swab greater than 20° from horizontal is deemed a positive outcome and implies a loss of anatomic support of the bladder neck and urethra.

The Pessary or Diaphragm Test. The pessary or diaphragm test is helpful in diagnosing stress incontinence (6). A suitable diaphragm or pessary is inserted in the vagina after the Marshall-Marchetti and Bonney tests have been carried out. If continence is reestablished, an anatomic weakness of the bladder neck and urethra is probably extant, and a successful outcome can be expected from a bladder-suspension surgery. It is believed that this procedure restores the urethra and bladder neck to their usual retropubic position (Fig. 19.2).

Differential Diagnosis

Urinary incontinence can be transient (i.e., be secondary to another disease, condition or drug). Chronic urinary incontinence may be divided into six types: 1) stress (anatomic), 2) urge (detrusor instability or hyperreflexic bladder), 3) reflex, 4) overflow, 5) mixed stress and urge, and 6) functional. The diagnosis is made based upon the history and physical examination. With the use of a few office tests, the diagnosis can be confirmed.

TRANSIENT INCONTINENCE

The initial history, physical examination, and laboratory evaluation may provide clues to possible cause(s) of transient incontinence (See Table 19.2) (7). Transient incontinence may be responsible for as much as a third of incontinence in elderly people living in the community and for half of incontinence in acutely hospitalized persons greater than 65 years of age; statistics for nursing home inhabitants are unavailable, but disorders related to transient incontinence in other milieus are frequent in these patients as well. Although the pathophysiology of each is different, the prevalence of each is not completely clear-cut, and in some cases the mechanism is poorly comprehended, each is amenable to therapeutic intercession. All causes should be meticulously sought and rectified before the physician goes further (7, 8). Approximately three quarters of patients who first develop incontinence in the course of hospitalization will be remedied through this approach (9). Ultimately, irrespective of their prevalence, transient causes should be meticulously searched for, since many are connected with morbidity outside the urinary tract.

STRESS INCONTINENCE

The most frequently diagnosed kind of incontinence in women is stress incontinence. Classical stress incontinence is typified by unexpected daytime leakage of small to moderate quantities of urine during actions that intensify intraabdominal pressure (i.e., coughing, sneezing, lifting, laughing, or exercising). Stress incontinence is associated with rare nighttime loss of urine, a sensation of heaviness in the pelvic area, and little post-voiding residual volume in the absence of a large cystocele. The prevailing cause is urethral hypermobility, i.e., distal displacement of the bladder neck and urethra from their usual anatomic location caudad to the pubic symphysis, due to pelvic-floor weakness. Other disorders, such as sphincter incompetence, urethral instability, or stress-induced detrusor instability, are infrequent etiologies.

URGE INCONTINENCE

Urge incontinence, possibly the most frequent kind in the elderly is typified by unintentional contractions of the bladder wall associated with complaints of urgency, frequency, and nocturia. Urge incontinence is caused by an unstable bladder (detrusor instability). The individual may leak moderate to large quantities of urine with an alteration in position (e.g., from lying down to standing up) or with

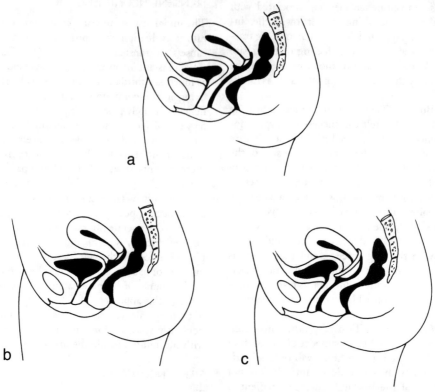

Figure 19.2. Use of diaphragm to test whether bladder-suspension procedure will correct urinary incontinence. a. Normal retropubic position of female bladder and urethra. b. Abnormal position of bladder and urethra seen in stress incontinence. c. Restoration of normal anatomy with insertion of diaphragm, suggesting anatomic weakness of bladder neck and urethra that will respond to surgery. Diaphragm can also be used to treat mild stress incontinence. (Adapted from Sloane B, Baum N. Urinary incontinence in women. Postgrad Med 1988: 84(5):254.)

auditory stimulation (e.g., dripping water). Unintentional micturition in urge incontinence is heralded by a forewarning of a few seconds to a few minutes. Sacral feeling and reflexes are intact, volitional control of the anal sphincter is preserved, and the post-voiding residual volume is small. The most common cause of urge incontinence is detrusor overactivity, a disorder in which the bladder eludes central inhibition and contracts reflexly. Nonneurologic etiologies of bladder instability include outlet obstruction, or a local bladder condition such as carcinoma-in-situ, bladder stones, lower urinary tract infection, radiation effects, or interstitial cystitis. If objective proof of neurologic damage is observed along with bladder instability, the individual is stated to have hyperreflexic bladder. Etiologies of hyperreflexic bladder are central nervous system injury secondary to stroke, Alzheimer's disease or other dementia, brain tumor, multiple sclerosis, or Parkinson's disease; or impedance

with spinal inhibitory pathways due to spinal cord injury, spondylosis, or metastasis.

REFLEX INCONTINENCE

Reflex incontinence is present when no stress or forewarning antedates intermittent unintentional micturition. Urinating is often, moderate in amount, and happens uniformly throughout the day and night. Sacral reflexes are intact, but voluntary sphincter control and perineal feeling may be damaged, and post-voiding residual volume may be enlarged. Typically, reflex incontinence is secondary to a suprasacral spinal cord injury (e.g., spondylosis or tumor). This not only impedes central nervous system inhibition, thereby causing hyperreflexia, but also impedes pathways coordinating detrusor contraction and outlet relaxation, producing detrusor sphincter dyssynergia and functional outlet obstruction (10). Interruption of sensory pathways prevents forewarning of imminent voiding.

OVERFLOW INCONTINENCE

Overflow incontinence happens when the weight of a large quantity of urine in an overdistended bladder overwhelms outlet resistance. In this disorder leakage of small amounts of urine is frequent during the day and night. The patient may also observe hesitancy, dribbling, decreased and interrupted flow, a need to strain to urinate, and a sensation of partial emptying. The bladder is generally palpable and the residual volume is great; if the difficulty is neurologically mediated, perineal feeling, sacral reflexes, and control of the anal sphincter are often damaged. Overflow incontinence is created by either outlet obstruction (which is infrequent in women), or by an underactive detrusor secondary to myogenic or neurogenic causes (e.g., a herniated disk, or peripheral neuropathy associated with diabetes mellitus, vitamin B12 deficiency, or tabes dorsalis).

MIXED INCONTINENCE

Particularly in the elderly, more than one kind of incontinence may be extant concomitantly. For example, it is not usual for females with stress incontinence to also have urge incontinence from detrusor instability. Thus, this type of incontinence is termed "mixed."

FUNCTIONAL INCONTINENCE

Functional incontinence is connected with the incapability to reach the bathroom at the proper moment or to position for toileting without help (e.g., environmental obstacles to toilets), and/or psychological resistance. It is observed in patients with impaired mobility, coordination, communication or cognitive abilities, and in demented, depressed, or contentious patients.

Management

The most practical management of urinary incontinence consists of fostering either bladder emptying or bladder storage, depending on the kind of condition that the patient has (11). Pharmacologic agents (Table 19.4) may be employed to prevent unintentional bladder contractions and to increase bladder outlet resistance. A small anatomic defect may respond to treatment with a mechanical device. More severe anatomic defects may necessitate surgical intervention. Various behavioral therapies can be useful in treating all kinds of incontinence except overflow.

PROMOTING BLADDER EMPTYING

Bladder emptying can be achieved by augmenting intravesical pressure or diminishing outlet resistance. The drug most frequently employed in increasing intravesical pressure in overflow incontinence associated with atonic bladder is bethanecol (Table 19.4). Outlet resistance can be diminished by employment of alpha-adrenergic blockers. Phenoxybenzamine has been helpful in patients with both functional and anatomic obstruction at the level of the bladder neck. More recently, prazosin has also been effective in treating both reflex and overflow incontinence (13). A relaxant of striated muscle (e.g., diazepam or baclofen) can be useful in reflex incontinence.

If pharmacologic therapy is unsuccessful in fostering bladder emptying, intermittent clean (nonsterile) self-catheterization can be employed safely and effectively by adults and the elderly as outpatients (15). Candidates for intermittent self-catheterization should be strongly motivated, have sufficient fine motor skills of the upper extremities, and have a normal urethra (i.e., no urethral strictures). The recommended schedule for self-catheterization is every three hours during the daytime and one or twice nightly (or frequently enough so that urine volume is less than 300 ml). A 14F clear plastic catheter made for this purpose (e.g., Mentor Self-Cath) can be employed. It can be cleaned with ordinary soap and water and can be introduced without lubrication. Most patients do not need antibiotics. For intractable incontinence, adjunctive measures such as pads and special undergarments are invaluable (8); insertion of a long-term indwelling urethral catheter or surgical diversion should be done only in extreme cases. In patients with reflex incontinence, bladder decompression can also be achieved mechanically, by suprapubic tapping, or stretching the anal sphincter (16); or surgically, by sphincterotomy.

PROMOTING BLADDER STORAGE

Bladder storage can be achieved by augmenting bladder outlet resistance or by diminishing intravesical pressure. Urethral hypermobility is ameliorated by weight loss if the patient is obese and by therapy of predisposing problems such as coughing or atrophic vaginitis. Estrogens are useful in the care of the postmenopausal woman with mild to moderate stress incontinence associated with

Table 19.4.
Drugs Used to Treat Urinary Incontinence

Drug	Mechanism	Uses	Side Effects	Dosage
Anticholinergics/spasmodics Propantheline (Proban-thine)	Inhibits involuntary bladder contractions; acts by competitive blockade of cholinergic receptors in the bladder wall	Urge incontinence associated with bladder instability	Dry mouth, blurry vision, drowsiness, constipation, increased heart rate. Contraindicated in patients with glaucoma and significant bladder outlet obstruction.	15–120 mg per day in three to four divided doses
Imipramine (Janimine, SK-Pramine, Tofranil)	Tricyclic anti-depressant. Exact mechanism is unknown. Has anticholinergic and adrenergic effects. Decreases bladder contractility and increases bladder outlet resistance.	Same as propantheline	Most common side effects are related to anticholinergic effects and are like those for propantheline. Contraindicated in patients receiving monoamine oxidase inhibitors and should be used with caution in patients with hypertension or cardiovascular disease.	50–150 mg per day in four divided doses, with a gradual increase to 150 mg as a night time dose
Oxybutynin (Ditropan)	Smooth muscle relaxant. Reportedly acts directly on smooth muscle at a site distal to the cholinergic receptor. Causes some anti-cholinergic activity and possesses local anesthetic properties as well.	Same as propantheline	Identical to those of propantheline.	5–20 mg per day in four divided doses
Flavoxate (Urispas)	See oxybutynin	Same as propantheline	See oxybutynin	300–800 mg per day in three divided doses
Alpha-adrenergic agonists Pseudoephedrine	Sympathomimetic drug. Acts by stimulating the alpha adrenergic receptors of the bladder, neck and proximal urethra.	Stress incontinence associated with sphincter weakness	Hypertension, anxiety and insomnia from central nervous system stimulation. Should be used with caution in patients who have hypertension, cardiovascular disease, or hyperthyroidism.	120–200 mg per day in four divided doses
Ephedrine	See pseudoephedrine	Same as pseudoephedrine	See pseudoephedrine	100–200 mg per day in four divided doses
Phenylpropanolamine	See pseudoephedrine	Same as pseudoephedrine	See pseudoephedrine	50–150 mg per day in three divided doses
Imimpramine	See above	See above	See above	See above

Drug	Action	Indication	Side effects/comments	Dosage
Conjugated estrogens: Oral	Improves the vascularity of the urethral mucosa and thus increases urethral resistance (17).	Stress incontinence associated with sphincter weakness	Changes in vaginal bleeding pattern and abnormal withdrawal bleeding or flow, reduced carbohydrate tolerance, increased risk of gallbladder disease, cholestatic jaundice, increased risk of gallbladder disease, cholestatic jaundice, increased risk of endometrial cancer if not used with a progestin. Should not be used in patients with known or suspected cancer of the breast.	.3–1.25 mg or more daily, depending upon the tissue response of the individual patient. Administer cyclically (e.g., 3 weeks on and one week off)
Topical	See oral	See oral	See oral	2 g inserted into vagina every other day. Can be reduced to 1 g after a response occurs
Cholinergic agonists Bethanechol (Duvoid, urecholine)	Promotes contraction of the detrusor muscle	Overflow incontinence associated with atonic bladder	Abdominal cramps, diarrhea, nausea, and sweating. Contraindicated in patients with asthma.	40–200 mg per day in four divided doses. Dosage is titrated by measuring the residual volume, which should be less than 10% of bladder capacity
Alpha-adrenergic blockers Phenoxybenzamine (Dibenzyline)	Blocks the sympathetic nerves to the internal sphincter at the level of the bladder neck and promotes bladder emptying	Functional and anatomic obstruction at the level of the bladder neck (i.e., reflex or overflow incontinence)	Orthostatic hypotension. Should be used only for a short period, because carcinogenic activity has been associated with prolonged use of the drug in laboratory animals (12).	20 mg per day in two divided doses.
Prazosin (Minipress)	Reduces outlet resistance at the bladder neck level by alpha adrenergic blockade	Same as phenoxybenzamine	Reflex tachycarcardia, nasal congestion, and retrograde ejaculation. Orthostatic hypotension is very common.	4–20 mg per day in two divided doses for reflex incontinence, 3–12 mg per day in two divided doses for overflow incontinence. A starter dose of 1 mg can be given before bedtime for several weeks before increasing to the therapeutic dose (14).

Adapted from Palmer MH. Urinary incontinence. Nurs Clin North Am 1990;25(4):926–927.

sphincter weakness. Drugs used to promote bladder storage are reviewed in Table 19.4. The two groups of medicines used for preventing unintentional bladder contractions are true anticholinergic drugs and smooth muscle relaxants. Propantheline is the most frequently employed anticholinergic drug. Smooth muscle relaxants include oxybutynin, flavoxate, and calcium channel blockers. Tricyclic antidepressants, such as imipramine, are also effective for fostering urinary storage.

Pharmacologic agents that augment bladder outlet resistance can ameliorate mild to moderate stress incontinence. These drugs include sympathomimetic agents such as ephedrine, pseudoephedrine, and phenylpropanolamine.

Vaginal devices (e.g., Habib pessary, Edwards spring device, or Bonnar balloon) have been used to treat conditions associated with pelvic relaxation, including stress incontinence (18). The device may relieve stress incontinence in women who have mild anatomic defects. One recent study (19) also showed a diaphragm to be effective in managing mild stress incontinence, particularly when the incontinence was extant only during exertion.

For women with stress incontinence secondary to urethral hypermobility, surgical procedures to reposition the urethra and bladder, and thus augment urethral resistance, are executed and are successful in the majority of elderly patients (8). If sphincter incompetence is discerned, it too can be rectified surgically in the majority of patients (8).

Behavior therapies are a disparate set of procedures used to change incontinence through systematic environmental modifications. These interventions are germane for two reasons: first, surgery for incontinence is often undesirable to patients or inappropriate because of other medical problems; and second, the side effects associated with pharmacologic therapy can sometimes effect considerable discomfort and result in noncompliance with the medical regimen. Behavioral therapies include sphincter training, bladder inhibition training, biofeedback, habit training, bladder retraining, contingency management, and staff management (Table 19.5). The only interventions which will be addressed in detail here are sphincter training (i.e. pelvic floor training), and biofeedback.

Pelvic floor training, or Kegel exercises (See Table 19.5) strengthen the pubococcygeal periurethral muscle fibers and increase bladder outlet resistance. The patient can be instructed to carry out these exercises; initially the patient is taught to practice the exercises by voluntarily initiating and terminating the urine stream. Once the patient knows what muscle groups are affected, she can practice the exercises when not urinating. The patient should contract the pubococcygeal muscle for three seconds, relax, and repeat the exercises ten times. (The pelvic floor muscle should be contracted without contracting the buttocks, thighs, and abdominal muscles). This sequence should be done five to ten times each day for several months. This is a useful and inexpensive way of controlling mild stress incontinence. Regrettably, many women neglect to stick to the exercises when they do not notice improvement after a few weeks.

Biofeedback (Table 19.5, Fig. 19.3) supplies a person with auditory or visual feedback of physio-

Table 19.5.
Behavioral Interventions for Urinary Incontinence

Intervention	Description	Types of Incontinence
Sphincter training (pelvic floor training)	Training to teach sphincter/pelvic floor contraction to prevent urine loss	Stress, Urge
Bladder inhibition training	Training to teach voluntary inhibition of detrusor contraction	Urge
Biofeedback	Feedback of physiologic responses to teach sphincter contraction or bladder inhibition	Stress, Urge
Habit training	Fixed or flexible toileting schedule, adjustable to accommodate patient's pattern of incontinence	Urge, Functional, Reflex
Bladder retraining	Toileting interval is gradually increased or decreased to achieve normal pattern	Urge, Stress, Reflex
Contingency management	Systematic reinforcement of appropriate toileting; Inappropriate toileting ignored or punished	Functional
Staff management	Systematic structuring and reinforcement of appropriate implementation of treatment by staff	Functional

From Burgio KL. Behavior therapies for urinary incontinence. Clinical Report on Aging 1988;2(6):10.

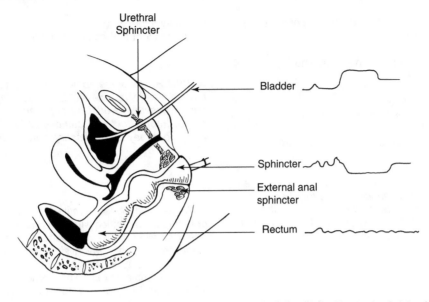

Urethral
Sphincter

Bladder

Sphincter

External anal
sphincter

Rectum

Figure 19.3. Diagram of female pelvic anatomy showing the devices used to provide biofeedback information to the patient. Sample polygraph tracings are shown at right. (Adapted from Burgio KL. Behavior therapies for urinary incontinence. Clinical Report on Aging 1988; 2(6):11.)

logic response of the bladder, pelvic floor muscle, and urethral sphincter to bladder filling during a cystometric procedure. During a biofeedback training session, pressure transducers are placed in the rectum to monitor anal sphincter activity and intra-abdominal pressure. The person is trained to watch polygraph tracings of changes in anal and abdominal muscle activity as the bladder is filled with sterile fluid via a catheter. Visual feedback of bladder activity during filling is also supplied to the individual, e.g., uninhibited contractions of the detrusor. The person is then taught to contract periurethral muscles while relaxing abdominal muscles. Polygraph tracings supply visual information about the efficacy of these efforts to regulate bladder function (20). This method necessitates both the cognitive ability to comprehend bodily feelings and biofeedback data, and the incentive to learn methods to regulate bladder and sphincter function.

ILLUSTRATIVE CASES WITH SELF-ASSESSMENT QUESTIONS AND ANSWERS

Case 1

A 42-year-old female comes to your office complaining of intermittent incontinence of moderate amounts of urine. She states that she urinates frequently, sometimes leaks urine upon standing, and that often when she feels the desire to urinate, she cannot get to the bathroom fast enough. She also has nocturia one to two times per night.

QUESTION: *What type of incontinence does she have?*

a. Stress
b. Urge
c. Reflex
d. Overflow
e. Mixed
f. Functional

ANSWER: b. *This patient has all the classical symptoms of urge incontinence. In addition, urge incontinence is the most common type for her age group.*

QUESTION: *What treatment(s) could you recommend for her?*

a. Bladder retraining, habit training
b. Biofeedback
c. Kegel exercises
d. Propantheline
e. Smooth muscle relaxant (e.g. oxybutynin, flavoxate)
f. Imipramine or other tricyclic antidepressant

ANSWER: *All of the above are options for treating urge incontinence. However, because all medicines have potential side effects, the three behavioral therapies should be tried before employing pharmacological treatment.*

Case 2

An 85 year-old-female nursing home patient is complaining of frequent incontinence of small amounts of urine, throughout the day and at night also. When she begins to urinate, sometimes the urine doesn't come out immediately, and when she finishes urinating, sometimes she has dribbling. She feels as if her bladder never completely empties. She also has "pins and needles" and numbness in her hands, and burning pains in her feet.

QUESTION: *What type of incontinence does she have?*

a. Stress
b. Urge
c. Reflex
d. Overflow
e. Mixed
f. Functional

ANSWER: d. *The answer is overflow incontinence. This patient has some sort of neuropathy as the cause of the incontinence, possibly secondary to diabetes mellitus, pernicious anemia or tabes dorsalis.*

QUESTION: *What treatment(s) would you recommend?*

a. Alpha blocker (e.g. prazosin)
b. Bethanechol
c. Treatment of underlying condition, if possible (i.e. good glucose control, B12 injections, etc.)

d. Phenoxybenzamine
e. Intermittent self-catheterization

ANSWER: *All of the above are correct choices, though clearly treatment of the underlying condition, if possible, would be of paramount importance. Intermittent self catheterization is a last resort, but may be necessary in some patients.*

Case 3

A 78-year-old obese female long-time smoker presents to your office with the complaint of leakage of small amounts of urine during the daytime when she coughs, which she frequently does. She also has a sensation of pelvic heaviness, and she complains of vaginal dryness on sexual intercourse. She has a history of breast cancer.

QUESTION: *What type of incontinence does she have?*

a. Stress
b. Urge
c. Reflex
d. Overflow
e. Mixed
f. Functional

ANSWER: a. *As could be predicted by her age group and sex, this patient has stress incontinence, perhaps secondary to her postmenopausal state and/or to her weight. It is aggravated by what sounds like chronic obstructive pulmonary disease (COPD) from her chronic tobacco abuse.*

QUESTION: *What treatment(s) would you recommend for her?*

a. Weight loss
b. Discontinue tobacco, treat COPD
c. Topical or oral estrogens
d. Alpha adrenergic agonist (e.g. phenylpropanolamine)
e. Imipramine or other tricyclic antidepressant
f. Sympathomimetic (e.g. ephedrine)
g. Insertion of pessary
h. Kegel exercises
i. Biofeedback
j. Bladder retraining

ANSWER: *All of the above are correct except estrogens, in this particular patient with stress incontinence. Estrogens are contraindicated in patients with a history of breast cancer either in themselves or a first degree relative (i.e., mother, sister). As with the previous patients, nonpharmacological management should be attempted before utilizing medications.*

MALE VOIDING PROBLEMS

Male voiding involves a complex array of neurologic and hormonal interactions which take place between the ureters, the bladder, the prostate, and the urethra. Patients with difficulty voiding most commonly present to the primary care clinician with symptoms of obstruction (hesitancy, nocturia, frequency, etc.) and perineal pain and tenderness. The differential diagnosis for these symptoms include: benign prostatic hypertrophy (BPH), prostate cancer, prostatitis, urethral stricture, neurogenic bladder, bladder calculi, bladder cancer and the various prostatitis syndromes (acute bacterial prostatitis, chronic bacterial prostatitis, nonbacterial prostatitis, and protadynia). Functional obstruction or worsening of a mild anatomic obstruction may also occur as a result of medications, chronic debilitating diseases, or from psychogenic causes.

Because BPH, prostate cancer, and prostatitis are the most commonly encountered problems related to male voiding, they will be addressed in detail in this chapter. The outpatient diagnosis and management of BPH and prostate cancer is an important aspect of primary care medicine since patients with these conditions are usually first encountered by generalists. Additionally, because these patients are typically older and often have multiple medical problems, the participation of a generalist becomes even more critical. Consequently, primary care clinicians need to familiarize themselves with the various presentations of BPH and prostate cancer, as well as the available diagnostic tests and treatment options (surgical and medical).

Pathophysiologic Correlation

The prostate is an accessory male sex organ situated between the base of the bladder and the external striated urethral sphincter. It produces between 15–30% of the normal ejaculate, thus providing the spermatozoa with transport medium. The prostate surrounds the proximal or prostatic urethra. The urethra courses through the prostate dividing it into the ventral fibromuscular segment and the dorsal glandular segment (Fig. 19.4). Histologically, the gland is divided into three zones; the transitional zone, the central zone, and the peripheral zone (Fig. 19.5). The peripheral zone is surrounded by the fibrous prostatic capsule. The majority of prostate cancers lie within the peripheral zone, whereas BPH occurs primarily within the transitional zone. Although the fact that prostate cancer occurs primarily in the peripheral zone is helpful in that it allows detection by digital rectal examination (DRE), regretfully this location is also responsible for the late onset of symptoms and hence the difficulty in detecting prostate cancer early.

At birth, the prostate weighs approximately 1 gram, about the size of a pea. At puberty, the gland grows rapidly secondary to the effects of testosterone. Growth slows around the age of 20 with the gland weighing about 20 grams. The gland remains that size until about the age of 40 when the microscopic changes of BPH begin to occur.

Throughout prostatic growth, the pituitary releases luteinizing hormone, which stimulates the production of testosterone by the testes. Testosterone is then converted by the prostate to its active form, 5-alpha dihydrotestosterone, which acts upon the prostate to stimulate protein synthesis and induce hypertrophy. Shrinkage or a halt in development may occur if the hypothalamic-pituitary-testes-prostate axis is disturbed (Fig. 19.6). For example, creating medical castration by giving a person a luteinizing releasing hormone (LHRH) agonist, results in regression of hyperplasia and shrinkage of the prostate size by 20 to 30 percent.

There are three different components involved in the pathophysiology of obstruction: mechanical obstruction, dynamic obstruction, and the bladder detrusor muscle response to obstruction. Mechanical obstruction in BPH occurs when the inner transitional zone hypertrophies. Unable to grow outwardly due to restriction by the prostatic capsule, it grows inward and compresses the prostatic urethra, thus creating an obstruction. Mechanical obstruction occurs in prostate cancer when the cancer, in the outer peripheral zone, grows large enough to compress the inner zone and urethra. Dynamic obstruction occurs due to changes in the tone of the prostatic smooth muscle fibers, which are under the control of the alpha-adrenergic system. Stimulation of these alpha receptors, which are located in the prostate and the bladder neck, cause compression of the gland and worsen mechanical obstruction (Fig 19.7). Detrusor muscle response to obstruction is a major cause for many symptoms

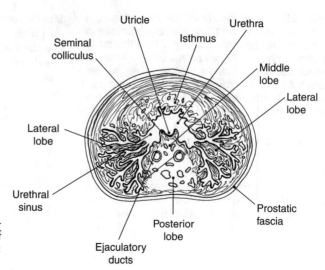

Figure 19.4. Cross section of the prostate. (Adapted from Netter FH. Atlas of human anatomy. Summit New Jersey: Ciba-Geigy Corporation, 1989:362.)

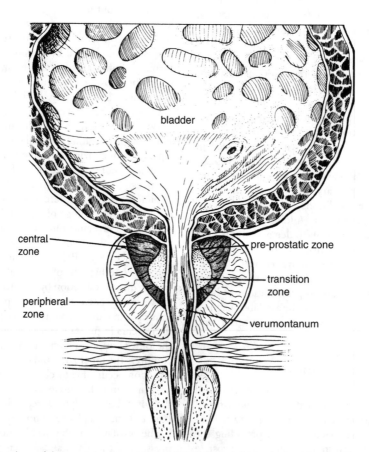

Figure 19.5. Histology of the prostate. (From Meares EM. Differential Diagnosis of Prostate Disorders. Merck and Co., Inc. 1993:4.)

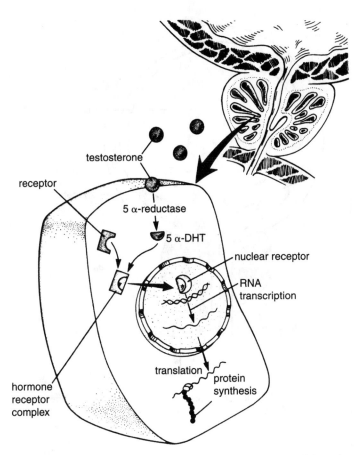

Figure 19.6. Conversion of testosterone to dihydrotestosterone by the enzyme 5-alpha-reductase in the prostatic epithelial cells. (From Meares EM. Differential Diagnosis of Prostate Disorders. Merck and Co., Inc. 1993:4.)

associated with obstruction. As obstruction worsens, the bladder's detrusor muscles initially hypertrophy, and then develop hyperplasia. Although the muscles hypertrophy to overcome the pressure of obstruction, they may lead to a loss of compliance and decrease in the functional capacity of the bladder if the obstruction goes untreated. Finally, chronic obstruction may result in collagen deposits within the bladder wall.

Clinical and Laboratory Evaluation

A comprehensive evaluation of patients with difficulty voiding involves: (a) classifying the nature of the symptoms (e.g., irritative, obstructive, perineal pain), (b) identifying the etiology of these symptoms (e.g., BPH, prostrate cancer, prostatitis) and, (c) finally, assessing symptom severity.

Obstructive symptoms are the most common complaints related to male voiding. BPH and pros-

tate cancer are the most commonly encountered etiologies of these symptoms, occurring most frequently among men over the age of 50. The second most commonly encountered complaint related to male voiding is perineal pain and discomfort. These symptoms are classically associated with prostatitis.

HISTORY

A thorough past medical history and medication use is critical in assessing the patient with complaints of voiding (Table 19.6). A history of diabetes, stroke, Parkinson's disease, multiple sclerosis, or any other CNS dysfunction may indicate a neurologic etiology for patients with obstructive symptoms, and hence may need to be ruled out. Knowledge of medication use is also important. Several medications may either worsen the symptoms of BPH or actually cause a BPH-like syndrome. For example, anticholinergics, calcium channel blockers, prosta-

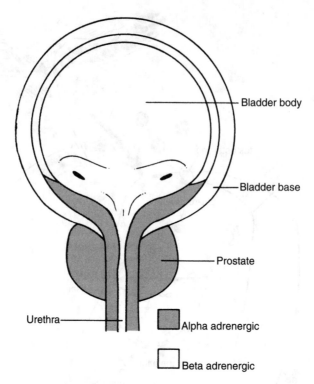

Figure 19.7. Neuropharmacology of the lower urinary tract. (From Meares EM. Differential Diagnosis of Prostate Disorders. Merck and Co., Inc. 1993:4.)

Table 19.6.
Pertinent History and Initial Evaluation in Patients with Difficulty Voiding

History		
Symptoms	Medication History	Past Medical History
Frequency	Anticholinergics	UTIs
Urgency	CA channel blockers	Urethral stricture
Hesitancy	Beta blockers	Hematuria
Nocturia	Alpha agonists	
AUA Symptom Index		

Initial Work up			
Physical Exam	Urinalysis	SMA-7	Prostate Specific Antigen
Digital rectal exam	To assess for	To assess renal	To evaluate for potential
Prostate size	UTI	function	prostate cancer
Consistency	Hematuria		
Tenderness			
Rectal tone			
Neurologic exam			

glandin inhibitors (e.g., ibuprofen), beta adrenergic agonists, and tricyclic antidepressants all decrease bladder contractility, and may, therefore, worsen symptoms of BPH. Another group of medications, the sympathomimetic drugs, e.g., pseudoephedrine or levodopa, may stimulate the prostatic alpha receptors and cause an increase in bladder outlet obstruction. Diuretics, a third group, may worsen the symptoms of BPH by simply increasing the volume of urine in the bladder.

When assessing past medical history, it is also important to pay close attention to any history of urinary tract infections (UTI), hematuria, or urethral manipulation which may have led to stricture. A history of urinary tract infections may indicate a severe obstruction or may indicate chronic bacterial prostatitis. The presence of hematuria may merely be an indication of a urinary tract infection but may also be a sign of malignancy, such as bladder cancer or renal cell cancer.

A history of present illness entails a thorough review of obstructive, irritative symptoms including perineal pain. Many of the symptoms classically encountered among patients who have difficulty voiding are often not volunteered by patients and directed questions may be necessary. Obstructive symptoms include hesitancy, dribbling, decreased force of stream, intermittency, and incomplete voiding. Irritative symptoms such as nocturia, frequency, urgency, and incontinence result from inappropriate bladder contraction, decreased bladder compliance and decreased bladder capacity. Perineal pain may be a sole complaint or may occur in conjunction with low back pain, fever, and in many cases, with obstructive or irritative symptoms.

If patients present with a primary obstructive and/or irritative type of symptomatology, the first consideration must be BPH, followed by prostate cancer. More unusual causes include urethral stricture, neurogenic bladder, and bladder cancer. Since patients with advanced prostate cancer often present with symptoms similar to BPH, it may be difficult to distinguish between the two on clinical presentation and a definitive diagnosis may only be ascertained following further testing. In cases of metastatic prostate cancer, patients may have associated bone pain and possibly compression fractures.

For patients presenting with perineal pain, the most likely diagnosis is prostatitis. Prostatitis is fundamentally a clinical diagnosis. Although the word, prostatitis, implies an infectious etiology, it actually comprises several different syndromes with varying etiologies. Some of the etiologies are infectious while the majority of cases of prostatitis are not clearly related to infection. Symptom duration can vary between days, months, and even up to a year. Perineal pain and low back pain are common features in all the prostatitis syndromes hence other related symptoms must be considered in narrowing the diagnosis. For example, patients with acute bacterial prostatitis (ABP) typically present with fever, chills, low back pain, and both irritative and obstructive symptoms. Alternately, chronic bacterial prostatitis (CBP), the most common cause of recurrent UTIs in men, can present in various forms but unlike patients with ABP, these patients rarely present with fever or chills.

PHYSICAL EXAMINATION

Vital Signs. Fever may indicate either a UTI or bacterial prostatitis. Urinary retention, which may occur in cases of severe obstruction, may present with an increase in blood pressure and heart rate. Increases in respiratory rate may also be observed, particularly if the bladder is distended.

Neurologic Examination. Frequently, patients with neurologic disorders develop a neurogenic bladder and then experience symptoms which may mimic obstruction. Therefore, close attention should be given to any signs of neurologic deficits in patients presenting with difficulty voiding. This is especially true for patients with a history of stroke or diabetes. Physical signs of peripheral neuropathy, for example in a diabetic patient, may be an indication of a neurogenic bladder and may require further diagnostic studies. The neurologic exam should, therefore, include a thorough evaluation of both sensory perception and muscle strength. The Romberg maneuver, where patients are required to stand with their feet shoulder length apart and eyes closed, is a quick and simple method for detecting subtle peripheral neuropathy and may be considered abnormal if significant imbalance is observed.

Digital Rectal Exam (DRE). The digital rectal examination is central to the evaluation of patients who present with difficulty voiding. Attention should be paid to the prostate size, consistency, tenderness, and the location of any discrete masses or nodules. Although prostate size should be evaluated, it is difficult to determine by DRE and estimates are often inaccurate. Further, since prostate size does not necessarily correlate with symptoms, size estimation is not a critical aspect of the DRE. The consistency of the prostate may be noted as either smooth, irregular, firm, boggy or containing discrete nodules.

For example, descriptions of prostate cancer detected by the DRE may contain the following information:

"The patient has a nontender, normal sized prostate with a firm, discrete nodule located in the anterior segment of the left lobe."

Alternately, the description of chronic bacterial prostatitis may classically be described as follows:

"The patient has a tender, boggy, slightly enlarged prostate with no discrete nodules."

Rectal tone should also be noted during DRE, with poor tone suggesting a neurologic etiology.

Abdominal Examination. Patients with urinary tract infections may have lower abdominal tenderness and fullness. Patients with significant obstruction may demonstrate lower abdominal fullness and dullness to percussion, signifying an enlarged and full bladder, possibly secondary to outlet obstruction.

LABORATORY EVALUATION

The initial evaluation of the patient presenting with obstructive or irritative symptoms should include a urinalysis and an SMA-7. Urinalysis is performed to check for the presence of red blood cells, white cells and bacteria, all of which may indicate a urinary tract infection. A baseline SMA-7 should be ordered to evaluate renal function, which although rarely affected in BPH or prostate cancer, may be damaged in severe and longstanding cases. Finally, a prostate specific antigen (PSA) level should be measured in patients suspected of BPH or prostate cancer. The PSA is not very accurate in patients

with BPH or prostatitis because of the high rate of false positive results. Therefore, caution should be taken in measuring this antigen (for evaluation of PSA, see section on PSA in prostate cancer screening).

The etiology of prostatitis can be determined by a complete history, physical examination, and examination of the urine and prostatic fluid. Prostatic fluid is obtained via urinalysis and/or bacterial localization by urethral urine (first voided 10 ml, VB1), midstream bladder urine (urine sampled after the first 200 ml have been voided, VB2) and prostatic expressate (obtained by prostatic massage, EPS) (Fig. 19.8).

There are several optional diagnostic studies that can be performed to help evaluate patients suspected of having BPH. While a generalist may not perform these studies, he or she should still be familiar with them and know when they are indicated. These studies may clarify the severity of the obstruction and the etiology of the symptoms. Uroflowmetry is a noninvasive recording of urine flow rate. The flow is measured in millimeters per second and the peak flow rate (Qmax) is the best discriminator of a decrease in flow. Uroflowmetry has demonstrated some utility as a predictor of treatment outcome. For example, patients with peak flow rates less than 12 ml/sec have a high response to surgical treatment. A drawback to the use of uroflowmetry is the lack of a clearly defined cutoff point in the Qmax to guide therapy. In addition, the flow rate is difficult to standardize because it naturally decreases with age and is dependant upon total urine volume. Uroflowmetry does not

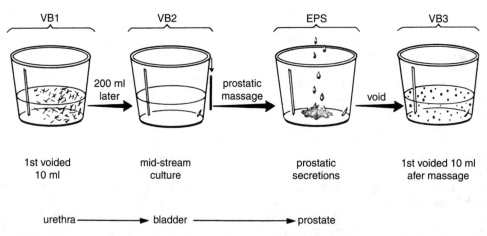

Figure 19.8. Bacteriologic localization of cultures in the diagnosis of chronic bacterial prostatis. (From Meares EM. Differential Diagnosis of Prostate Disorders. Merck and Co., Inc. 1993:4.)

distinguish between obstruction and detrusor muscle weakness (i.e., patients with BPH vs neurogenic bladder).

The post void residual (PVR) is a useful and simple diagnostic test which can also be performed on the patient suspected of having obstruction. The PVR is the volume of urine remaining in the bladder following completion of micturition. This is classically measured by placing a straight catheter in a patient's bladder after voiding, but can also be measured by sonography. The post void volume can assess severity in the initial workup of BPH and follow the progression of obstruction in a patient with known BPH. Any post void volume greater than 12 ml is considered abnormal whereas volumes greater than 50 ml are considered significant. Drawbacks to measuring PVR volumes are the lack of clearly defined cutoff points to guide therapy, a high variation in measurements when performed on the same patient, and the tests inability to clearly predict which patients will respond to surgery.

Finally, Pressure flow studies differentiate between those patients with obstruction and those patients with detrusor muscle weakness. These studies measure bladder pressure during voiding by introducing a transurethral measuring device and a transrectal device. The detrusor pressure, which is the difference between the intravesicular pressure and the intrarectal pressure, can be helpful in differentiating between bladder dysfunction and obstruction. Drawbacks to pressure flow studies include the discomfort of the tests themselves, and their inability to predict surgical outcomes or the need for surgery.

Other tests that are available but usually not indicated in uncomplicated cases of BPH are filling cystometry (CMG), urethrocystocopy, and imaging studies such as ultrasound and intravenous pyelograms. CMG measures the bladder capacity, compliance, and the presence of and the threshold of uninhibited detrusor muscle contractions. Urethrocystocopy is not recommended unless there is evidence of microscopic or gross hematuria. Finally, imaging studies are not part of the routine workup of patients with obstruction unless the patient has hematuria, recurrent urinary tract infections, renal insufficiency, or a history of renal stones.

Screening PSA for Prostate Cancer

As with all screening efforts, the goal in prostate cancer screening is to identify patients in early treatable stages of their disease in order to reduce mortality. Prostate cancer occurs primarily in the outer peripheral zone of the prostate and typically does not cause symptoms until it has grown outside its capsule, at which point it is very difficult to treat. For this reason, there have been many attempts to find markers to detect early treatable stages of the disease. Until the development of the prostate specific antigen (PSA), the only available test was the annual digital rectal examination, which has not proven to be a very sensitive screening tool.

The prostate specific antigen (PSA) is a protease produced by the prostatic epithelium and can be measured by immunoassay. PSA has been aggressively investigated for its potential as a screening device in prostate cancer and controversy surrounds its use in asymptomatic men. There are two central problems in the PSA controversy. The first problem is related to the test's lack of specificity. PSA is prostate specific and not prostate cancer specific and is therefore elevated in prostate cancer as well as in benign disorders such as prostatitis and BPH. Patients with PSA values in the normal range (0–4) typically need no further diagnostic workup while those with values in the high range (+10) typically need further diagnostic investigations such as biopsies. However, there are no clear guidelines for a large percentage of patients whose values lie within the intermediate range (4–10). The second problem in screening with PSA relates to recent studies that have been unable to demonstrate differences in mortality rates among screened populations who were treated versus not treated for early prostate cancer. These studies may suggest that a majority of organ confined prostate cancer identified during screening is slow growing and may never develop outside the organ, hence having no or minimal impact on mortality (1). At present, researchers do not clearly understand the natural history of prostate cancer and hence aggressive screening and therapy for organ confined prostate cancer cannot be recommended until more conclusive studies are performed. Currently, routine screening with an annual digital rectal examination is recommended for men over the age of 50. PSA remains controversial and there is no clear consensus on its utility in screening asymptomatic men. However, if the PSA is used, patients should first be made aware of the benefits and drawbacks associated with early detection and treatment.

Differential Diagnosis

The differential diagnoses for patients who present with difficulty voiding include BPH, prostate cancer, prostatitis, urinary tract infection, urethral stricture, neurogenic bladder, bladder cancer, and bladder calculi. Some of these diseases are discussed elsewhere in this book.

BENIGN PROSTATIC HYPERTROPHY

BPH is the most commonly encountered etiology of obstructive symptoms in men over the age of 50. Patients may present with both obstructive and irritative symptoms. The diagnosis is primarily a clinical one, based on history, a benign rectal examination, and initial laboratory evaluations.

Histologic proven BPH occurs in approximately 50% of men over the age of 50. By the age of 80, the prevalence reaches approximately 90%. However, it is important to note that the presence of microscopic BPH does not necessarily correlate with the symptoms of obstruction. For example, only a quarter of those with microscopic changes will eventually develop symptoms of BPH, and only one in four men above the age 80 will have required some form of treatment for symptomatic relief of obstruction.

The bulk of the patients who present with symptoms of obstruction are found to have uncomplicated BPH (i.e., no history of urinary tract infections (UTI), hematuria, or urinary retention). The Symptom Index, developed by the American Urological Association (AUA), is an accurate and inexpensive method that easily categorizes patients with obstruction secondary to BPH as having either mild (1–7), moderate (8–19), or severe symptoms (20 or more) (Table 19.7).

PROSTATE CANCER

Prostate cancer is the second most commonly diagnosed cancer among men in the U.S. In 1990, 30,000 men died from prostate cancer, making it the second most common fatal neoplasm in males and the leading cause of cancer death among men over the age of fifty-five. Ten to thirty percent of men between the ages of 50–60 and 50–70% of men above the age of 80 will have histologic evidence of prostate carcinoma. The prognosis is generally favorable when the disease is limited to the gland (stage A and B).

There are four basic stages of prostate cancer.

Stage A is clinically unsuspected prostate cancer, which is usually diagnosed after a TURP procedure for patients being treated for BPH. The cancer may be minimal or may diffusely involve the prostate. Once the diagnosis is made, further evaluation is needed with serum acid and alkaline phosphatase, PSA, and a bone scan. If these studies indicate

spread, the patient is excluded from stage A. Patients who remain within stage A are further subdivided into stage A1 and A2, depending on the grade and tumor mass. Patients with stage A1 are thought to be at little or no risk while patients with stage A2 are considered to be at similar risk to those with stage B.

Stage B cancer is localized to the prostate and is diagnosed either by history or digital rectal examination. Stage B is further subdivided into B1, in which only one lobe of the prostate is involved and stage B2, in which both lobes are involved.

Stage C is reserved for those cancers that have shown periprostatic spread but without evidence of metastases (normal acid and alkaline phosphatase) while stage D includes all cancers with evidence of distant metastases.

PROSTATITIS

Younger patients who present with perineal pain and low back pain are more likely to have one of the four prostatitis syndromes (acute bacterial, chronic bacterial, nonbacterial prostatitis, prostatodynia). Prostatitis occurs typically in men over the age of 18, with a mean age of forty-two. The symptoms of prostatitis are one of the most frequent reasons why male patients visit urologists and approximately 50% of all men will experience symptoms of prostatitis in their lives.

In acute bacterial prostatitis (ABP), there is classically an enlarged, boggy, tender prostate. The diagnosis is confirmed by positive urine culture. Patients suspected of acute bacterial prostatitis should not have prostatic massage, since it is painful and may induce bacteremia. The most common pathogens found in ABP are gram negative aerobes such as *Escherichia coli* and proteus, and gram positives such as *Staphylococcus aureus*. Chlamydia, ureaplasmas and mycoplasma are not thought to play a role in the etiology of ABP.

Chronic bacterial prostatitis (CBP) is a relatively rare cause of chronic prostatitis, accounting for less than 5% of cases. However, the diagnosis should be sought because it is treatable and there are sequela. As in ABP, it is important to isolate the pathogen when making the diagnosis of CBP. Pathogens can be isolated from cultures of prostatic secretions and urine. Bacterial growth in these cultures may be relatively low but all growth is considered significant. The most common pathogen implicated in CBP is *E. coli*.

Nonbacterial prostatitis (NBP) is the most common prostatitis syndrome. Although patients with

Table 19.7.
AUA Symptom Index

Questions to be Answered	AUA Symptom Score (Circle 1 number on each line)					
	Not at All	Less Than 1 Time in 5	Less Than Half the Time	About Half the Time	More Than Half the Time	Almost Always
1. Over the past month, how often have you had a sensation of not emptying your bladder completely after you finished urinating?	0	1	2	3	4	5
2. Over the past month, how often have you had to urinate again less than 2 hours after you finished urinating?	0	1	2	3	4	5
3. Over the past month, how often have you found you stopped and started again several times when you urinated?	0	1	2	3	4	5
4. Over the past month, how often have you found it difficult to postpone urination?	0	1	2	3	4	5
5. Over the past month, how often have you had a weak urinary stream?	0	1	2	3	4	5
6. Over the past month, how often have you had to push or strain to begin urination?	0	1	2	3	4	5
7. Over the past month, how many times did you most typically get up to urinate from the time you went to bed at night until the time you got up in the morning?	0 (None)	1 (1 time)	2 (2 times)	3 (3 times)	4 (4 times)	5 (5 times or more)

Sum of 7 circled numbers (AUA Symptom Score): _____

(From US Department of Health and Human Services, Public Health Service. Agency for Healthcare Policy and Research. Benign Prostatic Hypertrophy. Clinical Practice Guideline #8, 1992.)

NBP and CBP present with similar complaints, they differ in that NBP has no identifiable pathogen. However, the presence of white blood cells and fat laden macrophages is essential for the diagnosis. The etiology of NBP is unclear but several theories have been proposed, including anaerobic bacteria, fungi, autoimmune etiology or inflammation secondary to urinary reflux.

Patients with prostatodynia have symptoms of prostatitis but have no identifiable infectious etiology or history of urinary tract infections. Patients often complain of perineal pain, but have normal digital rectal examination, urine analysis, and prostatic fluid. The etiology of this disorder is unclear, but prostatodynia may result from intraprostatic and ejaculatory duct reflux.

FUNCTIONAL OBSTRUCTION

Older patients who take regular medications or who present with a history of chronic debilitating diseases may have a form of functional obstruction or worsening of mild anatomic obstruction. This is a diagnosis of exclusion.

Management

Treatment approaches vary depending upon the etiology of the patient's symptoms. Once the etiology of the symptoms has been determined, therapy should be guided accordingly.

BENIGN PROSTATIC HYPERTROPHY

The treatment of uncomplicated BPH depends on the severity of the symptoms and the patient's preference. Therefore, decisions are based not only on scientific evidence, but also on patient values. Because uncomplicated BPH is truly benign, the majority of decisions to be made in its management are "patient centered." In patient centered care, the provider acts as a source of information, allowing the patient to make the choices. The treatment of uncomplicated BPH depends upon the severity of the symptoms and the patient's preference. Therefore, decisions are based not only on scientific evidence but also on patient values. Quantification of symptoms by the Symptom Index helps to guide therapy and allows clinicians to follow the progress of symptoms more accurately. Patients with mild symptoms can be managed by simple "watchful waiting," i.e., following symptom scores and measuring PVRs. Patients with symptoms in the moderate range can be offered various medical and surgical options.

Medical therapies include alpha-adrenergic blockers and 5-alpha reductase inhibitors. Alpha-adrenergic blockers such as doxazosin (Cardura), prazosin (Minipress), and terazosin (Hytrin) inhibit alpha mediated contraction of the prostatic smooth muscle. High doses used in hypertension should be avoided in BPH since lower doses of these medications are equally effective among these patients, and higher doses merely increase their risk for side-effects such as orthostatic hypotension. 5-alpha reductase inhibitors (finesteride) have been recently developed as another therapeutic alternative for BPH. As mentioned earlier, testosterone is secreted by the testes and converted to its active form, 5-alpha dihydrotestosterone (5-HT), by the enzyme 5-alpha reductase which is present within the prostate. 5-HT is then capable of inducing hypertrophy within the prostate. Finesteride competes for 5-alpha reductase and, therefore, blocks the essential conversion of testosterone to its active form 5-HT at the organ site itself. The utility of finesteride was recently demonstrated in a large, double-blind placebo controlled study, where patients receiving finesteride demonstrated a significant decrease in prostate size, increase in urine flow rates, and mild changes in symptom scores as compared to those receiving placebo (2). Side effects of finesteride include decreased libido, which were experienced by approximately 3% of the study sample. The long-term benefits of finesteride are still unclear and are currently under investigation.

There are four surgical options available to the BPH patient: balloon dilatation, transurethral incision of the prostate (TUIP), transurethral resection of the prostate (TURP) and open prostatectomy. Surgery is indicated in patients with refractory urinary retention, recurrent urinary tract infections, recurrent gross hematuria, bladder stones, or renal insufficiency clearly due to BPH. However, surgery may also be considered for patients with moderate to severe AUA symptom scores who do not present with the above complications. Balloon dilatation is a transurethral procedure which compresses the prostrate and reduces obstruction without removing significant tissue. Although it has a very low side-effect profile, few outcome studies have been performed on this procedure, and those conducted indicate that benefits appear to diminish rapidly after therapy. Consequently, balloon dilatation cannot be currently recommended as an adequate treatment for BPH. Transurethral incision of the prostate (TUIP) is an endoscopic surgical procedure which is limited to patients with prostates less than 30 grams in size. This procedure entails passing an endoscope through the urethra and performing several incisions in the prostate to relieve the obstruction. TUIP has fewer side effects than the TURP. Transurethral resection of the prostate (TURP), also performed by passing an endoscope through the urethra, is a more invasive surgical procedure which removes the inner transitional zone of the prostate. It is indicated for patients with moderate to severe AUA symptom scores. Transurethral resection of the prostate which is performed to relieve the symptoms of severe obstruction is the second most commonly performed surgical procedure in the Medicare population, second only to cataract surgery. Open prostatectomy is the definitive surgical procedure since it removes the entire prostate thus eliminating any further risk for obstruction. However, it has the highest rate of side effects and is only indicated in very serious forms of obstruction. Table 19.8 summarizes the side effects and sequela of therapy for BPI).

PROSTATE CANCER

As indicated earlier, there is no clear consensus in the therapy of early stage organ confined prostate cancer because a large percentage of patients with early stage disease have a very good prognosis with-

Table 19.8.
Side Effects and Sequelae of Therapy for BPH

Therapy	Impotence (%)	Retrograde Ejaculation (%)
Alpha blockers	0	6
Finesteride	1–2	0
TUIP	11	25
TURP	13	73
Retropubic	16	77

TUIP = transurethral incision of the prostate; TURP = transurethral resection of the prostate. Percentages indicate mean probability. From the US Department of Health and Human Services Clinical Practice Guideline on Benign Prostatic Hypertrophy.

out treatment. Recent data from Scandinavia demonstrated that elderly men (ages 70–74) with low volume stage A1(T1) tumors who received no treatment had only a 6 percent disease specific mortality rate (3, 4). The majority of deaths in the Scandinavian study were in fact due to unrelated causes. Hence, there is little room for improvement in the mortality of patients with early stage prostate cancer. These facts underline the need for randomized trials comparing treatment with no treatment for these patients, without evidence of which, the radical treatment of early stage disease remains in an experimental phase.

Although there is no clear consensus on treatment, organ confined prostate cancer continues to be diagnosed using routine PSA screens on asymptomatic males, and TURPs performed on patients with BPH. Consequently, clinicians face difficult treatment decisions once patients are diagnosed. Based on a synthesis of current research, treatment recommendations are offered here to guide the clinician.

Stage A1. The recommended approach is surgery for younger patients with stage A1 and watchful waiting for patients over the age of 70, the latter because stage A1 has demonstrated an extremely slow progression in men over the age of 70. It is recommended that these patients instead be followed with occasional PSA values. Younger patients with early stage disease have a higher rate of progression because of the longer projected life span and, therefore, may benefit from definitive therapy. Regardless of the choice, central to the decision of treatment or no treatment are patient concerns and preferences.

Stage A2. Younger patients with higher grade or diffuse tumors should be offered definitive surgical therapy while older patients with concurrent life limiting disease can be offered external radiation therapy.

Stage B. Patients with stage B2 cancer can be offered definitive therapy with prostatectomy unless there are significant comorbid conditions or the patient is over the age of 75.

Stage C. Patients with stage C disease can be offered radiation therapy.

Stage D. Stage D disease is managed medically with androgen ablation therapy.

As discussed earlier, the prostate gland is sensitive to testosterone which stimulates growth. Medical therapy can reduce the symptoms of metastatic disease but has not demonstrated an ability to reduce mortality from prostate cancer. Although there is some controversy over whether to start therapy before or after symptoms begin, the current practice is to wait until symptoms begin. Both forms of therapy, surgical castration or medical castration, involve reduction in testosterone or its effect on prostatic tissue. The most commonly used medical therapy is the use of either estrogens or luteinizing hormone releasing hormone (LHRH) in combination with androgen-receptor antagonists. The principal effect of estrogens is the suppression of the release of luteinizing hormone (LH) from the pituitary, thereby reducing the secretion of testosterone. The LHRH agonists cause an acute increase in the release of LH and a rise in serum testosterone. However, chronic treatment with LHRH leads to a decrease in LH and eventually, a decrease in testosterone. Leuprolide was the original LHRH analogue studied and proven to be of benefit. Flutamide is a nonsteroidal anti-androgen that acts by inhibiting the binding testosterone.

Surgical castration, the alternative to medical anti-androgen therapy, has also been proven beneficial in the treatment of symptomatic stage D prostate cancer.

PROSTATITIS

Although therapy should be eventually directed at the identified pathogen, initial anti-bacterial therapy for acute bacterial prostatitis (ABP) is recommended before culture results are known. The most effective treatment, trimethoprim/sulfamethoxazole, should be to give two tablets b.i.d for 2 weeks unless culture results indicate resistance. Other suggested treatment options include clindamycin 150 to 300 mg every 6 hours and erythromycin 250 to 500 mg twice a day. For young sexually active males, chlamydia cultures and concurrent treatment with doxycycline may be indicated. The quinilones have not been effective therapy for ABP, possibly due to their poor penetration of the prostate. If fever and symptoms persist, the patient may have a prostatic abscess and further imaging studies such as a CT scan may be indicated.

Treatment of CBP consists of therapy with trimethoprim/sulfamethoxazole (Bactrim) two tablets twice a day for 1 month with repeat prostatic cultures performed after therapy has been completed. However, if cultures remain positive there is no evidence to support further treatment with antibiotics. For those patients whose cultures continue to be positive, prophylactic treatment with Bactrim one tablet at bedtime

may prevent or reduce symptoms and the number of urinary tract infections.

The treatment for NBP consists of a 2-week trial of antibiotic therapy with trimethoprim/sulfamethoxazole two tablets twice a day for 2 weeks. If there is no relief of symptoms, further urologic work up may be considered to rule out causes that could potentially mimic NBP, such as in situ bladder cancer. Although there is no clearly defined therapy, trimethoprim/sulfamethoxazole two tablets twice a day for 2 weeks is recommended for prostatodynia.

ILLUSTRATIVE CASES WITH SELF-ASSESSMENT QUESTIONS AND ANSWERS

Case 1

A 65-year-old man with no significant past medical history presents to your office. He complains that he gets up frequently in the middle of the night to urinate and has to wait for several seconds before he begins to urinate. He denies any history of urinary tract infections, hematuria, bladder or kidney stones, or previous urologic procedures. You perform a thorough physical examination, including a neurologic examination and prostate examination both of which appear normal.

QUESTION: *You suspect that he has BPH and want to investigate further. What test or tests should you order? (One or more answers may apply):*

a. SMA-7
b. PSA
c. Ultrasound
d. Biopsy
e. Post void residual
f. Urinalysis
g. All of the above

ANSWER: a, b, *and* **f.** *The initial evaluation of a patient suspected of having BPH should include a thorough history, physical, urinalysis, SMA-7, and a PSA. The PSA is optional and should be ordered with an understanding that many patients with pure BPH have abnormally elevated PSA values. Post void residual is an optional diagnostic test which may be performed and ultrasound is*

not indicated in patient with uncomplicated BPH. Your patient's initial workup is normal and you wish to initiate therapy.

QUESTION: *Which of the following studies will help you decide on which therapy to offer your patient? (One or more answers may apply).*

a. Filling cystometry
b. AUA symptom index
c. Patient preference
d. Flow cystometry
e. All of the above

ANSWER: b *and* **c.** *Treatment of BPH is "patient centered" and, therefore, the patient is the key to your treatment decisions. The AUA symptom index is now a standard part of the management of BPH. Depending on the Symptom index scores the patient can be offered various forms of therapy. Flow cystometry may be helpful in determining those patients who would benefit from surgery and is optional. Filling cystometry is not indicated in patients with uncomplicated BPH.*

Case 2

A 73-year-old man with a history of coronary artery disease and a MI which occurred approximately two years ago, comes to your office asking to be checked out for prostate cancer. He saw an advertisement in a magazine for a blood test for prostate cancer. He has no symptoms of obstruction and has a normal physical examination, including a normal rectal examination and urinalysis.

QUESTION: *Which of the following would you recommend?*

a. Annual DRE without a PSA
b. Annual DRE and PSA, with an understanding that if either are abnormal surgery would be indicated
c. Annual DRE and a PSA, with an understanding that surgery would not be an option if either were abnormal
d. Convince the patient there is no utility to performing either a DRE or a PSA.

ANSWER: a. *The patient presented is over the age of 70 and has a significant medical condition and would, therefore, be very unlikely to benefit from any definitive therapy for organ confined prostate cancer because of the slow growing nature of the disease. In addition, ordering PSA in this patient and possibly identifying a subclinical cancer would only create the perception in the patient's mind that he has a serious illness and would not benefit him in any way. This patient's age and history make the decision not to order a PSA an easy one. If the patient had been a healthy asymptomatic 60 year old man, it would be at the heart of the controversy over screening for prostate cancer. If patients insist on having their PSA values determined it must be done only after patients have received a complete understanding of the controversy regarding prostate screening.*

URETHRITIS AND GENITAL LESIONS

Urethritis and genital lesions are common symptoms encountered in patients with sexually transmitted diseases (STD). With the advent of the HIV virus, the prompt diagnosis, treatment, and prevention of STDs has become even more essential. This chapter will focus on the presentation, differential diagnoses, and treatment of male patients presenting with urethritis and genital lesions.

Sexually transmitted diseases (STD) are increasing at a dramatic rate among younger sexually active patients, particularly those living in the inner city. The incidence of STDs is approximately 12 million infections per year, with the total cost of treatment estimated at 3.5 billion dollars per year. One in four Americans will contract some form of STD in their lifetime.

Pathophysiologic Correlation

Urethritis and genital lesions are caused by various infectious agents that are transmitted from person to person, typically through sexual contact. Each infectious agent has a unique presentation causing a specific symptom complex. For example syphilis, a spirochete, causes an indolent infection which if left untreated may last for decades. Alternatively, gonorrhea, a gram negative diplococcus, has an abrupt onset and a typically discrete duration lasting six months when left untreated. Each organism causes infection when it invades the mucus membrane or skin of the patient, causing ulcers, vesicles, or purulent discharge.

Clinical and Laboratory Evaluation

With the exception of herpes, history and physical examination are not sufficient to diagnose urethritis or sexually transmitted disease. Laboratory confirmation is necessary. The history and physical examination of the infection can provide clues to diagnosis and help the clinician gauge the risks to the patient and his contacts.

HISTORY

It is critical to ascertain a thorough history, in particular, a sexual history, from patients complaining of urethritis or a genital lesion. Identifying patients who participate in high risk behaviors is especially important because therapy may have to be initiated prior to the confirmation of the diagnosis, i.e., presumptive treatment is often conducted before culture results are known.

Many clinicians are uncomfortable eliciting sexual histories from their patients and often miss opportunities for both therapeutic and educational interventions as well as opportunities for identifying patients at risk. Sexual history is best obtained by initially making open-ended, nonjudgmental statements (e.g., "to give you the best care possible I need to ask you some personal questions about your sexual history....") which allow patients the space to speak freely and create important opportunities to gather information that would have otherwise been missed. Open-ended statements can be followed by more specific questions to ensure that important aspects of the history have not been left out such as a history of multiple sexual partners, history of previous STDs, and having had a partner with an STD. Inquiries into sexual behavior should be gender neutral and should not assume a patient's sexual orientation. For example instead of asking if a patient has had sexual encounters with women, one should use the phrase sexual partners. An integral component of every sexual history is patient education about transmission of sexually transmitted diseases, including HIV.

The assessment of the patient with urethritis or genital lesions includes documenting the onset of genital symptoms, and the presence or absence of extragenital symptoms, systemic symptoms (fever, chills, nausea, and vomiting) as well as symptoms of tender lymphadenopathy. These symptoms may vary dramatically between patients, even amongst those infected with the same pathogen. For example, urethritis caused by gonorrhea may be associated with a purulent and persistent discharge, causing significant staining of the undergarments in one patient. In other patients, the discharge may be minimal and intermittent, present only during the early morning void. Depending on the pathogen, the discharge may be clear, white, yellow, brown, or green. Dysuria is a very common symptom.

Extra-genital manifestations also need to be fully investigated because patients may not relate them to their genital symptoms. Therefore, patients need to be questioned regarding any symptoms of discharge, rashes, or lesions located in the mouth, anorectum, or skin. Gonorrhea, for example, may disseminate in up to 20 to 30% of cases and involve the distal portions of the extremities, causing small pustules. It is also capable of infecting the oral mucosa where it may cause a purulent oral discharge.

Gonorrhea and chlamydia are the most common causes of urethritis in the United States, while ureaplasma, herpes simplex and trichomonas account for only a minority of cases. Chlamydia, Ureaplasma, herpes simplex and trichomonas are classified as nongonococcal urethritis (NGU). Patients with chlamydia typically present with mild to moderate symptoms of urethritis without discharge.

The presentations of different genital lesions may vary only slightly but can be differentiated clinically by focusing on several key characteristics such as a history of pain, the type of ulcer (multiple singular crusted, papular or pustular), and the presence of lymph nodes, either tender or nontender (Table 19.9). The most common causes of genital ulcers are herpes, syphilis, and chancroid, whereas lymphogranuloma venereum (LGV), and donovanosis occur in only a minority of cases in the U.S. Each of these have subtle differences in their clinical presentation. For example, herpes classically presents as multiple painful vesicles located on the shaft of the penis with tender inguinal lymph nodes. Primary syphilis on the other hand classically presents with a nontender singular lesion with or without lymphadenopathy. A history of travel may be of help in identifying those rare cases of chancroid and lymphogranuloma venereum, which are far more common in Africa and the Far East.

Physical Examination

Patients presenting with urethritis or a genital lesion should receive a detailed examination of the overlying skin, testes, penis, rectum, and all regional lymph nodes. It is recommended that patients be examined in the standing position with

Table 19.9.
Genital Lesions

Genital Lesion	Description	Nodes	Systemic Symptoms	Etiology
Herpes	Multiple painful vesicles	Bilateral	Present	Herpes
Syphilis	Nontender singular raised ulcer	Bilateral	None	T pallidum
Chancroid	Tender ragged edged papule	Unilateral painful	None	Hemophilus ducreyi
LGV	Small vesicular papule	Painful, matted large with fistulas groove sign	Present after lesion heals	C. trachomatis
Donovanosis	Painless indurated	Pseudo buboes	None	C. granulomatis
	Nodule progresses to heaped up ulcer	Weeping with crusty lesions		

the examiner seated. A strong examining lamp and magnifying lens are helpful in identifying lesions. The skin around the genital area should be thoroughly examined including retraction of the foreskin, the dorsum of the penis, the entire scrotum, and inspection of the hair follicles for co-infection with pubic lice. The inguinal nodes should be palpated while the patient is standing and noted for tenderness and size. The rectum should also be routinely examined in all patients, looking for any lesions, discharge, or rash.

LABORATORY EVALUATION

All patients suspected of having gonorrhea and or chlamydia should have urethral swabs taken. Gonorrhea is a gram-negative diplococcus, which needs to be plated and incubated immediately at 35 degrees C in an atmosphere containing 5–10% carbon dioxide. Chlamydia is an obligate intracellular parasite with a unique life cycle possessing both DNA and RNA, replicating via binary fission. Since it is difficult and expensive to grow in culture, most institutions use a relatively sensitive enzyme linked immunosorbent assay (ELISA) which is both less expensive and quicker than performing a culture.

Genital Lesions.   Diagnosis of genital lesions is frequently based on clinical presentation. Although several laboratory studies may be performed to help strengthen the clinical diagnosis, these tests are not mandatory for confirming the diagnosis. For example, while cultures for herpes and chancroid are considered the gold standard, they are rarely used to confirm the diagnosis since they are expensive and lack sensitivity. The Tzanck smear, performed by taking cells from the base of fresh vesicle and staining it with either Giemsa or Wright stain, is also helpful in identifying the classic multinucleated giant cells of herpes. However, this test is also not crucial for making the diagnosis, particularly since it lacks sensitivity. Gram stains of ulcer samples may also be performed to confirm the diagnosis of chancroid if the classic chains of gram negative streptobacilli can be identified. Finally, serum antibody titers are available to confirm the diagnosis of herpes but are also rarely used because they lack specificity and sensitivity.

Syphilis.   The clinical diagnosis of primary syphilis is confirmed by serologic testing first with a screening nontreponemal test such as the VDRL (Venereal Disease Research Laboratory) or the RPR (rapid plasma reagin). However, since the VDRL and the RPR can be very insensitive in the early stages of primary syphilis, it is wise to also send a treponemal test such as the FTA-ABS (fluorescent treponemal antibody absorption test) to confirm the diagnosis. Nontreponemal tests such as the VDRL are very useful screening tests for secondary and tertiary syphilis. However, they lack specificity and have a high rate of false positives in patients with collagen vascular disease, pregnancy, and acute viral illnesses. Therefore, a confirmatory treponemal test should always be performed in these cases to confirm the diagnosis of syphilis. Dark field microscopy can demonstrate treponemes in cell scrapings from the base and side of an ulcer. Finally, all patients with syphilis should be encouraged to be tested for HIV.

DIFFERENTIAL DIAGNOSIS

The differential of urethritis and of penile lesions is reviewed in this section. Only common etiologies are discussed. Remember if one STD is diagnosed, there is a good chance the patient has another.

GONORRHEA

Although the incidence of gonorrhea appears to be declining slightly, it still remains at epidemic proportions in certain populations, such as inner city teenagers. This continued epidemic is partly due to *N. gonorrhea's* high resistance rates to penicillin, secondary to penicillinase producing bacteria. Patients present with dysuria, with or without urethral discharge, a few days after intercourse. Gram stain of the discharge will show gram negative diplocci. In addition, while gonorrhea is a common cause of urethritis, it can also cause infections of the rectum, pharynx, and conjunctiva which may go unnoticed and untreated unless they concurrently occur with urethritis. Disseminated gonorrhea is characterized by pustular skin lesions on the extremities and arthralgia in one or more joints (most often the knee). Cultures of joint fluid or blood are positive less than half the time. Gram stain and culture of urethral discharge may clinch the diagnosis.

CHLAMYDIA

Recognized as the most common cause of STD in the 1980s, chlamydia continues to have high prevalence rates and is also the most common cause of urethritis in men. One of the reasons for chlamydia's high prevalence rates is related to the fact that many patients are asymptomatic carriers of *C. trachomatis* or only mildly symptomatic and often go untreated while continuing to spread the infection from partner to partner. Diagnosis is made by ELISA. A presumptive diagnosis can be made based on a gram stain of urethral discharge that shows polymorphonuclear leukocytes, but no bacteria.

OTHER CAUSES OF URETHRITIS

Ureaplasma, herpes simplex, and trichomonas account for only a minority of cases of urethritis. Their diagnoses should be pursued if treatment for gonorrhea or chlamydia fails.

HERPES

Herpes is currently the major cause of genital ulcers in the U.S. The classic presentation of herpes is multiple painful vesicles on the shaft of the penis. Typically, patients have tender lymphadenopathy and may have extragenital manifestations of fever, malaise, and anorexia. The patient is considered to have primary disease if it is his first lesion and there is no history of prior exposure to herpes. The majority of genital infections are caused by Herpes simplex virus type two. More than ninety percent of patients have recurrence by the end of the first year after the initial infection.

SYPHILIS

Syphilis is caused by the spirochete *T. pallidum*, which can be visualized by reflected light using dark field microscopy. The late 1980s and early 1990s saw a dramatic increase in the prevalence of syphilis. This rise was associated with certain epidemiologic factors such as inner city residence, drug abuse, and prostitution.

Syphilis presents in its early stage, primary syphilis, as a painless ulcer, called a chancre, which may go unnoticed. Patients may also develop bilateral nontender inguinal adenopathy. Secondary syphilis occurs approximately 3 to 6 weeks after the appearance of the chancre and is associated with a diffuse maculopapular rash notably on the palms, the soles of the feet, almost always involving the oral mucous membranes and the genitalia. Other symptoms associated with secondary syphilis are fatigue, malaise, generalized lymphadenopathy, and patchy alopecia. Latent syphilis is clinically silent and diagnosis is made only by serology. Latent syphilis is divided into "early latent" if diagnosed within a year of infection or "late latent" if diagnosed after a year following the initial infection. Tertiary or late syphilis may occur in up to one third of untreated patients. It may present with signs of cardiac involvement such as aortic insufficiency or as neurosyphilis which may include dementia or posterior

column disease resulting from tabes dorsalis. Diagnosis of primary syphilis is confirmed by darkfield microscopy or by VDRL and FTA positivity. The VDRL is nearly always positive in secondary syphilis. Latent and tertiary syphilis are diagnosed by VDRL and FTA tests.

CHANCROID

Although uncommon among residents of the United States, chancroid is a leading cause of genital ulcers in developing countries and has a high association with HIV transmission. Chancroid is caused by a gram negative rod *Hemophilus ducreyi*. Patients typically present with single or multiple painful ulcers located on the shaft of the penis, with jagged edges associated with painful inguinal adenopathy occurring in a majority of the cases. Clinical diagnosis is based on gram staining of ulcer specimens.

Management

Treatment should be instituted before culture results in all patients in whom there is a high index of suspicion, i.e., those who engage in high risk behaviors or who have clear symptoms. Equally crucial, the physician must arrange to inform and treat all sexual partners who may be involved. Patients suspected of having a sexually transmitted disease and who engage in high risk behavior should be counseled to the risk of HIV infection and possibly tested.

GONORRHEA

Recommended therapy for uncomplicated anogenital or pharyngeal gonococcal infection is ceftriaxone, 250 mg IM once. Ciprofloxacin 500 mg orally is an alternative therapy. Secondary infection with arthritis is treated on the inpatient setting. Patients are reminded to use a condom during intercourse for 2 weeks after treatment, as they may remain infected for that long.

CHLAMYDIA

The treatment for chlamydia is doxycycline 100 mg po twice a day for a total of 7 to 10 days. The current increase in the prevalence of chlamydia has not been due to antibiotic resistance but is instead related to the noncompliance, typical of young patients who receive the therapy. An alternative therapy, azithromycin in a single dose of 1 gram orally, has recently demonstrated a 98% eradication rate 4 weeks following therapy and has been approved by the Federal Drug Administration for the treatment of chlamydia (2).

OTHER CAUSES OF URETHRITIS

Standard treatment of all forms of urethritis entails treating both gonorrhea and chlamydia because 10 to 30% of heterosexual men and 40–60% of women with gonorrhea are infected with both organisms. The other forms of NGU are rarely cultured and only pursued if traditional therapy fails.

HERPES

Standard treatment for nonimmune compromised patients with herpes includes the use of either topical or oral acyclovir. The key to effective therapy is instituting treatment as soon as symptoms begin. The topical solution can be applied two times a day until the lesions begin to crust. Standard oral therapy is acyclovir 200 mg po five times a day for 7 to 10 days. Patients who suffer from frequent recurrences can be treated prophylactically with 200 mg two times a day for approximately 1 year. Special consideration should be given to patients with HIV and those on immunosuppressive therapy such as steroids and cyclophosphamide. These patients may benefit from more aggressive treatment and suppressive therapy.

SYPHILIS

Treatment for primary, secondary, and early latent syphilis consists of benzathine penicillin 2.4 million units I.M. times one (patients who are allergic to penicillin may be treated with doxycycline 100 mg po twice daily for 15 days). Latent syphilis is treated with an I.M. injection of 2.4 million units of penicillin given once weekly for 3 weeks. Doxycycline 100 mg twice daily is used for penicillin allergic patients. Neurosyphilis is treated with 12 to 24 million units of IV penicillin per day for 10 days. Follow up nontreponemal titers (VDRL) should be ordered 1 month and 6 months after therapy to assess the success of therapy. Nontreponemal titers should convert to normal several months after appropriate therapy while the treponemal test will remain positive.

CHANCROID

Treatment for chancroid consists of one IM injection with 250 mg of ceftriaxone. Erythromycin 500 mg po every 6 hours for 2weeks is the alternative choice for penicillin allergic patients.

ILLUSTRATIVE CASES WITH SELF-ASSESSMENT QUESTIONS AND ANSWERS

Case 1

A 27-year-old male comes to clinic complaining of burning on urination and intermittent discharge from his penis. He denies any significant past medical history, but does admit having intercourse with several sexual partners without the use of condoms. He has a history of one previous episode of gonorrhea for which he received treatment two years ago. His physical exam is completely normal including a normal genital exam and normal lymph nodes.

QUESTION: *Your initial work up and treatment for this patient should include which of the following?*

a. Urethral culture for gonorrhea
b. Urethral specimen for chlamydia assay
c. Treatment with ceftriaxone
d. Treatment with Azithromycin
e. Treatment of sexual partners
f. HIV counseling and testing
g. All of the above

ANSWER: g. *All of the above. Patients who are at high risk for sexually transmitted disease and who present with symptoms of urethritis consistent with either gonorrhea or chlamydia should be investigated and treated for both gonorrhea and chlamydia. The above patient has a history of practicing unsafe sex, a history of a STD and of dysuria and discharge, therefore presumptive therapy with both ceftriaxone for gonorrhea and azithromycin for chlamydia is indicated. It is also critical to treat all partners involved and counsel patients about HIV testing and safe sex.*

Case 2

A 19-year-old male comes to your office complaining of a painful lesion on the shaft of his penis which developed one day ago. The patient denies any history of previous genital infections but admits to having unprotected sex with his partner of 1 year. His partner has a history of recurrent genital herpes but has not had a genital sore for over 6 months. The patient states that the lesion is tender and that he just hasn't felt well over the past 2 to 3 days. His physical examination is significant for mild fever to 100.5 and small tender inguinal lymph nodes. On the shaft of his penis are several small 1-ml vesicles that are tender to touch. No other lesions or rash are noted.

QUESTION: *Your initial management should include which of the following? (you may choose more than one answer)*

a. Urethral swab for gonorrhea and chlamydia
b. Tzanck prep to investigate for herpes
c. Serum titers for herpes antibodies
d. Empiric therapy for Herpes simplex
e. Serum VDRL to test for syphilis
f. Empiric therapy for syphilis with I.M. PCN

ANSWER: d *and* **e.** *Herpes is fundamentally a clinical diagnosis. Based on this patient's exposure history and symptom complex he most likely is experiencing a primary infection with genital herpes. Serum antibodies and a Tzanck prep will be of little help in this situation. If they are positive they only confirm your clinical suspicion and if they are negative you will still treat on clinical grounds. Patients with primary infections may experience more serious systemic symptoms and their course may be shortened by therapy with acyclovir 200 mg five times a day. As this case demonstrates patients infected with genital herpes may shed the virus during the asymptomatic phase and infect their partners. Syphilis although unlikely in this case should be screened for, as in all sexually active patients suspected of having an STD.*

SEXUAL DYSFUNCTION IN MEN AND WOMEN

Sexuality is an integration of emotional, somatic, intellectual, and social aspects of an individual. It may involve intimacy with a partner, masturbation, integration of social or religious views, or conflict/definition of one's sexual identity and orientation. It is a skill that involves the complex performance of physical and emotional behaviors (1). In summary, sexuality is truly a biopsychosocial phenomenon.

Sexual problems are common. The prevalence of sexual dysfunction ranges from 20–63% in women and is about 40% in men (2). In one of the most cited prevalence studies, Frank and colleagues surveyed couples with a high degree of marital satisfaction and found that 63% of the women reported arousal or orgasmic dysfunction and 40% of the men reported erectile or ejaculatory dysfunction; and even a higher percentage (77% of the women and 50% of the men) reported "sexual difficulties" (3). Despite the frequency of sexual issues, practitioners rarely take sexual histories, as many are uncomfortable talking to their patients about sex or are not trained or experienced in the skills involved in sexual history taking. However, as demonstrated in one study in which clinic physicians were properly trained to take a screening sexual history, 53% of the patients reported a sexual problem or concern. Ninety-one percent of the patients said they considered questions about sexuality to be an appropriate part of the interview. In 50% of the encounters, physicians said they elicited medically relevant information and identified sexual problems (4). Thus this study demonstrates the importance and value of addressing sexual problems in the ambulatory setting.

Pathophysiologic Correlation

The human sexual response illustrated schematically in Figure 19.9 is governed by neurologic, vascular, and hormonal mechanisms. During arousal, arterial dilatation and genital vasocongestion is achieved via a local reflex pathway involving the pudendal sensory nerve fibers and parasympathetic fibers from S2-S4 ganglia and cortical influences initiated by psychic stimuli and mediated by T12-L1 parasympathetic and sympathetic fibers. Orgasm is achieved by skeletal muscle contractions via the pudendal nerve; autonomic (sympathetic) components play a role in men and probably in women. The subjective pleasurable sensation is purely cortical and psychic in nature. The genital blood supply is from the internal iliac arteries via the internal pudendal artery. Hormonal influences are predominantly those of the androgens, which in normal levels maintain sexual desire and function.

The human sexual response is best characterized by the four phases of the sexual response cycle: desire, excitement (arousal), orgasm, and resolution (Table 19.10). The ideal approach to sexual problems involves an analysis in terms of these phases. The classic sexual dysfunctions are described in Table 19.11. The sexual pain disorders include dyspareunia and vaginismus.

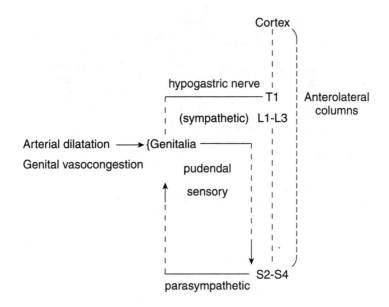

Figure 19.9. Functional anatomy of the sexual response.

Orgasm
  a. Emission: in men muscle contractions via sympathetic fibers. In women—? autonomic component.
  b. Skeletal muscle contractions via pudendal nerve: ejaculation in men
      rhythmic contractions of outer ⅓ vagina in women
Genital blood supply
  Internal iliac arteries to internal pudendal artery
Hormonal influences
  Androgens necessary to maintain sexual desire and function, levels within normal range adequate

The etiology of sexual dysfunction can be divided into "deep" and "immediate" causes. "Deep" causes include relationship difficulties, psychosexual conflicts, and job stress. "Immediate" causes are those reactions, feelings, and cognitions that impinge on sexual responsiveness such as performance anxiety or "spectatoring" (4).

The human sexual response is vulnerable to learned inhibition, which can occur if negative feelings become associated with sexual experiences. These negative feelings, called "negative contingencies," become the "immediate" causes which act as the final common pathway by which "deep" causes are translated into real sexual problems (4).

It is important to remember that sexual performance is a subjective experience with a wide variation in interpretation. While the classic sexual dysfunctions are less common, sexual problems and concerns are much more common. Individuals may have concerns about normalcy, adequacy, fantasy, timing, communication, knowledge or technique. Couples may have disparate needs or different attitudes or values. It is important in the ambulatory setting to develop an approach which incorporates an appreciation for this spectrum of sexual concerns, problems, and dysfunctions.

Clinical and Laboratory Evaluation

The sexual history, when accurately performed, can narrow the range of diagnostic possibilities. Physical examination must include the accessible sexual organs.

HISTORY

The sexual history is the most important aspect of the evaluation of sexual problems. One must become accustomed to incorporating sexual history taking into routine evaluations and to approaching sexual problems when they are brought up by the patient.

The standard techniques of data gathering should be applied with the following modifications. In introducing the sexual history, it is important

Table 19.10.
Sexual Response Cycle

Desire phase
  Fantasies or thoughts about sexual activity, and/or desire to have sexual activity.

Excitement phase
  A subjective sense of sexual pleasure with accompanying physiological changes related to pelvic vasoconstriction: erection in men and the lubrication-swelling response in women.

Orgasm phase
  A peaking of sexual pleasure associated with rhythmic contractions of the perineal muscles and pelvic organs and with emission and ejaculation in men.

Resolution phase
  A sense of physical relaxation and emotional well-being following orgasm. Men are refractory to further erection and orgasm for a variable period of time, whereas women are able to respond again almost immediately.

From Williams S. The sexual history. In: Lipkin M. The medical interview: clinical care, education, and research. Springer-Verlag, 1995:239.

Table 19.11.
Sexual Dysfunctions

Sexual desire disorders
  Hypoactive sexual desire disorder
  Sexual aversion disorder

Sexual arousal (excitement phase) disorders
  Female sexual arousal disorder (impairment of lubrication-swelling response)
  Male erectile disorder

Orgasm disorders
  Inhibited female orgasm
  Inhibited male orgasm (includes delayed ejaculation)
  Premature ejaculation

Sexual pain disorders
  Dyspareunia (genital pain in a man or woman before, during, or after sexual intercourse)
  Vaginismus (spasm of the vagina preventing intercourse)

Each disorder is further classified as either primary (being present since the patient became sexually active), or secondary (occurring after a period of normal sexual function).
From Williams S. The sexual history. In: Lipkin M. The medical interview: clinical care, education, and research. Springer-Verlag, 1995:244.

to explain the reasons for questions; for example, one might state: "I ask these questions of all my patients so that I might better understand their needs," or one might introduce the topic in the context of discussing risk factors. The open-ended approach may not be ideal initially; but rather patients may more easily volunteer information when asked specific questions about sexual function. For example, one might start with a question such as "do you use condoms when you have sexual intercourse?" Positive responses might then be followed up with more open-ended questions such as "can you tell me more about that?" The practitioner should model the level of explicitness with which he/she wishes the patient to answer. The closed to open-ended line of questioning and the use of specific language will help to overcome the barriers that usually interfere with accurate history taking (4).

The language used in the encounter should be clear and explicit. The practitioner should use language that puts the patient at ease and is appropriate to the patient's level of understanding and education. One should avoid both overmedicalization and forced informality, and euphemisms should be clarified. Language should be comfortable for the interviewer as well.

The practitioner should be careful to avoid assumptions about sexual activity, function, or orientation. It is preferable to ask directly about sexual orientation, i.e., "do you have sex with men, women, or both?" than to assume heterosexuality; as well, do not assume that elderly or disabled individuals are sexually inactive.

The sexual history can be introduced at several different points in the medical interview. When sexual problems are brought up by the patient, they should be discussed directly. Screening questions about sexual function may be introduced in the context of the social history when asking about the patient's relationships, as a part of HIV or other risk assessment, or as part of the GU or GYN review of systems. It is important not to assume that when a patient discusses a primary relationship, that this is his/her (only) sexual partner.

The discussion of sexuality in ambulatory settings should include an approach to screening for sexual problems and concerns (Tables 19.12, 19.13). Once a problem has been identified, one must obtain an accurate description of the problem. One useful approach is to use the phases of the sexual response cycle as a guide to questions. This history can be embellished by further questions about medical illness, psychologic factors, and the

Table 19.12.
Screening for Sexual Problems and Concerns

1. Are you sexually active?
2. Have you noticed any changes or problems in your sexual functioning lately?
3. If yes (to 1 or 2), proceed with specific questions as appropriate:
   a. *For men:*
      —Do you have any problems developing or maintaining an erection?
      —Do you have any trouble having an orgasm (ejaculating or "cumming": too soon, not soon enough, or in the wrong direction)?
   b. *For women:*
      —Do you have pain during intercourse?
      —Problems with lubrication or becoming excited?
      —Do you have difficulty having an orgasm?

From Williams S. The sexual history. In: Lipkin M. The medical interview: clinical care, education, and research. Springer-Verlag, 1995:237.

social context in which the problem developed. The practitioner should have an appreciation of issues relevant in different phases of the life cycle.

The practitioner should ask about medication use (prescribed and over the counter), drug and alcohol use, tobacco use, and psychiatric conditions such as depression, anxiety, and eating disorders. One should ask questions about symptoms of diabetes (polyuria, polydipsia, numbness in distal extremities), vascular disease (claudication), menstrual irregularities, and structural damage to the genitalia. History should be obtained regarding hypertension, cardiopulmonary disease, adrenal or thyroid disorder, pituitary disease, neurological conditions, and previous surgery.

Sexual problems are often complex and require simultaneous evaluation of all relevant factors. Patients may not be aware of the interplay of these often subtle factors or may not note temporally associated events with the onset of sexual problems. An effective history can help to uncover these associations.

Table 19.13.
Screening for Sexual Problems

—Has your illness (if applicable) affected your sexual functioning?
—What is your pattern of sexual activity (monogamy, serial monogamy, multiple or casual partners, etc.)?
—Do you have sex with men, with women, or with both?
—Do you have sex with people who are (or might be) in high risk groups (IV drug users, homosexual or bisexual men, prostitutes, unknown partners, etc.)?
—Are you using birth control? What type?
—If not for birth control, are you using condoms to prevent disease?
—Do you have any concerns about getting a sexual disease or AIDS?
—Do you have any other questions or concerns about sex?

From Williams S. The sexual history. In: Lipkin M. The medical interview: clinical care, education, and research. Springer-Verlag, 1995:237.

PHYSICAL EXAMINATION

As with any complex problem in ambulatory care, a thorough physical examination is indicated in the evaluation of sexual dysfunction. The practitioner should assess the general appearance of the patient, assessing the overall health as well as the patient's mood and grooming, which may offer clues to psychiatric disorders or social factors. Vital signs such as blood pressure and respiratory rate should be assessed for evidence of hypertension or other cardiopulmonary diseases. One should look for signs of endocrine disease, evaluating thyroid, adrenal, and pituitary function, as well as signs of diabetes and liver disease. Galactorrhea or visual field defects suggest hyperprolactinemia. Signs of peripheral vascular disease, such as peripheral pulses and skin changes, should be assessed. Neurologic function should be evaluated including detection of peripheral neuropathy and testing of sacral sensation, genital reflexes (anal, bulbocavernosus, cremasteric), and motor function (sphincter tone and perineal muscles). Men should be evaluated for signs of androgen deficiency such as gynecomastia, sparse body hair, and decreased beard growth. A testicular exam should be performed, looking for atrophy, hernia, or other structural problems. A penile exam for lesions or fibrosis (Peyronie's Disease) and a prostate exam for evidence of enlargement or infection should also be performed. In women, a pelvic exam will detect infection or structural problems that may be related to dyspareunia, such as atrophic vaginitis in post-menopausal women.

LABORATORY EVALUATION

The laboratory evaluation should include general screening for systemic disease (complete blood count, electrolytes, BUN, creatinine, lipids, liver function tests), a fasting blood sugar, prolactin level; and if indicated, TSH and free T4, LH, FSH, estradiol, and testosterone should be obtained. When infection is suspected, one should perform appropriate testing such as wet mount or KOH preparation of vaginal discharge, urinalysis and urine culture, chlamydia and gonorrhea cultures, and Tzank preparation for herpes simplex. Further evaluation should be performed for suspected or identified problems such as pelvic sonogram for suspected fibroid disease, pituitary imaging in the presence of hyperprolactinemia, and penile tumescence studies in men with suspected organic impotence.

Differential Diagnosis

Sexual problems should be approached with an appreciation for the multifactorial nature of their etiologies. This is particularly true in older patients with complex illnesses and complicated medication regimens. In younger patients the problem may be more clear-cut and amenable to an either/or approach, i.e., psychogenic or organic. However, the differential diagnosis of a more complex sexual problem is best understood in terms of its contributors.

DYSPAREUNIA

Dyspareunia is caused by organic factors in both sexes and in women is classified as superficial or deep (Table 19.14). Although causes are varied, pelvic examination will often provide the specific diagnosis. Infections and structural abnormalities are common causes. Atrophic vaginitis with loss of normal lubrication is common in post menopausal women.

VAGINISMUS

Vaginismus is synonymous with vaginal spasm. It is the result of a nonorganic, usually intrapsychic conflict, and may develop in the setting of early trauma. The history of spasm during intercourse suggests the diagnosis.

ORGANIC DISEASE

Organic problems affect all phases of the sexual response cycle. At least 50% of erectile dysfunction is primarily organic; thirty percent of surgical procedures result in temporary dyspareunia, and 30–40% of women seeking help for dyspareunia have pelvic pathology (5). Neurologic impairment can result from local structural damage, spinal cord injury, or from diseases affecting the peripheral nerves (diabetes, multiple sclerosis). Vascular dam-

Table 19.14.
Organic Factors That May Affect Sexual Function: Women Only

Dyspareunia
  Superficial
    Atrophic vaginitis
    Bartholins gland inflammation
    Clitoral phimosis
    Episiotomy scar
    Glomus tumor
    Human papilloma virus infection
    Imperforate/tender/rigid hymen
    Infections—chlamydia, herpes, candida albicans, trichomonas, bacterial vaginosis
    Irritants—contraceptives, douches
    S/P radiation
    Vulvar vestibulitis
  Deep
    Adhesions (surgical)
    Cervical cancer
    Ectopic pregnancy
    Endometriosis
    Fibroid uterus
    Hemorrhoids
    Infections—cervicitis, pelvic inflammatory disease
    Intrauterine device complications
    Ovarian cysts, tumors
    Pelvic tumors
    Posthysterectomy scarring
    Retroverted uterus
    Uterine prolapse

Miscellaneous
  Cystitis
  Cystocoele
  Rectocoele
  Urethritis

age can also occur locally and in large and small arterial vessel disease; vascular mechanisms are probably more important than neurologic in diabetics with impaired sexual function. Androgen deficiency, caused by panhypopituitarism, adrenalectomy, oophorectomy, or castration and liver disease in men, can significantly affect libido. Hyperprolactinemia can impair desire, arousal, and orgasm. Estrogen deficiency may lead to decreased vaginal blood flow and cause atrophic vaginitis; hyper and hypothyroidism can also contribute to sexual dysfunction. Pregnancy may interfere with sexual desire. In men, Peyronie's disease (fibrous plaque formation in the tunica albuginea layer of the penis) may contribute to dysfunction. Prostatectomy, diabetic neuropathy, and anticholinergic medications may lead to retrograde ejaculation; in this condition the ejaculatory fluid travels backward into the bladder, and the man may experience a diminished pleasurable sensation during orgasm. Structural abnormalities of the genitalia can be caused by factors such as surgery, radiation, scarring, infection, and congenital disorders. Organic causes also include endstage cardiopulmonary, renal or hepatic disease. (See Tables 19.14, 19.15, and 19.16) for a complete list of organic factors).

DRUGS

Drugs may affect sexual function by interfering with adrenergic function, by causing CNS depression or sedation, by their anticholinergic or antihistaminic effects, and by various other mechanisms. Common agents associated with sexual dysfunction include all classes of antidepressants, antihypertensives (i.e., beta blockers and centrally acting agents), cimetidine, L-dopa, spironolactone, benzodiazepines, and antipsychotics. Substances of abuse may interfere with sexual performance; alcohol and marijuana are associated with decreased libido and with erectile difficulty, and heroin users may experience difficulties in all response cycle phases. Tobacco use may affect the vascular system.

Table 19.15.
Organic Factors That May Affect Sexual Function: Men Only

Dyspareunia
  Abnormal penile anatomy
    Peyronie's Disease
  Penile skin infections
  Prostatic infections
  Testicular disease (orchitis, epididymitis, tumor, trauma)
  Urethral infections (gonorrhea, nonspecific)

Hypogonadal androgen—deficient states
  Klinefelter's, orchitis, hyperprolactinemia, testicular tumor, castration

Mechanical problems
  Hernia
  Hydrocoele

Surgical procedures
  Bowel resection
  Lumbar sympathectomy
  Prostatectomy

From Schmidt CW. Sexual disorders. In Barker LR, Burton RB, Zieve PD. Ambulatory medicine. 3rd ed. Baltimore: Williams & Wilkins; 1991.

Table 19.16.
Organic Factors That May Affect Sexual Function: Both Sexes

Angina pectoris, recent myocardial infarction
Chronic systemic disease—anemia, uremia, cirrhosis
Chronic obstructive pulmonary disease
Chronic pain
Degenerative arthritis
Disc disease of lumbosacral spine
Sickle cell disease
Diabetes
Hyperlipidemia
Hypertension

Endocrine disorders
  Hypo and hyperthyroidism
  Addison's Disease
  Cushing's Disease
  Hypopituitarism
  Hyperprolactinemia

Neurologic disorders
  Multiple sclerosis
  Peripheral neuropathy (alcoholic, diabetic)
  Cord lesions: low and high
  Temporal or cortical lobe lesions
  Neuromuscular disease
  Neurogenic bladder

Vascular disease
  Large artery vessel (Leriche Syndrome)
  Small artery vessel (Pelvic vascular insufficiency)
  Venous insufficiency

Pelvic fracture
Radical pelvic or urologic surgery
Pelvic radiation

Modified from Schmidt CW. Sexual disorders. In Barker LR, Burton RB, Zieve PD. Ambulatory medicine. 3rd ed. Baltimore: Williams & Wilkins; 1991:175.

PSYCHOSOCIAL CAUSES

Medical illnesses that do not have a direct effect on sexual function but that have symbolic implications may have a detrimental effect on sexuality. After a mastectomy, hysterectomy, myocardial infarction, or stroke, an individual may experience shame, guilt, diminished self esteem, or fear; all of which may impair sexual function. Systemic disease may impair function even without direct sexual organ involvement; examples include cardiopulmonary diseases, musculoskeletal deformities, and debilitating illnesses such as cancer, anemia, and uremia. Disabled individuals may have issues affecting sexual function such as poor self-image, neurologic impairments, other physical problems, and social

Table 19.17.
Screening for Organic Dysfunction

	Psychogenic	Organic
Onset	Usually abrupt	Usually gradual decline
Course	Selective, intermittent, episodic, or transient	Usually persistent, often progressive
Degree of Impairment	Partial: may respond to strong erotic stimulation, change of partner or of situation	Absolute, except in early stages
Nocturnal or Morning Erection	Generally present	Generally absent, or reduced in frequency and intensity
Associated Features	Onset temporally related to specific psychosocial stress(es)	Onset temporally related to symptoms of organic disease

Modified from Schmidt CW. Sexual disorders. In Barker LR, Burton RB, Zieve PD. Ambulatory medicine. 3rd ed. Baltimore: Williams & Wilkins; 1991:179.

concerns such as institutionalization and lack of privacy.

Even when an organic cause is identified, there are often complicating psychological factors; other sexual problems are primarily psychogenic in origin. Psychological factors which may impact on sexual function include depression, anxiety, diminished self-esteem, frustration, guilt, anger, infertility, conflict over sexual orientation, as well as strong internalized religious prohibition, strict upbringing, or a history of physical or sexual abuse. Psychiatric disorders such as major depression, anorexia nervosa and bulimia, and psychosis may present with sexual dysfunction. See Table 19.17 for hints on how to differentiate psychological from organic causes

Social factors can play a role in sexual dysfunction. Relationship issues, child rearing, and environmental factors such as time, job stress, or lack of privacy are important contributors. Homosexual men and lesbian women may be stigmatized in society, as well as suffer the consequences of internalized "homophobia." The AIDS epidemic has had an enormous impact on the sexual desires and behaviors of many individuals.

Management

As most problems do not have a singular etiology, a sensible approach is to evaluate for organic and psychogenic contributors and simultaneously address those that are amenable to intervention. For example, an HIV positive patient may have difficulties with sexual function as a result of overall debilitation, structural lesions such as genital herpes, depression and low self-esteem as a result of the diagnosis, and interpersonal issues that are a consequence of the nature of HIV transmission. An approach might include medical therapy and nutritional support, psychologic counseling, and education about transmission and safer sex.

Practitioners can address a substantial segment of sexual problems in the ambulatory setting. Some of the discomfort practitioners may have with approaching such problems may be related to their own thoughts, feelings, and values about sexuality. It is important that these reactions be understood and managed so that they do not interfere with the therapeutic relationship. It is useful to use a matter-of-fact, practical style in negotiating with the patient a plan for evaluation and treatment.

The role of the practitioner is to provide medical evaluation, education, counseling, medications, simple interventions, and referral, if appropriate. Treatment of contributing medical problems or symptoms can be extremely helpful, such as giving estrogen creme to treat the dyspareunia associated with atrophic vaginitis and testosterone injections to hypogonadal men; the pharmacologic agent yohimbine is now being used for male erectile dysfunction. Bromocryptine may improve sexual function in patients with hyperprolactinemia.

Open discussion of concerns can be therapeutic in resolving a minor or temporary problem, as can reassurance about adequacy or about the normalcy of aspects of sexuality. Education about HIV risk reduction, birth control, and condom and lubricant use can be helpful, as can technical advice and behavioral prescriptions. Some examples are the use of vibrators, Kegel exercises, and masturbation for anorgasmic women, "stop-start" exercises or squeeze technique for premature ejaculation, and suggestions about variation in the traditional "missionary" position in the setting of physical impairment. "Sensate focus" exercises are helpful for all categories of sexual dysfunction.

Supportive counseling may be helpful for working through emotional issues, for stress-related problems, or those with recent disfiguring surgery such as a hysterectomy or mastectomy. Vaginismus may be treated with desensitization or in vivo progressive dilator therapy. Men with organic (neurologic or vascular) impotence may be referred for urologic evaluation and possibly for erectile devices and penile implants.

Referral for psychiatric care or sex therapy is indicated when interventions such as those described are not helpful, when marital or family therapy is indicated, when psychiatric disease is present, or when history of past sexual trauma is identified.

ILLUSTRATIVE CASES WITH SELF-ASSESSMENT QUESTIONS AND ANSWERS

Case 1

A 25-year-old female comes to your office complaining of intermittent post-coital vaginal pain and tenderness for the past 2 months. She states she has had the problem since having sex with her new partner of 2 months. She claims his sex organ is "too big" for her; he assures her that all she needs to do is relax. The patient cannot enjoy sex because she is worried about the post-coital pain she experiences. Physical examination reveals superficial lacerations at 6 o'clock and 10 o'clock on the labia minora and is otherwise normal.

QUESTION: *What recommendations would you make?*

ANSWER: *The patient should be educated about the human sexual response and the importance of foreplay in promoting adequate arousal (lubrication-swelling response), which may alleviate some of the pain she experiences during intercourse. Lubricants should be suggested, and authoritative reassurance should be employed. If these interventions are unsuccessful, dilators may be considered.*

Case 2

A 56-year-old male with a past medical history significant for mild hypertension controlled by diet visits you in your office to have his blood pressure checked. The patient reveals upon further questioning that he not quite feeling himself and that he and his wife have not been able to have intercourse for the past month. He states that he doesn't have any interest in sex anymore. He is concerned that maybe his blood pressure has affected him and maybe he should be on some form of therapy. Upon further questioning the patient reveals that his feeling of decreased desire has been gradually worsening over the past 5 to 6 months. Over the past 2 weeks, he has been unable to maintain an erection even when directly stimulated. He denies any changes or difficulties in his relationship with his wife. They both appear very happy, and there do not appear to be any new stressors in his life. The patient has no history of neurologic disease, diabetes, heart disease, peripheral vascular disease, hyperlipidemia, or surgery. His physical reveals normal blood pressure, normal secondary sexual characteristics, normal genital and neurologic examination.

QUESTION: *What should the initial work-up and management of this patient include? (you may choose more than one answer)*

a. Nocturnal-penile tumescence testing
b. Thyroid function tests
c. Serum testosterone level
d. Psychiatric evaluation
e. Prolactin level
f. GU consult for possible prosthesis
g. CT scan of the head
h. Physical exam of peripheral vascular system

ANSWER: b, c, e, *and* **h.** *The patient presents with progressive decline in sexual desire and somewhat more sudden difficulty with arousal. It is possible this patient has an organic cause of his impotence, although psychogenic contributors may be exacerbating the problem. One would need to inquire further about social factors,* *such as job stress and the marital relationship. It is important, however, to begin the initial evaluation of organic causes of impotence, which includes physical examination for signs of peripheral vascular disease and prolactin, testosterone, and thyroid levels. If warranted, penile tumescence studies may be performed as a later step.*

REFERENCES

Female Voiding Problems

1. NIH Consensus Conference Urinary incontinence in adults. JAMA 1989;261:2685.
2. Jewett MAS, Fernie GR, Holliday PJ, et al. Urinary dysfunction in a geriatric long-term care population: prevalence and patterns. J Am Geriatr Soc 1981;29:211–214.
3. Long term care facility improvement study. U.S. Department of Health, Education, and Welfare, Office of Nursing Home Affairs. Washington, DC, Public Health Service, publication no. 588459, 1975.
4. Burgio LD, Jones LT, Butler F, et.al The prevalence of geriatric behavior problems in an urban nursing home. J Gerontol Nurs 1988;14:31.
5. Brazda JF, Washington report. Nation's Health. March 1983:3.
6. Bhatia NN, Bergman A. A pessary test in women with urinary incontinence. Obstet Gynecol 1985;65(2):220–226.
7. Resnick NM. Urinary incontinence in the elderly. Med Grand Rounds 1984;3:281–290.
8. Resnick NM. Voiding dysfunction in the elderly. In: Yalla SV, McGuire EJ, Elbadawi A, Blaivas JG, eds. Neurology and Urodynamics: principles and Practice. New York: Macmillan, 1988:303–330.
9. Resnick NM, Paillard M. Natural history of nosocomial urinary incontinence. International Continence Society Proceedings 1984;471–472.
10. Blaivas JG, Sinha HP, Zayed AAH, et al. Detrusor-external sphincter dyssynergia. J Urol 1981;125:542–544.
11. Wein A, Van Arsdalen KN. Nonsurgical management of neuropathic voiding dysfunction. Semin Urol 1985;3:216–237.
12. Mundy AR, Stephenson TP, Wein AJ. Urodynamics. New York: Longman (Churchill Livingstone), 1984:31.
13. Anserason K, Ek A, Hedlund H, et al. Effects of prazosin on isolated human urethra and in patients with lower motor neuron lesions. Invest Urol 1981;19:39–42.
14. Badlani GH, Smith AD. Pharmacotherapy of voiding dysfunction in the elderly Semin Urol 1987;5(2):120–125.
15. Bennett CJ, Diokno AC. Clean intermittent self-catheterization in the elderly. Urology 1984;24(1):43–45.
16. Low AI, Donovan WD. The use and mechanism of anal sphincter stretch in the reflex bladder. Br J Urol 1981;53:430–432.
17. Hilton P, Stanton SL. The use of intravaginal estrogen cream in genuine stress incontinence. Br J Obstet Gynaecol 1983;90(10):940–944.
18. Bergman A, Bhatia NN. Pessary test: a simple prognostic test in women with stress urinary incontinence. Urology 1984;24(1):109–110.
19. Baum NH, Suarez GM. The use of the diaphragm in the management of stress incontinence. Presented at the Southeastern section of Am Urological Assn. New Orleans: 1987.
20. Burgio K, Whitehead W, Engel B. Urinary incontinence in the elderly. Ann Intern Med 1985;103:507–515.

Male Voiding Problems

1. Thompson I. Observation alone in the management of localized Prostate cancer: the natural history of untreated disease. Urology 1994;43:41–46.
2. Gormley G, Stoner E, Bruskewitz RC, et al. The effect of finesteride in patients with benign prostatic hyperplasia. N Engl J Med 1992;327:1185–1191.
3. Johansson J, Adami H, Anderson S, et al. High ten year survival rate in patients with untreated prostate cancer. JAMA 1992;267:2191–2196.
4. Johansson J. Watchful waiting for early stage prostate cancer. Urology 1994;43(2):138–142.

Urethritis and Genital Lesions

1. Romanowski B, Sutherland R, Fick GH, et al. Serologic response to treatment of infectious syphilis. Ann Intern Med 1991;114:1005–1009.
2. Stamm WE. Azithromycin in the treatment of uncomplicated genital chlamydia infections. Am J Med 1992;91:3a-19s-3A-22S.

Sexual Dysfunction in Men and Women

1. Cheadle MJ. The screening sexual history. Clin Geriatr Med 1991;7:937.
2. Spector IP, Carey MP. Incidence and prevalence of the sexual dysfunctions: a critical review of the empirical literature. Arch Sexual Behavior 1990;19:389–407.
3. Frank E, Anderson C, Rubinstein D. Frequency of sexual dysfunction in normal couples. N Engl J Med 1993;299:111–115.
4. Williams S. The sexual history. In: Lipkin M. The Medical interview: clinical care, education, and research. Springer-Verlag. 1995:235–250.
5. Halverson JG, Metz ME. Sexual dysfunction, part I: classification, etiology, and pathogenesis. JABFP 1992;5:51–61.

SUGGESTED READINGS

Female Voiding Problems

Badlani GH, Smith AD. Pharmacotherapy of voiding dysfunction in the elderly. Semin Urol 1987;5(2):120–125.

Resnick NM, Yalla SV. Management of urinary incontinence in the elderly. N Engl J Med 1985;313:800–805.

Resnick NM, Yalla SV, Laurino E. The pathophysiology
of urinary incontinence among institutionalized elderly
patients. N Engl J Med 1989;320:1–7.

Male Voiding Problems

Barker LR, ed. Principles of ambulatory medicine:3rd ed.
Baltimore: Williams & Wilkins, 1990.

de la Rosette JJ, Hubregtse MR, Mueleman EH, Stolk-
Engelaar MVM, Debruyne FM. Diagnosis of 409 patients
with   prostatitis   syndrome.   Urology   1993;
41(4):301–307.

U.S. Department of Health and Human Services. Benign
prostatic hyperplasia guideline panel. Benign prostatic
hyperplasia: diagnosis and treatment. Clinical Practice
Guideline Number 8. February 1994.

Williams RD. Radical prostatectomy for early stage cancer of the prostate. Urology 1994;43(2):135–137.

Urethritis and Genital Lesions

Barker L, ed. Principles of Ambulatory Medicine. 3rd ed
Baltimore: Williams & Wilkins, 1990.

Hook EW, Marra CM. Acquired syphilis in adults (review
article). N Engl J Med 1992;326:16.

Kassler WJ, Cates W. The epidemiology and the prevention of sexually transmitted diseases. Urol Clin North
Am 1992;19:1–12.

Mandel GL, Bennett JE, Dolin R. Principles and Practice
of Infecious Diseases. 4th ed. New York: Churchhill Livingstone, 1995.

Reese R, ed. A practical approach to infectious diseases.
3rd ed. Boston: Little, Brown and Company; 1991.

Sexual Dysfunction in Men and Women

Halverson JG, Metz ME. Sexual Dysfunction part II:
diagnosis,   management,   and   prognosis.   JABFP
1992;5:177–192.

Kligman EW. Office evaluation of sexual function and
complaints. Clin Geriatric Med 1991;7(1):15–39.

Sadock V. Normal human sexuality and sexual disorders.
In: Kaplan HI, Sadock BJ, eds. Comprehensive textbook
of psychiatry. Baltimore, MD: Williams & Wilkins, 1991.

Stine CC, Collins M. Male sexual dysfunction. In: Primary care clinics. 1989;16:1031–1056.

chapter 20

GYNECOLOGY

Angela Astuto, Peggy P. Chou, Daisy Otero, Margaret Smirnoff

VAGINAL DISCHARGE

One of the most common reasons women see a health care provider is because of a gynecologic symptom such as vaginal discharge. Vaginal discharge is usually associated with other symptoms including pruritus, lower abdominal discomfort, dysuria and dyspareunia. This constellation of symptoms is known as vaginitis.

Pathophysiologic Correlation

Although the vagina is teeming with microorganisms, it is resistant to infection. Normal lubrication of the mucosa and maintenance of an acidic pH by lactobacillus and other bacteria help prevent mucosal invasion by bacteria, fungi, and protozoans. Changes in hormone levels, destruction of beneficial bacteria, and malfunction of the immune system predispose to infection. Some organisms that cause vaginitis have special characteristics that allow them to invade the mucosa.

Clinical and Laboratory Evaluation

Most cases of vaginitis can be presumptively diagnosed by a focused history and examination. Simple office microscopy confirms the diagnosis. Correct technique for pelvic examination and sample collection is reviewed in this section.

HISTORY

The evaluation of a patient with vaginal discharge begins with a thorough medical history. The patient should be specifically questioned about duration of symptoms, previous episodes, past treatments and response to those treatments. Ask for a description of the discharge including color, consistency and odor. A sexual history should be obtained with inquiry into recent change in partner. Obtain a complete list of the patient's medications.

PHYSICAL EXAMINATION

A complete physical examination should be performed including a pelvic examination which begins with inspection of the external genitalia. Observe the mons pubis, labia majora, and perineum for any abnormalities such as ulcerations, rashes, or erythema (Fig. 20.1). Separate the labia and observe the labia minora, clitoris, urethral orifice, and introitus (vaginal opening) for redness, swelling or discharge. To examine the cervix and vagina, a speculum is necessary. After lubricating the speculum with warm water, insert it into the vagina obliquely with a downward direction. Next, turn the speculum horizontally and open the blades. Visualize the cervix and note its appearance as well as any evidence of discharge or bleeding. Tighten the thumb screw on the speculum to keep the speculum open while collecting the pap smear. Collect one specimen using the wooden cervical scraper. Place the long end of the scraper into the cervical os and turn it in a circle. This will collect a specimen from the outer portion of the cervix. Smear a glass slide with the scraper and then spray the slide with a fixative. Collect a second specimen by using a brush or a cotton applicator. Place the applicator in the cervical os and turn it in a circle. This will collect a specimen from the inner portion of the cervix in the endocervical canal. Again, smear a glass slide with the applicator and spray it with a fixative (Fig. 20.2). While visualizing the cervix, collect specimens for evaluation of the presence of *Neisseria gonorrhoeae* and *Chlamydia trachomatis* with an applicator from a prepared culture system. Use a cotton applicator to swab vaginal secretions for further examination at a later time. Untighten the thumb screw on the speculum and remove it while observing the vagina. Now perform a bimanual examination in order to palpate the cervix, uterus and ovaries (Fig. 20.3). Insert the index and

443

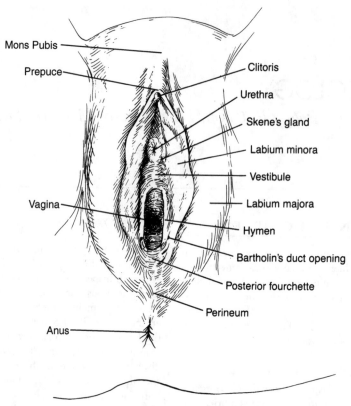

Figure 20.1. External Female Genitalia (From Burnett LS. Anatomy. In: Jones HW III, Wentz AC, Burnett LS, eds. Novak's textbook of gynecology. 11th ed. Baltimore: Williams & Wilkins, 1988:57.)

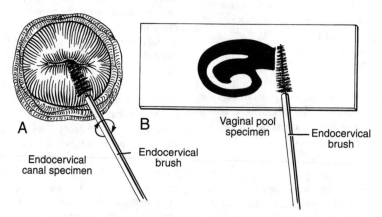

Figure 20.2. Collecting a Pap Smear. (A) Obtaining endocervical portion of Pap smear. (B) Strong specimen before fixation within 10 sec. (From Beckmann CRB, Ling FW, Barzansky BM, Bates GW, Herbert WNP, Laube DW, Smith RP. Obstetrics and Gynecology. 2nd ed. Baltimore: Williams & Wilkins, 1995:14.)

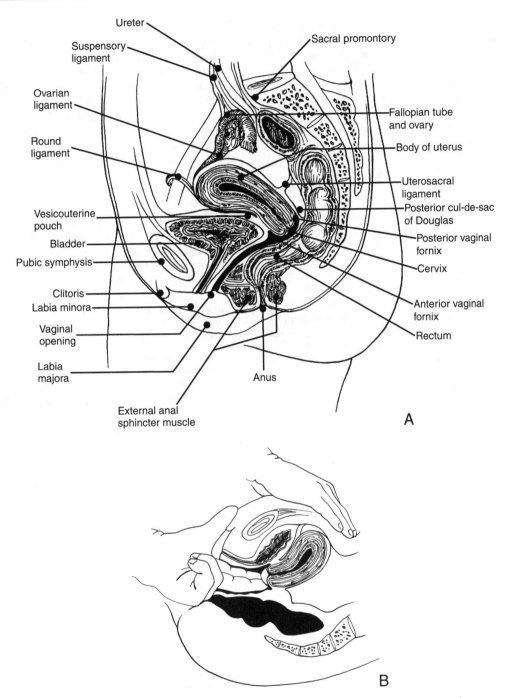

Figure 20.3. Internal female genitalia. (A) Midsagittal view of pelvic viscera and perineum. (B) Bimanual examination of the uterus and adnexa. (From Beckmann CRB, Ling FW, Barzansky BM, Bates GW, Herbert WNP, Laube DW, Smith RP. Obstetrics and Gynecology. 2nd ed. Baltimore: Williams & Wilkins. 1995:39, 14.)

middle fingers of one hand into the vagina after lubricating them with a water soluble lubricant. Note any abnormalities in the vagina then palpate the cervix. Examine it for shape, tenderness and mobility. Place the other hand on the patient's abdomen halfway between the umbilicus and the pubic symphysis. Try to palpate the uterus by pressing down with the abdominal hand and lifting the cervix upward with the pelvic hand. The uterus should be palpable between the two hands. Note its size, mobility, and the presence of tenderness or masses. Move the pelvic hand into the right lateral fornix which is the area on the right side of the cervix and move the abdominal hand onto the right lower quadrant. Try to palpate the adnexal structures by pressing down with the abdominal hand and moving the adnexa to the pelvic hand. Do the same on the left. It may be difficult to examine the adnexa in obese or poorly relaxed patients. If possible, note the size, shape and mobility of the adnexal structures as well as the presence of tenderness. Remove the pelvic hand, lubricate the fingers again and place the index finger in the vagina and middle finger into the rectum. This allows examination of the area behind the cervix and the recto vaginal wall. Remove fingers and then perform a rectal examination.

LABORATORY EVALUATION

Specimens collected after swabbing the vagina can now be examined. A sample of vaginal secretions from the swab can be diluted in a few drops of normal saline and examined under the microscope. Microscopy also allows for the identification of vaginal epithelial cells and the vaginal flora which are normally present. Normal vaginal flora appears as a moderate amount of rod-shaped organisms. Microscopy also allows for the observation of some of the possible causes of vaginal discharge including trichomonads, yeast, and the organisms responsible for bacterial vaginosis (Fig. 20.4). A specimen of vaginal secretions should be examined microscopically after addition of 10% KOH. The presence of a fishy odor after addition of 10% KOH is known as a positive whiff test and is found in association with some causes of vaginal discharge. The pH of vaginal secretions should also be determined by placing pH paper into the secretions.

Differential Diagnosis

About 90% of cases of vaginitis are classified as vulvovaginal candidiasis, trichomoniasis, or bacterial vaginosis. Bacterial vaginosis is the most common cause of vaginal infection, followed by vulvovaginal candidiasis and then by trichomoniasis (l). The remainder of cases are associated with a number of less frequent causes (Table 20.1).

BACTERIAL VAGINOSIS

Bacterial vaginosis is found as the cause of vaginal infection in 40–50% of cases. It affects women of reproductive age, pregnant, and nonpregnant equally. The incidence varies depending on the population studied; it is highest in patients attending sexually transmitted disease clinics and lowest in asymptomatic college students. Risk factors for infection are unclear. Bacterial vaginosis is more common in those patients over the age of 25 years, those patients with associated chlamydia infection or gonorrhea and those patients using a barrier method of contraception. Intrauterine devices are found more commonly in women with bacterial vaginosis. It is still controversial as to whether bacterial vaginosis is sexually transmitted.

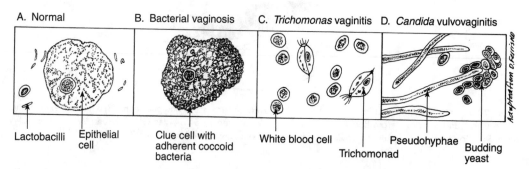

A. Normal   B. Bacterial vaginosis   C. *Trichomonas* vaginitis   D. *Candida* vulvovaginitis

Lactobacilli   Epithelial cell   Clue cell with adherent coccoid bacteria   White blood cell   Trichomonad   Pseudohyphae   Budding yeast

Figure 20.4. Microsopic examination of vaginal flora. (A) Normal vaginal flora. (B) Bacterial vaginosis. (C) Trichomonas vaginitis. (D) Candida vulvovaginitis. (From Beckmann CRB, Ling FW, Barzansky BM, Bates GW, Herbert WNP, Laube DW, Smith RP. Obstetrics and Gynecology. 2nd ed. Baltimore: Williams & Wilkins. 1995:99.)

Bacterial vaginosis is caused by the loss of the normal vaginal flora made up of lactobacilli and the overgrowth of anaerobic flora including *Gardnerella vaginalis*, Bacteroides species, and genital mycoplasmas. The reason for this overgrowth is unknown. However, no one species of bacteria is the cause for bacterial vaginosis.

Patients with bacterial vaginosis complain of foul smelling vaginal discharge especially noticeable after intercourse. There may be mild vulvar itching. It must be remembered, however, that up to half of those women with bacterial vaginosis will be asymptomatic. Physical examination usually reveals only a gray-white discharge that may be found on the labia, near the introitus, and adherent to the vaginal wall. Because signs and symptoms can be subtle, diagnosis is based on the presence of at least three of four criteria. These criteria are an adherent homogenous vaginal discharge, vaginal pH greater than 4.7, positive whiff test or amine odor test and the presence of clue cells. Vaginal pH can be determined by dipping pH paper into the discharge on the speculum. The whiff test or amine odor test is performed by adding 10% KOH to the vaginal discharge. The test is positive when a fishy odor is noted. The presence of clue cells can be determined by the microscopic examination of vaginal discharge diluted with normal saline. Clue cells are vaginal epithelial cells with an unclear cell border and granular appearance. Their appearance is secondary to the attachment of *Gardnerella vaginalis* and other bacteria to their surface. Further microscopic examination of vaginal discharge from a patient with bacterial vaginosis will demonstrate a lack of white blood cells and a bacterial flora consisting of mostly coccobacillary organisms instead of the usual rodlike organisms (See Fig. 20.4)

VULVOVAGINAL CANDIDIASIS

Following bacterial vaginosis, the next most common type of vaginitis is vulvovaginal candidiasis. The exact incidence is unknown since it is a nonreportable disease. However, approximately 13 million prescriptions were written in 1990 for products to treat candidiasis in the United States (2). About 75% of women of child-bearing age will have one episode of vulvovaginal candidiasis; 40–50% of these women will have a second episode. Approximately 5% of women will continue to have recurrent episodes of vaginitis.

Candida can be found in the genital tract of about 20% of asymptomatic women of reproductive age. About 85–90% of the yeast found in the vagina is *Candida albicans*. This candida originates from the perianal area. Candida can exist in the vagina either as a pathogen or as a commensal organism. What causes candida to become a pathogen is unclear. Several factors have been associated with increased asymptomatic vaginal colonization and/or vaginitis. These factors include pregnancy, diabetes mellitus, certain contraceptives, antibiotic and steroid therapy, HIV infection, and the use of tight synthetic underclothing. Pregnancy is presumed to cause increased vaginal colonization and vaginitis due to the high levels of reproductive hormones including estrogen. During the third trimester of pregnancy, the chance of developing vaginitis is greatest. Recurrence of symptomatic infection is more common after treatment throughout pregnancy. Diabetic women are more commonly colonized with candida and diabetic women with uncontrolled glucoses more commonly develop vaginitis. Among contraceptives, the IUD, the sponge, the diaphragm, and high-dose estrogen oral contraceptives are associated with increased rates of colonization with candida. Antibiotics especially the broad spectrum agents such as ampicillin and the cephalosporins are also associated with increased rates of vaginal colonization as well as symptomatic vaginitis. This effect is thought to be secondary to the disruption of the usual vaginal flora, which may be protective. The exact mechanism by which asymptomatic vaginal colonization is transformed into symptomatic vaginitis is unknown. It is evident that symptomatic vaginitis develops in the presence of factors that enhance candidal virulence or when local defense mechanisms are altered.

Women with vulvovaginal candidiasis present with complaints of vulvar itching and vaginal discharge. The discharge classically is described as cottage cheese-like although it can vary. It is not foul smelling. Vaginal soreness, dyspareunia, and dysuria may also be present. Symptoms are usually worse in the week before menstruation and improve with the beginning of menstruation. Physical examination reveals redness and swelling of the labia and vulva. A discrete rash, which is erythematous, with small, round, raised macular lesions involving the vulva and possibly the inguinal and perianal areas may be present. The vagina is also erythematous and is covered with a white discharge. The cervix is usually normal. Microscopic examination of vaginal secretions diluted with normal saline should be performed. This wet mount preparation allows for the identification of yeast and the possible identification of other causes of vaginal dis-

Table 20.1.
Causes of Vaginitis

	Symptoms	Signs	Treatment
Bacterial vaginosis	Foul smelling vaginal discharge, vulvar	Adherent vaginal discharge, pH 4.7, positive whiff test, presence of clue cells	See text for details
Candidiasis	White cottage cheese-like discharge, vulvar itching, dysuria, dyspareunia	Redness, swelling of labia and vulva, erythematous vagina with white discharge, yeast may be seen on wet mount or 10% KOH prep	See text for details
Trichomoniasis	Foul smelling, yellow-green discharge, vulvar itching, dysuria, dyspareunia	Vaginal erythema, strawberry cervix, trichomonads seen on wet prep, pH 4.5, positive whiff test	See text for details
Atrophic vaginitis	Blood-tinged vaginal discharge, vaginal dryness, urinary incontinence, dyspareunia, most common in women lacking estrogen—especially post-menopausal women	Thin, shiny skin with loss of fat and hair on vulva, pale vaginal mucosa with decreased folds and petechial hemorrhages, wet prep shows many WBC's and immature epithelial cells	Topical estrogen ½-1 applicator before bed for 1-2 weeks and then as needed, can also use oral estrogens if topical therapy not possible
Herpetic vaginitis	Fever, malaise, myalgias, vaginal discharge, itching, erythema and pain, dysuria, genital lesions	Genital lesions are erythematous vesicles or pustules found over labia majora, labia minora and mons pubis, cervical involvement occurs as well with resultant discharge	Primary genital herpes (infection without presence of antibodies to the herpes simplex virus) is treated with Acyclovir 200 mg 5 times a day for 10 days. Recurrent genital herpes (infection by the same virus as in the past) can be treated with Acyclovir if begun early, can also use Acyclovir as suppressive therapy in those with 6 episodes a year, 400 mg 2-3 times a day or 200 mg 3-5 times a day.

Condition	Symptoms	Signs	Treatment
Irritant and allergic vaginitis	Irritant vaginitis is associated with immediate erythema, edema, burning and itching, symptoms decrease without re-exposure, repeated exposure leads to chronic dermatitis, it is usually due to irritants in soaps, skin care products, tissues, etc. Allergic reactions develop later and last longer	Vulvar erythema and edema	Acute treatment involves elimination of irritants and allergens, soaks and baths can be useful, chronic dermatitis can be treated with topical corticosteroids such as hydrocortisone cream or ointment 1%.
Lichen simplex chronicus	Vulvar itching	Thickened, dry skin with excoriations on vulva	Determination of underlying cause, may be secondary to any condition which causes itching such as candidiasis, tinea, exposure to irritants and allergens. Treat the underlying cause. Can also use topical corticosteroids to control symptoms.
Vulvar vestibulitis	Dyspareunia, vulvar pain and burning	Severe pain is present upon vaginal entry at the time of exam and when cotton applicator is touched to the walls of the vestibule	This condition represents an inflammatory reaction of the vestibule and the area around the hymen and inferior to the urethra. Origin of reaction is unclear, may be some relation to human papilloma virus infection. Treatment is difficult and directed to relief of symptoms. Moisturizers are suggested as well as topical lidocaine. Surgical excision of the affected area or laser ablation may be necessary in order to control pain.
Foreign body	Vaginal discharge	Foreign body visible on exam	Removal of foreign body. Can use antibiotic cream if bacterial overgrowth has occurred.

449

charge. Large numbers of white cells should not be present (See Fig. 20.4). Vaginal secretions should also be examined after the addition of 10% KOH. The KOH disrupts cellular material allowing for easier visualization of the yeast. The vaginal pH should be normal. Finding a pH greater than 4.7 or large numbers of white cells or the presence of clue cells points to a mixed infection. Vaginal cultures are not routinely performed, but are reserved for those cases in which microscopic examination is negative but symptoms and signs are consistent with candidiasis.

TRICHOMONIASIS

The third most common cause of vaginitis is infection with *Trichomonas vaginalis*. Trichomonas is responsible for about 2.5 to 3 million cases of vaginitis a year in the United States. Trichomonal infection is acquired sexually. Therefore, its prevalence is higher in those populations at risk for sexually transmitted diseases. Risk factors for infection include a history of sexually transmitted disease, current infection with *Neisseria gonorrhoeae*, and the use of contraceptives other than barrier contraceptives or oral contraceptives. Transmission rates of infection are higher in women than men; a greater percentage of women contract the infection after exposure than men. Trichomonas will still be found, however, in 30–40% of male partners of infected women. The percentage of men infected appears to decrease with time indicating the infection may be more easily cleared in men.

Trichomonas is a anaerobic protozoan with several flagella which provide motility. It attaches to the epithelial cells of mucous membranes and destroys the cell through an as yet undetermined mechanism. It does provoke an inflammatory response involving neutrophils which are responsible for most of the body's defense against trichomonas.

One of the most common complaints of women with trichomoniasis is profuse vaginal discharge. In only about 10% of women, however, the classically described foul-smelling, frothy, yellow-green discharge is present. Other complaints include pruritus, dyspareunia, dysuria, and rarely lower abdominal pain. Symptoms may develop during or just after menstruation. On physical examination, vaginal erythema is usually present. Occasionally, a "strawberry cervix" can be seen. This term is used to describe the appearance of the cervix because of the small hemorrhages on its surface. This finding is more easily seen with colposcopy. Microscopic examination of the vaginal secretions in normal saline should demonstrate trichomonads. This wet prep examination will also show many polymorphonuclear cells and an absence of clue cells. Vaginal pH is greater than 4.5 in most cases. The whiff test may be positive in about half the patients.

Management

Once the cause of a vaginal discharge is identified, treatment can begin. The treatment regimens vary for bacterial vaginosis, vulvovaginal candidiasis, and trichomoniasis.

BACTERIAL VAGINOSIS

The recommended treatment for symptomatic women with bacterial vaginosis is metronidazole; the usual regimen is either 500 mg orally twice a day for 7 days or 2 g orally as a single dose. Overall cure rates are 95% for the 7-day regimen and 84% for the single dose regimen. Common side effects include gastrointestinal upset and metallic taste in the mouth. Patients given metronidazole should be warned not to drink alcohol because of the potential for a disulfiram-like reaction in which patients develop severe nausea, vomiting and abdominal pain after alcohol ingestion. Other alternative regimens include clindamycin 300 mg orally twice a day for 7 days, clindamycin cream 2%, one application intravaginally at bedtime for 7 days, and metronidazole gel 0.75%, one applicator intra vaginally twice a day for 5 days. Clindamycin is a useful alternative for patients who are allergic to metronidazole or cannot tolerate it and patients who have failed metronidazole therapy. Current guidelines from the Centers for Disease Control do not recommend treatment of sexual partners (5). Treatment for those with HIV infection is the same as those who do not have HIV infection. In pregnancy, clindamycin cream is the treatment of choice during the first trimester since metronidazole is potentially teratogenic. During the second and third trimester, oral clindamycin or metronidazole may be used, but clindamycin cream or metronidazole gel is preferable. Current Centers for Disease Control guidelines do not recommend treatment of asymptomatic women, pregnant or nonpregnant (7). However, bacterial vaginosis has been associated with pelvic inflammatory disease and endometritis following endometrial biopsy, hysterectomy, and other invasive procedures. For these reasons, the Centers for Disease Control recommend treatment of all women with bacterial vaginosis before surgical abortion procedures (4). At this time, it is unclear if treatment before other invasive procedures will decrease post-procedure morbidity. Bacterial vaginosis has also been associated with preterm labor, preterm delivery, and premature rupture of the membranes as well as postpartum endometritis. It is also unclear whether the benefit of treating asymptomatic pregnant women will outweigh the risks associated with treatment.

VULVOVAGINAL CANDIDIASIS

Vulvovaginal candidiasis can be treated with any one of several available antifungal agents. These agents are available as creams, vaginal tablets, and vaginal suppositories. The choice of specific product should depend on patient preference. Antifungal agents are broadly divided into two groups; the polyene derivatives (nystatin) and the azole derivatives (most other available agents). The Centers for Disease Control advise the use of azole agents because of a higher cure rate. The recommended regimens for treatment can be found in Table 20.2 (8). Single dose treatment should only be used for uncomplicated cases of candidiasis. Over the counter preparations of miconazole (Monistat) and clotrimazole (Mycelex and Gyne-Lotrimin) are available and are recommended for women who have recurrence of identical symptoms more than

Table 20.2.
Recommended Treatment for Vulvovaginal Candidiasis

Medications	Treatment Regimen
Clotrimazole	1% cream 5 g intravaginally for 7–14 days, or 100 mg vaginal tablet for 7 days, or 100 mg vaginal tablet, 2 tablets for 3 days, or 500 mg vaginal tablet as a single application
Miconazole	2% cream 5 g intravaginally for 7 days, or 200 mg vaginal suppository for 3 days, or 100 mg vaginal suppository for 7 days
Butoco-nazole	2% cream 5 g intravaginally for 3 days
Tioconazole	6.5% ointment 5 g intravaginally as a single application
Terconazole	0.4% cream 5 g intravaginally for 7 days, or 0.8% cream 5 g intravaginally for 3 days, or 80 mg suppository for 3 days

2 months after initial treatment. Oral antifungal agents have also been used to treat candidiasis. Although only fluconazole has been approved by the Food and Drug Administration for this use, other effective regimens include ketoconazole 400 mg once a day for 5 days, itraconazole 200 mg once a day for 3 days or 400 mg as a single dose and fluconazole 150 mg as a single dose (9). These drugs can be associated with significant side effects. Ketoconazole can cause gastrointestinal upset and hepatotoxicity in about one of every 15,000 women treated. Itraconazole and fluconazole are associated with similar, but less frequent side effects. Pregnant patients should only be treated with topical therapy. Clotrimazole, miconazole, terconazole and butoconazole have been found to be the most effective. Vulvovaginal candidiasis is difficult to treat during pregnancy and is associated with a slower response to therapy and with more recurrences after therapy. For these reasons, 7 days of treatment should be given. The potential for harm to the fetus during the first trimester of pregnancy must be kept in mind before treating the mother. Because candidiasis is not sexually transmitted, there is no need to treat sexual partners.

Management of recurrent vulvovaginal candidiasis demands special attention. It is defined as three or more episodes of candidiasis in a year. The exact pathogenesis of recurrent candidiasis is unclear. Its treatment should begin with confirmation of the diagnosis through vaginal culture. The next step involves the search for predisposing factors such as uncontrolled diabetes, the use of steroids or other immunosuppressive agents and the use of estrogens. Recurrent vaginal candidiasis has been associated with HIV infection, therefore, HIV testing should be performed in those women at risk. In most cases, a predisposing factor cannot be found. These women require long-term suppressive therapy. The recommended therapy is ketoconazole 100 mg daily by mouth for 6 months. Cessation of maintenance therapy is associated with a recurrence of symptoms in up to 50% of women. Alternative regimens under study include therapy with the other oral agents, fluconazole and itraconazole and intravaginal therapy with clotrimazole weekly. Those patients with HIV infection and recurrent candidiasis should be treated in the same way as those who do not have HIV infection.

TRICHOMONIASIS

All patients found to have trichomoniasis either symptomatic or asymptomatic, should be treated.

Their sexual partners should be treated concurrently. The recommended regimen is metronidazole 2g orally as a single dose or metronidazole 500 mg orally twice a day for 7 days (10). Patients who do not respond to either of these regimens are retreated with the 7-day regimen. Resistance of the trichomonads to metronidazole is possible and nonresponders should be treated with an increased dosage and/or an increased duration of treatment. Metronidazole gel is not effective treatment alone. Since there are no effective alternatives to metronidazole, the treatment of pregnant patients is difficult. During the first trimester, patients may be treated with clotrimazole cream intra vaginally for six days with some efficacy. Pregnant women can then be treated after the first trimester with metronidazole. Asymptomatic women might benefit from screening and treatment for trichomonas especially pregnant women who are at high risk for poor outcomes and women who have invasive gynecologic procedures. These women may benefit because of the association of trichomonas with preterm labor, premature rupture of the membranes, low birth weight, and upper reproductive tract infections after gynecologic surgery.

ILLUSTRATIVE CASES WITH SELF-ASSESSMENT QUESTIONS AND ANSWERS

Case 1

A 35 year-old woman with a history of non-insulin dependent diabetes mellitus complains of three days of white vaginal discharge with severe itching. She also complains of dysuria. She is sexually active and uses a diaphragm for contraception.

The pelvic examination of this patient reveals an erythematous macular rash on the vulva and in the inguinal area as well as labial swelling. Further examination demonstrates an erythematous vagina with white discharge and a normal cervix. Microscopic examination of the discharge diluted in normal saline shows yeast. The vaginal pH is normal.

QUESTION: *What is the most likely explanation for the patient's symptoms and findings?*

a. Trichomoniasis
b. Bacterial vaginosis
c. Vulvovaginal candidiasis

ANSWER: c. *Of the three most common causes of vaginal discharge, only vulvovaginal candidiasis is associated with an erythematous vagina, white vaginal discharge, normal cervix and these microscopic findings.*

QUESTION: *How should the patient be treated?*

a. Miconazole 100 mg vaginal suppository nightly for 7 days

b. Clotrimazole 100 mg vaginal tablet nightly for 7 days
c. Metronidazole 500 mg twice daily for 7 days

ANSWER: b *or* **c.** *The patient can be treated with either miconazole or clotrimazole as well as several other antifungal agents. Metronidazole is the appropriate treatment for bacterial vaginosis and trichomoniasis.*

PELVIC PAIN

Several organs lie in or near the pelvis. The uterus and adnexa, the bladder, the prostate, the intestine, and the pelvic nerves, bones and muscles can be responsible for pain. This chapter will focus on the uterine and tubovarian causes of pelvic pain.

Pathophysiologic Correlation

In the female reproductive tract, infection or inflammation, bleeding, or the effects of estrogens and progestins may cause pain. Prostaglandins and other vasoactive substances appear to have a role in menstrual cramps. Intrapelvic bleeding may cause symptoms due to the irritant nature of the components of the blood. The uterus, fallopian tubes, and ovaries can be affected. The lumenal surface of the uterus, the endometrium, or the muscular myometrium are the common sites of pain, as is the cervix, the opening of the uterus into the vagina.

Clinical and Laboratory Evaluation

The causes of acute pelvic pain are numerous. Not only can gynecologic disease result in pelvic pain, but gastrointestinal, urologic and infectious diseases may also result in pain (Table 20.3). Pelvic pain may also be chronic; that is, it has been present for at least 6 months. Chronic pelvic pain may also result from a number of different diseases and, therefore, presents some of the most difficult diagnostic and treatment dilemmas. The cause of pelvic pain, either acute or chronic, can be determined after a careful history and physical examination are performed as well as necessary supplemental laboratory tests.

HISTORY

A thorough history should include further questions about the location, quality, and duration of the pain. The presence or absence of associated

Table 20.3.
Causes of Acute Pelvic Pain

Diagnosis	Symptoms
Abortion (spontaneous)	Bilateral, crampy pain with vaginal bleeding and positive pregnancy test
Cervicitis	Pain is accompanied by vaginal discharge
Torsion of adnexa	Acute, crampy pain with right and left lower quadrant tenderness on exam
Pelvic inflammatory disease	See text for further details
Tuboovarian abscess	Similar to pelvic inflammatory disease
Ectopic pregnancy	See text for further details
Rupture of follicle or corpus luteum cyst	Sudden, severe pelvic pain
Endometriosis	See test for further details
Degenerating ovarian tumor	Acute onset of pain
Appendicitis	Right lower quadrant pain with nausea, vomiting, anorexia, fever
Diverticulitis	Left lower quadrant pain in older age group
Cystitis	Pain is accompanied by dysuria and suprapubic tenderness on exam
Renal calculus	Flank pain radiating to lower abdomen
Musculoskeletal disorders	Includes low back sprain and strain

symptoms such as fever, chills, anorexia, nausea, vomiting, or diarrhea must be determined. Also ask about the presence or absence of vaginal bleeding or vaginal discharge. As when evaluating a vaginal discharge, a sexual history should be obtained.

PHYSICAL EXAMINATION

Perform a complete physical examination while paying special attention to the abdominal examination. Inspect the abdomen for rashes, or scars indicating past surgery. Next, listen for bowel sounds. Determine liver and spleen size by percussion. Palpate the abdomen for areas of tenderness and for masses. Assess for the presence of rebound tenderness. Keep in mind that certain signs are consistent with specific diseases (See Table 20.3). For example, the patient with appendicitis classically presents initially as periumbilical pain which then localizes to the right lower quadrant. The physical examination should also include a pelvic examination with a Pap smear if it was not done within the last year and cultures for *Neisseria gonorrhoeae* and *Chlamydia trachomatis*. A rectal examination should be performed as well.

LABORATORY EVALUATION

A complete blood count, chemistry examination and pregnancy test should be sent on all women with pelvic pain. Examine a urine sample for white blood cells and/or bacteria. If a vaginal discharge is present, it should be examined microscopically after the addition of normal saline and after the addition of 10% KOH. A whiff test should be performed and the vaginal pH should be determined. Further diagnostic studies such as x-ray, an ultrasound or a CT scan may be necessary to determine the cause of the pain.

Differential Diagnosis

The differential diagnoses of pelvic pain are extensive. The more common gynecologic causes of pelvic pain are pelvic inflammatory disease, dysmenorrhea, endometriosis, uterine myoma, and ectopic pregnancy. These will be discussed in the following paragraphs.

PELVIC INFLAMMATORY DISEASE

Pelvic inflammatory disease is certainly a common cause of acute pelvic pain affecting more than one million women a year and costing about four billion dollars a year in the United States. The term refers to an infection of the upper genital tract including the endometrium, the fallopian tubes, the ovaries, the uterine wall, and the pelvic peritoneum. Risk factors for this infection are young age, multiple sexual partners, use of an IUD, residence in an area with a high prevalence of sexually transmitted diseases, and frequent vaginal douching. A history of pelvic inflammatory disease is a risk factor for repeat infection. Seventy-five percent of cases of pelvic inflammatory disease occur in women under the age of 25. It can be prevented by the use of barrier methods of contraception including condoms, diaphragms, and spermicides. The use of oral contraceptives has been associated with a decreased incidence of pelvic inflammatory disease.

Pelvic inflammatory disease begins most commonly as an infection of the cervix and vagina that ascends to involve the upper genital tract. It is usually a polymicrobial infection. The bacteria found are *Neisseria gonorrhoeae, Chlamydia trachomatis*, vaginal aerobic and anaerobic flora such as nonhemolytic Streptococcus, *Escherichia coli*, group B streptococcus, Bacteroides species, Peptostreptococcus, and peptococcus and genital Mycoplasma species. The two most important organisms are *N. gonorrhoeae* and *C. trachomatis*, and they are found together in 25–40% of infections. Infection with *N. gonorrhoeae* is associated with a severe inflammatory reaction in the fallopian tubes. This inflammation leads to destruction of the cells of the tubes and subsequent narrowing of the tubes. It has been estimated that 15% of women with cervical infection secondary to *N. gonorrhoeae* will go on to develop pelvic inflammatory disease. Infection with *C. trachomatis*, on the other hand, produces a milder inflammatory reaction. The organism can then remain in the fallopian tubes for months after initial exposure. Its presence results in chronic asymptomatic inflammation, which damages the tubes and leads to infertility and ectopic pregnancy.

Pelvic inflammatory disease has a wide spectrum of presentations from mild asymptomatic infection to life-threatening infection. The most frequent symptoms are abdominal and pelvic pain. The pain is usually bilateral, constant, and worsened by sexual activity or motion. It has been present for less than 7 days in most cases. Because there is an associated cervical infection in about 75% of patients, a vaginal discharge is present. Abnormal uterine bleeding, dysuria, nausea, vomiting, and fever may also be present. Gonococcal infections are noted to have a more abrupt onset a few days after the beginning of menstruation. Chlamydial infection, however, has a slow onset with less pain and fever.

Examination of women with pelvic inflammatory disease reveals lower abdominal tenderness upon palpation at times associated with rebound tenderness. There also is tenderness of the adnexa and cervical motion tenderness. An adnexal fullness may be palpated representing either an abscess or edema. An increased white blood cell count, elevated erythrocyte sedimentation rate, and elevated C-reactive protein can be present. In cases in which the diagnosis of pelvic inflammatory disease is not clear, further studies are obtained. Laparoscopy is the most accurate diagnostic test. It allows visualization of the pelvic organs. Culdocentesis, which is the removal of peritoneal fluid from the cul-de-sac by needle aspiration can also be helpful. The finding of an increased white blood cell count in the peritoneal fluid points to infection. Sonography is helpful in evaluating the presence of an adnexal mass.

DYSMENORRHEA

Dysmenorrhea can be simply defined as pelvic pain occurring at the time of menstruation. The pain is usually described as cramping. It may be accompanied by sweating, increased heart rate, nausea, vomiting, diarrhea, and headaches. Dysmenorrhea is usually divided into primary and secondary dysmenorrhea. Primary dysmenorrhea is found in women with cyclic pelvic pain, but no pelvic pathology. In secondary dysmenorrhea, pelvic pathology can be found which causes the pain. There are several features that help to distinguish between primary and secondary dysmenorrhea. Primary dysmenorrhea usually begins at the time of menarche or within 6 to 12 months of menarche while secondary dysmenorrhea begins later in a woman's life. The pain of primary dysmenorrhea begins shortly before or right after the start of menstrual flow. The pain lasts from 48–72 hours. The pain of secondary dysmenorrhea, on the other hand, lasts for the duration of the menstrual flow. Patients with primary dysmenorrhea typically have cramping pain in the suprapubic area with radiation to the inner thigh and back. Clues that point to a diagnosis of secondary dysmenorrhea include a history of recurrent pelvic inflammatory disease, menorrhagia, irregular menstrual cycles, use of intrauterine device or infertility. The physical examination including pelvic examination of women with primary dysmenorrhea is usually normal. However, the pelvic examination of women with secondary dysmenorrhea may reveal a cause for the pain such as the presence of an IUD or a uterine myoma.

The exact prevalence of primary dysmenorrhea is unknown, but a good estimate seems to be about 75% of women. Women who use oral contraceptives and women who have vaginally delivered a child are less likely to complain of dysmenorrhea. Women with an early menarche, heavy menstrual flow, and long duration of menstrual flow have more severe dysmenorrhea and usually have mothers and sisters with dysmenorrhea.

Primary dysmenorrhea appears to result from increased production and release of prostaglandins by the uterus. In fact, increased levels of prostaglandins have been found in the endometrium and menstrual fluid of women with dysmenorrhea. The prostaglandin usually found to be increased is prostaglandin FF. While there is an increase in prostaglandins, there is also a decrease in prostacyclin which is a vasodilator and smooth muscle relaxant. This causes marked uterine contractions and vasoconstriction leading to uterine hypoxia and pain. An increase in leukotrienes in the endometrium of women with dysmenorrhea has also been found. Leukotrienes act as vasoconstrictors and cause uterine muscle contractions. Increased levels of vasopressin resulting in abnormal uterine contractions have been linked to dysmenorrhea as well. The abnormal and increased uterine contractions are responsible for the cramping. Certain prostaglandins and leukotrienes may hypersensitize pain fibers in the uterus.

Unlike primary dysmenorrhea, secondary dysmenorrhea results from visible pathology. The causes of secondary dysmenorrhea are listed in Table 20.4. In patients suspected of having secondary dysmenorrhea either because their history does not fit the typical pattern associated with primary dysmenorrhea or because of a finding on pelvic examination further evaluation is necessary. Ultrasonography is helpful if uterine myoma or ovarian cyst is suspected. Hysterosalpingography (visualization of the uterine cavity and lumina of the fallopian tubes after injection of contrast material through the cervical canal by Xray imaging) is useful if congenital anomalies are possible. Hysteroscopy allows intrauterine lesions to be seen through the use of an endoscope. Laparoscopy may provide the best answers because the pelvic organs can be observed directly.

One of the causes of secondary dysmenorrhea is cervical stenosis. Cervical stenosis may be congenital or may result from previous injury such as operative trauma or past infection. The cervical canal becomes narrowed and menstrual flow is prevented. There is resultant increased pressure in the uterus and pain. Cervical stenosis should be suspected in patients with a history of minimal menstrual flow and pain throughout the duration of the flow. The diagnosis is confirmed by the inability to pass a thin probe through the cervix or by hysterosalpingography. Pelvic infections may result in scarring and adhesions that can cause pain at the time of menstruation and secondary dysmenorrhea. The pelvic congestion syndrome results from engorgement of the pelvic vessels for unclear reasons. The pain associated with this syndrome is burning or throbbing and is worse at night. Laparoscopy allows visualization of the engorged pelvic vessels and uterine vascular congestion.

ENDOMETRIOSIS

Endometriosis is a disease characterized by the aberrantly located growing stroma of the lining of the uterus. Its pathogenesis and manifestations are complex. The exact incidence of endometriosis is unknown. It is found in between five to fifteen percent of women of reproductive age undergoing laparotomy. In infertile women, the incidence is greater by about 30–45%. The course of endometriosis is extremely variable and difficult to predict.

There are a number of theories that explain the cause of endometriosis. One theory is based on the existence of retrograde menstruation. Endometrial cells enter the peritoneal cavity during menstruation, implant there and begin to grow. This results in areas of endometrial cells outside of the uterus. It is thought that the lymphatic and vascular systems transport the endometrial cells to distant parts of the body. This explains the occurrence of endometriosis in the lung for example. There is also a theory that suggests the disease results from the metaplasia of certain cells in the peritoneal cavity. These cells further differentiate into endometrial

Table 20.4.
Causes of Secondary Dysmenorrhea

Cervical stenosis
Pelvic inflammatory disease—acute or chronic
Pelvic congestion syndrome
Ovarian cysts or tumors
Uterine myomas
Endometriosis
Congenital malformations
Intrauterine devices

From Daywood MY. Dysmenorrhea. Clin Obstet Gynecol 1990:33;169.

cells. It has been postulated that the occurrence of endometriosis is related to changes in the immune system. Endometriosis seems to be affected by genetic factors as well since there is a familial predisposition. There is an increased incidence of the disease in relatives of women with endometriosis.

Endometriosis is found in a number of sites in the pelvis. The most common site in the pelvis is the ovary. Other sites include the peritoneum covering the uterus, the cul-de-sac, the ligaments of the uterus and the pelvic lymph nodes. Endometriosis can also involve the cervix, vagina and vulva. About ten percent of patients have involvement of the rectosigmoid. Uncommon sites of endometriosis are the abdominal wall, bladder, kidney, lungs, arms, and legs.

Most patients with endometriosis complain of pelvic pain. The pain is usually classified as secondary dysmenorrhea. It begins 24–48 hours before menstruation. It is usually constant and lasts for the duration of menstrual flow. The pain may be located on both sides or on one side of the pelvis and may radiate to the back and legs. There is often an inverse relationship between the extent of endometriosis and the severity of the pain. Women with large pelvic masses may have minimal pain whereas women with a few foci of disease may have severe pain. Patients with endometriosis also complain of dyspareunia. The pain occurs during deep penetration and can last for several hours after intercourse. About 15 to 20% of women have abnormal vaginal bleeding which includes menorrhagia and premenstrual spotting. Endometriosis is far more common before menopause. Women with endometriosis affecting the gastrointestinal tract complain of abdominal pain, constipation, diarrhea, and pain during defecation. When endometriosis affects the urinary tract dysuria and hematuria often occur. Patients will also give a history of infertility. It must be remembered, however, that one third of patients will be asymptomatic and their disease will have been found incidentally. The pelvic examination of a woman with endometriosis demonstrates a fixed retroverted uterus. There can be tenderness of the pelvic organs including the ovaries. The ovaries may also be enlarged and fixed to the pelvic wall. Nodularity of the uterosacral ligaments and cul-de-sac is often palpable. Laparoscopy establishes the diagnosis of endometriosis. There are a number of classification systems which are used to describe the extent of the disease based on laparoscopic findings.

UTERINE MYOMA

Uterine myomas also commonly called fibroids and fibromyomas are responsible for pelvic pain in a significant number of women. They are benign tumors originating from uterine muscle cells. They are found in one in four white women and in one in two African-American women. Not all of these women, however, become symptomatic from their myomas. The pain associated with myomas presents as a secondary dysmenorrhea. Pain can also result from degeneration of the fibroid once it outgrows its blood supply or from torsion of a pedunculated fibroid. Patients may also complain of a dull ache or a feeling of heaviness in the pelvis which probably results from edema of the myoma. Myomas can cause symptoms other than pelvic pain. About 30% of women with myomas have abnormal uterine bleeding. Usually, there is heavy and prolonged bleeding. Myomas may also press on the urinary bladder and cause urinary frequency. They can be responsible for infertility and difficulties during pregnancy. Myomas are found most commonly in the fifth decade of life. The size, number, and location of the myomas affect the severity of the symptoms as well as the type of symptoms present.

The majority of the time myomas are found in the body of the uterus. There may be one or many myomas and they may grow to enormous size. Myomas are classified according to their location in the uterus. They can be intramural, within the wall of the uterus; subserosal, just below the serosal surface; or submucosal, just below the endometrium. The location of the myoma is responsible for the symptoms which develop. For example, submucosal myomas may be associated with uterine bleeding and may cause infertility or difficulties with pregnancy because they protrude into the uterine cavity. Subserosal myomas may grow into the peritoneal cavity and cause pain. The growth of myomas seems to be dependent on estrogen. They develop after menarche and decrease in size after menopause. They also increase in size during pregnancy and during use of oral contraceptives. Fewer than one of one thousand myomas develop into malignant sarcomas.

The diagnosis of myoma in a patient with symptoms consistent with its presence is confirmed by pelvic examination. The examination reveals an enlarged, nodular uterus. Extremely large myomas may be palpable even during abdominal examination. The diagnosis can be further confirmed by ultrasound.

ECTOPIC PREGNANCY

The occurrence of a pregnancy anywhere outside the uterine cavity is known as an ectopic pregnancy. The exact incidence of ectopic pregnancy in the United States is difficult to determine, but it was estimated to be 17 per 1000 pregnancies in 1987. Its incidence has been increasing for the last several years probably because of the increased incidence of pelvic inflammatory disease and improved diagnostic capabilities. About half of the ectopic pregnancies in the United States occur in women between the ages of 25 to 34 years. Ectopic pregnancy is also more common in women who have had three or more pregnancies. It occurs twice as often in nonwhite women as in white women. Ectopic pregnancies cause profound hemorrhage. Ectopic pregnancy is a significant cause of maternal mortality resulting in 40 to 50 deaths per year in the United States. It is responsible for most of the maternal deaths occurring in the first half of pregnancy. The risk of death associated with ectopic pregnancy is about three times higher in African-American women. The risk of death from ectopic pregnancy has been estimated to be about ten times greater than the risk from childbirth. Those women with a history of ectopic pregnancy are at increased risk for having another ectopic pregnancy.

Ectopic pregnancy is usually caused by the complications of pelvic inflammatory disease. Salpingitis results in the destruction of the folds of the fallopian tubes which prevents the normal passage of the blastocyst. The blastocyst then implants in the fallopian tube or another site outside of the uterus. Almost half the women with ectopic pregnancy have a history of salpingitis or have histologic changes in their tubes consistent with a past episode of salpingitis. Ectopic pregnancy has also been found to occur in women who have had a tubal sterilization procedure performed. Depending on the procedure used, it is still possible for conception to occur and the blastocyst to implant in the fallopian tube. Ectopic pregnancy occurs more commonly in women who become pregnant while using an IUD or progestin-only oral contraceptives. Women who become pregnant while using combination oral contraceptives or diaphragms are at no increased risk for ectopic pregnancy. However, women using any method of contraception are at much less risk of developing an ectopic pregnancy than women who use no contraception at all.

Most ectopic pregnancies occur in the oviduct. A small number also occur in the peritoneal cavity, ovary, and cervix. Once implanted in the oviduct, the blastocyst grows in the area between the lumen of the tube and the tube's peritoneal covering. This growth results in stretching of the peritoneal covering and pain as well as destruction of blood vessels and bleeding. Rupture of the fallopian tube occurs when the peritoneal covering has been maximally stretched.

The most common symptom associated with ectopic pregnancy is abdominal pain. It may be unilateral or bilateral and becomes most intense after rupture of the fallopian tube has occurred. About one quarter of patients complain of shoulder pain probably secondary to diaphragmatic irritation. Patients also give a history of a missed period and irregular vaginal bleeding. Other symptoms include breast tenderness, nausea, and dizziness. Patients may notice the passage of a decidual cast which is the lining of the endometrial cavity. On examination, women with an ectopic pregnancy will have abdominal and adnexal tenderness. About half the patients may have a palpable adnexal mass and about one third may have uterine enlargement of less than 8-week size. Fever is an uncommon finding. Hypotension and tachycardia are present if rupture of the fallopian tube has occurred with significant blood loss.

Further testing is necessary to make the diagnosis of ectopic pregnancy. All patients should have a sensitive serum assay for human chorionic gonadotrophin hormone. A negative serum radioimmunoassay for b-HCG makes ectopic pregnancy very unlikely. Women with an ectopic pregnancy have a lower level of HCG than women with a normal pregnancy at a similar gestational age. In normal early pregnancies, the HCG level doubles about every 2 days while in ectopic pregnancies and pregnancies destined to abort this rate of increase does not occur. Therefore, following serial HCG measurements and their rate of increase can be used to help make the diagnosis of ectopic pregnancy in a stable patient. Ultrasonography is extremely useful in making the diagnosis. In women with an ectopic pregnancy, ultrasonography using a transvaginal probe will demonstrate the absence of a gestational sac in the uterus or an adnexal mass. This technique is accurate when the HCG level is greater than 2500 mIU/ml. In women with symptoms of ectopic pregnancy, a HCG level below 2500 mIU/ml and no evidence of a gestational sac on ultrasound, serial HCG measurements and serial ultrasound examinations can be used to establish the diagnosis. Culdocentesis may also be of assistance. The finding of nonclotting blood with a hematocrit above 15% is consistent with ectopic pregnancy. Ultimately, the diagnosis can be definitively made by laparoscopy. There is, however, a 2–5% false positive or false negative rate probably due to difficulties visualizing the pelvic organs because of adhesions, obesity, or bleeding.

CHRONIC PELVIC PAIN

Chronic pelvic pain is one of the more complicated problems faced by the health care provider. Patients with chronic pelvic pain should be evaluated by the gynecologist. The pain may result from dysmenorrhea, either primary or secondary, endometriosis, pelvic infections, pelvic adhesions, urinary tract diseases, and gastrointestinal diseases. A significant number of patients have no cause for the pain. In one series of 100 patients with pelvic pain in the same location for at least 6 months, 83% of women had abnormal pelvic findings during laparoscopy. About 17% of the women with pain had no abnormalities found during laparoscopy (11).

The workup for chronic pelvic pain should be thorough. The history should include attention to the patient's daily life. A relationship exists between a history of physical or sexual abuse and chronic pelvic pain. Patients with chronic pelvic pain have a greater prevalence of major depression, substance abuse, and somatization. Physical examination, of course, includes a pelvic examination. Laboratory evaluation begins with a complete blood count, erythrocyte sedimentation rate, a test for syphilis, and urinalysis. Further studies of the urinary tract or the gastrointestinal tract may be necessary depending on the patient's complaints. Laparoscopy is eventually performed to complete the evaluation.

Management

Once the etiology of a patient's pelvic pain has been found, treatment can begin. Each of the common causes of pelvic pain: pelvic inflammatory disease, dysmenorrhea, endometriosis, uterine myoma, and ectopic pregnancy, is managed differently.

PELVIC INFLAMMATORY DISEASE

The diagnosis of pelvic inflammatory disease should be considered in all women of reproductive age with pelvic pain. It is associated with several serious sequelae. Ectopic pregnancy is six to ten times more common in women who have had pelvic inflammatory disease. Women with a history of this infection are four times more likely to develop chronic pelvic pain. The risk of developing infertility after infection is not insubstantial. Infertility developed in 8% of women after a single episode of infection and then increased to about 20% after two episodes and then to 40% after three or more episodes (12). It is because of these sequelae of infection that the Centers for Disease Control recommends empiric treatment with antibiotics for women who present with lower abdominal tenderness, adnexal tenderness, and cervical motion tenderness without another cause for these symptoms. Patients diagnosed with pelvic inflammatory disease can be treated as inpatients or outpatients depending on the clinical situation. The CDC has provided certain guidelines to determine the need for hospitalization. These guidelines state that the patient should be hospitalized if the diagnosis is uncertain and the possibilities of appendicitis or ectopic pregnancy cannot be excluded, if the patient is pregnant, is an adolescent, or has HIV infection, if a pelvic abscess is suspected, if the patient is too ill to go home, if it is unclear that the patient will be compliant with the medications, if the patient has failed to respond to outpatient therapy, or if follow-up within 72 hours of starting treatment is not possible (13). The treatment regimens for pelvic inflammatory disease are designed to cover a number of bacteria since the responsible organism is usually unknown at the time of starting treatment. There are two outpatient regimens recommended by the Centers for Disease Control. One regimen uses cefoxitin 2 g IM with probenecid 1 g orally as a single dose or ceftriaxone 250 mg IM or another third generation cephalosporin in a single dose plus doxycycline 100 mg twice a day for 14 days orally. The alternative regimen is ofloxacin 400 mg orally twice a day for 14 days plus clindamycin 450 mg four times a day orally or metronidazole 500 mg twice a day orally for 14 days. The regimens for patients hospitalized for pelvic inflammatory disease recommend intravenous antibiotic therapy with either cefoxitin or cefotetan plus doxycycline. The alternative regimen is clindamycin plus gentamicin intravenously (14). The antibiotics are usually given intravenously for 48 hours after the patient has improved substantially. The doxycycline should then be continued at a dose of 100 mg orally twice a day for a total of 14 days. The detailed regimens for inpatient treatment and outpatient treatment can be found in Table 20.5. The Centers for Disease Control suggests sending repeat cultures for *C. trachomatis* and *N. gonorrhoeae* 7–10 days after treatment is completed and possibly 4–6 weeks after treatment as well. Women

Table 20.5.
Treatment Regimens for Pelvic Inflammatory Disease

	Regimen A	Regimen B
Outpatient treatment	Cefoxitin 2 g IM with probenecid 1 g orally at the same time **or** Ceftriaxone 250 mg IM **or** Another third-generation cephalosporin (ceftizoxime or cefotaxime) IM **with** Doxycycline 100 mg orally twice a day for 14 days	Ofloxacin 400 mg orally twice a day for 14 days **with** Clinamycin 450 mg orally four times a day for 14 days **or** Metronidazole 500 mg orally twice a day for 14 days
Inpatient treatment	Cefoxitin 2 g IV every 6 hours, **or** Cefotetan 2 g IV every 12 hours **with** Doxycycline 100 mg IV or orally every 12 hours	Clindamycin 900 mg IV every 8 hours **with** Gentamicin initial loading dose of 2 mg/kg IV or IM followed by a maintenance dose of 1.5 mg/kg every 8 hours

with HIV infection may be at risk for more serious infections and may be more likely to develop pelvic abscesses and to require surgery. For these reasons, as already mentioned, women with HIV infection should be hospitalized for intravenous therapy. The sex partners of women with pelvic inflammatory disease should be treated whether they are symptomatic or asymptomatic for *C. trachomatis* and *N. gonorrhoeae*. The recommended Centers for Disease Control guidelines for the treatment of uncomplicated endocervical infection with *N. gonorrhoeae* or *C. trachomatis* are given in Table 20.6.

DYSMENORRHEA

The management of dysmenorrhea depends on making the distinction between primary and secondary dysmenorrhea. Primary dysmenorrhea is treated effectively with either prostaglandin synthetase inhibitors (nonsteroidal anti-inflammatory drugs) or oral contraceptives. If the patient wishes to use oral contraceptives for birth control and there are no contraindications, a combination estrogen-progestin pill may be given. This will relieve the pain in about 90% of women treated. If the pain is not relieved, a nonsteroidal anti-inflammatory drug may be added after an adequate trial of oral contraceptives for three to four months. Oral contraceptives seem to work by causing a decrease

in menstrual fluid volume and by producing an environment in which prostaglandin levels are low. The prostaglandin synthetase inhibitors decrease the production and release of uterine prostaglandins. These drugs also have analgesic properties as well. The drugs should be started as soon as menstrual flow and pain starts. They should be continued for the first 48–72 hours at regular intervals instead of on an as needed basis. Prostaglandin release seems to be maximal during this time. Nonsteroidal anti-inflammatory drugs should not be given to patients with a history of gastrointestinal ulcers or bleeding, those with a history of hypersensitivity to these drugs and those with renal disease. Common side effects are gastrointestinal upset, headache, and dizziness. Table 20.7 lists the more commonly used prostaglandin synthetase inhibitors. Patients who do not respond to oral contraceptives and/or prostaglandin synthetase inhibitors after a trial of 4 to 6 months of therapy should be evaluated for causes of secondary dysmenorrhea.

The treatment for secondary dysmenorrhea is dependent on the cause. Cervical stenosis is treated with dilation of the cervix. Dysmenorrhea thought to be secondary to the presence of an intrauterine device should be treated with nonsteroidal anti-inflammatory drugs because of their ability to decrease prostaglandin production. In other cases such as uterine polyps or ovarian cysts, surgery may be necessary.

Table 20.6.
Treatment Regimens of Uncomplicated Endocervical Chlamydial and Gonococcal Infection

	Treatment Regimens	Alternative Treatment Regimens
Chlamydia infection	Doxycycline 100 mg orally 2 times a day for 7 days **or** Azithromycin 1 g orally as a single dose	Ofloxacin 300 mg orally twice a day for 7 days **or** Erythromycin base 500 mg orally 4 times a day for 7 days **or** Erythromycin ethylsuccinate 800 mg orally 4 times a day for 7 days
Gonococcal infection	Ceftriaxone 250 mg IM as a single dose **or** Cefixime 400 mg orally as a single dose **or** Ciprofloxacin 500 mg orally as a single dose **or** Ofloxacin 400 mg orally as a single dose **with** Treatment regimen for chlamydial infection (see above)	

ENDOMETRIOSIS

The goals of treatment of endometriosis are to relieve pelvic pain and to restore fertility if possible. About 25% of patients experience spontaneous remission of their endometriosis while in the majority of patients the disease persists unchanged or progresses. Treatment should be individualized according to the patient's age, symptoms, extent of disease, and plans for future fertility. Therefore, the treatment of endometriosis is complex and best left to the gynecologist.

The treatment of endometriosis can be broadly divided into medical therapy and surgical therapy. Medical therapy is based on the use of several drugs

Table 20.7.
Prostaglandin Synthetase Inhibitors Used to Treat Dysmenorrhea

Ibuprofen (Motrin)	400–800 mg orally every 6 hours
Naproxen (Naprosyn)	250–500 mg orally every 6 hours
Naproxen Sodium (Anaprox)	275–550 mg orally every 6 hours
Piroxicam (Feldene)	20 mg orally 1 or 2 times a day
Indomethacin (Indocin)	25 mg orally 3–6 times a day
Ketoprofen (Orudis)	50 mg orally 3 times a day

which influence the hormonal environment of the body. These drugs induce amenorrhea and inhibit the growth of the ectopic endometrium. The drug most commonly used is Danazol. It is a synthetic steroid that is mildly androgenic. It produces endometrial atrophy as well as atrophy of ectopic endometrium by inducing a hypoestrogenic and hypoprogestational state. The drug is associated with several side effects due to its androgenic activity. These side effects include weight gain, oily skin, facial hair, acne, and deepening of the voice. It also decreases high density lipoprotein levels and increases low-density lipoprotein levels. Patients are usually treated for 6 to 9 months. The use of the drug results in symptomatic improvement and regression of the disease in about 85% of patients. However, from 15–30% of patients will have a symptomatic recurrence within 2 years after completion of therapy. Medroxyprogesterone acetate, a progestin, has also been used to treat endometriosis. It has the same effect on endometrial tissue as Danazol and has been found to work as well as Danazol. However, medroxyprogesterone acetate is associated with less frequent and severe side effects than Danazol. Gonadotropin-releasing hormone agonists can be used to treat endometriosis. These drugs suppress anterior pituitary gonadotrophin secretion and thereby stop ovarian hormone production. These drugs have been compared with Danazol in treating endometriosis. Gonadotropin-releasing hormone agonists are associated with a different set of side effects. These drugs produce a hypo-estrogenic state and cause side effects similar to menopausal symptoms including hot flushes and vaginal dryness. For this reason, estrogens, progestins, or combinations of these two hormones are sometimes added to gonadotropin-releasing hormone therapy.

Surgical therapy has also been used to treat endometriosis. The decision between medical and surgical therapy is based on the patient's symptoms, the extent of the disease and the patient's desire for future fertility. Surgical therapy is the therapy of choice in the treatment of women with moderate to severe endometriosis affecting organs other than the genital tract such as the colon and urinary tract. When it has been decided to treat endometriosis of the genital tract with surgical therapy, a conservative approach can be used in those women who want children. Laparoscopy allows the removal of all the visible areas of endometriosis using either a laser or electrocautery. In patients who fail medical therapy and/or conservative surgical therapy and are not interested in fertility, a total abdominal hysterectomy and bilateral salpingo-oophorectomy are performed along with removal of all visible areas of endometriosis. It is not yet decided if the addition of medical therapy preoperatively or postoperatively improves the outcome of patients.

UTERINE MYOMA

Women with asymptomatic myomas are best managed with close follow-up. Patients should have repeat pelvic examinations in 4 to 6 months to assess the further growth of the myoma. The management of patients with symptomatic or large myomas can be complicated. Women with persistent symptoms are considered for surgical therapy, either hysterectomy or myomectomy (removal of the myoma only). The decision between the two procedures is broadly based on the patients plans to have children. Myomectomy is usually performed in patients with heavy persistent uterine bleeding, persistent pain, or a rapidly growing myoma, and in patients with difficulties with fertility, and/or a history of previous miscarriages thought to be secondary to the myoma. Myomectomy should not be performed in pregnant patients because of the risk for increased bleeding and in those patients in which removal of the myoma would result in significant loss of the endometrium so that the uterus would be nonfunctional. Hysterectomies are performed for the above indications in patients who no longer desire children or are in an older age group. Hysterectomies are also performed in pa-

tients with asymptomatic myomas whose uteri have reached a 12–14 week size. Patients with myomas that increase in size after menopause are considered candidates for hysterectomy because of the possibility of sarcoma. Myomas can also be treated medically using drugs that decrease the amount of estrogen and therefore decrease the size of the myomas. Two such drugs currently being investigated are the gonadotropin-releasing hormone agonists and gestrinone which is an anti-estrogen, anti-progesterone derivative of testosterone. Neither drug is currently approved by the Food and Drug Administration for this use.

ECTOPIC PREGNANCY

Most of the management of ectopic pregnancy involves surgical therapy. Occasionally, ectopic pregnancies may regress spontaneously and no further treatment is necessary. The surgical procedure chosen depends on the patient's plans for future pregnancies and the clinical situation. If there is rupture of the fallopian tube or the ectopic pregnancy involves the entire tube and the patient does not desire future fertility, salpingectomy (removal of the fallopian tube) with or without oophorectomy (removal of the ovary) is performed. Those patients with an unruptured ectopic pregnancy who want future pregnancies can have one of several surgical procedures performed to salvage the tube. Future ectopic pregnancy rates seem to be the same regardless of whether the patient is treated with salpingectomy or a more conservative procedure which saves the fallopian tube. Conservative procedures benefit women with a history of infertility or evidence of contralateral tube damage the most. Medical therapy for ectopic pregnancy is still experimental and involves the use of methotrexate.

The further management of ectopic pregnancy involves counseling the patient on future fertility. The overall conception rate after ectopic pregnancy is 60%. About half of these pregnancies end in either another ectopic pregnancy or miscarriage. The fertility rate is higher in women under the age of 30 years if this is not their first pregnancy, women with a high parity and in women with an unruptured ectopic pregnancy. Women who develop an ectopic pregnancy while using an IUD have a normal fertility rate and are not at increased risk for further ectopic pregnancies if the IUD is removed. The fertility rate is lower in women with a past history of pelvic inflammatory disease or with evidence of damage to the opposite tube because of the previous infection. The fertility rate decreases with further episodes of ectopic pregnancy.

ILLUSTRATIVE CASES WITH SELF-ASSESSMENT QUESTIONS AND ANSWERS

Case 1

A 17-year old woman with no past medical history complains of several months of lower abdominal pain. It is crampy and radiates to the back. She occasionally has diarrhea with the pain. She has noticed that the pain begins right before her period. She is sexually active and uses condoms for contraception. Her last period was 2 weeks ago. A physical examination including pelvic examination is normal. A pregnancy test is negative.

QUESTION: *The most likely diagnosis in this patient is:*

a. Endometriosis
b. Primary dysmenorrhea
c. Pelvic inflammatory disease

ANSWER: b. *The patient's history is typical for primary dysmenorrhea. A normal pelvic examination makes endometriosis and pelvic inflammatory disease unlikely. Therefore, primary dysmenorrhea is the most likely diagnosis.*

QUESTION: *The appropriate treatment for this patient is:*

a. Prostaglandin synthetase inhibitors
b. Oral contraceptives
c. Either of the above

ANSWER: c. *The patient may be treated with either prostaglandin synthetase inhibitors or oral contraceptives. The patient should then be re-evaluated after an adequate trial of 3 to 4 months.*

Case 2

A 19-year-old woman with no past medical history complains of 2 days of lower abdominal and pelvic pain. She also complains of a vaginal discharge and fever of 102°F. Today, she has felt nauseous and vomited three times. She is sexually active with one partner and does not use a barrier method of contraception. Physical examination is significant for an ill-appearing young woman and right and left lower quadrant pain. On pelvic examination, there is adnexal tenderness and cervical motion tenderness. A pregnancy test is negative. The diagnosis of pelvic inflammatory disease is made.

QUESTION: *The patient should be hospitalized if which of the following is true?*

a. She is willing to take medications and return in 72 hours.
b. She is HIV positive.
c. She is unable to take oral medications.
d. B and C.

ANSWER: d. *The indications for hospitalization include patients who are pregnant, HIV positive or are adolescents, patients whose diagnosis is uncertain and an appendicitis or ectopic pregnancy is possible, patients who are too ill to go home and patients with a suspected pelvic abscess. The indications also include patients who may not be compliant with medications and those patients who cannot return in 72 hours. Patients who have already failed outpatient therapy should be hospitalized.*

QUESTION: *Proper outpatient treatment includes which of the following?*

a. Ceftriaxone 250 mg IM as a single dose with Doxycycline 100 mg twice daily for 14 days orally
b. Ofloxacin 400 mg twice daily and Clindamycin 450 mg four times a day for 14 days orally
c. Cefoxitin 2g IM as a single dose with probenecid 1 g orally as a single dose and Doxycycline 100 mg twice a day orally for 14 days
d. A, B, and C

ANSWER: d. *All of the above regimens are used to treat pelvic inflammatory disease in outpatients.*

PRE-CONCEPTION CARE OF THE MEDICAL PATIENT

In the last century, advances in prenatal care have led to decreased maternal and fetal morbidity and mortality. More recently, clinicians have begun to focus on pre-conception care; that is, preparing the patient for pregnancy before the pregnancy has actually occurred. This form of preventative health care is noteworthy for several reasons. Since most organogenesis in the embryo occurs between the 17th and 56th day of conception, at a time when most women do not yet realize they are pregnant, maximizing a women's health before conception ensures that the environment in which vital organs develop is optimal. Additionally, because of advances in medical care, many women with congenital and chronic diseases are surviving into their reproductive years. Pre-conception care helps to assess what impact a pregnancy could have on a woman's medical condition and also what impact such medical condition(s) would have on her fetus (15).

Pathophysiologic Correlation

This section will cover basic physiological changes that occur with pregnancy in the cardiovascular, pulmonary, and endocrine/metabolic systems. The various effects these changes could have on the pregnant woman and her fetus will also be discussed. The interested reader should consult one of the textbooks listed in the reference section for a more detailed discussion.

CARDIOVASCULAR SYSTEM

The cardiac output (CO) increases by about 40% in pregnant women. Since CO is the product of stroke volume (SV) and heart rate (HR), either the SV or HR must increase if CO is increased. Early in pregnancy, most of the increase in CO is due to an increase in the SV rather than to an increase in the heart rate. There is also about a 40% increase in the blood volume, mostly due to an increase in the plasma volume. The net effect of the increased blood volume is a physiologic anemia of pregnancy.

During early pregnancy, there are changes in the blood pressure (BP) also. The relationship between BP and CO is as follows: BP is the product of CO and systemic vascular resistance (SVR). Thus, because CO is increased, there must be a decrease in the SVR to maintain a normal BP. This is exactly what happens during early pregnancy. In fact, the decreased SVR is more than would be expected, leading to an overall decrease in the BP during early pregnancy, as illustrated by Figure 20.5. Women who have chronic hypertension may not need medication during early pregnancy. Women who have chronic hypertension and do not show

a decreased blood pressure early in pregnancy may be at a higher risk of a more complicated course.

The exact mechanism by which these changes occur is not known. There is speculation that increased steroid hormones may contribute to the decreased SVR. During early pregnancy there is resistance to the effects of Angiotensin II. There are also other complex neurohormonal changes involving aldosterone, atrial natriuretic factor, and prostaglandins that may remodel the heart to allow for the increased SV without a concomitant increase in filling pressures (16). These changes also result in the tendency for salt and water retention during pregnancy. Because of these physiological changes, many pregnant women experience symptoms such as easy fatigability, dyspnea on exertion, and edema. These symptoms could easily be mistaken for symptoms of heart disease. On the other hand, because of the potential for the development of these symptoms, women who have structural heart disease may be at an increased risk for decompensation.

As pregnancy progresses, blood pressure slowly increases, about 10 mm of Hg in diastolic blood pressure during the third trimester (Fig. 20.5). Also, later in pregnancy, the SV decreases to pre-pregnancy levels and the increased CO is a result of an increased HR. Again, women with structural heart disease, especially certain types of valvular disease such as mitral stenosis, may be at increased risk of decompensation in the face of increased HR.

There may be increased risk of fetal mortality and intrauterine growth retardation when the diastolic blood pressure is greater than 90 mm Hg. The American College of Obstetrics has determined that any increases of more than 30 mm Hg systolic or 15 mm Hg diastolic during pregnancy be considered abnormal (17). However, there is controversy regarding what the upper limit of normal blood pressure should be. Most experts agree that the cutoff of blood pressure should be 140/90, but clinicians should use their judgment because for certain patients, for example women with a previous history of pre-eclampsia/eclampsia and women who have previously had fetal demise, a lower cutoff may seem prudent. Risks to the patient of having increased blood pressure during pregnancy include pre-eclampsia/eclampsia, placental abruptio, stroke, and heart failure. Of course, any of these would also have grave consequences for the fetus.

PULMONARY SYSTEM

As pregnancy progresses and the uterus enlarges, there are changes that occur in pulmonary function.

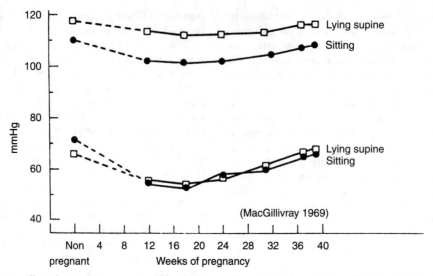

Figure 20.5. Effect of pregnancy on postural blood pressure. (From MacGillivray I, Rose GA, Rowe B. Blood pressure survey in pregnancy. Clin Science 1969;37:399.)

As the gravid uterus pushes against the diaphragm, the resting position of the diaphragm and thorax changes. However, the function of the diaphragm is not changed significantly, and measured lung volumes are only affected slightly. There is no change in lung compliance, diffusing capacity, or in measurements of forced vital capacity (FVC) so the changes imposed by the gravid uterus are not thought to have much clinical significance (18).

Because of the increased demands placed by fetal and placental needs for nutrition and oxygen, maternal physiology accommodates by several mechanisms. There is an increase in overall maternal work which increases the oxygen consumption by 20–30%. The basal metabolic rate (BMR) thus also increases. Additionally, there is also an increase in the resting minute ventilation which is out of proportion to the increases in oxygen consumption and BMR. Because the respiratory rate has not been observed to increase during pregnancy, the increase in minute ventilation must be due primarily to increases in the tidal volume (TV). These changes may be mediated by the action of progesterone (18). Progesterone is also thought to stimulate the respiratory center. The net effect is a physiological dyspnea of pregnancy and a mild respiratory alkalosis.

The most common pulmonary condition clinicians will likely encounter in young women is asthma. Most women with asthma will tolerate pregnancy well with little risk of any adverse consequences to the fetus. However, any conditions which may impose hypoxemia to the mother could be detrimental to the fetus. Blood is preferentially shunted away from the fetus and placenta to preserve maternal cerebral and coronary circulation during any maternal stress such as hypotension or hypoxia. Potential complications to the fetus include intrauterine growth retardation, preterm birth, and death.

ENDOCRINE AND METABOLIC SYSTEM

During pregnancy, there is resistance to the glucose lowering effects of insulin. This causes pancreatic beta cell hyperplasia. Estrogen, progesterone, and placental hormones also contribute to pancreatic beta cell hyperplasia and insulin resistance. Women who have limited pancreatic reserve may not be able to compensate for the insulin resistance during pregnancy and may manifest signs and symptoms of diabetes for the first time during pregnancy. Other important metabolic changes during pregnancy occur to ensure that there is enough fuel for both the growing fetus and the mother. As the placenta matures, a hormone called human placental lactogen is made which promotes lipolysis over gluconeogenesis from skeletal muscle amino acids during maternal fasting periods so that there is enough fuel in the form of ketone bodies for maternal brain function, and any glucose is reserved for fetal use (19). As the fetus grows and requires more glucose, maternal fasting glucose levels decrease. In patients who have pre-existing diabetes, hypoglycemia may occur.

Despite improvements in medical care for pregnant diabetic women, there is still at least a three-fold greater incidence of congenital malformations (Table 20.8). Hyperglycemia has been implicated in the cause. Additionally, hyperglycemia greater or equal to 130 mg/dl has increased the risk of fetal macrosomia and its risks for traumatic birth injury and shoulder dystocia (19).

Because of increased levels of estrogen during pregnancy, there is an increase in the thyroxine-binding globulin. Thus, total T4 is increased; however, the free T4 remains normal or is only slightly elevated. Early in pregnancy, there may be a slight decrease in TSH because human chorionic gonadotropin (HCG), which increases early in pregnancy, has intrinsic TSH-like activity. There is also a slight increase in the maternal T4 requirement, not explained entirely by placental transfer of T4 for fetal use (20).

Clinical and Laboratory Evaluation

Clinicians should not greatly alter their approach to the patient who presents for pre-conception care. There is no substitute for a thorough history and physical examination, especially in young women

Table 20.8.
Congenital Malformations in Infants of Diabetic Mothers

Cardiovascular
   Transposition of the great vessels
   Ventricular septal defect
   Atrial septal defect
   Hypoplastic left ventricle
   Situs inversus
   Anomalies of the aorta
Central nervous system
   Anencephaly
   Encephalocele
   Meningomyelocele
   Microcephaly
Skeletal
   Caudal regression syndrome
   Spina bifida
Genitourinary
   Absent kidneys (Potter's syndrome)
   Polycystic kidneys
   Double ureter
Gastrointestinal
   Tracheoesophageal fistula
   Bowel artesia
   Imperforate anus

From Laudon MB, Gabbe SG. Diabetes mellitus. In: Barron WM, Lindheimer MD, eds. Medical disorders during pregnancy. St. Louis: Mosby-YearBook, Inc. 1991:78.

who may not have had close medical contact before. There is always the potential for making a new diagnosis and being able to make an early intervention.

HISTORY

A comprehensive history should be obtained for all women who present for pre-conception care. The non-obstetrical clinician who may later serve as medical consultant should pay particular attention to any underlying medical conditions the patient may have. For each medical condition brought out by the history, the clinician should attempt to assess its severity and its impact on any previous pregnancies.

Patients may present for pre-conception care because of the fear that medications they take for various conditions will cause birth defects. The clinician should thoroughly review all the over-the-counter and prescription medications the patient currently uses and assess whether any could be discontinued or changed to a drug which has been proven safe in pregnant women. Unfortunately, not much is known regarding the safety of many drugs during pregnancy, and most medications used today have not been thoroughly studied in pregnant women. Table 20.9 shows the current classification of drugs based on risk to pregnant women.

Clinicians need to make a nutritional assessment of the patient. Nutritional deficiency is not a problem for most patients in the Western world. However, those who practice in areas where there are indigent and immigrant populations may encounter nutritional deficiencies. Clinicians need to ask patients about what they eat and whether they will make any changes in diet during pregnancy. Anyone who mentions any restrictions on diet should be questioned further. For example, for patients who say they are vegetarians, clinicians need to assess whether that means that milk and/or eggs are consumed. It is also important to asses whether there is a history of lactose intolerance. Attention should be made to whether enough foods are being consumed that supply adequate amounts of iron, calcium, and folic acid. Finally, clinicians should familiarize themselves with diets from other cultures of their patients so that any nutritional advice given to patients can be easily understood.

As part of the comprehensive history, clinicians should also inquire about past legal and illegal substance use and assess whether there is any ongoing substance abuse. It may be easier to first question the patient about tobacco and caffeine use, two "socially accepted" legal substances, before inquir-

Table 20.9.
Food and Drug Administration Pregnancy
Risk Classification

Category A: Controlled studies in women fail to demonstrate a risk to the fetus in the first trimester (and there is no evidence of a risk in later trimesters), and the possibility of fetal harm appears remote.

Category B: Either animal-reproduction studies have not demonstrated a fetal risk, but there are no controlled studies in pregnant women, or animal-reproduction studies have shown an adverse effect (other than a decrease in fertility) that was not confirmed in controlled studies in women in the first trimester (and there is no evidence of a risk in later trimesters).

Category C: Either studies in animals have revealed adverse effects on the fetus (teratogenic or embryocidal effects, or other) and there are no controlled studies in women, or studies in women and animals are not available. Drugs should be given only if the potential benefit justifies the potential risk to the fetus.

Category D: There is positive evidence of human fetal risk, but the benefits from use in pregnant women may be acceptable despite the risk (e.g., if the drug is needed in a life-threatening situation, or for a serious disease for which safer drugs cannot be used or are ineffective). There will be an appropriate statement in the "warnings" section of the labeling.

Category X: Studies in animals or human beings have demonstrated fetal abnormalities, or there is evidence of fetal risk based on human experience, or both, and the risk of using the drug in pregnant women clearly outweighs any possible benefit. The drug is contraindicated in women who are or may become pregnant. There will be an appropriate statement in the "contraindications" section of the labeling.

From Federal Register 1980;44:37434.

ing about alcohol and illicit drug use. The clinician should attempt to quantify the amount of each substance used so that the magnitude of risk to the fetus can be estimated. Some patients can become evasive when asked specific questions about substance use, and often a patient's account of quantity falls short of actual use. To promote an open discussion and to retain the patient's acceptance of care, clinicians should always use a non-judgmental approach when questioning patients about substance abuse. Sometimes, the history can provide clues that point to a potential problem with substance abuse, as illustrated in Table 20.10.

PHYSICAL EXAMINATION

A comprehensive physical examination should be done for all patients who present for pre-conception care. Depending on any existing medical condition(s), the clinician will want to pay particular attention to the organ system(s) involved. Additionally, all patients should have a thorough pelvic examination.

LABORATORY EVALUATION

Clinicians will want to obtain basic laboratory tests, a Pap smear, and any other additional laboratory tests warranted given the individual patient. Basic laboratory tests include a complete blood count, urinalysis, VDRL, hepatitis B screen, and rubella titers. These are important because iron deficiency anemia, common in young women, should be addressed prior to pregnancy when the increases in blood volume will further exacerbate the anemia. All women should have adequate titers for Rubella to prevent the congenital TORCH syndrome. Similarly, all women should be screened for syphilis and hepatitis B. Treatment for syphilis can be given to avoid congenital transmission. In the case of hepatitis B, knowledge that a woman could potentially transmit the disease to her fetus is obtained and appropriate treatment of the newborn can be planned. Some women will also want to have HIV testing done prior to conception, especially since new data suggests that intravenous zidovudine given during delivery may prevent transmission of the HIV virus to the newborn.

Other laboratory tests that are needed depend on any specific medical conditions the patient may have. Patients who have hypertension should have an evaluation of electrolytes and renal function. If creatinine is elevated, a 24-hour urine should be obtained for creatinine clearance. If suspected by the clinical history, secondary causes of hypertension should be ruled out (see Chapter 13). If secondary causes of hypertension, for example pheochromocytoma, or renal artery stenosis, are left untreated, the morbidity to the patient and unborn child is high.

Patients who have diabetes should also have laboratory tests for electrolytes and renal function and a 24-hr urine collection if needed. Additionally, clinicians should obtain glycosylated hemoglobin (Hgb A1c) measurements to assess overall glycemic control. Studies have shown that the level of Hgb A1c correlates with the risk of congenital malformations (21), the most common cause of poor outcome today among pregnant diabetic patients.

Table 20.10.
Clues to Substance Abuse

Medical	Obstetric	Social
History of multiple injuries	History of multiple pregnancy loss,	Noncompliance: missed appoint-
Requests for analgesics, tranquiliz-	premature labor, placental abrup-	ments
ers, sedatives, stimulants	tion, IUGR, inadequate prenatal	Multiple emergency room visits
Infections: HIV, hepatitis B, endo-	care	Problems with law enforcement
carditis, skin infection, multiple	History of neonatal abstinence syn-	Marital and custodial disputes
STDs, unusual sites of infection	drome	Family history of substance abuse
Suicide attempts, insomnia	Current pregnancy complicated by	
Withdrawal syndrome or symptoms	poor nutrition, unexplained fetal	
Body decorations	tachycardia, labile maternal	
	blood pressure, IUGR	

HIV = human immunodeficiency virus, IUGR = intrauterine growth retardation, STDs = sexually transmitted diseases. (From Lee RV. Drug Abuse. In: Burrow GN and Ferris TF eds. Medical complications during pregnancy. 4th ed. Philadelphia: WB Saunders Co., 1995:584.)

When a patient who has thyroid disease presents for pre-conception care, the clinician should obtain thyroid function tests. Patients who have a history of Grave's disease, even though euthyroid, should have determinations of thyroid stimulating immunoglobulin done. These antibodies may still be present and could cross the placenta and affect the fetus. The presence of these antibodies can alert the clinician that more aggressive fetal monitoring is needed during the pregnancy.

Differential Diagnosis

Clinicians who prepare women for pregnancy need to be aware of when to advise against pregnancy. Ideally, most medical conditions should be stable and optimally managed before conception. This section will briefly mention some common medical conditions clinicians are likely to encounter in an ambulatory setting and provide guidelines on when to advise against pregnancy or to advise that pregnancy be postponed.

Hypertensive patients should have well-controlled blood pressures. Any patient who has hypertension on the basis of a secondary cause (See Chapter 13) should be advised to have that condition treated before attempting to become pregnant. Pregnancy is not advised for patients who are hypertensive and have creatinine clearance less than 30mg/min or blood urea nitrogen (BUN) of greater than 30mg/dl (1). Diabetic patients who also have ischemic heart disease should be advised against pregnancy (15). Some women who have congenital and valvular heart disease should have the lesion repaired before attempting to become pregnant. Pregnancy is not advised for patients who have

primary or secondary pulmonary hypertension. Patients who have undergone treatment for Graves disease with radioactive iodine should not become pregnant within 12 months of receiving the treatment. Ideally, a patient with a substance abuse problem should undergo detoxification and substance abuse treatment prior to becoming pregnant.

Sometimes despite a health care provider's best intentions, the patient chooses to become pregnant even though there is a medical condition which is not being optimally managed. This is often the most frustrating situation a clinician will encounter. If the patient has understood the counseling regarding the risks of pregnancy, there is little that the clinician can do. The principle of patient autonomy prevails. The role of the pre-conception counselor is to offer recommendations based on medical knowledge as they relate to the patient's situation, not to make decisions for the patient, nor to coerce the patient into what he/she considers to be an acceptable course of action.

Management

Clinicians should address any particular medical condition(s) the patient may have and should not only provide advice regarding the medical management but also counsel the patient about the risks to herself and to her fetus. This section will emphasize the more common conditions clinicians are likely to encounter in an ambulatory setting.

GENERAL NUTRITION ISSUES

Women who take vitamin supplements containing 0.4 mg folic acid have a decreased risk of having a fetus with a neural tube defect (22,23). The CDC now recommends that all women of childbearing age who could become pregnant take 0.4 mg folic acid per day. However, because the effect of high doses of folic acid is not known, the CDC further recommends that women not consume more than 1 mg folic acid per day (23). Folic acid is found in raw green leafy vegetables, seeds, whole grains, and legumes. Therefore, women may not need a supplement to obtain 0.4 mg folic acid per day (22,23). Women on special diets may need vitamin supplements to correct any potential nutritional deficiencies. Women who are lactose intolerant or who are strict vegetarians will need supplementation of vitamin B12, calcium, and vitamin D. All women who do not consume meat will need iron supplementation.

Obese patients present a challenging problem to clinicians. Obstetrical risks associated with obesity, defined as 20% above standard weight for height, include hypertension, pre-eclampsia, and gestational diabetes. Women gain about 27–30 lbs during pregnancy. Marked caloric restriction to achieve weight loss is not advised during pregnancy, nor is there much evidence that over the long term weight reduction is maintained. Therefore, clinicians should encourage patients to undergo a sensible program of weight reduction before pregnancy that includes caloric restriction and exercise. Often it takes at least a year to achieve substantial weight loss, and many patients may not be willing to wait such a long time before conception.

SUBSTANCE USE/ABUSE

Caffeine. Human studies have not shown evidence that caffeine has major teratogenic effects. About 80% of women consume caffeine during their first trimester, probably before they realize they are pregnant. Studies of rats consuming the equivalent of 12–24 cups of coffee a day did show a dose response teratogenic effect (24). Thus, it is probably prudent to advise women planning a pregnancy not to consume more than the equivalent amount of caffeine in 1–2 cups of coffee.

Tobacco. Women contemplating pregnancy should not smoke. Studies consistently demonstrate that smoking is associated with perinatal mortality and morbidity. Smoking is thought to cause increased placental vascular resistance, which may impair oxygen exchange. The increased carbon monoxide levels in women who smoke further impair oxygen delivery to the fetus. Consequences include increased risk for placenta abruptio, placenta previa, premature rupture of membranes,

preterm births, and spontaneous abortions. There has also been an association between smoking and development of sudden infant death syndrome. Long-term effects of nicotine exposure in utero include the increased risk of subsequent development of leukemia and Wilm's tumors.

Alcohol. Alcohol use during pregnancy brings on confusion and anxiety. There is an association between heavy consumption of alcohol and what is known as the Fetal Alcohol Syndrome. This is a constellation of neurological and morphological characteristics. However, what has not been well characterized is how much alcohol constitutes "heavy consumption." Even within the medical profession, there is controversy whether there is such a thing as a "safe" level of alcohol consumption. Most clinicians reassure patients that an occasional drink at a special celebration will not harm the fetus. However, there are also those clinicians who advocate complete abstinence of alcohol during pregnancy and pre-conception. They argue that it is impossible to predict which patients will be adversely affected by alcohol because the exact mechanism of the development of Fetal Alcohol Syndrome is not known. It is probably prudent to encourage patients planning a pregnancy to limit their alcohol intake to no more than one drink at any given event. Patients who the clinician suspects may have an alcohol abuse problem should be encouraged to be abstinent.

Cocaine. The clinician should advise women not to use cocaine during the pre-conception period. Referral for appropriate substance abuse treatment in this period may be necessary. There are many adverse effects associated with cocaine use during pregnancy. There is a high incidence of spontaneous abortion, intrauterine growth retardation, and placental abruptio. These are thought to be mediated by the vasoconstrictive effects of cocaine. There is also a higher incidence of congenital malformations such as limb reduction, gastrointestinal atresia, and cardiac anomalies. The clinician needs to make the patient aware of these potential complications.

Opiates. Opiate withdrawal is potentially life-threatening to the fetus. The best course of action in active narcotic users is to suggest a methadone maintenance program. The patient would then receive narcotics in a controlled setting which minimizes the negative effects the illicit drug culture has on the patient and avoids the erratic use pattern which could easily potentiate withdrawal. However, methadone treatment of narcotic addiction still subjects the fetus to opiate withdrawal upon birth. Therefore, in selected highly motivated patients, withdrawal from methadone can be attempted prior to conception. The clinician needs to make it clear to the patient that adequate contraception should be used during the withdrawal period and that attempts to conceive should not be made until withdrawal is complete.

Marijuana. This is the most common illicit drug used by women of childbearing age, especially during the first trimester when its anti-emetic properties are welcomed. Clinicians need to inform patients that the safety of marijuana during pregnancy has not been defined. Studies in monkeys have shown increased embryonic death and spontaneous abortions. However, these effects have not been documented in humans (24).

HYPERTENSION

Patients whose blood pressures are well controlled can remain on their medications. The exception is angiotension converting enzyme (ACE) inhibitors. There is a high incidence of fetal loss in animal studies. Limited human experience with ACE inhibitors in women who were unaware they were pregnant showed a high incidence of fetal acute renal failure. There is controversy regarding the use of diuretics in pregnancy. Theoretically, diuretics would blunt the normally increased circulating volume during pregnancy which may lead to retarded fetal growth. This has not been shown in studies, and patients who have been taking diuretics can remain safely on them during pregnancy. However, clinicians might not want to start diuretics during pregnancy. There has also been limited experience with calcium channel blockers in pregnant women. Hydralazine can cause fetal tachycardia and distress. Its use during pregnancy is limited to the intravenous form for rapid blood pressure control. Thus, if a pregnant patient expresses concern about her medications, an alternative plan to keeping her on her current medications (assuming an ACE inhibitor is not involved) would be to switch her to an agent with more clinical data. The drug that has been the most widely studied in pregnancy and subsequently in children exposed in utero is methyldopa (Aldomet). Beta blockers have been less studied but still have a long history of efficacy and safety. Either methyldopa or a beta blocker can be substituted for women on an ACE inhibitor or for women who do not wish to remain on their current regimen.

DIABETES

Much tighter glycemic control is needed during pregnancy to prevent the increased incidence of congenital malformations and macrosomia. Thus, diabetic women contemplating pregnancy should undergo intensified management. Hgb A1c should be checked monthly, and a woman should be advised not to become pregnant until Hgb A1c has been normal for 2 months. All patients should be taken off of oral hypoglycemic agents and placed on insulin therapy. Oral hypoglycemic agents cross the placenta and can result in fetal beta cell stimulation, leading to fetal hyperinsulinemia. The clinician should review home glucose monitoring techniques and good dietary practices with the patient. During the periconception period, patients should keep fasting glucose at more than 100 mg/dl and 2 hr post-prandial glucose no more than 120 mg/dl.

ASTHMA

Clinicians should inform patients that the course of asthma during pregnancy is unpredictable. However, if there have been previous pregnancies, the course of asthma is likely to be similar. About a third of patients will experience an improvement in asthma, a third will experience no change, and a third will have worsened asthma during pregnancy. Unfortunately, there are no other predictors of who will likely have worsened asthma. Patients who give a history of triggers that exacerbate their asthma should be counseled to avoid the known triggers. About 75–80% of patients have an allergic component to their asthma. Many patients receive immunotherapy ("allergy shots"). Patients who have been receiving immunotherapy can continue during pregnancy. The major risk is anaphylaxis which can induce uterine contractions. However, patients should not begin immunotherapy during pregnancy or contemplate starting immunotherapy while trying to conceive (25).

Patients may have concerns regarding the safety of their asthma medications during pregnancy (Table 20.11). The clinician should reassure patients that all asthma medications should be continued during pregnancy. Medications administered by inhalation act locally and have minimal systemic effects; therefore, there is theoretically very minimal risk to the fetus. Although the absolute safety of oral medications such as theophylline and corticosteroids are not known, the risk of hypoxia to the fetus outweighs the risks of the medications.

THYROID DISEASE

Clinicians should counsel women who are hypothyroid to continue thyroid hormone replacement. Patients should be euthyroid prior to conception.

Table 20.11.
Drugs and Dosages for Asthma and Associated Conditions Preferred for Use During Pregnancy*

Drug Class	Specific Drug	Dosage
Anti-Inflammatory	Cromolyn Sodium	2 puffs qid (inhalation) 2 sprays in each nostril bid-qid (intranasal for nasal symptoms)
	Beclomethasone	2–5 puffs bid-qid (inhalation) 2 sprays in each nostril bid (intranasal for allergic rhinitis)
	Prednisone	Burst for active symptoms: 40 mg a day, single or divided dose for 1 week, then taper for 1 week. If prolonged course is required, single a.m. dose on alternate days may minimize adverse effects.
Bronchodilator	Inhaled Beta-Agonist	2 puffs every 4 hours as needed
	Theophylline	Oral: Dose to reach serum concentration level of 8–12 µg/mL
Antihistamine	Chlorpheniramine	4 mg by mouth up to qid 8–12 mg sustained-release bid
	Tripelennamine	25–50 mg by mouth up to qid 100 mg sustained-release bid
Decongestant	Pseudoephedrine	60 mg by mouth up to qid 120 mg sustained-release bid
	Oxymetazoline	Intranasal spray or drops up to 5 days for rhinosinusitis
Cough	Guaifenesin	2 tsp by mouth qid
	Dextromethorphan	
Antibiotics	Amoxicillin	3 weeks therapy for sinusitis

*This table presents drugs and suggested dosages for the home management of asthma and associated conditions. Source and dosages for the treatment of exacerbations in the emergency department or hospital are presented in the full report of the working group. (From Report of the working group on asthma and pregnancy. NIH publication No. 93-3279 A. 1993.)

Women who are hypothyroid and not treated often have difficulty conceiving.

The most common thyroid disease clinicians are likely to encounter in young women is Grave's disease. Women should be counseled not to become pregnant until the hyperthyroidism is treated. There may be an increased risk for neonatal mortality, low birth weight, and congenital malformations. The three treatment options are thionamides, radioactive iodine, and partial thyroidectomy. The thionamides (see Chapter 18) interfere with the iodination of tyrosine. There are two drugs that are commonly used today, propylthiouracil (PTU) and methimazole. There may be an association between methimazole and a congenital scalp disorder called aplasia cutis. Therefore, PTU is the drug of choice for use in women who are contemplating pregnancy. There have been some studies that have shown no increased risk of hypothyroidism in children exposed in utero to PTU (26). Women who elect to have radioactive iodine should not become pregnant for 12 months afterwards. The fetal thyroid has a much higher affinity for iodine. Also, fetal tissues are much more sensitive to radiation. Women who did not know they were pregnant and received radioactive iodine had fetuses with higher incidences of microcephaly, mental retardation, and malignancies (26). Partial thyroidectomy is

done before conception or if the patient has already become pregnant, delayed until after the first trimester to decrease the risk of spontaneous abortions. The risks of this type of surgery to the patient are hypoparathyroidism and recurrent laryngeal nerve paralysis. Thus, today, surgery is done only after all other treatment options have failed.

SEIZURE DISORDERS

Clinicians should inform patients that the effect of pregnancy on seizure frequency is variable. Women who have few seizures can expect that during pregnancy their seizures will remain few. However, women whose seizures are not controlled tend to have increased seizure frequency during pregnancy. Risks to the fetus during a seizure are minimal unless the patient has status epilepticus. Then, there is a 50% risk of fetal loss, probably due to fetal hypoxia.

The major concern for many patients is whether taking anti-seizure medications will cause adverse effects for the fetus. All anticonvulsants have the potential for altering the absorption of folic acid. Therefore, women contemplating pregnancy should be taking folic acid supplements to decrease the risks of neural tube defects in their fetuses. Table 20.12 shows the major anti-convulsant drugs

Table 20.12.
Anticonvulsant Drugs Associated with Malformations in Infants

Drug	Minor Anomalies	Major Anomalies and Complications	Comment
Diphenylhydantoin[14,25,63] (Dilantin)	Craniofacial and digital; "fetal hydantoin embryopathy"	Cleft lip and palate; delay in growth and cognitive development	Causal determinants also include genetic and environmental factors
Carbamazepine[41] (Tegretol)		Risks similar to diphenylhydantoin	
Trimethadione[30,64,65] (Tridione) and Paramethadione	Fetal trimethadione syndrome; craniofacial	Congenital heart defects; perinatal mortality rate; delayed growth and psychomotor development; neural tube defects; spina bifida	CONTRAINDICATED IN PREGNANCY
Valprorate[66] (Depakene or Depakote)	Not described		CONTRAINDICATED IN PREGNANCY
Phenobarbital[67,68]	Case reports of facial anomalies and minor anomalies		Limited information
Diazepam[69-72] (Valium)	Eight fold increase in frequency of facial clefts		Limited studies
Primidone[73,74] (Mysoline)	Case reports of malformations congenital heart defects, growth and developmental retardation when used along or with other anticonvulsants		Limited information
Ethosuximide[75,76] (Zarontin)	Inadequate data		No information
Clonopin[75,76] (Clonazepam)	Inadequate data		No information

From Wiederholt WC. Neurologic disorders. In: Hollingsworth DR, Resnick R, eds. Medical counseling before pregnancy. New York: Churchill Livingstone, 1988:421.

and associated congenital abnormalities. Women should continue their anti-convulsants unless they are taking valproic acid or carbamazepine. In that case, a neurologist should be consulted for advice regarding the next best agent. Phenobarbital may have fewer teratogenic effects so a trial of it may be warranted. Clinicians should review the seizure history with all patients to determine if anti-convulsant medications are really needed. If a patient has been seizure free for 2 years or more, the clinician should consider tapering off the medications, usually in consultation with a neurologist.

CONGENITAL HEART DISEASE

Most patients with a history of congenital heart disease who present for pre-conception care have had the lesion(s) repaired. If this has not been the case, the clinician should advise the patient to undergo surgical correction prior to planning a pregnancy. Repair of the lesion will improve the hemodynamics of the maternal circulation and provide a better environment for the fetus (27).

Several congenital cardiac lesions go unnoticed until the patient is well into adulthood. The most common is an asymptomatic atrial septal defect (ASD). Clinicians can tell patients that pregnancy is usually well tolerated. However, if the ratio of blood flow between the pulmonary and systemic circulations, as determined by echocardiography, is greater than 1.5, increased pulmonary arterial pressures could reverse the left to right shunt. These patients should be advised to have the ASD repaired before pregnancy. Patients should also be informed that there is a 15% incidence of fetal loss and that correction of the ASD does not necessarily improve this statistic. Also, there will be a higher incidence of ASD in the patient's children.

Patients with interseptal hypertrophic subaortic stenosis (IHSS) also need to be advised of the increased risk of IHSS in their children. Pregnancy is often difficult because there could be increased outflow obstruction necessitating bedrest. However, pregnancy itself is not contraindicated. The patient needs to be informed of these risks and of the potential for a more complicated course of pregnancy.

ILLUSTRATIVE CASES WITH SELF-ASSESSMENT QUESTIONS AND ANSWERS

Case 1

A 29-year-old woman who was diagnosed with diabetes mellitus 3 months ago when she presented with diabetic ketoacidosis necessitating a 2-wk hospital admission now presents for regular medical care. The patient takes 20 units of NPH insulin in the morning and 10 units of NPH insulin in the evening. During her hospitalization, she learned how to do home glucose monitoring and received diet counseling. However, her blood glucose values are all above 200 mg/dl, sometimes even in the 300 mg/dl range. She is recently married and is eager to start a family soon.

QUESTION: *What do you advise this patient?*

ANSWER: *Inform the patient that her diabetes is not in good control and that the risks of congenital malformation and macrosomia are increased because her diabetes is not yet optimally managed. The patient should also be informed that much tighter control of glucose will be needed during*

the periconception period, that ideally, fasting glucose should be less than or equal to 100 mg/dl and 2 hour post-prandial glucose should be less than or equal to 120 mg/dl. This will necessitate the patient monitoring her glucose at least 7 times per day, before each meal, 2 hours after each meal and at bedtime. Recommend that she delay pregnancy until her diabetes is under better control. Referral to a nutritionist would also be a good idea to reinforce dietary management of diabetes.

Case 2

The same patient in Case 1 returns to the clinic 3 weeks later now on 30 units of NPH insulin in the morning and 15 units of NPH insulin in the evening. She says that she is finding it difficult to monitor her glucose even 4 times a day. Although her glucose control is better, her morning fasting glucose still remains above 200 mg/dl. She also says that she has been thinking about your previous discussion and that she and her husband are not using any contraception because they are trying to conceive. She states that even though there is increased risk of congenital malformation, she is willing to take the risk knowing that it still amounts to a less than 5% risk. Afterall, she says that means that there is still a greater than 90% chance of having a healthy baby.

QUESTION: *How would you respond to this patient?*

ANSWER: *Reinforce the previous discussion but realize that in the end, the choice of whether to delay pregnancy is up to the patient and her husband, even though the clinician may not necessarily agree with the decision. Make sure the patient understands the risks, although it seems clear that she does.*

Case 3

The practice has recently become affiliated with a managed care plan. One day, a 26-year-old woman comes into the office to seek general medical care. However, she immediately says that she thinks she is pregnant and wants a referral to a gynecologist so that she can have an abortion. When asked why she desires an abortion, the patient states that she and her partner attend regular social functions and drink alcohol, mostly wine. She is afraid that because she has been drinking, she has already harmed her fetus. She states that had she been planning to get pregnant, she would have abstained completely.

QUESTION: *What do you tell the patient?*

ANSWER: *Tell the patient that although the decision to have an abortion is hers and that a referral to a gynecologist will be made if she wishes, her fears may be too magnified. An assessment of the patient's degree of alcohol consumption to rule out a substance abuse problem should be done. Assuming that no clinical suspicion of substance abuse exists, the patient should be told that although a "safe" level of alcohol consumption has not been determined for pregnant women, many more women drink during pregnancy than there are babies born with Fetal Alcohol Syndrome. Thus, her decision to have an abortion should not rest solely on the fact that she has been consuming wine.*

CONTRACEPTION

Control of fertility is a major issue throughout most of a woman's life. A woman's reproductive life cycle can be divided into three parts: the time from first sexual intercourse to the birth of her first child, the time from her first to her last child, and the time from her last child to menopause. On average, a woman will spend about 8 1/2 years in the first stage, 4 years in the second, and 18 1/2 years in the last. Thus, she may spend about 27 years of her reproductive life trying to avoid pregnancy. That is more than three-quarters of her entire reproductive life span of 35–40 years (28).

Patients often turn to their primary care clinicians for information and advice regarding contraception issues. Unfortunately, many clinicians do not discuss these issues with their patients. Reasons for this are many and have as much to do with the scientific controversies surrounding the safety and efficacy of currently available contraception as well as the ethical, moral, and religious issues any discussion about contraception can evoke. Unfortunately, the current political climate in the United States has tied contraception to the more controversial issue of abortion. Women often obtain contraceptive services in the same place that abortions are being performed. As the number of such clinics declines because of violence and terrorism, women are at increased risk of being denied contraception, making them more at risk for needing an abortion.

A woman's decision to actively control her fertility has many beneficial aspects. A woman's health is placed at more risk if she does not desire pregnancy, but leaves contraception to chance. Contraception can reduce the risk of death from pregnancy-related causes. Even though there may be inherent risks to the contraceptive method itself, these are far outweighed by the benefits of decreased pregnancy-related mortality. Furthermore, many contraceptive methods have non-contraceptive benefits associated with their use, as illustrated in Table 20.13. For example, barrier methods can reduce the incidence of sexually transmitted diseases (STD) including HIV, and hormone related contraceptive methods have been shown to decrease the incidence of certain cancers. Clinicians who ignore a discussion of contraception with their female patients are not providing optimal care.

Pathophysiologic Correlation

MENSTRUAL CYCLE

The menstrual cycle is divided into two phases, follicular and luteal, that are based on changes that occur in the ovary. However, these two phases also correspond to simultaneous changes that occur in the endometrium and the cervical mucous. The

Table 20.13.
Major Methods of Contraception and Some Related Safety Concerns, Side Effects, and Noncontraceptive Benefits

Method	Dangers	Side Effects	Noncontraceptive Benefits
Pill	Cardiovascular complications (stroke, heart attack, blood clots, high blood pressure, hepatic adenomas)	Nausea, headaches, dizziness, spotting, weight gain, breast tenderness, chloasma	Protects against PID, some cancers (ovarian, endometrial) and some benign tumors (leiomyomata, benign breast masses) and ovarian cysts; decreases menstrual blood loss and pain
IUD	Pelvic inflammatory disease, uterine perforation, anemia	Menstrual cramping, spotting, increased bleeding	None known except progestin-releasing IUDs which may decrease menstrual blood loss and pain
Male Condom	None known	Decreased sensation, allergy to latex, loss of spontaneity	Protects against sexually transmitted diseases, including AIDS; delays premature ejaculation
Female Condom	None known	Aesthetically unappealing and awkward to use for some	Protects against sexually transmitted diseases, including on the vulva
Implant	Infection at implant site	Tenderness at site, menstrual changes	May protect against PID; lactation not disturbed; may decrease menstrual cramps, pains and blood loss
Injectable	None definitely proven	Menstrual changes, weight gain, headaches	May protect against PID; lactation not disturbed; may have protective effects against ovarian and endometrial cancers
Sterilization	Infection	Pain at surgical site, psychological reactions, subsequent regret that the procedure was performed	None known; may have beneficial effects vis a vis PID
Abstinence	None known	Psychological reactions	Prevents infections including AIDS
Abortion	Infection, pain, perforation, psychological trauma	Cramping	None known
Barriers: Diaphragm, Cap, Sponge	Mechanical irritation, vaginal infections, toxic shock syndrome	Pelvic pressure, cervical erosion, vaginal discharges if left in too long	Protects somewhat against sexually transmitted diseases
Spermicides	None known	Tissue irritation	Protects against many sexually transmitted diseases
Lactational Amenorrhea Method (LAM)	None known	Mastitis from staphylococcal infection	Provides excellent nutrition for infants under 6 months old

From Hatcher RA, Trussel J, Stewart F et al. Contraceptive technology 16th ed. New York: Irvington Publishers Inc. 1994:129.

cycle is regulated by complex interactions between hormones at the hypothalamic, pituitary, and ovarian levels. Figure 20.6 illustrates these complex interactions.

The hypothalamus secretes gonadotropin releasing hormone (GnRH) in a pulsatile manner, which serves to regulate the overall function of the menstrual cycle. The pulsatile release of GnRH signals the pituitary to make follicle stimulating hormone (FSH) and luteinizing hormone (LH)

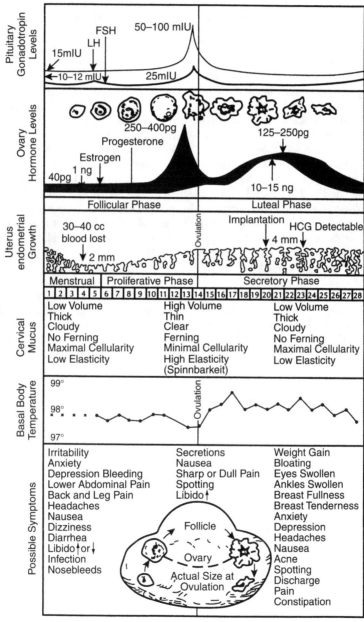

Figure 20.6. Menstrual cycle events: hormone levels, ovarian and endometrial patterns, and cyclic temperature and cervical mucus changes. (From Hatcher RA, Trussel J, Stewart F et al. Contraceptive technology 16th ed. New York: Irvington Publishers Inc. 1994:41.)

which in turn act on the ovary to produce estrogen and progesterone. Estrogen and progesterone have the potential to exert negative or positive feedback depending on the place in the menstrual cycle, upon the pituitary gland and hypothalamus to regulate the amount of FSH and LH.

The first day of the menstrual cycle is the first day of a woman's menses. The endometrium sheds its lining because at this point in the cycle levels of estrogen and progesterone are low. This is also the beginning of the follicular phase. At the beginning of this phase, many ovarian follicles begin to grow. Because there are low amounts of estrogen and progesterone, the hypothalamus releases GnRH to stimulate the release of FSH from the pituitary right about the time menses cease. As an increase in FSH occurs, follicles at the right stage to be stimulated by FSH begin to release estrogen. Other follicles that were not at the right stage of development to respond to FSH stimulation die. Eventually, one follicle becomes the dominant follicle, secreting increasing amounts of estrogen. The endometrium responds to the increased estrogen by proliferation of its lining. The cervix responds to the increased estrogen by production of thin, watery, cervical mucous.

At about mid cycle, ovulation occurs. As sustained increased amounts of estrogen are being produced by the dominant follicle, the pituitary responds by increasing production of LH. The increased LH stimulates the ovary to produce progesterone and androgens. Many women note increased sexual desire during this time which coincides with the increased androgenic activity. When the peak amount of estrogen is produced by the dominant follicle, a surge in LH production occurs. This sets into action a series of events that culminates in ovulation within 34–36 hours. The LH peak temporarily inhibits production of estrogen by the ovary resulting in a slight dip in the amount of estrogen. This is responsible for the mid cycle spotting some women experience.

The Luteal phase begins after ovulation when the ruptured follicle becomes the corpus luteum. The corpus luteum secretes estrogen, progesterone, and androgens. The increased levels of estrogen and progesterone affect the endometrium by causing its maturation making implantation of an embryo possible should the ovum become fertilized. The cervical mucous responds to increased progesterone by becoming scant and thick. The basal body temperature increases after ovulation probably due to the increased amount of progesterone. The peak amount of estrogen and progester-

one occur at about mid-luteal phase. These increased levels of estrogen and progesterone exert a negative feedback on the pituitary and cause the decreased release of LH and FSH. Decreased levels of LH and FSH cause the corpus luteum to degenerate and stop secreting estrogen and progesterone. Estrogen and progesterone levels fall so that eventually, at their lowest point, menses begins and the next cycle starts.

The life span of the ovum is 1–3 days. Sperm can remain viable in the female reproductive tract between 2–7 days. Fertilization occurs in the Fallopian tubes when the sperm attaches to a receptor on the zona pellucida, the halo that surrounds the oocyte. The sperm releases enzymes to penetrate the zona as the zona undergoes changes to make it impervious to other sperm. Eventually, the sperm and oocyte cell membranes fuse, and chromosomal fusion also occurs. Once the oocyte has been fertilized, it begins to make human chorionic gonadotropin (HCG) which supports the corpus luteum to maintain secretion of estrogen and progesterone so that endometrial shedding does not occur. The newly created embryo, called a blastocyst, remains in the fallopian tube for 2 days actively undergoing cell division. At the third day, the blastocyst travels to the uterine cavity and sheds the zona pellucida and comes into direct contact with the endometrial surface. A complex process occurs which allows the embryo to grow into the endometrium. This is known as implantation and begins at about day 6 and is completed by the 12th day.

MECHANISMS OF CONTRACEPTION

Conception can be disrupted by providing a physical barrier between sperm and the female reproductive tract so that the probability of sperm reaching the Fallopian tube to fertilize the ovum is greatly decreased. These methods are among the oldest known to mankind, and today are still being used as the diaphragm, cervical cap, and condom. Alternatively, conception can also be prevented by means of spermicides which kill the sperm before it can reach the Fallopian tube. Spermicides that are available in the U.S. act as surfactants to cause increased cell permeability resulting in leakage of sperm cell components and eventual disruption of cell membranes.

Other forms of contraception rely on hormonal manipulation of the menstrual cycle. The combined oral contraceptives use estrogen and progesterone to make conception theoretically impossible. Doses of estrogen and progesterone used in the oral contraceptives suppress FSH and LH to inhibit the emergence of a dominant follicle and to inhibit ovulation by inhibiting the LH surge. Furthermore, progesterone makes the endometrium unsuitable for implantation by making the tissue atrophic. Estrogen stabilizes this atrophic endometrium so that breakthrough bleeding does not occur. Progesterone also makes the cervical mucous thick and impenetrable to sperm, as in the luteal phase of the menstrual cycle. Progesterone may also inhibit the enzymes that allow sperm to penetrate the ovum. Progesterone can be used by itself as a contraceptive agent. Its effects would be on the cervical mucous, endometrium, and enzymes, but ovulation would not necessarily be inhibited without the presence of exogenous estrogen to completely inhibit FSH and LH.

Finally, contraception can theoretically be achieved by following the menstrual cycle and limiting sexual activity to the luteal phase, 3 days after ovulation to ensure that the ovum is no longer viable. Women can predict ovulation by charting their menstrual cycles, noting the quality of the cervical mucous, and/or recording basal body temperatures.

Clinical and Laboratory Evaluation

Counseling patients about contraception should be part of the general evaluation of all female patients in their reproductive years. The history, physical examination, and laboratory evaluation are no different from what would be ordinarily provided by the thorough primary care clinician. Contraceptive choices can change with time and thus should be evaluated yearly or whenever the patient has undergone a major life change, e.g., marriage, pregnancy, divorce.

HISTORY

A thorough history should be obtained from every patient. Particular attention should be paid to any pre-existing medical conditions such as diabetes, heart disease, breast disease, malignancies, and hypertension, as these can limit contraceptive choices. The patient should also be asked about any current medications she is taking because there might be important drug interactions with certain contraceptives. A thorough menstrual history should be obtained which includes information on menarche, presence of dysmenorrhea, previous pregnancies, and previous experiences with contraception. A good sexual history should also be obtained. Many clinicians are uncomfortable with asking patients

such detailed questions and often omit this part of the history. However, information about the number of sexual partners, previous history of STDs, and possible HIV risk factors are all relevant to the choice of a contraceptive and thus need to be obtained. Clinicians should be nonjudgmental and professional in their approach to the patient. Do not assume that every patient is heterosexual or assume that every married patient is monogamous. Examples of questions that can be asked are: "In the past year, have you had sex with another person?" "How many people?" "Did you have sex with men, women, or both?" "What do you do to protect yourself from AIDS?" "What do you do to protect yourself from an unplanned pregnancy (28)?"

Other relevant information to be elicited includes any family history of cancer, diabetes, coronary artery disease, or cerebral vascular disease. Patients should also be asked about tobacco, alcohol, and drug use. Finally, clinicians need to get a sense from the patient about her future plans for pregnancy, i.e., how many children she currently has, whether she has had all the children she wants, or whether at some point in the future she will want fertility to return.

PHYSICAL EXAMINATION

A thorough physical examination should be performed on all patients. All patients should also have a pelvic examination. Occasionally, a patient will ask that the pelvic be deferred. Reasons include current menses or discomfort at the first visit with a new clinician. Certain types of contraception (oral contraceptives, progestin only methods, spermicides, condoms) can still be discussed and prescribed if the clinician feels comfortable that the patient is at low risk for a STD (29). However, the patient should return within 3 months for the pelvic examination.

LABORATORY EVALUATION

In a healthy nonsmoking patient, no specific laboratory tests need to be obtained before prescribing contraception. Patients should always have a PAP smear done as part of the pelvic examination. Pregnancy should always be excluded before any contraceptive method is started. If a patient has irregular periods or is not sure whether she could be pregnant, the clinician should obtain a pregnancy test before advising the patient to begin contraception. Patients who are at risk for STD should be screened for gonorrhea and chlamydia. Women who are contemplating using an intrauterine device (IUD) for contraception should also be screened for cervical infection prior to IUD insertion.

Differential Diagnosis

There are many contraceptive choices, but some may be more appropriate for a particular patient. The role of the clinician is to provide the patient with information about each method and its safety and efficacy. The patient should also be counseled regarding which methods might be more appropriate for her. The following section will outline the basic ideas behind each method, advantages and disadvantages, and appropriate candidates for the method (See Table 20.13). Some of these methods may require skills beyond that of a primary care clinician for initiation and maintenance. Referral to a gynecologist is then recommended, but clinicians who provide primary care to women should be comfortable discussing all contraceptive methods.

Table 20.14 shows the available contraceptive methods and their efficacy. Data on the efficacy of

Table 20.14.
Failure Rates of Methods of Contraception During the First Year of Use

	Percent of Women with Pregnancy	
Method	Lowest Expected	Typical
No method	85.0	85.0
Combination pill	0.1	3.0
Progestin only	0.5	3.0
IUDs		3.0
Progesterone IUD	2.0	<2.0
Copper T 380A	0.8	<1.0
Norplant	0.2	0.2
Female sterilization	0.2	0.4
Male sterilization	0.1	0.15
Depo-Provera	0.3	0.3
Spermicides	3.0	21.0
Periodic abstinence		20.0
Calendar	9.0	
Ovulation method	3.0	
Symptothermal	2.0	
Post-ovulation	1.0	
Withdrawal	4.0	18.0
Cervical cap	6.0	18.0
Sponge		
Parous women	9.0	28.0
Nulliparous women	6.0	18.0
Diaphragm and spermicides	6.0	18.0
Condom	2.0	12.0

From Speroff L and Darney PD eds. A clinical guide for contraception. Baltimore: Williams & Wilkins. 1992:5.

various methods are usually obtained from rigorous studies before the method has been approved by the FDA. These failure rates are among the lowest quoted for that particular method. Once the method is in general use however, failure rates typically run higher than with controlled studies. That is because not everyone who uses a particular method uses it correctly every time. This is especially true for patient-initiated methods such as oral contraceptives and barrier methods, which require the patient to actively make an intervention to prevent conception. Patients should understand that individual circumstances can make typical failure rates higher or lower than expected. When counseling patients, clinicians need to bring out aspects obtained from the medical history that may make a certain method less efficacious for that patient.

BARRIER METHODS

Currently available barrier methods in the U.S. include the diaphragm, the cervical cap, and both male and female condoms. The cervical sponge has recently been discontinued by its manufacturer and will probably no longer be available (30). These methods all act to form a barrier between sperm and the female reproductive tract, thereby decreasing the chance that fertilization will occur. The diaphragm and cervical cap are used with spermicide, which adds yet another mechanism of contraception.

The major advantage to barrier methods is that they can protect against transmission of STDs and therefore, protect a woman's reproductive tract against the consequences of PID. The male latex condom protects against the transmission of HIV, but studies have not been done to show this for the diaphragm and cervical cap. However, the diaphragm can protect against cervical cancer, which is transmitted by the human papilloma virus (HPV) so theoretically, it should also be protective against transmission of HIV. The female condom is made of polyurethane which is stronger than the latex that male condoms are made from and theoretically should provide protection against STDs and HIV.

Risks associated with the use of barrier methods are minimal. Some women may experience vaginal irritation associated with spermicide use. This may be more common with the diaphragm as larger amounts of spermicide are used than with the cervical cap. The spermicide may also be responsible for the increased incidence of urinary tract infections among diaphragm users. It is thought that the spermicide alters the normal flora of the vagina and makes the environment more favorable for the growth of urinary pathogens. Spermicide may also play a role in the observed increased incidence of abnormal pap smears in women who use the cervical cap. Perhaps the spermicide enhances early neoplastic changes in women who are already infected by HPV (31).

Besides protection against STDs, another major advantage to the use of barrier methods is that they do not have any systemic effects. This is especially important for the patient who has medical conditions that may be worsened by the use of hormonally derived forms of contraception. This is true for some women with diabetes. Barrier methods should be recommended first to diabetic patients (32).

The female condom is sold over the counter so that patients do not need to visit a health care practitioner to obtain it. Thus, along with the male condom, it is among some of the cheaper contraceptive methods available. Patients however, need to be fitted for both the diaphragm and cervical cap. There are many sizes and types of diaphragms available in the United States so that more women are able to use this method. There is only one type of cervical cap available in the U.S, only 4 sizes; therefore, some patients may not be able to be fitted with the cap. Even though a visit to a clinician is required to obtain the diaphragm or cervical cap, both are still relatively inexpensive. After the initial expense of the office visit and the purchase of the diaphragm or cap, the patient subsequently only has the costs associated with obtaining the spermicide.

All barrier methods require the patient's active participation. They must be used each time intercourse is to take place. Some patients may feel that spontaneity during lovemaking is important and may not be able to tolerate having to insert a contraceptive device before each act of intercourse. However, the diaphragm can be inserted up to 6 hours before intercourse, the cervical cap 24 hours. Some partners are not able to tolerate the presence of these devices and may pressure the patient not to use these methods of contraception. This is especially true of the male condom. Female patients have to rely on their partner's willingness to use a condom for this method to be effective. The aforementioned disadvantages are responsible for the failure rates associated with the use of these barrier methods. Other reasons that patients may have higher than quoted failure rates include age less than 30, frequent intercourse (more than 3 times a week), and a lifestyle that suggests use of the method will be inconsistent.

The only contraindication to the use of the female condom is allergy to the polyurethane material from which it is made. Patients who express unwillingness to learn how to insert either the condom, cervical cap, or diaphragm correctly or who seem squeamish about having to insert anything are probably not good candidates for any of the barrier methods. The cervical cap is more difficult to learn how to insert than the other methods. Women who have latex allergy or allergy to spermicides are not candidates for the diaphragm or cervical cap. Women who have had a history of toxic shock syndrome are also not advised to use either the diaphragm or cervical cap because these are left in place 6–24 hours post intercourse and may serve as a nidus for development of toxic shock syndrome. Because there has been an association between abnormal PAP smears and cervical cap use, clinicians should avoid recommending the cervical cap to a patient with a history of abnormal PAP smears. Lastly, patients with anatomical abnormalities may not be candidates for the diaphragm or cervical cap because they may not be able to be properly fitted. Similarly, multiparous women sometimes are unable to be fitted for the cervical cap, and those who manage to be fitted experience higher failure rates.

SPERMICIDES

Spermicides can be used alone for contraception. They are sold over the counter so pose little barriers for the patient to obtain them. Table 20.15 shows currently available spermicides. They are also inexpensive because a visit to the clinician is not needed. The only contraindication to spermicide use is a history of allergy to the spermicide.

The spermicide Nonoxynol-9 inactivates Herpes simplex virus (HSV) and HIV. It also offers protection against chlamydia and gonorrhea. However, there is some controversy surrounding the use of spermicides and protection against STDs. There is concern that frequent use of spermicides, which can be irritating to the vaginal mucosa, could actually increase transmission of HIV by the disruption of the vaginal mucosa.

Women may be concerned that the use of a spermicide may pose potential harm to their unborn children. Women should be counseled to visit their clinician if they suspect they are pregnant and to avoid using spermicides until pregnancy has been confirmed or denied. Patients should be counseled that the inadvertent use of spermicides during early pregnancy has not been shown to cause congenital abnormalities or miscarriages. Clinicians should

Table 20.15.
Available Spermicides

Product (Manufacturer)	Form	Spermicide
Conceptrol gel (Ortho)	Jelly	Nonoxynol-9, 4%
Conceptrol inserts (Ortho)	Suppositories	Nonoxynol-9, 8.34% 150 mg
Delfen (Ortho)	Foam	Nonoxynol-9, 12.5%
Emko (Schering)	Foam	Nonoxynol-9, 8%
Encare (Thompson Medical)	Suppositories	Nonoxynol-9, 2.27%
Gynol II extra strength (Ortho)	Jelly	Nonoxynol-9, 3%
Koromex (Schmid)	Foam	Nonoxynol-9, 12.5%
Koromex (Schmid)	Jelly	Nonoxynol-9, 3%
Koromex (Schmid)	Suppositories	Nonoxynol-9, 125 mg
Ramses (Schmid)	Jelly	Nonoxynol-9, 5%
Semicid (Whitehall)	Suppositories	Nonoxynol-9, 100 mg
Today Sponge (Whitehall)	Sponge	Nonoxynol-9, 1,000 mg
VCF (Apothecus)	Suppositories (film)	Nonoxynol-9, 72 mg
Gynol II original formula (Ortho)	Jelly	Nonoxynol-9, 2%
Koromex (Schmid)	Cream	Octoxynol, 3%
Koromex crystal clear (Schmid)	Jelly	Nonoxynol-9, 2%

Table 20.15.
Continued

Product (Manufacturer)	Form	Spermicide
Ortho-Creme (Ortho)	Cream	Nonoxynol-9, 2%
Ortho-Gynol (Ortho)	Jelly	Octoxynol-9, 1%
VCF (Apothecus)	Suppositories (Film)	Nonoxynol-9, 72 mg

FDA categorizes the film as a suppository because it is rolled up and inserted. (From Creinin M, Keith LG. Spermicides. In: Corson SL, Derman RJ, Tyrer LB, eds. Fertility control, 2nd ed. Ontario: Goldin Publishers, 1994;238.)

advise women to use an alternative method of contraception, e.g., the male condom, until their visit.

Appropriate candidates for use of spermicides alone are women who have infrequent intercourse who need a method that is inexpensive. The long shelf life of available spermicides is ideal for this situation. The woman who chooses to use a spermicide as the sole method of contraception should be at low risk for STDs. Clinicians should recommend the concomitant use of a barrier method if the patient may be at risk for PID/STDs. Table 20.16 summarizes important instructions for patients regarding spermicide use.

COMBINED ORAL CONTRACEPTIVE PILLS

Exogenous estrogen and progesterone inhibit ovulation, make changes in the endometrium to inhibit implantation, and render the cervical mucous impenetrable to sperm. For a more detailed discussion of the mechanisms of estrogen and progesterone, please refer to the Pathophysiologic Correlation section. The formulations of oral contraceptive pills which are available in the U.S. today are listed in Table 20.17. Most of the oral contraceptives in use currently contain much lower doses of estrogen than previously. Much of the controversy surrounding the use of oral contraceptives is based on studies that were done at the time when women were taking higher dosed estrogen oral contraceptives. Unfortunately, there has not been as much data obtained from women on the lower dosed estrogen oral contraceptives. Nevertheless, oral contraceptives are among the most well-studied medications in existence. The clinician needs to

Table 20.16.
Essential Instructions for the Use of Spermicides

- If a couple chooses spermicide as their method of contraception, the spermicidal preparation must be used with each and every act of intercourse to be effective. Additional acts of intercourse require repeated applications of spermicide.
- For maximal effectiveness, the spermicide should be combined with a condom, diaphragm, or cervical cap.
- The spermicide must be applied high in the vagina in order to cover the cervical os.
- Foams, creams and jellies are immediately effective after application and may be applied up to one hour before intercourse. Suppositories should be inserted 10–15 minutes before intercourse and also may be applied up to one hour before intercourse. Contraceptive film requires 5 minutes to dissolve after application and is effective for 2 hours.
- Douching, if performed, should not be done until at least 8 hours after intercourse. If the combination of spermicide and ejaculate becomes too messy, let the excess drain into the toilet or a cloth and wash the external genitalia with a damp cloth.
- If minor burning or irritation develops, the user should switch to another brand or, if irritation is experienced with many different products, use an alternative method of birth control.
- The cervical cap minimizes the amount of spermicide exposed to the vagina or penis. The use of condoms will also protect the male from exposure to spermicidal agents and thus help him to avoid any undesired side effects. The spermicidal preparations designed for use with a diaphragm or cervical cap have lower concentrations of spermicide and should not be used alone.

From Creinin M, Keith LG. Spermicides. In: Corson SL, Derman RJ, Tyrer LB, eds. Fertility control, 2nd ed. Ontario: Goldin Publishers, 1994;244.

emphasize to appropriate patients that currently available oral contraceptives are both very safe and very effective.

Oral contraceptives contain a synthetic estrogen, ethinyl estradiol or mestranol combined with a progestin. Ethinyl estradiol is the biologically active synthetic estrogen. Mestranol is converted into ethinyl estradiol by the liver. It has not been used in any new oral contraceptives introduced since 1968 (1), although formulations containing mestranol are still available. There is a range of progestins available with some that are more androgenic than others. More androgenic progestins have the potential to alter the lipid profile in patients and also may be more responsible for side

effects such as weight gain and acne. In general, levonorgestrel is more androgenic than norethindrone. There are three newer progestins that have become recently available, desogestrel, gestodene, and norgestimate which are weaker androgens and may affect lipid and carbohydrate metabolism less (6).

There are many benefits associated with the use of oral contraceptives besides that of fertility control. Women taking oral contraceptives are at decreased risk for endometrial and ovarian cancers and may be at decreased risk for PID, although the mechanism is unclear (7). Because the monthly withdrawal bleeding associated with oral contraceptive use is much less than a regular period, women who have a history of menorrhagia have improved symptoms and less anemia. Similarly, women with irregular periods benefit from oral contraceptive use. Women with a history of dysmenorrhea will often find that their symptoms are improved on oral contraceptives, probably because regular ovulatory cycles have been inhibited.

As Table 20.17 shows, the cost of oral contraceptives is about $30 per month. Often, this cost is not reimbursed by third party payers, but the cost compares favorably to other methods such as Norplant or Depo-Provera, which are much more expensive. Though barrier methods are cheaper, oral contraceptives are still affordable for most patients.

There has been a lot of concern regarding the risks of cardiovascular disease and stroke among women who use oral contraceptives. Although some of the more androgenic progestins can increase LDL and decrease HDL, it is unknown what clinical significance this has. There is currently no evidence to suggest that the low dosed estrogen oral contraceptives used today are associated with an increased risk of cardiovascular death (6), and in otherwise healthy young women who do not have any risk factors for cardiovascular disease, oral contraceptives are very safe. With the new progestins, alterations in lipid levels should no longer be of concern. For women who smoke, there is a synergistic effect between oral contraceptives and smoking to increase the risk of thrombosis, which could become clinically significant, especially in older women. Women who have other risk factors for cardiovascular disease, such as diabetes, are also at increased risk of thrombosis while taking oral contraceptives.

The progestin component of oral contraceptives can sometimes impair glucose tolerance. However, the newer progestins desogestrel, norgestimate,

Table 20.17.
Some Currently Available Oral Contraceptives

Drug	Estrogen (μg)[a]	Progestin (mg)[b]	Cost[c]
COMBINATION			
Loestrin 1/20 21, 28 (Parke-Davis)	Ethinyl estradiol (20)	Norethindrone acetate (1)	$25.24
Loestrin 1.5/30 21, 28 (Parke-Davis)	Ethinyl estradiol (30)	Norethindrone acetate (1.5)	25.24
Levlen 21, 28 (Berlex)	Ethinyl estradiol (30)	Levonorgestrel (0.15)	20.58
Nordette-21 (Wyeth-Ayerst)[d]	Ethinyl estradiol (30)	Levonorgestrel (0.15)	25.29
Lo/Ovral (Wyeth-Ayerst)[d]	Ethinyl estradiol (30)	Norgestrel (0.3)	26.21
Desogen (Organon)	Ethinyl estradiol (30)	Desogestrel (0.15)	19.55
Ortho-Cept 21 (Ortho)[d]	Ethinyl estradiol (30)	Desogestrel (0.15)	22.20
Tri-Levlen 21, 28 (Berlex)	Ethinyl estradiol (30, 40, 30)	Levonorgestrel (0.05, 0.075, 0.125)	19.73
Triphasil-21 (Wyeth-Ayerst)[d]	Ethinyl estradiol (30, 40, 30)	Levonorgestrel (0.05, 0.075, 0.125)	25.03
Ortho Tri-Cyclen (Ortho)[d]	Ethinyl estradiol (35, 35, 35)	Norgestimate (0.18, 0.215, 0.25)	22.20
Ovcon 35 21, 28 (Mead Johnson)	Ethinyl estradiol (35)	Norethindrone (0.4)	24.63
Brevicon 21, 28 (Syntex)	Ethinyl estradiol (35)	Norethindrone (0.5)	22.08
Genora 0.5/35 28 (Rugby)	Ethinyl estradiol (35)	Norethindrone (0.5)	9.06
Modicon 21 (Ortho)[d]	Ethinyl estradiol (35)	Norethindrone (0.5)	24.17
Nelova 0.5/35E 21 (Warner-Chilcott)[d]	Ethinyl estradiol (35)	Norethindrone (0.5)	13.90
Tri-Norinyl 21, 28 (Syntex)	Ethinyl estradiol (35, 35, 35)	Norethindrone (0.5, 1.0, 0.5)	21.38
Ortho-Novum 7/7/7 21 (Ortho)[d]	Ethinyl estradiol (35, 35, 35)	Norethindrome (0.5, 0.75, 1.0)	22.20
Nelova 10/11 21 (Warner-Chilcott)[d]	Ethinyl estradiol (35)	Norethindrone (0.5, 1)	13.90
Ortho-Novum 10/11 21 (Ortho)[d]	Ethinyl estradiol (35, 35)	Norethindrone (0.5, 1.0)	24.17
Jenest-28 (Organon)	Ethinyl estradiol (35)	Norethindrone (1)	16.93
Genora 1/35 21, 28 (Rugby)	Ethinyl estradiol (35)	Norethindrone (1)	12.10
N.E.E. 1/35 21, 28 (Lexis)	Ethinyl estradiol (35)	Norethindrone (1)	10.25
Nelova 1/35 21 (Warner-Chilcott)[d]	Ethinyl estradiol (35)	Norethindrone (1)	12.38
Norethin 1/35E 21, 28 (Roberts)	Ethinyl estradiol (35)	Norethindrone (1)	11.65
Norinyl 1/35 21, 28 (Syntex)	Ethinyl estradiol (35)	Norethindrone (1)	21.41
Ortho-Novum 1/35 21 (Ortho)[d]	Ethinyl estradiol (35)	Norethindrone (1)	22.06
Ortho-Cyclen (Ortho)[d]	Ethinyl estradiol (35)	Norgestimate (0.25)	22.20
Demulen 1/35 21 (Searle)[d]	Ethinyl estradiol (35)	Ethynodiol diacetate (1)	23.32
N.E.E. 1/50 21, 28 (Lexis)	Mestranol (50)	Norethindrone (1)	10.25
Genora 1/50 21, 28 (Rugby)	Mestranol (50)	Norethindrome (1)	12.10
Nelova 1/50 21 (Warner-Chilcott)[d]	Mestranol (50)	Norethindrone (1)	12.38
Norethin 1/50M 21, 28 (Roberts)	Mestranol (50)	Norethindrone (1)	11.00
Norinyl 1/50 21, 28 (Syntex)	Mestranol (50)	Norethindrone (1)	21.41
Ortho-Novum 1/50 21 (Ortho)[d]	Mestranol (50)	Norethindrone (1)	22.06
Ovral (Wyeth-Ayerst)[d]	Ethinyl estradiol (50)	Norgestrel (0.5)	35.79
Ovcon 50 21, 28 (Mead Johnson)	Ethinyl estradiol (50)	Norethindrone (1)	26.38
Demulen 1/50 21 (Searle)[d]	Ethinyl estradiol (50)	Ethynodiol diacetate (1)	26.00
PROGESTIN ONLY			
Ovrette (Wyeth-Ayerst)	None	Norgestrel (0.075)	23.82
Nor-QD (Syntex)	None	Norethindrone (0.35)	26.07
Micronor (Ortho)	None	Norethindrone (0.35)	27.84

[a]Ethinyl estradiol and mestranol are not equivalent on a milligram basis; the results of some studies indicate that 35 μg of ethinyl estradiol are equivalent to 50 μg of mestranol.
[b]Different progestins are not equivalent on a milligram basis.
[c]Cost to the pharmacist for one month's use, based on wholesale price (AWP) listings in *Red Book* 1994 and January 1995 *Update*.
[d]Also available in 28-day regimen at slightly different cost.
From Abramowicz M, ed. The medical letter. New Rochelle, The medical letter. 1995;37:10.

and gestodene have not altered carbohydrate metabolism significantly. Thus, oral contraceptives can safely be prescribed to diabetics who do not smoke. However, there may be increased insulin requirements for diabetic women taking oral contraceptives. These patients should be followed closely initially. Taking oral contraceptives will not make a non-diabetic patient acquire diabetes.

There still exists controversy regarding the use of oral contraceptives and breast and cervical cancer. Large populations of women from many countries who have taken oral contraceptives have been studied. Overall, there does not appear to be an increased risk of breast cancer in women who have taken oral contraceptives. However, data exists which suggests that for women under the age of

46 who took oral contraceptives at least 10 years, there is an increased incidence of breast cancer (33). However, based on surveys of different national cancer registries, there is not an increase in breast cancer attributable to the use of oral contraceptives (33).

The relationship between oral contraceptives and cervical cancer is less clear. The use of oral contraceptives has been associated with a higher incidence of cervical cancer, but the studies that have shown this did not control for frequency of sexual activity as a possible confounder (33). Furthermore, women who take oral contraceptives visit clinicians more often to renew their prescriptions, and this probably leads to higher screening rates for cervical cancer. The increased incidence in cervical cancer could merely be a result of lead time bias (34).

Other possible side effects that could occur in oral contraceptive users are varied. There has been an increased incidence in benign liver tumors known as hepatic adenomas but no increased incidence of malignant tumors. Some women on oral contraceptives develop elevations in blood pressure, which resolve upon discontinuation of the oral contraceptive. Some women report other bothersome side effects such as weight gain, acne, depression, breast tenderness, and decreased libido. Some women with a history of migraine headaches have increased headaches while taking oral contraceptives; however, other women, especially those whose migraines are related to their menses, have improvement in their headaches.

Table 20.18 reviews the major contraindications to oral contraceptives. Women who are older than age 35 and who smoke, women who have had a history of thrombosis or myocardial infarction, and women who have had a history of stroke should not take oral contraceptives because they could be at increased risk for a thrombotic event. Women with previous cancers of breast and cervix also should not take oral contraceptives. Clinicians should use their judgment in women who have hypertension, diabetes, or migraine headaches whether to prescribe oral contraceptives. These patients will need close follow-up. Additionally, women who are breast feeding should not take oral contraceptives as there can be a shortened duration of lactation.

Most women, however, can safely take oral contraceptives. Oral contraceptives remain one of the most effective contraceptives available. For most healthy, young women, oral contraceptives should be the first choice of contraception. Women who have multiple sexual partners and who are at risk for STDs may wish to combine an oral contraceptive with a barrier method to obtain both highly effective contraception with protection against STDs. This may be especially true for adolescents.

PROGESTIN ONLY METHODS

The currently available progestin preparations in the U.S. include the progestin only "minipill," injectable long acting progesterone (Depo-Provera), and implantable slow released progesterone (Nor-

Table 20.18.
Major Contraindications, Side Effects, and Sequelae of Oral Contraceptives

Method	Major Contraindications	Serious Sequelae	Reported Side Effects
Combination oral contraceptives	Thromboembolism—current or past Stroke Coronary heart disease Lipodystrophy Estrogen dependent tumor Breast or endometrial cancer Estrogen-related liver tumor Impaired liver function Cholestasis of pregnancy Smokers age 35 and older • Vascular or migraine headaches • Gallbladder disease • Lactation	Thromboembolism Stroke Myocardial infarction Hypertension (reversible upon discontinuation) Benign liver tumor Cholelithiasis	Irregular bleeding Amenorrhea Nausea Weight gain Breast tenderness Acne Mood changes Heachaches

From Andrews WC. Principles of oral contraception. In: Corson SL, Derman RJ, Tyrer LB, eds. Fertility control, 2nd. ed. Ontario: Goldin Publishers, 1994;70.

plant). These methods utilize progesterone to make the endometrium inhospitable for implantation and render the cervical mucous impenetrable to sperm. Additionally, in many women using Depo-Provera, ovulation is inhibited. The long acting progesterone available in Depo-Provera is able to inhibit FSH and LH to keep estrogen levels low so that the LH surge is inhibited and ovulation prevented. Ovulation is not inhibited to the same degree among users of Norplant and the minipill. This is probably due to the fact that these two methods use a constant release of physiological amounts of progesterone rather than sustained high levels.

By taking advantage of the progesterone effects on the normal menstrual cycle, these methods offer women a highly effective yet estrogen-free method of contraception. This is especially advantageous for women who have contraindications to the use of estrogen, e.g., those over 35 who smoke, those with previous thrombosis, and diabetics. The minipill is less effective than Norplant or Depo-Provera (See Table 20.14) and is only used in 2 special situations: women who are breast feeding, and women over the age of 35 with waning fertility. The other two methods, Norplant and Depo-Provera, provide excellent contraceptive efficacy, especially where patient compliance is an issue. With Norplant, once the implants are inserted, contraception is achieved for 5 years. The patient doesn't have to remember to do anything. With Depo-Provera, the patient only has to return to the clinic or office every 3 months for another injection.

There have been no studies to assess the long-term effects of these methods. Nevertheless, these methods are considered very safe. There is no data to suggest increased risk of breast, ovarian, or cervical cancer in women on Depo-Provera, which can probably be extrapolated to the other progesterone only methods. However, because some breast cancers are sensitive to progesterone, the manufacturers of Norplant advise against prescribing it to women with known or suspected breast cancer. There have not been any changes in blood pressure or glucose tolerance associated with the use of these methods.

These methods are among the more costly ones. Norplant implantation is a minor surgical procedure done in the outpatient office. To discontinue the Norplant, patients must go through another minor surgical procedure. Depo-Provera entails regular visits to the clinician for injections. Not all of these costs are reimbursed by third party payers.

Inherent disadvantages to these methods are minor. Some women who have used Norplant report that the implants are sometimes noticeable under the skin or that the area where the Norplant has been placed is more sensitive to accidental bumps. Depo-Provera has the disadvantage of being an injection that some women will object to. The minipill must be taken at the same time every day in order for maximum efficacy, and many women have difficulty doing this. Perhaps the biggest disadvantage to these methods is that they offer little protection against STDs, only through thickened cervical mucous, which may make infection harder to acquire.

The most common side effect reported with these methods is irregular bleeding. Progesterone alone makes the endometrium atrophic. Without cyclical estrogen in the milieu to support the endometrium, the atrophic endometrium can shed, and breakthrough bleeding/spotting can occur. Breakthrough bleeding usually improves or even resolves within the first year of use. In spite of this, many women discontinue these methods, citing irregular bleeding as the cause. Women may be less bothered by irregular bleeding if appropriate counseling is given before the initiation of one of these methods. Clinicians should also tell women that many users of Norplant and Depo-Provera become amenorrheal with long-term use. Despite breakthrough bleeding, overall, blood loss is much less than a regular menses, and women with anemia secondary to menorrhagia will have improved hematocrits on one of these methods.

Other side effects that women report with these methods include acne, weight gain, mood changes, and breast tenderness. Weight gain seems to be more common among Depo-Provera users. Some women have concerns about being able to quickly conceive once a method has been stopped. Fertility may take longer to return in women using Depo-Provera, the average about 4 ½ months. Fertility returns more quickly upon discontinuation of Norplant.

There are few contraindications to prescribing either Norplant or Depo-Provera. These are listed in Tables 20.19 and 20.20. Medications such as

Table 20.19.
Major Contraindications to Norplant

Pregnancy
Undiagnosed vaginal bleeding
Acute liver disease
Known or suspected breast cancer
Anti-convulsant medications
Long-term treatment with Rifampin
Active thromboembolic disease

Table 20.20.
Major Contraindications to Depo-Provera

Pregnancy
Undiagnosed vaginal bleeding

anticonvulsants and rifampin induce hepatic microsomal enzymes and can cause increased metabolism of progesterone. Because Norplant is the slow release of physiological amounts of progesterone, it could become less effective if metabolized faster. There is less chance of increased metabolism affecting the efficacy of Depo-Provera because of its higher levels of progesterone (28).

Ideal candidates for Norplant or Depo-Provera are those women who want effective long-term contraception and who want a method that requires minimal maintenance. These methods are especially useful in women who are taking medications that are potential teratogens, e.g., chemotherapy for cancer, Accutane, because of their excellent efficacy. The ideal candidate might also be someone who has a contraindication for estrogen. Adolescents would also seem to be ideal candidates because these methods don't rely on the patient to remember anything. Adolescents sometimes forget to take pills and are often too squeamish to learn proper insertion of diaphragms and cervical caps. Ideally, the clinician should encourage the adolescent to combine condom use with Norplant or Depo-Provera.

INTRAUTERINE DEVICE (IUD)

In carefully chosen candidates, the IUD is a very safe and effective method of contraception. Unfortunately, many patients have not forgotten the controversy and media attention over the Dalkon Shield and equate all IUDs with horrible effects. Similarly, many pharmaceutical companies stopped making IUDs because of the potential for legal action in the aftermath of the Dalkon Shield lawsuits. Today, there are only two IUDs available to U.S. patients, a copper containing IUD and a progesterone releasing IUD.

The endometrium mounts a sterile inflammatory response to an IUD which helps to prevent implantation. The addition of copper to the IUD increases its efficacy. The exact mechanism of how copper prevents conception is not known. It has been postulated that copper interferes with sperm motility or fertilizing ability, or even is spermicidal. Progesterone-releasing IUDs combine the inflammatory response of the endometrium with the local effects progesterone has on the endometrium to make it atrophic and unsuitable for implantation.

IUDs need to be inserted by specifically trained clinicians. The copper containing IUD should be replaced every 7 years. The progesterone IUD needs to be replaced annually.

The major risk in the use of an IUD is infection. This risk is higher immediately after insertion. Therefore, patients should be free of infections before insertion of an IUD, and clinicians who insert IUDs must use strict sterile techniques. The copper IUD should be used whenever possible (28) because the manipulation needed for insertion and removal need only occur every 7 years. There may be an increased risk of infection with the use of the progesterone IUD because of the need to have it replaced yearly. Patients who may be at high risk for STDs are probably not good candidates for the IUD. Also, patients with underlying medical conditions that may make them more susceptible to infection are not candidates for an IUD. Examples of medical conditions associated with immunosuppression include sickle cell anemia, AIDS, malignancy, diabetes, and steroid use. Women at increased risk for endocarditis, that is those with valvular heart disease or who are intravenous drug users, are also not candidates for the IUD. Obviously, women with Wilson's disease should not have the copper IUD.

In addition to those patients who are at increased risk for infection, others who should not receive the IUD include those who have anatomical abnormalities of the uterus that would make proper insertion of an IUD impossible. In cases in which pregnancy were to occur during use of an IUD, there is an increased risk of the pregnancy being ectopic. Some clinicians would also not prescribe an IUD to any woman with a previous history of ectopic pregnancy.

The most common side effects with IUD use are an increase in menstrual blood flow and menstrual pain. These effects may be lessened with the use of the progesterone containing IUD because the progesterone released curbs menstrual blood flow and decreases cramping. Therefore, patients with a history of dysmenorrhea who choose an IUD as their method of contraception should be recommended to have the progesterone IUD.

Most clinicians recommend the IUD to women involved in stable monogamous relationships who have already had most of their children. The potential for infection, though small in selected candidates, makes some clinicians uneasy to prescribe the IUD to someone who is still nulliparous. Other patients who could benefit from the IUD are those who have contraindications to estrogens, and those who desire an almost permanent form of contraception.

TUBAL LIGATION

Tubal ligation is a surgical procedure done under anesthesia to permanently interrupt the fallopian tubes. This virtually ensures permanent sterilization. Patients who choose this method should desire no more children. They need to be counseled that the procedure is NOT reversible, even though there are cases where reversal of the procedure has been done. Procedures to reverse tubal ligations are very complicated and are not always successful. Patients who might be at increased risk to want reversal of tubal ligation in the future are those who have had a loss of a child, have undergone a divorce or remarriage, or who are choosing tubal ligation because of unhappiness with their present method of contraception (28). In these cases, it would be more prudent for the clinician to help the patient find another method of contraception.

PERIODIC ABSTINENCE

Patients who use this method learn to determine when the luteal phase of their menstrual cycle has begun. Theoretically, 3–4 days after ovulation, the ovum is no longer viable and intercourse can be presumed to be "safe." There are different methods to determine the timing of the menstrual cycle. Women may be able to chart their menstrual cycles and predict when ovulation has occurred to determine when intercourse could theoretically be "safe." A woman can also learn how to characterize her cervical mucous, and during the period that the mucous is thick and scant, allow intercourse. Women also can chart the basal body temperature to determine when ovulation has occurred. Still other women combine charting of cervical mucous and basal body temperature with awareness of symptoms of ovulation such as mittelschmerz pain.

These methods offer patients whose culture or religion forbids the practice of contraception some control of fertility. For these methods to be effective, there must be cooperation between partners. These methods leave little room for error. With the most careful practice of this method, the failure rate is similar to spermicides and the female condom. However, the failure rate increases rapidly with the slightest deviance from the practice or with any difficulty with use of this method. Not all women are able to learn these techniques, and some women whose cycles are very irregular may not be able to practice periodic abstinence. Most of these methods leave about 2 weeks or less each month when it may be "safe" to have intercourse. Some couples may find this to be too limiting.

The primary advantage to periodic abstinence is that it is absolutely safe. There are no pills, injections, or anything to insert. There are no side effects other than psychological ones from having to refrain from intercourse during certain periods.

Women who choose to use periodic abstinence need to invest a lot of time to properly learn the techniques. Many clinicians are not trained to teach patients how to chart cervical mucous or basal body temperatures, nor do they often have enough time to help a patient thoroughly master these techniques. Clinicians should become familiar with groups and agencies in their area which offer training to patients in the methods of periodic abstinence.

Management

Clinicians who care for women in their reproductive years should be able to answer questions patients may have about their contraceptive methods. Frequently, primary care clinicians will be able to manage simple problems that arise. In some cases, referral to an obstetrician-gynecologist may be warranted.

BARRIER METHODS

Unless the clinician has been specifically trained to size the diaphragm or cervical cap, he/she should probably refer patients who choose these methods for correct fitting. Nevertheless, the clinician can remind patients to have the fit checked annually and after major weight changes or vaginal delivery. Patients should also be reminded to check the diaphragm or cervical cap periodically for leaks and to use another method of contraception if any are found.

Women using the diaphragm should not insert the diaphragm more than 6 hours before intercourse. After intercourse, the diaphragm should be left in place for at least 6 hours but no longer than 24 hours. If during this time period there are additional acts of intercourse, the patient should be reminded to use additional spermicide.

Patients using the cervical cap can insert it up to 8 hours before intercourse. The cervical cap should be left in place at least 8 hours after intercourse for a maximum time of 48 hours. No additional spermicide is needed for multiple acts of intercourse.

The most important information clinicians can give patients using condoms is to avoid mineral oil based lubricants such as contained in petroleum jelly or in sexual aids sold in adult novelty stores. These can rapidly decrease the strength of the latex and can cause the condom to fail. If patients desire extra lubrication, they should be advised to use only water based lubricants which can be purchased from most pharmacies.

All patients should have yearly pelvic exams and PAP smears. Patients who are using the cervical cap should have a PAP smear done after the first 3 months of use. If normal, the patient can be followed thereafter with yearly PAP smears. Patients who develop abnormal PAP smears while using the cervical cap should be advised to discontinue use. Switching to the diaphragm may be desirable.

SPERMICIDES

Patients may complain of vaginal irritation from use of a spermicide. This reaction may not necessarily indicate intolerance to the active ingredient, but intolerance to the base. Sometimes changing brands may relieve the irritation.

COMBINED ORAL CONTRACEPTIVES

After a patient has been determined to be a good candidate for oral contraceptives, the clinician must decide which one to prescribe. The clinician should start with the lowest dose of estrogen, 20–35 μg. Women who still have breakthrough bleeding after a few cycles of the oral contraceptives or who have amenorrhea should then have the estrogen dose increased provided that pregnancy is ruled out. Women who are experiencing estrogen-related side effects such as nausea and breast tenderness may need a lower dose of estrogen. The choice of a progesterone can be varied. The newer progesterones desogestrel, gestodene, and norgestimate tend to have fewer androgenic effects and therefore may have less bothersome side effects like acne, breast tenderness, weight gain. There are also triphasic oral contraceptives that vary the dose of estrogen and progesterone to more closely mimic natural physiology. These however, offer no advantages over the monophasic, fixed-dose varieties (33).

Patients can be instructed to take the pills in two ways. They can start on the 5th day of menses, regardless of whether they are still bleeding. They will take one pill each day for 21 days then take placebo if prescribed a 28-day pack or have 7 pill free days if prescribed a 21 day pack. During the placebo or pill-free days, the patient should have withdrawal bleeding. Alternatively, patients can start the pill pack on the Sunday following the first day of their menses, even if this means starting the very next day. This way of taking oral contraceptives minimizes the chance of having withdrawal bleeding on the weekends. Patients who miss a pill should take the pill as soon as they remember, even if that means taking two pills on a certain day. If a patient misses two pills in the first 2 weeks of beginning oral contraceptives, she should be instructed to take two pills for the next 2 days and then continue with the rest of her pills. She should also be advised to use another method of contraception for the next 7 days. If a patient misses two pills at any other time, she should be advised to start a new package, or if she utilized the Sunday start method, she should be advised to continue taking one pill every day until the following Sunday and then to start a new package. In both cases, the clinician needs to advise the patient to use another method of contraception for the next 7 days.

Patients who are beginning oral contraceptives should be scheduled for a follow-up visit within the next 3 months so that the clinician can answer any questions. Blood pressure should also be obtained during the follow-up visit and each time the patient is seen thereafter. Between 9–16% of patients have elevations in blood pressure while taking oral contraceptives (33), which is reversible upon discontinuation. All patients should have yearly pelvic examinations and PAP smears.

Management of other side effects involves reassurance and in some cases, changing oral contraceptives or even discontinuing oral contraceptives. Clinicians need to involve patients in the decision making process. Even though a side effect may be considered trivial by the clinician, it may be so bothersome for the patient that she wishes to discontinue taking the pills. Whenever possible, clinicians should try to point out to the patient the benefits of taking oral contraceptives, but in the end, only the patient will be able to make the decision whether to continue taking the oral contraceptive.

Side effects such as nausea, breast tenderness, and mood changes may resolve with prolonged use. Occasionally patients complain of depression or decreased libido while taking oral contraceptives. It may be possible to alleviate some of the symptoms by changing the progesterone to a less androgenic one or increasing the estrogen dose so that there is increased sex binding globulin and therefore less free testosterone circulating.

Patients may experience breakthrough bleeding during the first few months of use of oral contraceptives. They should be counseled that this is normal and will most likely resolve by the third pill pack. Patients who later present with breakthrough bleeding may need to take a short course of estrogen while continuing to take the oral contraceptive in order to stabilize the endometrium. Before doing this, clinicians should exclude pregnancy in the patient.

Some women may experience amenorrhea. The clinician should always first exclude pregnancy before doing any other work up. Once pregnancy is excluded, the cause of the amenorrhea is most likely due to insufficient estrogen to stimulate endometrial growth resulting in insufficient endometrial build-up. Management of this problem involves either increasing the dose of estrogen or changing the progesterone component to a more potent one, or doing nothing. The amenorrhea is not harmful to the patient.

Side effects such as elevated blood pressure or worsening headaches require that the patient discontinue the oral contraceptive. Because of the theoretical increase in the risk of thrombotic events, patients who continue to take oral contraceptives despite these signs/symptoms may be placing themselves at an increased risk of stroke.

Because of the theoretical increased risk for thrombotic events, patients who are about to undergo elective surgery should be advised to stop the oral contraceptive 1 month before the surgery and to use another method of contraception during that time. An alternative management strategy might be to continue taking the oral contraceptive, and prescribe subcutaneous heparin during the postoperative period.

Clinicians often overlook drug interactions with oral contraceptives. Any drug that induces hepatic microsomal enzymes could theoretically increase clearance of oral contraceptives from the circulation with resulting decreased contraceptive effect. Table 20.21 shows common drugs that can decrease the effectiveness of oral contraceptives. Antibiotics can theoretically increase hepatic circulation and increase clearance of oral contraceptives, making them less effective. However, there are very few reports of women taking antibiotics and accidentally conceiving. Oral contraceptives themselves can interfere with other medications making them less effective. An important example is Warfarin. Patients who require other medications for a short period, e.g. antibiotics, should be advised to use another method of contraception while taking the

Table 20.21.
Drugs That Decrease Effectiveness of Oral Contraceptives

Ampicillin
Barbiturates
Carbamazepine
Griseofulvin
Phenytoin
Rifampin
Tetracycline

medication in question. A barrier method is often a good choice under these circumstances. Patients who require long-term treatment with a medication that is known to have important drug interactions with oral contraceptives will need to change to another method of contraception.

PROGESTIN ONLY METHODS

Patients who choose the Norplant method should be referred to a clinician who has been specifically trained to insert and remove the implants. Patients who choose to begin the progestin only pill should begin the pill on the first day of menses and take each pill at the same time every day. Patients will need to use an alternative method of contraception during the first week. If a patient forgets to take the pill or takes a pill more than 3 hours later than scheduled, she should be counseled to use a back-up method of contraception for the next 2 days while continuing to take the pills. Patients who choose to have medroxyprogesterone injections should receive the first injection within the first 5 days of the onset of menses. The dose of medroxyprogesterone is 150 mg injected intramuscularly in the gluteal or deltoid muscle. Patients visit the clinician for follow-up injections at 3-month intervals. Since the efficacy of Depo-Provera remains for 14 weeks, patients have a 2 week safety zone in which to schedule visits. If a patient presents for an injection more than 14 weeks later, pregnancy should be ruled out prior to receiving the injection.

Breakthrough bleeding is a common side effect in women using any of the progestin only methods. Clinicians need to counsel patients to expect breakthrough bleeding during the first few months of use. Anticipation of this problem can go a long way towards making the patient feel comfortable using these methods. If a patient later complains of breakthrough bleeding, the clinician should check a pregnancy test, and then perform an examination to rule out the presence of vaginitis or cervicitis. If no cause other than the progesterone can explain the breakthrough bleeding, the clinician can reassure the patient. However, some patients are extremely distressed by breakthrough bleeding. If estrogens are not contraindicated, a trial of 7 days of estrogen can be prescribed.

Patients with no history of any medical problems do not need any special monitoring other than annual pelvic examinations and PAP smears. Diabetic patients may need to be followed more closely. Though the progesterones used in Norplant and Depo-Provera do not significantly affect serum glucose, individual patients on these methods should have glucose levels followed closely initially to make sure that diabetic medications do not have to be altered. With the progestin only pill, the effect of the pill on glucose depends on the progesterone, and clinicians should probably monitor glucose closely initially.

INTRAUTERINE DEVICE (IUD)

Patients who opt for this method should be referred to a clinician who has been trained to insert and remove these devices. Clinicians can help remind their patients who use the IUD of the need for regular follow-up to assess the placement. Also, patients should be reminded that the copper containing IUD should be replaced every 7 years and the progesterone containing IUD annually. Clinicians should make sure patients receive annual pelvic exams and PAP smears.

PERIODIC ABSTINENCE

Unless the clinician is knowledgeable about using periodic abstinence, he/she should refer patients who choose this method to various organizations that have resources and programs to help people learn the different techniques. Organizations like Planned Parenthood can help clinicians locate groups in their area which offer detailed programs for patients. Clinicians who care for patients using this method should perform yearly pelvic examinations and PAP smears.

ILLUSTRATIVE CASES WITH SELF-ASSESSMENT QUESTIONS AND ANSWERS

Case 1

A 28-year-old woman with insulin-dependent diabetes mellitus for 1 year presents for advice regarding contraception. She is married and has five children, but none of her children were fathered by her current husband. She is monogamous with her husband and has no prior history of STDs. She states that because of her diabetes she often finds it difficult to give as much attention to her five children as they require and therefore does not desire any more children. Her glucose control has been sub-optimal and on review of her current fingerstick logbook, she is noted to have glucose values mostly in the 200s.

QUESTION: *Which contraceptive methods should be recommended for this patient?*

ANSWER: *Because the patient does not desire any more children, she is a good candidate for a highly effective method of contraception. However, because of her underlying diabetes, she would not be a good candidate for oral contracep-* *tives because she could be at a higher risk for a thrombotic event. Furthermore, some diabetic patients taking the oral contraceptive have an increased insulin requirement. Usually, a simple adjustment of insulin is needed, but in this patient whose glucose is not optimally controlled, placing her on oral contraceptives could worsen the situation. However, if at some point her glycemic control were improved, a trial of oral contraceptives, if the patient wishes, could be undertaken. This patient is also not a good candidate for the IUD because her diabetes could place her at increased risk for infection. This patient would be a candidate for Norplant or Depo-Provera. Neither has been shown to interfere with glucose metabolism. Both would give this patient long-term fertility control. The progesterone in Norplant has been associated with decreased HDL. Whether this is clinically significant remains to be seen. However, in this patient who is a diabetic, decreased HDL could contribute theoretically to her risk of cardiac disease. This may make Depo-Provera a little better choice. Also, since she is not concerned with the return of fertility, concerns that ovulation is not restored until 4–9 months after discontinuation of Depo-Provera do not* apply to her. This patient is also a candidate for a barrier method. The diaphragm would be a better choice than the cervical cap because cervical caps are not as effective in multiparous women.

One obvious choice for this patient to consider is surgical sterilization. However, given that she has married a man whom she has not fathered any children with, this patient should receive extensive counseling prior to having surgical sterilization. Her husband should also be encouraged to participate in the counseling process and the ultimate decision. They could be at risk for later requesting a reversal of this procedure. However, if after counseling, this patient still wishes to use this method for contraception, she should be allowed to proceed.

Case 2

A 33-year-old woman with no significant past medical history who takes oral contraceptives presents to the clinic with symptoms of dysuria and frequency of urination. A diagnosis of urinary tract infection is made. The patient has no known drug allergies.

QUESTION: *What antibiotics can be prescribed for this patient?*

ANSWER: *Any antibiotic has the potential to interfere with oral contraceptives by causing increased hepatic circulation and increased clearance of the oral contraceptive. Ampicillin can induce hepatic microsomal enzymes to increase metabolism of oral contraceptives. However, there are many more women taking oral contraceptives together with antibiotics than there are anecdotal reports of unplanned pregnancies. This patient should be prescribed an appropriate antibiotic to treat the urinary tract infection, e.g., trimethoprim-sulfa. Perhaps the most prudent course of action would be to recommend that the patient use a back-up method of contraception, e.g., a barrier method, while she is taking the antibiotic. Some clinicians increase the estrogen dose to 50 g for patients taking antibiotics to counter any increased metabolism drug interactions produced. However, for an uncomplicated urinary tract infection, only a 3-day course of antibiotics is needed. Changing preparations of oral contraceptives for a 3-day course of antibiotics is excessive when another method of contraception, or even abstinence, could be used.*

MENOPAUSE

Menopause is the cessation of a woman's menstrual cycle. It signifies closure of reproductive capacity that commenced with menarche. A woman is considered to have achieved menopause 2 years after her last period. The "climacteric" refers to the transitional period of time, from the onset of irregular menses to their cessation, that may last months or years. During the climacteric the body adjusts to massive changes in the hormonal balance.

This phase of life may be accompanied by a complex of symptoms; hot flashes, night sweats, vaginal atrophy, and emotional lability, ranging from mild to debilitating. There is also an association with increased risks of heart disease and osteoporosis that contribute significantly to post menopausal morbidity and mortality. Coincident with the major shifts in hormonal balance many women also experience changes in their personal lives.

Menopause is a natural and universal event that is experienced physically and emotionally in different cultures. The societal context in which a woman undergoes menopause will greatly affect her perception of the event, her response and to a great extent, the outcome. Thus the approach to the patient with menopause must be rooted in medicine, but supported by emotional and cultural awareness to help her achieve her maximum potential in the years that follow.

Pathophysiologic Correlation

Menopause is not pathophysiologic, rather it is a normal process in female physiology. Its concomitant symptomatology and the long-term effects of hormone depletion may lead to pathology. The physiology of menopause, the physiology of its more severe sequela and epidemiologic perspective will be considered.

The menopause concludes a stage begun in the female fetus. The primordial ova, covered with a layer of epithelioid granulosa constitute a primordial follicle. At birth the female carries 750,000 primordial follicles in her ovaries, by puberty only 400,000 remain. Through the reproductive years only 450 follicles develop successfully to release ova, the remainder become atretic. During the menstrual cycle, there are regular changes in hormonal secretion. In response to hypothalamic releasing hormones the anterior pituitary produces follicle-stimulating hormones (FSH) and luteinizing hormone (LH) which stimulate ovarian production of estrogen and progesterone. The negative feedback loop is complete when the unfertilized ovum degenerates, and estrogen levels decrease and there is stimulation for the production of releasing hormones for FSH and LH.

The principal and most potent human estrogen is 17b estradiol, produced in the ovaries. Another, less potent estrogen, estrone, is secreted by the adrenals. Estrogen causes proliferative changes in the endometrium in preparation for the fertilized ovum, increased osteoblastic activity and a myriad of effects on secondary sexual characteristics. Progesterone prepares the uterus for the fertilized ovum via secretory changes in the endometrium and preparation of the breasts for lactation. All progesterone production ceases with the last period.

The classical definition of menopause is ovarian failure. By the mid-forties the body has expelled most of the viable primordial follicles. Fewer follicles stimulate less ovarian estrogen production and there is no negative feedback of FSH and LH to cause cycles. Estrogen production is tremendously reduced by menopausal ovarian shutdown although a small amount continues to be produced by the adrenals and stored in fatty tissue. Women with extra adipose may have fewer symptoms of estrogen withdrawal.

The most prevalent symptom of estrogen withdrawal, the hot flash, is common to 80% of women. Hot flashes range from infrequent to upwards of 20 a day. They last 3–5 minutes and persist for 3–5 years although they may persist for many years in some women. Hot flashes increase with stress, hot ambient temperature, and intake of highly spiced foods, alcohol and caffeine. Both hot flashes and their related night sweats originate from vasomotor instability caused by an increase in hypothalamic activity stimulated by lack of ovarian feedback. There are also age related alterations in the hypothalamus that can potentiate the thermoregulatory disruption. Hot flashes and night sweats can significantly interrupt sleep over an extended period of time to cause difficulty in wakeful concentration, irritability and emotional vulnerability.

Osteoporosis is a process by which a decrease in bone mass and its resultant changes in structure lead to increased risk of fractures. The incidence of osteoporosis increases with age and is usually preceded by a long, asymptomatic period of bone loss. There are 1.5 million osteoporotic fractures a year. The most commonly occurring fractures are of the vertebrae, hip and wrist. Eighty percent of all hip fractures are in women, two times the risk in men. It is not yet known how changes in ovarian hormones effect osteoporotic changes. Observational studies demonstrate increased skeletal turnover, however, no direct control of skeletal homeostasis by estrogen has been shown. There are other contributing factors to the development of osteoporosis including Caucasian race, family history, fair complexion, thin body type, sedentary lifestyle, cigarette smoking, alcohol and caffeine ingestion, and high animal protein intake. Genetic factors have a strong role in determining peak bone mass in young women, it is believed genetics have less of a role in later life. Childhood milk consumption correlates with post menopausal bone density. Rate of bone loss from a peak value in the mid 30s declines slowly (3%/decade) until 45 or 50 when there is accelerated bone diminution (9%/decade) until age 75. After age 75, rates of decline drop down to 3–4%/decade, the same as in men. As bone mass is tantamount to bone strength, lifetime projections of osteoporotic changes can be made from bone density studies.

Coronary heart disease (CHD) is the leading cause of death in the United States. Womens' rates for CHD increase sharply in the immediate post menopausal years. This has led to speculation about hormonally induced cardiotonic effects for women in their reproductive years. One proposed theory is based on estrogenic action on lipid metabolism (see section on Hormone Replacement Therapy). As yet, no mechanism of action has been proven and some authors consider the post menopausal CHD prevalence rates to be a result of age and lifestyle, particularly smoking.

SURGICAL MENOPAUSE

Thirty seven percent of American women have hysterectomies by the age of 60. Women who are left with their ovaries intact will have a slightly earlier onset of menopause, but their experience will be similar to women who have not had hysterectomies. Women who have hystero-oophorectomies will undergo sudden menopause. Their body is deprived of the gradual process of adjustment to hormonal changes. They may suffer overwhelming depression and lethargy and have a greater risk of heart disease. Osteoporotic changes begin at the time of hysterectomy, no matter at what age it occurs and proceed at a faster rate. It is usually recommended that these women immediately receive estrogen replacement.

EPIDEMIOLOGY

The age at which menopause occurs is genetically predetermined, unlike menarche, which is related to body mass. The only environmental factor that affects the age of menopause is cigarette smoking, which decreases the age by 2 years. The current average age at menopause is 51 years, as it has been for hundreds of years. In 1900 the life expectancy for women was 50 years. In the United States, the current life expectancy for a woman is 78.3 years. However, if a woman lives to be 65, she can expect to live to 83.6 years. Thus, one third of a woman's life may be in the post-menopausal phase.

With so many women living to an older age the health and social concerns of this group become a major public health concern. Inequities caused by sexism and racism that have led to the feminization of poverty will have ramifications on the aging process. The poverty rate for women older than 65 is twice that of males. Impoverishment often leads to inadequate nutritional intake, substandard and unsafe housing, reduced access to medical care and stress (35).

Many women at this age experience disequilibrium caused by their changing roles in society. Those involved in the maternal role may feel a great loss as children grow and move out of the home. There may be the care burden of aged parents or dealing with their death. Some couples learn to cope with the life changes and find renewed satisfaction in relationships, others may undergo the dislocation of divorce or widowhood. Underlying the individual woman's experience is the cultural context in which she makes sense of her life.

Clinical and Laboratory Evaluation

Presentation of an age appropriate (43–55) woman with a characteristic constellation of symptoms is a strong indicator of menopause. Laboratory tests are confirmatory.

HISTORY

A sympathetic elicitation of symptoms and review of systems will help clarify the severity of symptoms and the degree to which they interfere with activities of daily living. Relevant family history may help predict the risk of developing heart disease or osteoporosis. Contraindications to hormone replacement or other therapies should be identified.

Family History. Ask at what age her mother reached menopause. Also at what age did her sister reach menopause? Is there any family history of heart disease? Is there a family history of osteoporosis? Is there any family history of breast cancer?

Personal History. Has she had breast cancer or endometrial cancer? Has she had a uterine fibroid? Does she have diabetes? Has she had any type of heart disease? Does she have liver disease?

Has she experienced thrombophlebitis? What is her cigarette smoking history?

Social History. What are her children's ages and status? Is she in a relationship? What is the status of her partner? What are her parents' status? Does she have financial security? Does she have a supportive social network?

Review of Symptoms. Has she experienced hot flashes? How frequent are they, what are their duration and precipitating factors? Has she had night sweats? How frequent are they and has she had to change the bed clothes? Has there been a change in sleep patterns? How much sleep a night does she get? Has she experienced a change in weight or had signs of bloating? Has she felt a decrease in energy level? Does she exercise regularly? When was her last menstrual period? Have her periods been regular? Has there been a change in the quantity or caliber of flow? Has she had dysmenorrhea or pre-menstrual syndrome? Has she felt a change in mood? Has she noted irritability, lability, crying spells, memory loss, depression or feeling "out of sorts"? Has there been a change in sexual activity or interest in sex? Has she had dyspareunia? Has she had vaginal itching? Has this impacted on her intimate relationship(s)?

PHYSICAL EXAMINATION

The focused examination assesses for interventions for symptomatic relief. Areas of potential risk must also be evaluated. Blood pressure should be checked to evaluate for risk of heart disease. Breasts are examined because the risk of breast cancer increases with age and may limit treatment options. Examine for lumps, discharge, dimpling and work up any abnormal findings. Breast self exam should be taught and encouraged. In the pelvic exam, lack of moisture, thinning of vaginal walls, decreased elasticity, narrowing and foreshortening of the vault are all normal menopausal findings. A bimanual examination should be performed for uterine fibroids.

LABORATORY EVALUATION

The reduction in ovarian production of estradiol leads to an increase in gonodotropins. FSH levels >50 IU/ml and LH levels >35 IU/ml are diagnostic of menopause in the absence of underlying disease. Lipid profile/cholesterol levels may be helpful to determine cardiovascular risk. Pap Smears should be done annually to screen for cancer of the cervix or vagina. Mammograms should be done annually after the age of fifty for early detection of breast cancer. Bone density evaluation is optimal, if available. It may benefit a woman who uses the information to assess her risk of osteoporosis.

Differential Diagnosis

In an age appropriate woman with classic symptoms and supportive lab values the search for other causes is unnecessary. However, several primary "rule outs" must be kept in mind. Pregnancy can cause abnormal menstrual bleeding, amenorrhea, bloating and mood swings. It should be considered in all sexually active women. Endometrial cancer can cause excessive bleeding that may be confused with the "flooding" menses that occasionally accompany normal menopause. An endometrial biopsy is indicated for abnormal bleeding. Changes in sex steroid hormones may also be caused by polycystic ovarian syndrome or radiation therapy. Endocrine disorders, metabolic dysfunction, eating disorder and overwhelming infectious disease may cause abnormal menses or secondary amenorrhea. If suspected their work up can be found elsewhere. Emotional upheaval frequently disrupts the cycle and should be pursued via history for possible counseling and support.

Management

There is a continuum of response possible to menopause. It is the provider's responsibility to assess the patient's current clinical status and risk of developing deleterious sequela and provide balanced, current information. Some women may not consider menopause a problem to be "managed" but a normal life process to experience without intervention. Many women wish to ameliorate the uncomfortable symptoms and reduce long term risks by relying on natural methods that would limit interventions to lifestyle changes, but not drugs. Some women, because of severity of symptoms, risk of sequela or even in an attempt to hold back the aging process, choose hormone replacement therapy (HRT).

SUPPORTIVE THERAPIES

Exercise maintains bone mass and attenuates bone loss. Regular exercise, emphasizing weight bearing bones, 3–4 times a week for 30 minutes is recommended. Increasing intensity of the exercise and bone stress over time maintains effectiveness. Exercise may also help prevent fractures by maintaining muscle strength, eye hand coordination and a sense of balance, thereby reducing falls. It has enhancing

cardiovascular effect, assists in weight control, and imparts a sense of well being by endorphin production. Eating a balanced diet is the best nutritional plan. Possible supplements of vitamins C and D for bone formation, vitamin B to decrease edema, vitamin E for leg cramps and hot flashes, may be beneficial. A calcium-rich diet (1500 mg/day) or calcium supplements for those without adequate nutritional intake may help maintain bone mass. Calcium supplementation does not improve bone density status in the early menopause, but has a beneficial effect 5–10 years later. Calcium supplements are best absorbed when taken with food. In buying over-the-counter, the amount of elemental calcium in the product is what should be considered. Avoid alcoholic beverages, caffeine, and chocolate to ameliorate hot flashes. Water soluble vaginal lubricants available over-the-counter can alleviate vaginal drying. They are most effective if used daily rather than only prior to intercourse. Smoking cessation or at least reduction, should be encouraged to reduce the risks of heart disease and osteoporosis. Patient education should include the need for annual mammogram and Pap smears, as well as monthly breast self examination. Women who are sexually active should be advised to use birth control, if they wish to avoid pregnancy, for 2 years after their last menstrual period. The prudent provider should caution those patients without contraindications that there is sufficient evidence of a significant reduction in morbidity and mortality from heart disease and osteoporosis in women who use HRT to warrant the risk of its use.

HORMONE REPLACEMENT THERAPY

HRT seeks the minimum effective replacement dose to relieve deficiency induced pathology and avoid unwanted side effects. The literature on harmful side effects including endometrial and breast cancer and on the protective health effects on CHD and osteoporosis are reviewed. Available commercial hormone compounds are presented. Current treatment regimens are described as well as appropriate patient follow up.

In the 1970s, there was an increase in the incidence of endometrial carcinoma that was attributed to estrogen replacement therapy that was then the standard of care. Studies showed estrogen users had 1.7- to 20-fold increased relative risk for development of endometrial cancer. The rates increased with length of use and greater dosages (36). Endometrial hyperplasia is believed to be a precancerous condition. Unopposed estrogen causes incomplete shedding of the endometrium. When progestogen is added there is more complete shedding, leaving behind fewer glands and cells for potential proliferation. Progestogen was added to regimens and risks rapidly declined. Gambrell (1986) in a prospective study found women on combined estrogen progesterone therapy had the lowest incidence of cancer (49/100,000) those on unopposed estrogen had the highest (390.6/100,000) and those without any HRT had an incidence of 245.4 (37).

Breast cancer occurs in one of nine American women at an increasing frequency correlated with age. A causal relationship between estrogen use and breast cancer has not been found. It is also still undetermined if estrogens act as a cofactor to facilitate neoplastic changes in cells already sensitized. Stienberg (1991) in a meta-analysis of 16 studies found no risk up to 5 years of estrogen use but after 15 years of use the relative risk of developing breast cancer rose to 1.3. There was a significant relative risk of 3.4 among women with a family history (38). However, another analysis of 28 published studies of estrogen risk found all results to average around 1.0 or no increased risk (39). The effect of progesterone on breast cancer incidence has not been determined. It would appear the risk of developing breast cancer associated with HRT may be small, if any. Yet with the high disease prevalence any increase in risk can affect thousands of women annually.

The role of estrogen in counteracting the morbidity associated with menopausal osteoporosis has been studied by several investigators. In a study of women who had undergone oophorectomies, Linday et al. determined estrogen reduced the rate of cortical bone loss and the risk of fractures. Bone mass remained stable in estrogen treated women for at least 10 years while bone mass declined in non-users. Circulating estrogen levels were equal in either oral or parenteral routes of administration. Efficacy was enhanced by treatment initiated early in the climacteric that continued for the long term (40). Estrogen replacement has also been helpful to women with significant skeletal compromise and fracture to reduce continuing bone loss into the eighth decade. Ettinger et al. found bone loss ameliorated by low dose estrogen (0.3 mg/day) supplanted by 1,000 mg/day of calcium. There was no protective effect on the calcium only arm of the study (41).

The effect of estrogen on heart disease has been the subject of several long term studies. The Nurses Health Survey followed 48,000 post menopausal women for 10 years and found the relative risk of major coronary disease in women currently taking estrogen to be 0.56 independent of duration of use. The relative risk of current and past users compared to non-users was 0.89 for total mortality and 0.72 for mortality from cardiovascular disease. They concluded estrogen is associated with a reduction in the incidence of CHD as well as mortality from cardiovascular disease (42). This contrasted with the Framingham study that found a correlation between estrogen use and heart disease that has since been refuted by several other studies (43). A 3-year prospective, double blind, placebo-controlled study of 875 post menopausal women, the Post Menopausal Estrogen/Progestin Intervention Trial, compared cardiotonic efficacy of several different HRT regimens. They identified as a cardiotonic mechanism of action increasing high density lipoproteins (HDL) and decreasing low density lipoproteins (LDH). HDL levels are more closely related to cardiovascular disease in women. Also noted were lowered fibrinogen levels. The treatment group taking unopposed estrogen alone had the greatest enhancing effect on HDL. However, the women who took estrogen alone who had intact uteri had significant rates of endometrial hyperplasia and endometrial cancer. Women with intact uteri on estrogen with progesterone had no significant endometrial pathology. Women on conjugated equine estrogen (CEE) with micronized progesterone (MP) had higher HDL levels than those who took CEE with medroxyprogesterone acetate (MPA). They found CEE for women without a uterus and CEE with MP for women with a uterus to provide maximum protective cardiovascular effect (44). Unopposed CEE is recommended for women without a uterus and a combination of CEE with either MP or MPA, either cyclic or daily doses for women with a uterus. If progesterone is absolutely contraindicated for the individual woman with a uterus CEE alone may be tried with regular endometrial biopsy. Table 20.22 summarizes current hormone replacement therapies.

A prospective study of 8,800 postmenopausal female residents of a retirement community, the Leisure World Study, found the women with a history of estrogen use had 20% lower all-cause mortality from acute and chronic heart disease than lifetime non-users. Mortality decreased with increasing duration of use and was lower among current users than those who had used only in the past (45). Replacement estrogen often contributes to a generalized sense of well being, positive outlook and increased energy.

The primary type of estrogen used in the United

States is conjugated equine estrogen (CEE) derived from the purified urine of pregnant mares. It is a combination of several naturally occurring estrogenic compounds. When used in the standard oral dose of 0.625 mg/day, it produces a normal low level of estrogen as in a normal ovarian cycle. Estradiol in a micronized form is also effective and is used predominantly outside the United States. Other estradiol derivatives are not commonly used due to decreased efficacy. The estrogens can be administered via oral or parenteral routes. Oral treatments undergo metabolism before entry into the circulation. They are conjugated and excreted by the liver. Because of dependence on the liver for metabolism, in liver failure there is increased estrogenic activity. Parenteral HRT may be administered via injection, subcutaneous pellets or dermal patch. Parenteral administration allows for use of 17b estradiol which is the endogenous estrogen. It provides time released levels of absorption directly into the blood stream at predictable levels without intermediate metabolism. Some patients prefer a skin patch rather than taking medications by mouth. This also allows for a predictable amount of drug to be administered. A disadvantage of implantables is the inability to stop treatment immediately if desired. Topical vaginal creams are also available. They may be messy and give erratic doses of medication.

Progesterone compounds replicate the effects of endogenous progesterone on the endometrium. They frequently counter the mood uplift of estrogen and may cause bloating, headaches and "the blues". There are both naturally occurring and synthetic compounds, the most commonly used being medroxyprogesterone acetate (MPA). Usual doses of MPA range from 2.5–10 mg/day and micronized progesterone (MP) 200–300 mg/day.

There are several different schedules for administration. Unopposed estrogen is contraindicated in women with a uterus because of the risk of endometrial hyperplasia or cancer. Some providers use cyclic estrogen but daily doses are more easily remembered than cyclic and mimic more closely normal ovarian activity. Normal doses are CEE 0.625 mg/day or transdermal patches of 0.05 or 0.1 mg patch dose.

Continuous estrogen plus cyclic progestin is recommended for women with a uterus to prevent endometrial hyperplasia. In these regimens, estrogen is taken orally or by patch daily plus progestin MPA 5 or 10 mg/day from day 1–12 of each calendar month or MP 200 mg/day for 12 days of the month. Vaginal bleeding after day 10 is normal withdrawal bleeding.

Continuous estrogen plus continuous progesterone given as a regular daily combined dose has enhanced compliance. The patient no longer undergoes monthly withdrawal bleeding after the first 6 months of treatment although there may be some breakthrough bleeding. However, if a patient poorly tolerates progesterone she will have relief taking it intermittently. A common daily combined dose is CEE 0.625 mg plus MPA 2.5 mg (46).

HRT is contraindicated for some women. Absolute contraindications include a personal history of breast cancer or a current diagnosis of endometrial cancer. A history of cured endometrial cancer is not a contraindication. Other absolute contraindications are any estrogen dependent neoplasm, active thromboembolic disease or clotting disorder, active liver or renal disease, unexplained bleeding or pregnancy. The degree of contraindication posed by a family member with breast cancer is still problematic. To be considered are proximity of relationship, age at disease onset and if it is bilateral. Breast cancer with onset in the perimenopausal period afflicting primary family members, mother or sister, would be considered as an absolute contraindication. Disease occurring to any family member at seventy or eighty years would be considered less strongly than disease occurring at a younger age. More remote relatives are categorized as a relative contraindication. Bilateral breast disease, as it is indicative of genetic tendency, strengthens the contraindication. Other relative contraindications include a personal history of recurrent thromboembolic disorders, severe endometriosis and enlargening fibroids. Relative contraindications must weigh the degree of risk versus the woman's symptomatic suffering or risk of severe sequela. The degree of risk versus benefit must be clearly explained to the patient (47).

Duration of Treatment. Considerable debate still exists about the appropriate time, if any, to stop HRT. The determination to discontinue HRT should reflect the reason the woman is on HRT originally. If the reasons were protective, studies show acceleration of bone loss after HRT is stopped. Mortality from heart disease was shown to be least among long-time users and current users. This encourages long term use. Most researchers would support a duration of treatment of up to twenty years. If the reasons for HRT were to relieve the uncomfortable symptoms of vaginal atrophy and dyspareunia, the need for that may not always exist. Symptoms of night sweats and hot flashes will normally not return after cessation of long-term HRT.

Follow-up Care. All patients on HRT should be advised to report any unusual vaginal bleeding for which endometrial sampling is recommended. They should be seen every 6 months with a careful history taken for side effects and difficulties with compliance. Height for vertebral compression, weight for hormone induced bloating and blood pressure for CHD screening should be assessed. Breast and pelvic exams should be performed at each visit. Pap smears and mammograms (for women over 50) should be done annually. The need for continuation of HRT should be reviewed regularly.

ILLUSTRATIVE CASES WITH SELF-ASSESSMENT QUESTIONS AND ANSWERS

Case 1

A 62-year-old woman widowed 2 months ago, on estrogen therapy for twelve years, has an episode of bleeding.

QUESTION: *Which is the most correct provider response?*

a. Have the patient keep a diary of bleeds and make a follow-up visit in 6 weeks.
b. Spend extra time with patient to reassure her, suggest a widows' support group, follow up visit in 3 months.
c. Schedule for an endometrial biopsy.

ANSWER: c. *Emotional support is very important and a diary may provide helpful information, but a timely rule out of endometrial hyperplasia and/or carcinoma must be performed.*

Case 2

A 51-year-old menopausal woman seeks guidance on treatment. She has disabling hot flashes, lack of concentration and emotional lability that interfere significantly with her work. Her grandmother developed breast cancer around age 58. She has tremendous fear about developing breast cancer herself, but her severe symptoms are making her miserable. She requests HRT.

QUESTION: *What is the appropriate response to this patient?*

a. She should seek a second opinion from an experienced gynecologic oncologist.
b. Given the family history, HRT is absolutely contraindicated, alternative therapies should be pursued.
c. Consider the family history a relative contraindication, explain to the patient all of the risk data, and if she chooses, offer her HRT under a program of careful monitoring and quarterly visits.

ANSWER: c *responds to the patient's present need and attempts to aggressively prevent any harm. Answer a should also be encouraged when possible as each case is so individualized.*

Case 3

A 52-year-old menopausal woman is seen for her annual exam. She denies any discomforting symptoms and states she does not wish any intervention for her menopause as it is a natural process.

QUESTION: *What constitutes a prudent approach to the patient?*

a. Respect the patient's wishes to follow a natural course and do not bring up any interventions.
b. Despite patients stated belief, explain the potential for increased morbidity and mortality without HRT.

ANSWER: b. *Frequently, people make choices on the basis of inadequate knowledge and are entitled to the facts whatever their eventual choice. The health benefit from HRT is so strong that the provider would be negligent to not inform even a disinterested patient.*

BREAST LUMPS

Most women, at one time or another, experience some swelling, discomfort or lumpiness of their breasts. Others will have a suspicious lump in their breast discovered by their clinician or significant other. The role of the clinician should be two-fold. One, begin the process of evaluation to determine the etiology of the breast lump. Second, address the patient's fears and concerns. Every woman is at risk: one of every nine women will develop breast cancer in her lifetime. The fear of cancer alone can keep some women away from their provider and a diagnostic evaluation.

Pathophysiologic Correlation

The complex breast structure and the extreme sensitivity to endocrine influences predispose it to various benign and pathologic conditions. The breast is often considered to be a large, single, secretory gland, when in reality it is composed of five to nine separate branching glands. Each is autonomous and without anatomic connection to another. These glands drain through lactiferous ducts into the nipple. The mammary gland consists of 20 lobes subdivided into lobules. Commonly, there is a long process of breast tissue, known as the axillary appendage, extending into the anterior axilla. Disease or tumors of this tissue can be mistaken for involvement of axillary lymph nodes. The female breast, as the endometrium, is under the influence of the ovarian hormones causing histologic changes with each menstrual cycle. The proliferation of the ductal epithelium and bland bud epithelium is related to estrogen levels. With the progressive rise of estrogen, the ducts and glands become dilated and hypertrophied. During the last half of the menstrual cycle, with progesterone influence, stromal growth and edema begins. This combined effect on the intralobular breast elements accounts for the sense of fullness commonly experienced by women during the premenstrual phase of the menstrual cycle. With the decrease in estrogen and progesterone levels during the menstrual period, there is desquamation of epithelial cells, atrophy of intralobular connective tissue, loss of interstitial edema and shrinkage in the size of ducts and glands (48). The breast may feel lumpy in response to these hormonal fluxes.

Clinical and Lab Evaluation

An accurate history assessing the state of the breast lump throughout the menstrual cycle and risk factors for cancer is essential. Detailed physical examination and, some laboratory tests, if indicated, complete the evaluation. The clinician's foremost question is, "Could this be cancer?"

HISTORY

Most benign lumps are found either by the woman during breast self-examination, by her partner, or by her clinician. It is important to determine how long the mass has been present, if it is painful or if its size, consistency or the associated symptoms change with the menstrual cycle. The history must also include risk factor assessment for breast cancer. There are many risk factors associated with the development of breast cancer (Table 20.22). The strongest risk factor is a positive family history. There is a two-fold increase in breast cancer among women with a first-degree relative and a three-fold increased risk in women with two first-degree relatives with breast cancer. Other important risk factors are early menarche, late menopause, delayed child bearing, increased dietary fat, and possibly estrogen use.

PHYSICAL EXAMINATION

The clinician should examine the breasts carefully as the woman's arms are raised over the head and then lowered to her sides while she is sitting up and again while she is lying down. Having the woman flex her chest muscles with her hands pressed down on her hips, look for skin changes (pea de orange, dimpling) or puckering of the

Table 20.22.
Risk Factors for Breast Cancer

High risk
  Older age
  Personal history of breast cancer
  Family history of premenopausal bilateral breast
    cancer
  Breast biopsy with proliferative disease with atypia
Moderate risk
  First-degree relative with breast cancer
  Age greater than 30 at first full-term pregnancy
  Nulliparous
  Obesity in postmenopause
Low risk
  Menarche before age 12
  Menopause after age 55
  Moderate alcohol intake
  Greater than 15 years of estrogen replacement
    therapy

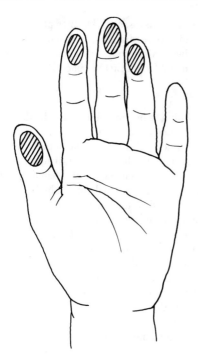

Figure 20.7. The portion of the finger tips that should be used during examination of the breast are indicated.

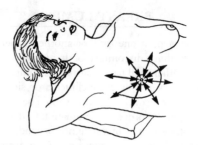

Figure 20.9. Alternatively, the breast may be examined in this pattern. (From Beckmann CRB, Ling FW, Barzansky BM, Bates GW, Herbert WNP, Laube DW, Smith RP. Obstetrics and Gynecology. 2nd ed. Baltimore: Williams & Wilkins. 1995:9.)

breasts. During the examination the provider must concentrate on feeling any lumps, knots, or thickening of the breasts, while looking for skin discoloration, dimpling, puckering or nipple inversion. Using the palmar surface of two or three extended fingers (Fig. 20.7) gently palpate the breast tissue in a circular pattern (Fig. 20.8) starting at the nipple and moving around the breast, or palpate the breast starting at the nipple and extend outward covering

each part of the breast (Fig. 20.9). Then, gently squeeze each nipple looking for a discharge. Examine under each arm in both the sitting and lying positions, palpating for lumps or thickening. During the examination, the clinician should teach the woman how to examine her own breasts (Fig. 20.10).

LABORATORY EVALUATION

A palpable breast mass requires evaluation if it is suspicious. Benign lumps and cysts are usually recognizable on examination because of the lobulated consistency of the underlying tissue, bilateral symmetry, increased tenderness, changes with the menstrual cycle and lack of secondary signs of malignancy (skin retraction, etc.). Ultrasound can determine if a palpable breast lump in a young woman or a benign-appearing mass seen on mammogram represents a cyst or a solid lesion. Ultrasound is 98 to 100% accurate in distinguishing a cyst from a solid mass (49). However, ultrasound should never be used for breast cancer screening.

Needle aspiration also is used to determine if a lump is a cyst. It is quick and less painful than a surgical biopsy. If the mass does not yield any fluid, it may still be a cyst or other benign growth. If a palpable mass is not proved to be a cyst by ultrasound or aspiration, then a biopsy or fine needle biopsy is required to rule out malignancy.

A biopsy is indicated if mammography shows a suspicious mass or calcification, if aspiration fluid is thick or bloody, if there are other symptoms (hard, swollen lymph node, nipple discharge, dimpling), if the lump remains after aspiration, if echoes are seen on ultrasound, or if a cyst recurs after aspiration. The biopsy then involves surgical removal of all of the lump (excisional), part of the

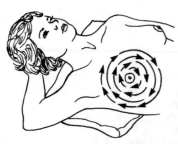

Figure 20.8. The breast can be examined in circular motion. (From Beckmann CRB, Ling FW, Barzansky BM, Bates GW, Herbert WNP, Laube DW, Smith RP. Obstetrics and Gynecology. 2nd ed. Baltimore: Williams & Wilkins. 1995:9.)

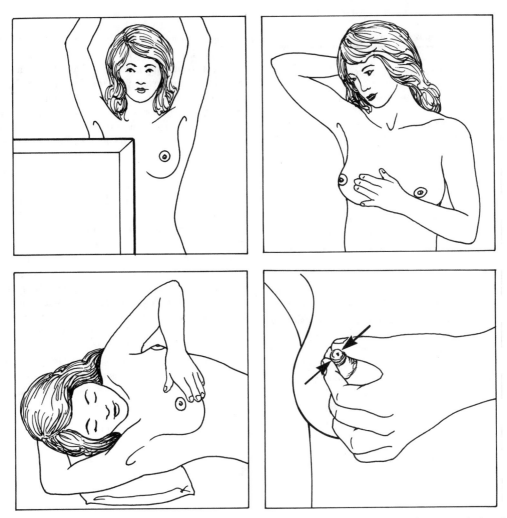

Figure 20.10. Breast self-examination. Instruct the patient to begin her examination in front of the mirror looking for retractions, dimpling or discoloration. The patient is to examine each breast with the opposite hand, either while in the shower or while lying down with a small pillow or rolled towel under her shoulder. The fingers should be held straight while the hand is held flat and gently presses against the breast with small circular motions making sure to palpate the entire breast. The nipples should be gently squeezed with the thumb and index finger. If a lump, dimpling, discharge or any abnormality is detected, she should contact her health care provider for re-examination and possibly diagnostic tests.

lump (incisional), or just removing some cells (needle biopsy). Core needle biopsies, also called Trocar, can be done as an office procedure. It is now common practice to perform incisional or excisional biopsy on an out-patient basis under local anesthesia (50). The results of any incisional biopsy can only be helpful if they are positive. There is always a possibility that an incisional biopsy has missed the malignant part of the lump.

The role of mammography in the work-up of a palpable breast lump is to exclude carcinoma or other suspicious tissue that should be biopsied as well in another part of the breast or in the opposite breast. A normal mammogram result does not change the original recommendation to biopsy a solid lump. Mammogram recommendations vary as to how often (every 1 vs 2 years) and at what age to begin screening, but there is concensus that mammography helps detect non-palpable cancers an average of 2 years before they are palpable (Table 20.23). It is considered to be less accurate in premenopausal women because of increased paren-

Table 20.23.
Mammographic Signs of Cancer

Irregular mass
Mass smaller on mammogram than on physical exam
Nipple retraction
New density or increased stromal density on sequential exams
Localized or clustered calcifications

chymal density of the breast. Mammary calcifications are easily seen on mammogram; most represent a benign process, but localized or clustered calcifications are viewed as indicative of breast carcinoma. A new density or any local area of increased parenchymal density on sequential studies suggests malignancy and should be biopsied. Benign mammographic findings include well circumscribed masses, e.g., intra-mammillary lymph nodes or fibroadenomas with characteristic coarse calcification. Multiple small, round calcifications scattered throughout suggests benign adenosis. The false negative rate for mammogram is between five and twelve percent; most are related to dense parenchymal tissue obscuring the presence of a mass (50). The advantages of mammography are that it can detect cancer before it is palpable, needles can be inserted as markers for the surgeon, and baseline mammograms can be used for comparison of suspicious changes.

Differential Diagnosis

The differential diagnosis of a breast lump is the most important clinical problem that arises with this organ. All suspicious lumps must be considered as a possible cancer until proven otherwise. This is particularly important for women older than 50.

FIBROCYSTIC BREAST CONDITION

In women under the age of fifty the fibrocystic breast condition is the most common cause of breast abnormalities. The fibrocystic breast, the most common benign condition is a non-descript lumpiness with numerous, well-delineated, mobile nodules having a firm, elastic consistency. This condition is the result of an exaggerated response of the cyclic breast changes that occur normally in the menstrual cycle. The fibrocystic breast demonstrates a variety of morphologic changes including fibrosis, cyst formation, sclerosing adenosis and duct epithelial hyperplasia (48). Sclerosing adenosis is characterized by intralobular fibrosis and lob-

ular epithelial proliferation without premalignant changes. Epithelial hyperplasia, on the other hand, may predispose to carcinoma. The fibrocystic breast is hormonally induced with cyclical pain and lumpiness. It can start with the first menstrual period or develop later. During ovulation and just before menstruation hormone levels change that can cause the breast to retain fluid, often developing cysts. Most of these will be tender and will decrease or disappear within 1 or 2 days of the onset of menses. Symptoms may vary from month to month, vary among women and usually disappear with menopause. Some women have progressive soreness to sharp pain and persistent lumpiness. With this hormonally induced condition there is a reduction in cyst size and pain with menopause, oral contraception use and pregnancy. A decrease in the ingestion of methylxanthines contained in coffee, tea, cola and chocolate also can alleviate the symptoms of the fibrocystic breast. Mastodynia, pain in the breast, in young women is usually suggestive of fibrocystic breasts. Many processes can cause mastodynia, including the fibrocystic breast, papillomas, sclerosing adenosis, duct ectasia, mastitis, breast lipomas, fat necrosis and galactoceles.

FIBROADENOMA

Eighty to eighty-five percent of breast lumps discovered are not cancers. The most common benign tumor of the female breast is the fibroadenoma. It is a new growth composed of fibrous and glandular tissue (48). The cause is unknown. Fibroadenomas are more common in women under the age of 30. These breast lumps are very mobile, without any attachment to underlying fascia or overlying skin; they are solid, firm and rubbery. The fibroadenoma is asymptomatic and does not change in size with the menstrual cycle. They often feel like cancer, but are not associated with an increase risk of breast cancer. Distinction from a solitary cyst is difficult.

GALACTOCELE

A galactocele is a cystic dilatation of a duct during lactation. The palpable nodules are tender and contain a milky fluid within their thin ductal walls. These cysts can become firm or superinfected.

INTRADUCTAL PAPILLOMA

Intraductal papillomas are neoplastic papillary growths within a duct or a cyst. They occur at any age, but are primarily seen in women between the ages of 30 and 50. They present clinically as a nipple discharge, serous or bloody, as a small areolar tumor or rarely as nipple retraction.

MASTITIS/BREAST ABSCESSES

Mastitis is accompanied by local and systemic signs of inflammation making the diagnosis fairly straightforward.

FAT NECROSIS

Fat necrosis is an uncommon innocuous lesion and is seen in the patient who has a history of trauma. It is without clinical significance except for possibly being confused with a tumor when fibrosis has created a palpable mass.

MAMMARY DUCT ECTASIA

Mammary duct ectasia is characterized by dilated ducts, breast secretions and marked chronic granulomatous inflammatory reaction. This disorder occurs in the fifth decade of life and is much more common in women who have had children. This lesion can produce pain and firmness of the peri- or subareolar region with skin fixation, nipple retraction or discharge which can cause it to be mistaken for a neoplasm (48).

CARCINOMA

In women over age 50, carcinoma is the most common cause of an abnormal lump. The most common sign of breast cancer is a lump or thickening that does not seem to change. Unilateral pain in the breast of a postmenopausal woman is suggestive of a malignant process. Breast cancer causes significant morbidity and mortality. Classically, breast carcinomas are firm or hard, irregular, nontender single nodules. Often, they seem fixed to surrounding tissues, but only a biopsy can distinguish a benign growth from a carcinoma.

Management

Non-palpable masses seen on mammogram are subjected to biopsy or followed based on radiographic criteria (See Table 20.23). A spiculated or irregularly marginated mass requires biopsy, no matter what the size. A well circumscribed solid mass between 5 and 10 mm can be followed with serial mammograms every 6 months up to a total of 3 years to ensure no change in size, or a biopsy can be obtained. Solid masses greater than 1 cm should be biopsied (49).

Palpable breast lumps must be differentiated as solid or cystic. Ultrasound and/or needle aspiration can accomplish this. If clear, or greenish, non-bloody fluid is obtained, a cyst is confirmed. If the cyst collapses and does not recur after several months, the evaluation is complete. All solid masses require incisional or excisional biopsy. Totally excised lesions should be sent for estrogen and progesterone receptor determination, along with routine pathology evaluation. Fine needle aspiration biopsy has a role only when used by an experienced clinician. The sample obtained is smeared on a slide and examined by the Papanicolaou technique, but it may not provide the histologic cell type or tumor architecture required to diagnose a carcinoma. An incisional or excisional biopsy should always be done in spite of a negative cytologic aspiration biopsy, if the pre-biopsy clinical diagnosis was cancer. If cancer is diagnosed, survival is related to the stage of the disease at the time of diagnosis. This is determined by the size of the tumor and the presence of metastases to axillary lymph nodes or more distant metastases (52).

ILLUSTRATIVE CASES WITH SELF-ASSESSMENT QUESTIONS AND ANSWERS

Case 1

Mary Morgan, a 57-year-old nurse, comes to your office because she found a lump in her left breast. The lump spans one centimeter, is irregular in shape, hard and mobile. The overlying skin appears normal and there is no axillary adenopathy. Her last mammogram was done 5 years ago, at menopause.

QUESTION: *What test is most important for diagnosis?*

ANSWER: *Biopsy is the most important diagnostic test. A mammogram should be obtained prior to biopsy, as other suspicious areas requiring biopsy may be discovered.*

QUESTION: *What lesions produce masses?*

ANSWER: *Many breast processes can produce a palpable mass. These include the fibrocystic breast condition, fibroadenomas, breast abscesses, benign cysts, fat necrosis and carcinomas.*

QUESTION: *What is the role of breast self-exam (BSE)?*

ANSWER: *Although BSE has not been proven to decrease mortality, it has helped detect cancers at an earlier stage. It is not the best primary screening test for breast cancer, but it is a valuable technique for women to take an active role in their health care (4).*

A screening mammogram provides an asymptomatic woman a fast and convenient examination of the breast tissue. The study is limited to two views, the mediolateral oblique and the cranial caudal views. The American Cancer Society, American College of Radiology, American Medical Association and other national health associations have issued a concensus for screening guidelines that specify that every women older than forty years old have an annual breast physical examination by a health professional; that non-symptomatic women between the ages of 40 and 49 have annual or bi-annual mammograms and that non-symptomatic women older than 50 years have annual screening mammograms. Women should have a baseline mammogram done between the ages of 35 and 40 (2).

REFERENCES

Vaginal Discharge
1. Sobel JD. Vaginal infections in adult women. Med Clin North Am 1990;74:1573.
2. Sobel, JD. Candidal vulvovaginitis. Clinical Obstet Gynecol 1993: 36:153.
3. Sobel JD. Candidal vulvovaginitis. Clinical Obstet Gynecol 1993: 36:156.
4. Heine P, McGregor JA. Trichomonas vaginalis: a reemerging pathogen. Clin Obstet Gynecol 1993;36:138.
5. 1993 Sexually transmitted diseases treatment guidelines. MMWR 1993;42 (RR14):69.
6. 1993 Sexually transmitted diseases treatment guidelines. MMWR 1993;42 (RR 14):70.
7. 1993 Sexually transmitted diseases treatment guidelines. MMWR 1993;42 (RR 14):69.
8. 1993 Sexually transmitted diseases treatment guidelines. MMWR 1993;42 (RR 14):75.
9. Sobel JD. Candidal vulvovaginitis. Clin Obstet Gynecol 1993:36:163.
10. 1993 Sexually transmitted diseases treatment guidelines. MMWR 1993;42 (RR 14):71.

Pelvic Pain
11. Kresch A, Seifer DB, Sachs LD, et al. Laparascopy in 100 women with chronic pelvic pain. Obstet Gynecol 1984;69:672.
12. McCormack WM. Pelvic Inflammatory Disease. N Engl J Med 1994;330:115–119.
13. 1993 Sexually transmitted diseases treatment guidelines. MMWR Morb Mortal Wkly Rep. 1993;42 (RR 14):75–81.
14. 1993 Sexually transmitted diseases treatment guidelines. MMWR Morb Mortal Wkly Rep. 1993;42 (RR 14):75–81.

Pre-conception Care of the Medical Patient
15. Cefalo RC, Moos MK. Preconceptional health care a practical guide, 2nd ed. St. Louis: Mosby-Year Book, Inc. 1995.
16. McAnulty JH, Metcalfe J, Ueland K. Cardiovascular disease. In: Burrow GN and Ferris TF, eds. Medical complications during pregnancy. 4th ed. Philadelphia: W.B. Saunders Company. 1995:123–154.
17. Barron WM. Hypertension. In: Barron WM and Lindheimer MD, eds. Medical disorders during pregnancy. St. Louis: Mosby Year Book, Inc. 1991:1–32.
18. Weinberger SE, Weiss ST. Pulmonary diseases. In: Burrow GN and Ferris TF, eds. Medical complications during pregnancy. 4th ed. Philadelphia: W.B. Saunders Company. 1995:439–483.
19. Buchanan TA, Coustan DR. Diabetes Mellitus. In: Burrow GN and Ferris TF, eds. Medical complications during pregnancy. 4th ed. Philadelphia: W.B. Saunders Company. 1995:29–61.
20. Burrow GN, Fisher DA, Larsen PR. Maternal and fetal thyroid function. N Engl J Med 1994;331:1072–1078.
21. Greene MF, Hare JW, Cloherty JP, et al. First-trimester hemoglobin A1 and risk for major malformation and spontaneous abortion in diabetic pregnancy. Teratology 1989; 39: 225.
22. Werler MM, Shapiro S, Mitchell AA. Periconceptional folic acid exposure and risk of occurrent neural tube defects. JAMA 1993;269:1257–1261.
23. Anonymous Recommendations for use of folic acid to reduce number of spina bifida cases and other neural tube defects. JAMA 1993;269(10):1233–1238.
24. Lee RV. Drug abuse. In: Burrow GN and Ferris TF, eds. Medical complications during pregnancy. 4th ed. Philadelphia: W.B. Saunders Company. 1995:579–598.
25. Anonymous Executive summary: management of asthma during pregnancy. Report of the working group on asthma and pregnancy. NIH Publication No. 93–3279A. 1993.
26. Burrow GN. Thyroid disease. In: Burrow GN and Ferris TF, eds. Medical complications during pregnancy. 4th ed. Philadelphia: W.B. Saunders Company. 1995:155–187.
27. Whitmore R, Hobbins JC, Engle MA. Pregnancy

and its outcome in women with and without surgical treatment of congenital heart disease. Am J Cardiol 1982;50:641–651.

Contraception

28. Hatcher RA, Trussell J, Stewart F, et al. Contraceptive technology. 16th ed. New York: Irvington Publishers, Inc. 1994.
29. Tyrer LB. Oral contraceptive practice. In: Corson SL, Derman RJ, and Tyrer LB, eds. Fertility control. 2nd ed. Ontario: Goldin Publishers. 1994:97–114.
30. Abramowicz M, ed. The medical letter. New Rochelle: The Medical Letter, Inc. 1995;37:9–12.
31. Bernstein GS. Cervical caps and female condoms. In: Corson SL, Derman RJ, and Tyrer LB, eds. Fertility control. 2nd ed. Ontario: Goldin Publishers. 1994:221–232.
32. Buchanan TA, Coustan DR. Diabetes mellitus. In: Burrow GN and Ferris TF, eds. Medical complications during pregnancy. Philadelphia: W.B. Saunders Co. 1995:1–28.
33. Baird DT, Glashier AF. Hormonal contraception. N Engl J Med 1993;328:1543–1549.
34. Speroff L, Darney PD. A clinical guide for contraception. Baltimore: Williams & Wilkins, 1992.

Menopause

35. The Boston: Women's Health Book Collective The new our bodies, our selves. New York: Simon and Schuster, 1992:516–553.
36. Gambrell RD. Complications of estrogen replacement therapy. In: Swartz DP, ed. Hormone replacement therapy. Baltimore: Williams & Wilkens, 1992:194.
37. Gambrell RD. Prevention of endometrial cancer with progestogens. Maturitas 1986; 8:159.
38. Steinberg KK, Thatcher SB, Smith SJ, et al. A meta-analysis of the effect of estrogen replacement therapy on the risk of breast cancer. JAMA 1991;265:1985–1990.
39. Gambrell RD. Complications of estrogen replacement therapy. In: Swartz DP, ed. Hormone replacement therapy. Baltimore: Williams & Wilkins, 1992: 200.
40. Lindsay R, Cosman F. Osteoporosis: The estrogen relationship. In: Swartz DP, ed. Hormone replacement therapy. Baltimore: Williams & Wilkins, 1992:17–64.
41. Ettinger B, Genant HK, Cann CE. Postmenopausal bone loss prevented by treatment with low dosage estrogen with calcium. Ann Intern Med 1987; 106:40–45.
42. Stampfer MJ, Coldetz GA, Willett WC, et al. Post menopausal estrogen therapy and cardiovascular disease: ten year follow up from the nurses health study. N Engl J Med 1991;325:756–62.
43. Wilson PWF, Garrison RJ, Castelli WP. Postmenopausal estrogen use, cigarette smoking, and cardiovascular morbidity in women over 50:the Framingham study. N Engl J Med 1985;313:1038–43.
44. The Writing Group for the PEPI Trial Effects of estrogen or estrogen/progestin regimens on heart disease risk factors in postmenopausal women: the postmenopausal estrogen/progestin interventions (PEPI) trial. JAMA 1995;273:199–208.
45. Henderson BE, Pajanini-Hill A, Ross RK. Decreased mortality in users of estrogen replacement therapy. Arch Intern Med 1991;151:75–78.
46. Stumph P. Estrogen replacement therapy: current regimens. In: Swartz DP, ed. Hormone replacement therapy. Baltimore: Williams & Wilkins, 1992: 171–190.
47. Wallis LA. Hormone replacement therapy: decision making in an age of uncertainty. JAMA 1992;47: 225–229.

Breast Lumps

48. Robbins S, Cotran R. Pathologic basis of disease, 3rd ed. W.B. Saunders, 1984:1165–1191.
49. Berman CG, Clark RA. Diagnostic images in cancer; primary care clinics 19:4, Dec. 1992;677–697.
50. Walker GM, Foster RS, McKegney CP, et al. Breast biopsies: comparison of outpatient and inpatient experience. Arch Surg 1978;113:942.
51. Warner EA. Breast cancer screening; primary care clinics 19:3, Sept. 1992;575–588.
52. Henderson IC. Carcinoma of the breast; office practice of medicine. 3rd ed. Philadelphia: W.B. Saunders Co. 1991:926–944.

SUGGESTED READINGS

Pelvic Pain

Dawood MY. Dysmenorrhea. Clin Obstet Gynecol 1990;33:168–177.

Droegmueller W. Endometriosis and adenomyosis. In: Herbst AL, Mishell DR, Stenchever MA, Droegemueller W, eds. Comprehensive gynecology:2nd ed. St. Louis: Mosby Year Book, 1992:556–559.

McCormack WM. Pelvic inflammatory disease. N Engl J Med 1994;330:115–119.

Vaginal Discharge

Reed BD, Eyler A. Vaginal infections: diagnosis and management. J Fam Pract 1993;47:1805–1816.

Sobel JD. Vaginal infections in adult women. Med Clin North Am 1990;74:1573–1576.

Preconception Care of the Medical Patient

Anonymous. Recommendations for use of folic acid to reduce number of spina bifida cases and other neural tube defects. JAMA 1993:269:1233–1238.

August P, Peterson LF, et al. Management of medical problems in pregnancy. In: Carr PL, Freund KM, Somani S, eds. The medical care of women. Philadelphia: W.B. Saunders Company, 1995:335–452

Barron WM, Lindheimer MD, eds. Medical disorders during pregnancy. St. Louis: Mosby Year Book, 1991.

Burrow GN, Feris TF, eds. Medical complications during pregnancy. 4th ed. Philadelphia: W.B. Saunders Company, 1995.

Contraception

Bengston J. Hormonal contraception. In: Carr PL, Freund KM, Somani S, eds. The medical care of women. Philadelphia: W.B. Saunders Company, 1995:226–236.

Corson SL, Derman RJ, Tyrer LB, eds. Fertility control. 2nd ed. Ontario: Goldin Publishers, 1994.

Hatcher RA, Trussel J, Stewart F, et al. Contraceptive technology. 16th ed. New York: Irvington Publishers, Inc. 1994.

Thabault P, Carr PL. Nonhormonal contraception. In: Carr PL, Freund KM, Somani S, eds. The medical care of women. Philadelphia: W.B. Saunders Company, 1995:236–243.

Menopause

Sheehy G. The silent passage. New York: Pocket Books, 1993.

Sherwin B. Menopause: myths and realities. In: Stewart D, Stoddard N, eds. Psychological aspects of women's health care. Washington, DC: American Psychiatric Press, 1993:227–247.

Schwartz DP, ed. Hormone replacement therapy. Baltimore: Williams & Wilkins, 1992.

Breast Lumps

Barker RL, Burton JR, Zieve PH. Principles of ambulatory medicine. 3rd ed. Baltimore: Williams & Wilkins, 1991.

Cotran RS, Kumar V, Robbins SL. Pathologic basis of disease. 5th ed. W.B. Saunders, 1994.

chapter 21

DERMATOLOGY
Matthew A. Berger, Rosemarie Conigliaro

RASH

Skin rash is a common reason why patients present to the health care provider in the ambulatory setting. The last National Ambulatory Care Survey reported that 42 million patient visits per year or 7.3% of all visits to physicians were for dermatologic complaints. The economic cost of skin disease in this country was estimated to be 1.5 billion dollars in 1985 (1). Harder to measure, though comparable in impact are the physical, psychological, and emotional costs to patients who have these potentially disabling and disfiguring conditions. The adolescent with severe cystic acne can become withdrawn and isolated just at a time when social acceptance is of the utmost importance. The chronic and unremitting pain of post-herpetic neuralgia can permanently corrupt a patient's sense of well-being. Fortunately, many skin rashes are either self-limited, curable, or readily controlled once an accurate diagnosis is made and appropriate therapy applied. Those that are more severe, chronic in nature, or are manifestations of underlying systemic illness will challenge the diagnostic skill and therapeutic armamentarium of the primary care clinician. While in most instances the generalist will be able to diagnose and treat many skin conditions, consultation with the dermatologist should be sought when the diagnosis is uncertain (raising the potential need for skin biopsy), the patient does not respond to treatment (Is the diagnosis correct?), or the appropriate treatment requires special equipment or skills (surgical excision, phototherapy).

Pathophysiologic Correlation

The functions of the skin stem directly from its position as the boundary between the internal milieu and the environment. These include the maintenance of structural integrity, thermoregulation, sensory function, and protection against microorganisms and injurious physical agents (radiation, heat). One can readily appreciate the impact that the skin's appearance has on psychodynamics and human social behavior. As it contains elements of the nervous, vascular, exocrine and immune systems, skin pathology often reflects generalized disease processes involving these tissues.

Clinical and Laboratory Evaluation

The word *rash* is a term in common usage referring to any cutaneous eruption. It has little diagnostic specificity given the enormous variety and etiologies of skin lesions. However, unlike other nonspecific chief complaints (e.g., dizziness or fatigue), in which the physician relies on the patient's ability to translate bodily sensations into words, a rash can be viewed directly. The only barrier to disclosure of the rash is the patient's clothing. Much of the emphasis in making a diagnosis will therefore be based on physical diagnosis, the visual aspects of the skin rash. The appearance of certain skin rashes is so characteristic that inspection alone is sufficient to diagnose accurately. When the findings are less specific, the account of the rash's appearance and its evolution combined with the patient's medical history will greatly narrow the possibilities. In some circumstances selected laboratory testing, including histologic examination, may be required to settle a diagnostic dilemma.

HISTORY

Once the rash has been examined, pertinent history should be elicited:

When was the rash first noted?
Where did the lesions first appear?
How did the lesions progress both in their
  appearance and distribution?

With what symptoms is the rash associated (itching, burning, pain)?

What treatment has already been used and with what response?

What medications does the patient take including over-the-counter and "health food store" preparations?

What skin products does the patient use?

What activities preceded the onset of the rash (e.g., gardening, sun bathing, housework, crafts)?

What work does the patient perform and with what skin contact?

Are there any systemic symptoms (fever, arthralgias, malaise) associated with the rash?

Does the patient have any chronic illnesses?

Does the patient have any known allergies?

What sexual contact has the patient had?

PHYSICAL EXAMINATION

The examination of a rash should address four questions about its visible features:

1. How are the lesions distributed over the body?

    By body location: face; scalp; neck; trunk; limbs; palms and soles

    Extensor vs. flexor surfaces

    By extent: localized to one body region; generalized to all body regions

    Universal: involving the entirety of the skin surface

    By predilection: sun-exposed areas; intertriginous areas (between skin folds); dependent areas; areas of thick vs thin skin

2. How do individual lesions group together?

    As an isolated lesion vs. multiple lesions randomly scattered in an area

    Arranged in a ring (annular), in a line (linear), like a net (reticular)

    As a crop of vesicles (herpetiform), as a band of vesicles (zosteriform), as a coalescence of maculopapules, (morbilliform, which means "like measles")

3. What is the shape of individual lesions?

    Round; oval; curved (arcinate); linear; annular; dimpled (umbilicated)

4. What type of lesion(s) is present?

    Macule: a circumscribed, flat lesion which differs from the surrounding skin by its color, e.g., the lesion of vitiligo which is a white macule devoid of melanin pigment

    Papule: a solid, visibly raised lesion less than 1 cm in diameter (large enough to see),

e.g., an insect bite which produces an erythematous papule at the site of the bite

Nodule: a solid, palpable, rounded lesion (large enough to feel), e.g., a lipoma which is a soft, subcutaneous nodule composed of adipose tissue

Plaque: a flat, raised lesion often with an overlying scale, e.g., the well circumscribed silvery plaque of psoriasis

Crust: an accumulation of dried serum, blood or pus exuded by the underlying lesion, e.g., the dried vesicular fluid that forms a crust over varicella lesions.

Wheal: a raised erythematous lesion, of varied shape and size, seen primarily in allergic reactions. They tend to appear and disappear within hours, e.g., the urticarial reaction associated with shellfish allergy.

Vesicle: a fluid filled, raised lesion. A large vesicle is called a bulla, e.g., the crop of vesicles produced by herpes simplex virus.

Pustule: a pus-filled, raised lesion, e.g., the pustule that forms around a hair shaft (folliculitis)

Erosion: a depressed lesion where there is loss of only superficial layers of skin, e.g., the lesion that forms after the rupture of a bulla

Ulcer: a lesion where deeper layers of skin and underlying tissue have been lost, e.g., the venous stasis ulcer that forms due to high venous pressure in the leg

Telangiectasia: a blood vessel sufficiently dilated as to be visible with the unaided eye, e.g., the "spider veins" that form on the lower extremities of pregnant women.

When examining a skin rash it is important that the patient be completely disrobed and gowned to permit a complete inspection of the skin. Not only will this disclose the full extent of the rash but also permits the examiner to screen the patient for potentially deadly pigmented lesions. The patient should be viewed both close up and from a distance of several feet; the former to reveal the detail of individual lesions, the latter to show the distribution of the rash. While conducting this examination, the physician must at all times remain aware of the patient's sensitivity and modesty. The examiner should be sure not to overlook "hidden areas" such as the scalp, under folds of skin, between the buttocks and thighs, and the mucous membranes. The examiner should be gloved before touching affected skin to prevent transmission from infectious lesions.

LABORATORY EVALUATION

Certain basic laboratory tests are valuable in confirming the diagnosis of a dermatologic condition. They can be carried out by the examining physician with standard equipment and supplies.

KOH Smear. This technique permits identification of fungal hyphae and budding yeasts in dermatophytoses and Candidal infections. Using a scalpel, collect scrapings from the edge (the location of proliferating organisms) of a suspected lesion onto a glass microscope slide. Apply several drops of 10% KOH solution, top with a cover slip and heat briefly. This will dissolve the keratin from the skin cells and reveal the fungal elements under light microscopy. The addition of ink to the KOH solution (Swartz-Lampkin solution) makes the organisms stand out more distinctly.

Tzanck Smear. When a herpes virus (Herpes simplex, Varicella-Zoster) infection is suspected, the vesicle should be carefully unroofed, the base of the lesion scraped, applied to a slide, allowed to dry, then stained with Wright's or Giemsa stain. The presence of multi-nucleated giant cells is evidence for the presence of herpes virus, though the specific type must be confirmed with either viral culture or serologic testing.

Skin Biopsy. This minor surgical procedure done under local anesthesia can be invaluable in dermatologic diagnosis. Knowing the indications for skin biopsy and selecting the site most likely to have the greatest diagnostic yield should be the province of the dermatologist. Accurate diagnosis will also depend on the availability of a skilled and experienced dermatopathologist.

The next section of this chapter will describe four common entities: eczema, acne, psoriasis, and viral exanthematous diseases, which present as a skin rash in the ambulatory setting.

Differential Diagnosis

ECZEMA

The term eczema connotes a nonspecific inflammatory reaction of the skin to a variety of endogenous and exogenous factors. In its acute form, eczematous skin is characterized by a coalesced papular eruption, which forms erythematous and edematous plaques (Fig. 21.1). With a more intense inflammatory reaction, there may be vesiculation, weeping of the skin, fissuring, and crusting. The lesions may become secondarily infected with bacterial or fungal organisms (impetigination) and exude purulent material. With chronicity, eczematous skin can thicken and develop prominent

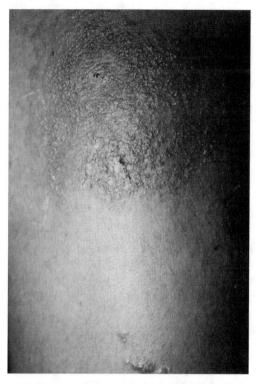

Figure 21.1. Allergic contact dermatitis. The forearm skin of this patient exposed to poison ivy demonstrates an acute eczematous reaction marked by erythema, edema and a coalesced papular eruption.

furrows (lichenification) or become hyperpigmented (Fig. 21.2). Histologic examination of an acute eczematous lesion shows intercellular epidermal edema (spongiosis); the chronic lesions exhibit epidermal hyperplasia and a mononuclear cell infiltrate. Like the macroscopic appearance, the findings on microscopy do not distinguish the varieties of eczematous dermatitis. Only by placing this otherwise undifferentiated skin reaction into the proper clinical perspective can the different forms and etiologies be separated.

Atopic Dermatitis. Atopic dermatitis, also termed atopic eczema, is the cutaneous syndrome of individuals with a personal or family history of other atopic diseases such as asthma, hay fever, and allergic rhinitis. It occurs most commonly in childhood, decreasing in prevalence with increased age (2). A variety of physical, immunologic and psychological factors have been described including elevated IgE levels, decreased T suppressor cell function, enhanced antigen induced histamine release, altered cutaneous vascular reactivity, de-

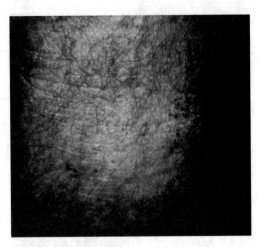

Figure 21.2. Lichenification. This patch of chronic eczema demonstrates prominent skin furrows, a thin white scale and excoriation.

creased itch threshold, excessive dryness of the skin, and a personality trait of inhibited emotional expression (3-6).

The most prominent features of the clinical presentation are the itching and dryness of the skin. Secondary manifestations, promoted by scratching and rubbing, may include papules, linear excoriations, weeping and crusting, bacterial skin infection (particularly with Staphylococcus aureus) and lichenification. Typical areas of involvement are the popliteal and antecubital fossae, the wrists, back of the neck, and face. Itching of the anogenital region is common in adults with this condition who may report that scratching provokes a pleasurable sensation. Uninvolved skin from an atopic displays white dermatographism, the appearance of pallor (vasoconstriction) in response to a gentle stroke with the thumbnail or a blunt instrument. Atopic eczema may be confused with allergic/irritant contact dermatitis or both may occur in the same patient. A careful search for environmental skin exposures can help to distinguish the two. In addition, any itchy, scaly lesion should be scraped and examined for fungal organisms.

Irritant and Allergic Contact Dermatitis. The eczematous reaction may stem from skin contact with either an irritant substance or an allergen that provokes a delayed hypersensitivity reaction. (In contrast, acute hypersensitivity of the skin is more likely to manifest urticaria.) The most common form of irritant dermatitis, hand eczema, is caused by frequent hand washing or the use of cleaning agents (detergents and spirits) that dry and irritate the skin. A very large variety of substances contained in consumer products, industrial materials and in the natural environment can provoke an allergic response in individuals who have been previously sensitized. Nickel plated jewelry can produce an eczematous reaction of the ear lobes, neck or wrists. The resins in nail care products, the preservatives in cosmetics, the curing agents in rubber goods (including latex gloves), the organic compounds in fragrances and other topical products can cause an eczematous reaction. Topical medications (containing neomycin, diphenhydramine, benzocaine, propylene glycol) and transdermal drug delivery systems may provoke an irritant or allergic contact dermatitis. The oleoresin urushiol is responsible for the plant dermatitis of poison ivy, poison oak, and poison sumac.

Acute contact dermatitis is manifested by an erythematous papular eruption that may include vesiculation or bullous formation. The more delicate areas of skin (face, flexor limb surfaces, dorsa of the hands, and feet) are more prone to irritant/allergic dermatitis than skin with a thicker stratum corneum (elbows, knees, palms, and soles). An allergic reaction is more likely to be pruritic whereas irritants tend to cause burning or pain. The distribution and arrangement of the lesions corresponds to manner and location of skin contact. For example, the patient who gardens in a patch of poison ivy will be left with a rash of linear streaks on the exposed skin that was brushed by the plant. Accurate diagnosis of allergic/irritant contact dermatitis will often require a careful and exhaustive inventory of all potential cutaneous contacts including personal articles, products from the home and materials from the work environment. In some circumstances, patch testing will be required to identify which specific agent(s) the patient should avoid. A testing kit of 20 common contact allergens has been recommended by the North American Contact Dermatitis Group (7).

Stasis Dermatitis. Stasis dermatitis can occur in the lower extremities of patients with venous insufficiency or chronic edema. In response to high venous pressures and edema the skin becomes reddened, scaly and itchy. Over time, extravasation of erythrocytes will lead to hemosiderin deposition and produce a speckled, brown discoloration of the medial lower leg and ankle. Brawny edema, extensive erythema, scaling, and ulceration can develop in more severely affected patients. The ulcers may become secondarily infected and extend over large areas of the leg necessitating debridement, systemic antibiotics, and potentially skin grafting. Fungal superinfection, which will intensify the eczema, may complicate this condition in diabetic patients and should be looked for in scrapings of the lesions.

Seborrheic Dermatitis. In seborrheic dermatitis a yellow, greasy plaque forms on the scalp, behind the ears, beneath the eyebrows, and in the nasolabial folds. Other intertriginous areas that may be involved are the axillae, the gluteal folds, and the groin. The lesions can flake copiously producing significant dandruff.

Nummular Eczema. Nummular eczema is characterized by the presence of coin shaped eczematous lesions on the dorsal surfaces of the hands, the shins and the trunk. The efficacy of treatment with antibiotics suggests a hypersensitivity reaction to bacterial colonization of the skin as the etiology.

Asteototic Eczema. Asteototic eczema is seen in the elderly and produces an eczematous patch on the legs particularly during the dry winter season.

Lichen Simplex Chronicus. Lichen simplex chronicus describes a longstanding eczematous patch of lichenified skin that stems from chronic scratching and rubbing. Common sites are the base of the neck and the ankles.

ACNE

The two major forms of acne are acne vulgaris (teenage acne) and acne rosacea (adult acne).

Acne Vulgaris. This condition, primarily affecting adolescents and young adults, is characterized by the presence of comedos, pustules, nodules, cysts, and scars on the face, chest, and upper back (Fig. 21.3). The age of onset as well as the type and distribution of lesions is so characteristic that the diagnosis is usually straightforward. Although the underlying cause remains unknown, the pathogenesis of the lesions involves the interaction of three factors: increased sebum production, abnormal keratinization of the skin follicle; and the action of the skin's microflora.

The pilosebaceous unit or skin pore (hair follicle and its associated sebaceous glands) is the site of the primary lesion of acne, the comedo. Sebum, the oily product of the sebaceous gland, appears to cause a build up of keratin in the follicular canal. This results in the open comedo (blackhead) with its dilated follicular opening filled with an oxidized, dark keratin plug. This lesion is usually noninflammatory. When the abnormal keratinization occurs at a deeper level, the duct orifice does not dilate and a closed comedo (whitehead) results. Further secretion of sebum into the obstructed follicle and the release of free fatty acids by bacteria (notably *Propionibacterium acnes*), cause rupture of the comedo into the adjacent dermis. An inflammatory reaction ensues forming red papules and pustules. With more intense activity, large inflammatory nodules may develop in the deep dermal layers of the skin. They may become cystic over time or may rupture producing subepidermal lakes and sinuses of pus that ultimately heal with significant scarring.

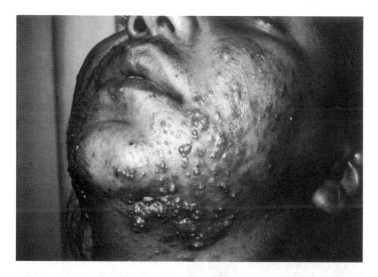

Figure 21.3. Acne vulgaris. This severe eruption displays the variety of lesions including open and closed comedos, extensive pustules, and nodules, some of which have coalesced. The skin has an oily sheen typical of increased sebum production.

Acne is a common condition that has affected most individuals at some time in their lives. As many as one-third of people age 15 to 44 report moderately to severely disfiguring acne. There is a slightly increased incidence ratio (1.5:1) of men to women. Androgen hormones play an important permissive and modulating role in the development of acne. The rising levels of gonadal and adrenal androgens at puberty stimulate the formation and growth of sebaceous glands and coincide with the onset of acne. Other states of androgen excess associated with acne are Cushing's disease, polycystic ovarian disease, and congenital adrenal hyperplasia. Certain non-hormonal factors may also stimulate comedo formation such as the use of skin products containing lanolin, petrolatum, butylstearate, lauryl alcohol and oleic acid. Excess friction and rubbing on existing comedos may cause their contents to rupture inducing inflammation.

The first appearance of acne in the adolescent is usually on the forehead followed by the cheeks, chin and nose. More extensive outbreaks can involve the upper back and chest. Lesions tend to progress through the typical stages and heal spontaneously without scarring. The more severely affected patient will manifest large inflammatory nodules, cysts and ultimately extensive, pitted scars that carry a significant cosmetic morbidity.

Acne Rosacea.　Acne rosacea differs from acne vulgaris in that it primarily affects adults (onset during 3rd decade of life) and is not associated with an increased production of sebum or the presence of comedos. The lesions are primarily papulopustules occurring on the central areas of the face (Fig. 21.4). A cutaneous vascular hyperreactivity is prominent, especially in women. A variety of vasoactive stimuli such as emotional arousal, alcohol, extremes of heat and cold, spicy food, and certain drugs cause an intense erythematous flushing of the face and neck. Initially, flushing is transient but over time telangiectasias form and the erythema becomes persistent. Inflammatory papules and pustules arise in proportion to the degree of vasodilation. In a subset of cases, a granulomatous reaction forms larger, nodular lesions. Rhinophyma, seen primarily in men with acne rosacea, results from hyperplasia of the soft tissue and sebaceous components of the nose. W.C. Fields not withstanding, rhinophyma is not a sign of alcoholism.

The differential of acne rosacea includes acne vulgaris, which differs by the age of onset and distribution of lesions (central face vs. entire face, chest, and back). Perioral dermatitis, a rosacea-like reaction around the mouth and chin may occur after long-term use of topical fluorinated corticosteroids. The flush of rosacea may be confused with the malar rash of lupus erythematosus. The two can be distinguished by the sparing of the nasolabial fold (non-sunexposed) in lupus. Other granulomatous diseases, such as sarcoid, may involve the face. Carcinoid, which also causes facial flushing, may be confused with rosacea.

PSORIASIS

Psoriasis is a chronic papulosquamous disorder characterized by the presence of erythematous plaques covered by a silvery scale. The lesions ap-

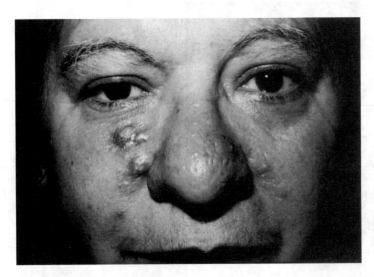

Figure 21.4.　Acne rosacea. Papules and nodules over the central face with an erythematous flush and rhinophyma.

pear to arise from an accelerated proliferation of the epidermis and abnormal keratinocyte maturation. Like acne vulgaris, significant cosmetic disfigurement is a common and important clinical feature of this disease.

The worldwide incidence is approximately 2% and is found more commonly in peoples of temperate and northern climates. The disease may begin at any time in life but is rare under the age of two and has a mean age of onset of about 27 years (8). There is no gender predisposition. The fundamental cause remains unknown, although a number of genetic, immune, and environmental factors have been identified that influence the disease. As many as one-third of patients with psoriasis report having at least one affected family member. Several HLA haplotypes (HLA-B13, HLA-Bw16 and HLA-B17) have been linked to psoriasis. The interaction of T-lymphocytes with a variety of immunomodulating substances has been shown to play a role in the regulation of disease activity. The well known Koebner phenomenon, the development of a psoriatic lesion at the exact site of previous physical trauma to the skin, strongly relates immune reaction to disease pathogenesis. Patients infected with the human immunodeficiency virus may develop extensive psoriatic lesions when the number of T-helper cells decreases below 400 μl. The environment is another important modulator of psoriasis as the disease tends to improve in sunny, humid seasons and worsen during cold, dry ones. A number of drugs including chloroquine, lithium, indomethacin and beta-blockers have been associated with exacerbations of psoriasis.

The initial lesion is an erythematous papule with an overlying scale. These papules coalesce to form sharply demarcated erythematous plaques covered by a silvery scale. Scraping off the scale leaves behind a moist, pink area that will bleed from several punctate sites (Ausptiz's sign). On microscopy there is exuberant epidermal proliferation and a greatly thickened stratum corneum. Studies of cellular kinetics demonstrate an eight-fold increase in the rate of epidermal turnover suggesting that psoriasis is a disorder of the regulation of cell replication. The psoriatic plaques can range greatly in size from small coin lesions to those which cover entire body surfaces. They tend to distribute symmetrically and are common on the scalp, knees, elbows, and lower back although any area of skin can be affected (Fig. 21.5). Nail involvement is common and may be of great diagnostic value in uncertain cases. Typical nail findings are tiny pits, yellow discoloration and thinning of the nail plate, and the build up of kerti-

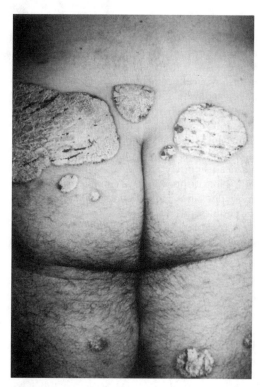

Figure 21.5. Psoriasis. Large, well-circumscribed plaques with dense silvery scale and an erythematous border.

naceous material, especially under the toenails. Some variants in the patterns of psoriasis are as follows:

Guttate–The eruption of tiny erythematous papulosquamous lesions on the trunk, often seen in children with streptococcal infections.

Pustular–Extensive pustule formation occurring over erythematous skin of the trunk, limbs, palms and soles associated with systemic signs. It may occur in patients with psoriasis who are withdrawn from systemic steroids.

Inverse–The psoriatic lesions occur in areas of skin folds such as the axillae, the groin and under the breasts. The location of lesions may confuse this variant with tinea.

Exfoliative erythroderma–A generalized form of the disease affecting all body sites with diffuse erythema and scaling. It may develop in response to the injurious effect of treatments with ultraviolet light or harsh topical preparations. It resembles a generalized drug reaction or severe atopic dermatitis.

The rapid proliferation and shedding of epidermal cells can lead to a number of non-cutaneous manifestations in patients with psoriasis. A mild anemia may result from the loss of iron and folate in shed skin cells combined with the increased requirement for folic acid generated by cellular hyperproliferation. High cell turnover can cause negative nitrogen balance or increase uric acid to levels that could precipitate gout or nephrolithiasis. The marked increase in blood supply to psoriatic lesions (particularly in erythroderma) could induce heart failure in patients who have an underlying cardiomyopathy. Fever and profound weakness is seen in the pustular and erythrodermatous variants. Psoriasis is associated with a seronegative inflammatory spondyloarthropathy termed psoriatic arthritis.

VIRAL EXANTHEMS

Skin rash is a prominent feature of a number of viral illnesses. The next section will focus primarily on the cutaneous manifestations of these entities. For a more detailed discussion, one should consult a textbook of Internal Medicine or Infectious Diseases.

Measles (Rubeola). Measles (or Rubeola), the archetype of exanthematous diseases, is an acute febrile illness with a prominent eruption, upper respiratory tract symptoms and uncommonly, severe involvement of the lung and central nervous system. Outbreaks occur primarily in the winter and spring spreading rapidly among nonimmune contacts. In the United States most cases occur within clusters of unvaccinated individuals or in vaccine recipients who failed to establish or maintain immunity. This is more likely to occur if the vaccine was administered before 1 year of age. Current recommendation calls for a two dose primary immunization with attenuated live measles vaccine. It is particularly important to ensure that groups of young people living in close quarters (students and military recruits) have been immunized. Measles vaccine is not contraindicated for patients infected with HIV although vaccine failures are common.

The illness begins with an asymptomatic incubation period of 7 to 10 days followed by a prodrome of fever, malaise, rhinitis (coryza), conjunctivitis and cough. By day 3, the typical maculopapular erythematous rash begins at the forehead and behind the ears. It descends down the face, neck, trunk then to the extremities. The lesions tend to coalesce on the face, neck, and upper trunk,

remaining discrete on the lower extremities. Lasting approximately 4 days in total, the rash darkens, fades and lightly desquamates in the order it appeared. One to two days before the onset of the rash, pathognomonic Koplik spots appear (named for New York pediatrician Henry Koplik). They are bright red, irregular lesions with blue/white centers appearing on the buccal mucosa. A variant of measles termed atypical measles may develop in individuals who received the killed measles vaccine available between 1963 and 1967. Here the prodrome of fever, headache, myalgias, and abdominal pain is followed by a rash that begins at the hands and feet and progresses toward the head. It may manifest a variety of forms including maculopapules, vesicles, wheals, and purpura which are especially prominent in skin creases. While the entirety of the clinical presentation of measles is fairly specific, the rash may be mimicked by a variety of other viruses (rubella, adenovirus, enterovirus), bacteria (secondary syphilis, scarlet fever, toxic shock syndrome), and allergic drug reactions. The rash of atypical measles may be confused with that of Rocky Mountain Spotted Fever.

Rubella (German Measles). Rubella (or German Measles) is a milder exanthematous illness whose major health impact is the fetal damage it causes during maternal infection. The live attenuated virus vaccine produces life-long immunity in most persons vaccinated after the age of 1 year. Although congenital rubella syndrome is not known to occur as a result of inadvertent immunization during pregnancy, it is recommended that women avoid conception for 3 months after receiving the vaccine. The illness begins two to three weeks after infection with a prodrome of fever, headache, conjunctivitis, pharyngitis, and lymphadenopathy. A light pink maculopapular rash begins on the face, quickly spreads to the trunk and extremities, coalesces, then fades by the third day.

Varicella-Zoster Virus. Varicella-Zoster Virus is the agent that causes varicella (chicken pox) as a primary infection and as herpes zoster (shingles), its reactivation form. An effective attenuated virus vaccine has been available for the past twenty years although its use in this country has been restricted primarily to immunocompromised children.

The incubation period of acute varicella is approximately 10 to 14 days after which moderate fever and a rash appear. Adults may experience a prodrome of fever, malaise and headache for several days. The rash, which is often pruritic, starts on the face and spreads onto the trunk with sparse involvement of the extremities. The lesions begin as light red macules that rapidly progress to papules, to vesicles, to pustules that crust over and usually heal without scarring. Crops of lesions erupt successively so that, at any one time, lesions of all stages are present. Vesicles may appear on the mucous membranes especially the palate. Viral particles are present in vesicular fluid rendering the patient contagious until all lesions have crusted and no new crops appear. The illness tends to be more severe in adults and may by complicated by pneumonia or meningoencephalitis.

Herpes zoster is a disease caused by reactivation of latent Varicella-Zoster virus from sensory root ganglia which become infected during the primary illness. A number of factors are associated with the development of herpes zoster including advanced age, underlying malignancy and immunosuppression. Skin trauma may herald an outbreak of zoster. The rash is an erythematous papulovesicular eruption which appears in a unilateral dermatomal pattern, most commonly on the trunk. Moderate to severe dysesthetic pain at the involved site is a hallmark finding that often precedes the rash by a day or two. During this gap period the pain may be confused with other pathogenic processes as varied as renal colic, pleurisy or acute myocardial infarction. The vesicles ultimately crust and heal over a one to two week period. Pain that may persist for weeks or months after the rash has healed (postherpetic neuralgia) is the most common complication of herpes zoster and may affect up to 15% of patients. Zoster that involves an extremity may lead to frank neuritis and subsequent motor paralysis. Herpes zoster of the ophthalmic branch of the trigeminal nerve may affect the eye and should prompt consultation with the Ophthalmologist. Immunosuppressed patients may experience a severe varicella-zoster reactivation with cutaneous and visceral dissemination.

Management

ATOPIC ECZEMA

Therapy should include avoidance of irritants that promote dryness and itching (primarily hot water and standard soaps); the use of lukewarm water and lotions (e.g., Cetaphil) for washing; the use of low to medium potency topical glucocorticoid creams and ointments (Table 21.1) to moisturize and reduce inflammatory reactivity; anti-histamines to relieve itching; and systemic antibiotics when secondary bacterial infection has developed.

ALLERGIC AND IRRITANT CONTACT DERMATITIS

The first step in treatment should of course be the removal of the irritant or allergen from contact with the skin. Patients should expect one to three weeks for complete healing to occur. Cool compresses of tap water or Burow's solution as well as soaking in an Aveeno (oatmeal) bath will reduce pruritis. Antihistamines are helpful adjuncts to control itching. Topical lotions containing calamine or zinc oxide can be soothing, drying and antipruritic. Glucocorticoid creams and ointments are effective anti-inflammatory agents. Systemic glucocorticoid therapy may be indicated in particularly severe cases.

STASIS DERMATITIS

General steps in therapy are aimed at reducing the underlying venous stasis and edema including the use of leg elevation, compression stockings, diuretics and exercise. Patients whose jobs entail prolonged standing or sitting should be encouraged to take periodic walking breaks followed by leg elevation throughout the day.

SEBORRHEIC DERMATITIS

Treatment consists of the use of shampoos containing coal tar, selenium, or salicylate and medium to low potency topical steroid preparations.

NUMMULAR ECZEMA

The same general principles of anti-itch and anti-inflammatory treatment applies here as well. In addition, anti-staphylococcal antibiotics may be of particular value.

ASTEOTOTIC ECZEMA

Moisturizers and low to medium potency topical corticosteroids are the primary modes of treatment.

LICHEN SIMPLEX CHRONICUS

Treatment consists of interruption of the itch-scratch cycle with the use of high potency corticosteroid topicals, sometimes under occlusive dressings.

ACNE VULGARIS

Treatment is aimed at preventing comedo formation, removing them once they occur, and reducing

Table 21.1.
Topical Corticosteroid Preparations Grouped by Potency

Group	Generic Name/Brand Name	
I (highest potency)	Betamethasone diproprionate in optimized vehicle 0.05% *Diprolene Ointment*	Clobetasol propionate 0.05 *Temovate cream, ointment* Diflorasone diacetate 0.05% *Psorcon ointment*
II	Amcinonide 0.1% *Cyclocort ointment* Betamethasone dipropionate 0.05% *Diprolene AF cream* Betamethasone diproprionate 0.05% *Diprosone ointment* Mometasone furoate 0.1% *Elocon ointment*	Diflorasone diacetate 0.05% *Florone ointment* *Maxiflor ointment* Halcinonide 0.1% *Halog cream* Fluocinonide 0.05% *Lidex cream, ointment* *Topsyn gel* Desoximetasone 0.25% *Topicort cream, ointment*
III	Triamcinolone acetonide 0.5% *Aristocort HP cream* Betametasone dipropionate 0.05% *Diprosone cream*	Diflorasone diacetate 0.05% *Florone cream* *Maxiflor cream* Valisone ointment 0.1% *Betamethasone valerate*
IV	Triamcinolone acetonide 0.1% *Aristocort ointment* *Kenalog ointment* Betamethasone benzoate 0.025% *Benisone ointment*	Mometasone furoate 0.1% *Elocon cream* Flucocinolone acetonide 0.025% *Synalar ointment* Flurandrenolide 0.05% *Cordran ointment*
V	Betamethasone benzoate 0.025% *Benisone cream* Flurandrenolide 0.05% *Cordran cream* Fluticasone propionate 0.05% *Cutivate cream* Betamethasone dipropionate 0.02% *Diprosone lotion*	Triamcinolone acetonide 0.1% *Kenalog cream, lotion* Hydrocortisone butyrate 0.1% *Locoid cream* Fluocinolone acetonide 0.025% *Synalar cream* Betametasone valerate 0.1% *Valisone cream, lotion* Hydrocortisone valerate 0.2% *Westcort cream*
VI	Aclometasone dipropionate 0.05% *Aclovate cream* Desonide 0.05% *Tridesilon cream, ointment*	Flumethasone pivalate 0.03% *Locorten cream* Fluocinoline acetonide 0.01% *Synalar solution*
VII (lowest potency)	Hydrocortisone 1.0, 2.5% *Hytone cream, lotion, ointment* *Synacort, Cort-Dome*	

the inflammatory reaction. Open comedos may be emptied of their keratin plugs through careful use of a comedo extractor. Cleansing with abrasives, astringents and desquamatives also helps to remove blackheads but may irritate the skin if used excessively. Topical lotions, creams and gels containing benzoyl peroxide in concentrations of 2.5 to 10% are commonly prescribed to dry out pustules and accelerate healing. Topical antibiotic preparations

of erythromycin or clindamycin can inhibit the growth of skin bacteria that contribute to pustule formation. Retinoic acid is highly effective in small papulopustular acne and acts by loosening the contents of comedos and drying out inflammatory lesions. It is usually applied nightly in increasing strengths. Excessive skin dryness, irritation, erythema and sunsensitivity may complicate its use.

Acne with a more extensive and intense inflammatory component may require systemic therapy. Oral antibiotics have long been a mainstay in the treatment of pustular acne. Drugs of the tetracycline class (tetracycline, doxycycline, and minocycline) along with erythromycin have been most extensively used for their broad spectrum of activity, low incidence of side effects, and safety in long term usage. The tetracyclines may cause upper gastrointestinal irritation and photosensitivity as well as being contraindicated in pregnancy. Vaginal candidiasis or pseudomembranous colitis may complicate the long term use of any antibiotic. The treatment of nodulocystic acne has been revolutionized by a class of drugs derived from Vitamin A, the retinoids. Isotretinoin administered in dosages of 1 to 2 mg/kg/day over several months has resulted in complete clearing of severe acne lesions in a large proportion of affected individuals. Its mechanism of action appears to be related to a marked reduction in sebum production and inhibition of keratin formation. Because of serious potential side effects, this drug should be reserved for severely affected patients who have failed other modalities of treatment. When this highly teratogenic drug is prescribed to female patients, a negative pregnancy test should be obtained and the patient must be informed about the necessity to employ a highly reliable form of birth control. The drug may cause excessive skin dryness, conjunctival irritation and hyperlipidemia. In long-term use changes in night vision, calcification of the anterior spinal ligament and other skeletal hyperostoses may occur.

ACNE ROSACEA

Treatment should include avoidance of the environmental and pharmacologic factors that promote vasodilation. The inflammatory papulopustules and nodules respond to the same topical and systemic antibiotics used in acne vulgaris. Metronidazole, an antibiotic with excellent coverage for anaerobic bacteria, is highly effective as a topical agent for the treatment of rosacea. Topical and systemic retinoids have been also successfully used in selected patients.

PSORIASIS

Treatment modalities are highly varied and require a fair degree of expertise to prescribe. Most moderately to severely affected patients are best managed by the dermatologist. Scalp involvement is treated with shampoos containing anti-mitotic and anti-inflammatory coal tar preparations (e.g., T-Gel, Zetar) and keratinolytic salicylates (e.g., T-Sal).

Localized plaques respond to topical glucocorticoid preparations although their use should be guided by a number of principles:

1. High-potency topical steroids should not be used on delicate skin such as the face, the axilla or the groin as skin atrophy and striae may result.
2. High-potency topical steroids applied to large body surface areas or under occlusive dressings may be absorbed in sufficient quantity to suppress the pituitary-adrenal axis.
3. Better drug penetrance into a thick psoriatic plaque is achieved using ointment bases rather than creams or lotions and by softening the plaque first by soaking in warm water or coal tar bath.
4. Allergic reactions to the vehicle base should be considered if the lesions worsen with treatment.
5. The minimum effective potency and strength should be employed for long-term use.

Topical anthralin used in graded strengths is effective in psoriasis although it can cause irritation and may stain the patient's clothing. Phototherapy using long and short wave (UVA and UVB) ultraviolet radiation in a variety of regimens, sometimes with photosensitizing agents, is a highly effective form of treatment for more extensive body involvement. It requires specialized equipment and must be administered under close supervision. An increased incidence of skin cancer may result from this form of therapy. Severely affected patients who have failed other modalities may respond to systemic drug therapy with either methotrexate, an anti-metabolant with significant hepatotoxicity or etretinate, another retinoid compound similar in action and side-effects to isotretinoin. Cyclosporin, a potent immunosuppressive drug, can treat severe, recalcitrant psoriasis.

VIRAL EXANTHEMS

There is no specific therapy for most of the viral illnesses described (Table 21.2). Important exceptions are severe and disseminated forms of varicella-zoster virus infection, which respond to the intravenous administration of acyclovir, a specific anti-herpes virus agent. The duration of varicella and herpes zoster is shortened by several days if treatment with high dose oral acyclovir is employed. Prevention of post-herpetic neuralgia remains elusive; the value of corticosteroids and acyclovir for this purpose are to date unproven (10–14).

Table 21.2.
Selected Viral Illnesses Associated with Cutaneous Manifestations

Clinical Entity	Causative Agent	Cutaneous Manifestation
Erythema Infectiosum	Parvovirus B19	Fiery red cheeks followed by a maculopapular eruption on the trunk and upper arms
Common Warts	Papilloma virus	Verrucous, scaly papules usually on the hands or genitalia
Gingivostomatitis and Genital Herpes	Herpes Simplex	Crops of vesicles that form erosions and crusts on the vermillion of the lip and the anogenital region
Varicella	Varicella-zoster virus	Successive crops of pruritic maculopapules which vesiculate then crust
Shingles	Varicella-zoster virus	Unilateral dermatomal distribution of a painful vesicular rash
Hand-Foot and Mouth Disease	Coxsackie A16	Cutaneous and oral mucosal vesicles which may ulcerate
Herpangina	Coxsackie type A	White papulovesicles with a surrounding red halo on the palate
Molluscum Contagiosum	Poxvirus	Umbilicated flesh colored papules on the genital regions, head and trunk
Infectious Mononucleosis	Epstein-Barr virus	Erythematous maculopapular rash on the trunk and upper extremities. A generalized rash may result from the simultaneous use of ampicillin
Acute Respiratory Disease	Adenovirus	A morbilliform erythematous maculopapular rash
Acute HIV infection	Human Immunodeficiency Virus	A maculopapular/urticarial rash occurring 3 to 6 weeks after primary infection with HIV
Measles	Paramyxovirus	A maculopapular eruption associated with conjunctivitis and coryza
Rubella	Togavirus	A maculopapular eruption with mild systemic symptoms and short course

ILLUSTRATIVE CASES WITH SELF-ASSESSMENT QUESTIONS AND ANSWERS

Case 1

A 19-year-old woman presents to your office complaining of a rash on her hands and eyelids. She tells you that it began as dryness and itching over the dorsal surface of her fingers. They became reddened and scaly and then the rash spread over the entire hand. More recently her eyelids have become itchy, red, and puffy. Two weeks before coming to see you, she tried a bottle of Itch-Be-Gone lotion that she bought at a flea market but the rash has worsened. The itching is so severe that it keeps her awake at night. Her history includes frequent bouts of bronchitis and sinusitis especially in the cooler months. As a child she had hives after eating certain foods. She takes no medications and has no chronic illnesses. She recently began working as a manicurist in a nail salon. On examination you find an intensely erythematous maculopapular eruption over the entire dorsal surface of the hands extending into the web spaces between the fingers. There is fine scaling, scattered vesicles and innumerable linear excoriations with some yellow crusting. The hands are somewhat puffy. There is some mild erythema of the eyelids and slight periorbital edema.

QUESTION: *The most likely diagnosis is:*

a. Pustular psoriasis
b. Allergic contact dermatitis
c. Psychogenic dermatitis with secondary impetigination
d. Asteototic eczema

ANSWER: b. *There are a number of allergen/ irritant contacts from the patient's job as well as the hand lotion. By touching the eyes patients may transfer allergens from the hands. This patient may be an atopic and is probably predisposed to contact dermatitis.*

QUESTION: *Appropriate therapeutic interventions should include all the following except:*

a. Continue the Itch-Be-Gone lotion for its soothing properties.
b. Prescribe hydroxyzine (an oral antihistamine) at bedtime.
c. Advise the patient not to touch her eyes after applying nailpolish.
d. Prescribe lukewarm Aveeno soaks and a medium potency topical corticosteroid.

ANSWER: a. *Hand lotions often contain fragrances, topical anesthetics and other compounds that may be sensitizing and should be discontinued.*

Case 2

An 80-year-old man complains of severe pain over his left eye for 2 days. He has been in very good health all his life and "never even took an aspirin for a headache." He awoke yesterday morning with a tingling feeling over the left forehead that progressed to a more intense burning pain centered over the eye. His daughter, who suffers from migraines, gave him some of her headache medicine but it has not helped. His past medical history and review of symptoms are remarkably negative. On examination the left eye is slightly reddened and he is unable to read newsprint with the right eye closed. There is no tenderness on palpation of the globe or the face. You note an erythematous vesicular lesion on the tip of the nose and several more on the left cheek.

QUESTION: *What is the most likely diagnosis?*

a. Atypical measles
b. Trigeminal neuralgia
c. Herpes simplex ophthalmitis

d. Herpes zoster

ANSWER: d. *The distribution of pain and vesicles points to herpes zoster of the ophthalmic branch of the trigeminal nerve.*

QUESTION: *The most specific confirmatory diagnostic test would be:*

a. A serum varicella titer
b. Tzanck smear of scrapings from the base of an unroofed vesicle
c. Viral culture of the vesicular fluid
d. MRI of the cervical root ganglia

ANSWER: c. *Only the viral culture will specifically identify varicella zoster virus from the active lesions. A serum titer for varicella is likely to be positive in most patients older than 80 years given the ubiquity of primary varicella infection. A Tzanck smear that shows multinucleated giant cells could suggest a herpes virus infection but does not indicate the species. An MRI is of no value in making this diagnosis.*

HAIR LOSS

Alopecia (absence or loss of hair) is a common problem affecting both men and women. Although it may be secondary to an underlying systemic disease, most patients with alopecia who present to primary care providers will have one of three common non-systemic disorders: androgenetic alopecia, alopecia areata, and telogen effluvium. This section will review the stages of the hair cycle, discuss the most common causes of alopecia, and outline a clinically oriented approach to the patient with alopecia.

Pathophysiologic Correlation

Because common causes of alopecia are not diseases, a brief review of normal hair growth is presented here. Humans have a heterogeneous pattern of hair growth. Hair grows in three phases. The anagen phase is the growth phase, catagen is the transitional phase when growth slows down and then stops, and telogen is the resting phase. Approximately 85 to 90% of hairs are in the anagen phase, 3% in catagen, and 10–15% in the telogen phase. Because individual hairs can be in any of the three phases, hair loss is continuous, unlike the seasonal shedding seen in other mammals. Daily normal hair loss is approximately 25 to 100 telogen hairs but may be more on days the hair is shampooed.

Clinical and Laboratory Evaluation

Most causes of alopecia are not associated with a systemic illness. However, a thorough history and physical examination should be undertaken in any person presenting with a complaint of hair loss. Pay special attention to the signs and symptoms of those systemic conditions. Table 21.3 lists the most pertinent aspects of the history and physical that should differentiate a localized from a systemic process.

HISTORY

For the majority of cases of hair loss the history will provide many clues to the underlying cause. An active process can be established by demonstrating hair looseness. Knowing if the hair seems to be breaking versus coming out from the roots helps

Table 21.3.
Evaluation of Hair Loss

History
　Hair loss (active or stable process)
　Hair breakage or "coming out by the roots"
　Location (local or diffuse)
　Onset (acute or gradual)
　Duration (ongoing or limited)
　Precipitating events
　Medication use
　Previous episodes
　Previous treatments
　Thyroid disease
　Family history
　Menstrual history (females only)
Physical
　Distribution of hair loss
　Pattern of hair loss
　Hair looseness
　Hair breakage vs. hair cycle abnormality
　Exclamation mark hair
　Eyebrows
　Thyroid
　Acne/hirsutism (females only)
Laboratory
　Thyroid function
　Iron studies/ferritin
　Anti-nuclear antibody (ANA)
　Dehydroxyepiandrosterone sulfate (DHEA-S)
　Serologic tests for syphilis (RPR, VDRL)
　Fungal culture

Adapted from Bertolino AP. Clinical hair loss: diagnosis and treatment. J Dermatol 1993;20:608.

distinguish hair fragility from a hair cycle abnormality. Do not underestimate the importance of a recent history of hair treatments (permanents, dyes, braidings).

PHYSICAL EXAMINATION

To differentiate an active process from a stable process, a "pull test" may be performed. This is accomplished by applying mild tension with fingers to groups of hair throughout the scalp. Removal of more than six to eight hairs is indicative of hair looseness, and thus, an active process (15). Loss of lateral eyebrow density may be seen in hypothyroidism.

LABORATORY EVALUATION

Selected laboratory studies are often not necessary in the evaluation of alopecia. They may be helpful to confirm the presence of a systemic process if there is evidence elsewhere. In such cases, studies should be directed towards the particular process.

Differential Diagnosis

Other causes of alopecia include trichotilloma, a self-inflicted hair pulling disorder, traumatic or cosmetic alopecia, which is caused by traction from certain hairstyles, and infectious causes particularly fungal (Tinea capitis) and treponemal (secondary syphilis). The diagnosis can be made either from the history or appropriate laboratory studies (potassium hydroxide [KOH] slide and fungal culture, serological tests for syphilis [VDRL or RPR]). Treatment is specific to the underlying cause.

ANDROGENETIC ALOPECIA

Androgenetic alopecia accounts for the vast majority of cases of alopecia. It is also known as common baldness, male-pattern baldness, genetic hair loss or diffuse hair loss. It is believed to be an androgen-mediated process in genetically predisposed persons. Terminal hair follicles (thick pigmented hair) are transformed into vellus-like follicles (fine, "peach fuzz" hair) and then shed. This occurs on androgen-sensitive follicles such as those on the top of the scalp. The pattern in men is usually that of a receding hairline, with further loss at the vertex, and eventual merging of the balding areas (Fig. 21.6). In women there is usually sparing of the anterior hairline with the crown affected most predominantly (Fig. 21.7). Although there is a clear genetic component to this disorder, the mode of

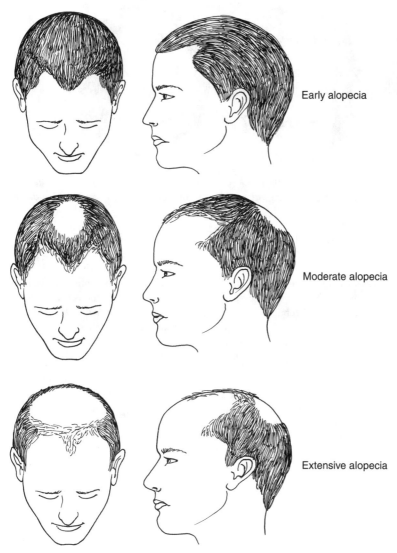

Figure 21.6. Typical patterns of androgenetic alopecia in the male. (Redrawn from Hamilton JB. Patterned loss of hair in man: Types and incidence. Ann NY Acad Sci 1951; 83:712.)

inheritance is not known. Prevalence approaches 100% in whites, is less common in African-Americans, and is uncommon and of later onset in Asians.

The diffuse hair loss of androgenic alopecia should be differentiated from the alopecia caused by senescence, which is nearly universal in the elderly. This may be difficult. Both processes will be stable, of gradual onset and long duration, and without evidence of an underlying systemic process. The major clue in addition to the patient's age at onset is whether the hair-loss is diffuse or follows one of the patterns described.

ALOPECIA AREATA

Alopecia areata (Fig. 21.8) is a common disorder characterized by the rapid onset of total hair loss in a sharply defined, usually round area. These areas may be single or multiple. Many cases are familial. The etiology is unknown but may be autoimmune in origin. It is seen more commonly in patients with atopic dermatitis, autoimmune thyroid disease and vitiligo, but may less commonly accompany such systemic disorders as Addisons disease, systemic lupus erythematosus, ulcerative colitis, and Down syndrome. Most patients

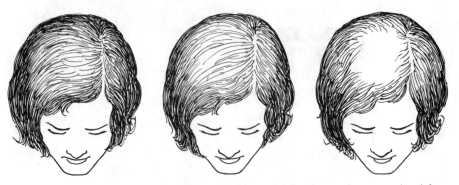

Figure 21.7. Typical patterns of androgenetic alopecia in the female. Grades I, II, and III (left to right). (Redrawn from Ludwig E: Classification of the types of androgenetic alopecia (common baldness) occurring in the female sex. Br J Dermatol 1977;97:251.)

are young (<40), and otherwise asymptomatic. The diagnosis of alopecia areata is usually made on clinical grounds although the pathognomonic finding is the "exclamation point" hair. These affected hairs at the periphery of the lesion are thicker distally and thinner near the scalp, resembling an exclamation point (!).

TELOGEN EFFLUVIUM

Telogen effluvium is a reversible, non-scarring hair loss seen more commonly in women than in men. It is characterized by rapid and diffuse hair shedding. The history is important in this disorder as the hair loss usually occurs about 8–16 weeks after an acute incident. The most common precipitating event is parturition but other known precipitating events

include use of oral contraceptives, high fever, "crash" dieting, drugs or other physiologic stress (e.g., major surgery). The mechanism is unknown but the result is an increase in hair follicles shifting into the telogen phase, which then shed in a synchronized manner. Patients will usually have a positive "pull test."

Management

ANDROGENETIC ALOPECIA

In a male with a typical pattern of androgenetic alopecia, and without scarring or other evidence of systemic disease, reassurance and education should be given. Current available treatment options include topical minoxidil, hair transplantation, scalp

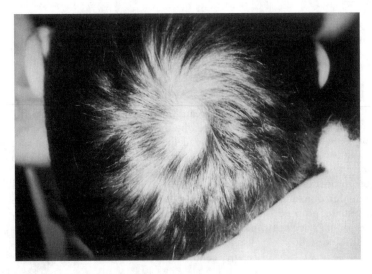

Figure 21.8. Alopecia areata.

reductions and scalp flaps. These have had various success and usually require multiple sessions (surgery) or life-long therapy (minoxidil). A female exhibiting the distinct pattern of central scalp alopecia described may have an adrenal androgenic pattern of alopecia secondary to increased levels of the adrenal androgen dehydroepiandrosterone sulfate (DHEA-S). These women usually have other evidence of androgen excess such as acne and hirsutism, and should undergo further investigation including determination of serum DHEA-S, total and free testosterone, and prolactin levels. Depending on these results, treatment may be undertaken with cyproterone acetate (CPA) an antiandrogenic progestin, spironolactone, or flutamide.

ALOPECIA AREATA

The prognosis for the patient with alopecia areata is usually excellent for hair regrowth, which usually begins in 1 to 3 months. Treatment consists entirely of reassurance. Young patients, and patients with more extensive hair loss including total loss of scalp hair (alopecia totalis) and total body hair loss (alopecia universalis) have a poorer prognosis for hair regrowth. Fortunately these two conditions are rare. Patients who opt for treatment can undergo intralesional injections of triamcinolone acetonide, or topical treatment with minoxidil, cyclosporine, or nitrogen mustard. None of these alter the course of the disease and hair may be shed again once treatment is terminated.

TELOGEN EFFLUVIUM

Telogen effluvium can be very alarming to the patient, who may feel she is going bald "overnight." If the history is consistent with an incident within the appropriate time course, the patient should be reassured that the process is entirely self-limited. However it may take up to a year for the hair cycle to readjust and for the hair to return to its former thickness. An exception to this is chronic telogen effluvium, which is seen almost exclusively in menstruating women and is caused by iron deficiency, with concomitant protein insufficiency. The diagnosis should be entertained in any woman with persistent hair shedding and a serum ferritin level less than 40 nanogram/millileter (ng/ml). Treatment consists of daily iron replacement. If hair shedding persists after the serum ferritin level has increased above 70 ng/ml for 3 months or more, further endocrinologic studies should be undertaken (17).

ILLUSTRATIVE CASES WITH SELF-ASSESSMENT QUESTIONS AND ANSWERS

Case 1

A 44-year-old man presents with a complaint of thinning hair. He first noticed this in his mid- twenties, and it has been a steady and continuous process. His medical and family history are unremarkable. His physical examination does not reveal any evidence of systemic disease. His scalp examination reveals normal texture hair, with thinning at the vertex, and a receding hairline. His pull test is negative.

QUESTION: *What is his likely diagnosis? Are confirmatory blood tests needed? What is his prognosis?*

ANSWERS: *The most likely diagnosis in this patient is androgenetic alopecia. His hair loss is diffuse, on-going and gradual yet he does not have evidence of hair looseness or abnormality.*

Because there is no evidence for a systemic process, no laboratory evaluation is indicated. He can expect continued, gradual hair loss with eventual balding unless he decides to undergo treatment to slow or prevent this process.

Case 2

A 25-year-old female presents with a complaint of hair falling out. She states this began rather abruptly several weeks ago and is continuing. When she brushes her hair, she notes the brush is full of loose hairs, and this is very upsetting to her. She is afraid she is rapidly going bald. Her medical and family history are unremarkable, but you hear her 3-month old crying in the waiting room. Her physical examination reveals a normal mature female pattern of hair distribution. Her scalp examination reveals no focal areas of hair loss, and her pull test is markedly positive.

QUESTIONS: *What is her likely diagnosis? Are confirmatory blood tests necessary? What is her prognosis?*

ANSWERS: *The clinical picture and time course are consistent with telogen effluvium secondary to childbirth. No confirmatory studies are indicated at this time and the patient should be reassured that this process is self-limited. However should her hair loss not abate over the next several weeks, consideration should be given to evaluate her for chronic telogen effluvium.*

SKIN CANCER

Skin cancer is a common problem that should be recognized by primary care providers. Nonmelanoma skin cancer (basal cell and squamous cell carcinoma) is the most prevalent malignant condition in the United States today, with more than 700,000 new cases diagnosed each year. Cutaneous melanoma, although not as common, is the eighth most prevalent cancer in the United States. The importance of early recognition and treatment cannot be overemphasized. These cancers, if detected early, can be completely cured but, if detected later, can have devastating consequences. Thus, any thorough screening or surveillance evaluation should include a complete examination of the skin, especially in a high risk patient.

Pathophysiologic Correlation

All skin cancers have been increasing in prevalence over the past 50 years, probably as a direct result of increased sun exposure. With the increase in outdoor leisure activity, change in clothing fashions allowing for greater skin exposure, and depletion of the ozone layer, the lifetime exposure to ultraviolet radiation has increased. Ultraviolet B (UVB) radiation (wavelengths 290–320 nanometers) is most important in the induction of skin cancer, by causing damage to skin DNA and its repair system. Longer wavelength ultraviolet A (UVA), the radiation used in tanning salons, has only been shown to be carcinogenic in animals. However, UVA causes DNA damage similar to that of UVB, and it is not clear that this wavelength carries any less risk to humans (18). Patients receiving UVA radiation as part of treatment for psoriasis (psoralens and UVA = PUVA) have a dose-dependent increased risk of squamous cell carcinoma. Thus, it would seem prudent that any ultraviolet radiation exposure be viewed as potentially harmful, and measures to decrease or avoid exposure altogether should be recommended.

Despite increased public awareness of the dangers of prolonged sun exposure, most people do not comply with simple measures designed to minimize their risk. These measures include avoidance of sun exposure during the hours of 10 a.m to 2 p.m., wearing of protective clothing, and regular use of sunscreens. Current recommendations are to use a sunscreen with a sun protective factor of at least 15. The sun protective factor (SPF) is the ratio of the length of exposure to the sun required to produce a given level of erythema after the application of sunscreen to the length of exposure required to produce the same degree of erythema before the application of sunscreen. Sunscreens with an SPF of 15 will block about 93% of UVB radiation, while those with an SPF of 30 will block about 96%. Because the risk of skin cancer may be related to either the cumulative lifetime exposure to UV radiation or to severe intermittent sun exposure, it is prudent to recommend that sunscreen protection be used on a regular and consistent basis.

Clinical and Laboratory Evaluation

The diagnosis of skin cancer is based on a clinical picture in which particular features of the history and physcial examination reveal a patient who is at risk. Table 21.4 lists these features. It is imperative

Table 21.4.
Factors Associated with an Increased Risk of Skin Cancer

Historical
  Prolonged frequent or episodic severe sun exposure (including use of tanning salons)
  Arsenic exposure or ingestion (nonmelanoma)
  Ionizing radiation (occupational or therapeutic)
  Hydrocarbon exposure (nonmelanoma)
  Tobacco use (squamous cell only)
  Residence in areas of lower latitudes
  Immunosuppression
Physical
  Older age (nonmelanoma)
  Fair skin or skin that tans poorly, burns easily
  Blue or green eyes
  Blond or red hair
  Freckles
  Nevi (melanoma)
Genetic
  Xeroderma pigmentosum
  Albinism
  Vitiligo

From Preston DS, Stern RS: Nonmelanoma cancers of the skin. N Engl J Med 1992;327:1650.

for primary care providers to have a high index of suspicion in these patients, and to refer them for appropriate management.

HISTORY

Prolonged exposure to sunlight is the single greatest risk factor for the development of skin cancer; thus these cancers are seen more commonly in persons who reside in geographic areas where ultraviolet radiation is strongest (Florida, Texas, Southern California). For nonmelanoma skin cancer, prevalence is higher in persons whose occupations or leisure activities involve prolonged sun exposure. Evidence suggests that a person's risk is reflected by the total or cumulative sun exposure over a lifetime. Other less common predisposing factors for the development of nonmelanoma skin cancer include exposure to ionizing radiation, inorganic arsenic, and industrial tar compounds. Squamous cell carcinoma is also commonly seen in immunosuppressed persons. Initially, renal transplant patients had a much higher than expected incidence of squamous cell carcinoma, but now immunosuppression from any cause confers a risk. Other associations have been noted with human papilloma virus. Both cigarette smoking and use of chewing tobacco are associated with an increased risk of squamous cell carcinoma of the lip and mucous membranes. Certain genetic disorders are also associated with an increased risk.

The single most important risk factor for the development of cutaneous melanoma is exposure to sunlight, particularly UVB radiation. Unlike basal cell and squamous cell carcinomas in which the risk is related to the cumulative exposure over a lifetime, the risk for melanoma development is related to intermittent, severe, blistering sunburns, particularly in childhood and adolescence. Surprisingly, persons with outdoor occupations are at lower risks, perhaps because their chronic exposure provides some protection through tanning. Persons at highest risk are indoor workers of higher socioeconomic, usually professional class, whose sun exposure consists of short, intense periods during leisure activities, such as skiing, golf, and sailing. Despite this association, however, melanoma can occur anywhere on the surface of the skin, including areas not subject to ultraviolet radiation exposure. Other risk factors for the development of cutaneous melanoma include Caucasian race, family history of melanoma, and immunosuppression. Because most melanomas arise in preexisting moles or nevi, a history of pre-cancer lesions, such as giant congenital nevi and the dysplastic nevi syndrome (familial or sporadic) confer additional risk.

PHYSICAL EXAMINATION

Risk factors for skin cancer are related to the physical characteristics listed in Table 21.4. Persons with these characteristic features may exhibit evidence of chronically sun-damaged skin known as actinic keratoses. These superficial, erythematous, scaling lesions with wrinkling and loss of elasticity may be seen on sun exposed areas and are a marker of chronic sun exposure. These lesions may have malignant potential.

LABORATORY EVALUATION

Because skin cancer is a clinical diagnosis confirmatory blood tests are not necessary. All suspicious lesions should have a pathologic confirmation. Suspicious lesions requiring a tissue diagnosis warrant referral to a specialist.

Differential Diagnosis

BASAL CELL CARCINOMA

Basal cell carcinoma is the most common skin cancer, with approximately 600,000 new cases diagnosed annually. Basal cell cancer usually affects older persons in the fifth and sixth decade; however, it is being seen increasingly in younger individuals. Men and women are equally affected. Dark-skinned persons are rarely affected.

The vast majority of basal cell carcinomas occur on the head and neck, particularly the eyelids, nasolabial folds, and scalp. It is much less common on the trunk and extremities (<10 percent) and almost never seen on the palms and soles. Basal cell carcinomas are usually asymptomatic and rarely metastasize. They come to attention only if they bleed or invade underlying structures (subcutaneous tissue, bone, cartilage, and nerve) and cause deformity or destruction.

The most common type of basal cell carcinoma is the nodular ulcerative form (Fig. 21.9). This form presents as a flesh-colored or pink nodule or papule with a waxy, pearly, or translucent appearance, and characteristic rolled or sloping borders. There are usually telangectatic vessels throughout the lesion. As the lesion grows, central ulceration and crusting are common. The superficial basal cell carcinoma usually presents as multiple, erythematous, or lightly pigmented, sharply demarcated macules or papules that generally occur on the trunk and extremities. These lesions spread out as they grow

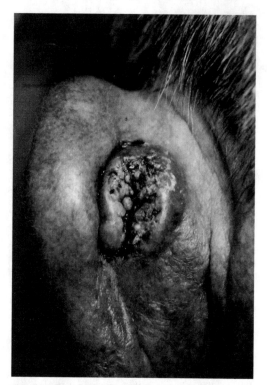

Figure 21.9. Nodular ulcerative form of basal cell carcinoma.

and may form scaly or crusted patches or plaques. Telangectatic vessels may be seen along the periphery of the lesion. Superficial basal cell carcinoma is often mistaken for a patch of inflammatory dermatitis, eczema, or psoriasis. The diagnosis should be considered when such a lesion does not respond to topical corticosteroid therapy. Cystic basal cell carcinoma is similar to the nodular form except the appearance is more cystic. It usually occurs on the face. Sclerosing basal cell carcinomas are infiltrating, slightly pigmented flat lesions with indistinct borders. Except for location, sclerosing basal cell carcinoma does not share other characteristic features of basal cell carcinoma (nodularity, telangiectasias, "pearly" appearance) and so may be difficult to diagnose. The pigmented type of basal cell carcinoma is commonly mistaken for malignant melanoma. It usually presents as a brown or black nodule, more commonly seen in darker skinned persons.

SQUAMOUS CELL CARCINOMA

Squamous cell carcinoma is much less common than basal cell carcinoma, accounting for approxi-

mately 20% of nonmelanoma skin cancers. However, it has a much greater tendency to metastasize, causing morbidity and mortality equal to that of melanoma. Squamous cell carcinoma is a disease of the elderly. The average patient age at the time of diagnosis is 70 years. Squamous cell carcinomas are twice as common in men than in women. Dark-skinned persons and persons of Asian ancestry are rarely affected.

The most common sites for the development of squamous cell carcinoma are the head and neck, particularly the scalp, superior surface of the pinna, lower lips, and the trunk and extremities, particularly the dorsum of the hands. It can also occur on the palms of the hands and soles of the feet. Sites at risk usually show signs of radiation damage such as wrinkling, telangectasia, hyper or hypopigmentation, and chronic inflammation (erythema and scaling). Squamous cell cancer also occurs at sites of previous skin damage, such as burns, scars, chronic ulcers, and sinus tracts. Squamous cell carcinomas that develop at sites of chronic skin irritation or injury may be difficult to diagnose. In addition, squamous cell carcinomas arising in areas of chronic injury act more aggressively and are more likely to metastasize than those arising in sun or radiation damaged skin. Radiation-induced squamous cell carcinoma typically presents as an erythematous, solitary lesion, usually a nodule or papule, that slowly enlarges and develops an indurated base (Fig. 21.10). The borders may be elevated and the margins indistinct. As the lesion grows, scaling, erosion, and central ulceration are common. Squamous cell carcinomas may exhibit the pearly, rolled border characteristic of basal cell carcinoma, may contain telangiectasias, or may be deeply pigmented, resembling melanoma. Squamous cell carcinomas may develop overlying conical protrusions of keratinized material known as cutaneous horns. Squamous cell carcinomas arising on the lower lips often develop at sites of chelitis; the fissures thicken over time, finally forming a nodule. Lesions of the lips and mucous membranes tend to be extremely aggressive. Squamous cell carcinomas arising at sites of chronic injury, scar, or inflammation usually present with pain, pruritus, bleeding, or ulceration, and any change or rapid growth at one of these sites should be a cause for concern.

Bowen's disease is squamous cell carcinoma-in-situ. In Bowen's disease, the entire epidermis is involved without invasion of the basement membrane. This pre-malignant lesion usually presents as an asymptomatic, sharply circumscribed patch of erythema and scaling in an exposed area.

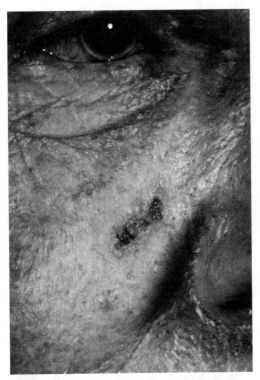

Figure 21.10. Radiation-induced squamous cell carcinoma.

MELANOMA

Melanoma is the eighth most common cancer in the United States, but its incidence has been increasing dramatically over the past 40 years. Melanoma is a disease of middle aged persons. The median age at diagnosis is 45. Whites are affected much more than African-Americans. Men and women are equally affected although women tend to have a better prognosis. Roughly 50% of lesions are discovered by the patients themselves, and 50% during physical examination by a health care provider. Many lesions are not found on sun-exposed areas including the scalp, axilla, palms and soles, back, subungual areas, interdigital web spaces, genitalia, perineum, and perianal areas.

Because melanoma may arise de novo or in a pre-existing lesion, it is important to be able to recognize both. The two most common lesions that cause confusion are benign nevi and seborrheic keratoses. Benign nevi or moles have a more uniform appearance; they tend to be round or oval in shape, the color may be tan, brown, or black, but tends to be homogeneous, the borders are regular, and tend to be symmetric. They are usually flat and not very large (diameter < 6 mm). Most benign moles appear in childhood, adolescence, and early adulthood. They may grow, darken, or increase in number during puberty or pregnancy, or with hormonal treatment. During such times, all nevi in a person should change together, reflecting the systemic process in contrast to the autonomous influence of a single malignant lesion.

Seborrheic keratoses (Fig. 21.11) are extremely common in elderly patients. These lesions resemble warts, with a characteristic "stuck on" appearance. Seborrheic keratoses are usually elevated, greasy, brown or black, and of various sizes. They may be single or multiple. They are usually found on the face, back, and chest of darker-skinned persons who have greasy or oily skin. Unlike actinic keratosis or senile keratosis, seborrheic keratosis usually causes no symptoms, and has no malignant potential.

For primary care providers to better recognize the signs that may suggest development of a melanoma, an ABCD rule has been established (Table 21.5). Changes in shape and color are important early warning signs, while bleeding and ulceration are late signs and confer a poorer prognosis.

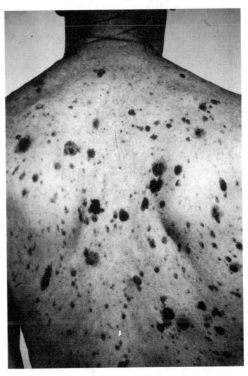

Figure 21.11. Seborrheic keratoses.

Table 21.5.
Clinical Signs of Malignant Melanoma

A	**A**symmetry in shape
B	**B**order irregularity
C	**C**olor variation including change in color, heterogeneity of color, and surrounding erythema
D	**D**iameter greater than 6 mm or increase in diameter

Changes in color include deepening of the pigmentation, as well as hypopigmentation in areas of regression. Color changes may also include erythema from vasodilatation and inflammation. Other ominous signs include the appearance of satellite lesions, and the development of symptoms such as pain or pruritus.

There are four major types of melanoma. Superficial spreading melanoma (Fig. 21.12) is the most common type, accounting for about 70% of all melanoma. These usually arise in pre-existing nevi. Superficial spreading melanomas are usually found on the upper back in men and on the upper back and legs in women. They are flat, and grow by spreading out horizontally with areas of regression resulting in hypopigmented patches within the lesion. This stage of radial growth may last months to years. Lesions detected in this stage are curable with surgery. Later, the vertical phase occurs resulting in penetration into the dermis. This is evident clinically by elevation of the lesion, which at this point may resemble a papule or nodule. Once the vertical stage has begun, metastatic potential is greatly increased and curative potential diminished.

The second most common form of melanoma is the nodular form, accounting for about 15% of all lesions. It is twice as common in men than in women. Nodular melanoma may arise in pre-existing nevi or in previously uninvolved skin, and has no site predilection. It also has no discernible

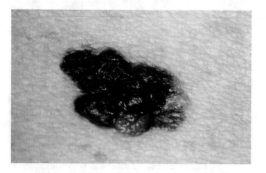

Figure 21.12. Superficial spreading melanoma.

radial growth phase. Nodular melanomas present as pigmented nodules that grow rapidly over weeks to months. Because they may be round with discrete borders, uniformly blue-black or dark gray in color, or amelanotic, nodular melanomas cannot accurately be assessed by the ABCD rule. Thus, any rapidly growing lesion must raise suspicion.

Acral-lentiginous melanoma accounts for about 5% of all melanoma. It is uncommon in Caucasians and found mainly in persons of African, Asian, or Hispanic descent. It usually occurs on the palms, soles, and subungual regions. Other commonly affected areas include the mucous membranes, perineum, rectum, and vagina. The lesions of acral-lentiginous melanoma usually appear as irregularly shaped and pigmented papules, or pigmentation in the nailbed or nail plate. They may be difficult to diagnose, either because they resemble normal pigmentation in the hands and feet of dark-skinned persons, or because they occur in areas not readily examined by either the patient or health care provider. Because of this difficulty, acral-lentiginous melanomas tend to be more advanced at the time of diagnosis.

Lentigo maligna melanoma accounts for about 10% of melanoma and is a disease of the elderly. It arises from lentigo maligna, a macular pigmented lesion usually found at sites of chronic sun exposure. The face and hands are the most common areas affected, but lesions may be found on the arms and legs. The lesions of lentigo maligna have a very long radial growth phase that may last 10 or 20 years. They resemble superficial spreading melanoma, appearing as tan or brown macules with irregular, notched borders, pigment irregularity, and hypopigmentation. Lentigo maligna lesions are considered melanoma-in-situ until they develop a vertical phase, representing lentigo maligna melanoma.

Management

BASAL CELL CARCINOMA

The diagnosis of basal cell carcinoma should be confirmed by biopsy in any patient with a suspicious lesion. Treatment options include curettage and electrodesiccation, surgical excision, cryotherapy, radiotherapy, and Mohs microscopic surgery. All of these confer advantages and disadvantages. The choice of treatment modality is based upon type, size, and location of the lesion, patient age and cosmetic preference, likelihood of scarring or recurrence, and physician skill. Patients can expect a 95% cure rate in uncomplicated cases. However, recurrences are common, particularly with lesions on the face and lesions greater than 6 mm. Most recurrences occur within 1 to 3 years after initial treatment. Recurrent lesions often lack the characteristic appearance of the initial tumor and, therefore, may be difficult to diagnose. Because they are usually associated with scarring and erosions, recurrent basal cell carcinomas are more difficult to treat. Since basal cell carcinomas rarely metastasize, however, the prognosis is usually good. Basal cell carcinomas that do metastasize are usually found in regional lymph nodes but may also invade bone, lungs, and liver. The prognosis in such cases is poor.

SQUAMOUS CELL CARCINOMA

All suspicious or questionable lesions should be biopsied. Treatment options are similar to those for basal cell carcinoma: curettage and electrodesiccation, surgical excision, cryosurgery, radiation therapy, and Mohs microscopic surgery. Other modalities include topical fluorouracil (for superficial lesions only), intralesional interferon alpha and photodynamic therapy, which are investigational, and laser therapy, which is expensive. Treatment type depends on the same characteristics described above for treatment of basal cell carcinoma.

The cure rate for a primary lesion is excellent with standard therapy. However, as with basal cell carcinoma, recurrences are common (average, 10%). The majority occur within 2 years from the time of initial diagnosis. Recurrent squamous cell carcinomas are usually treated with Mohs microscopic surgery for a better cure rate. Lesions of the lips, mucous membranes, trunk, and lower extremities, as well as those in immunocompromised patients, are more likely to recur. The rate of metastasis for squamous cell carcinoma has been between 2 and 10%. Lesions associated with areas of chronic inflammation and radiation damage, scars, or in immunocompromised hosts are more likely to metastasize. Other strong predictors of metastatic potential include tumor thickness and level of invasion rather than degree of differentiation. Most metastases are found within six months of initial diagnosis. The most common site for metastasis is the regional lymph nodes. If lymph nodes can be palpated, surgical excision must be undertaken. Distant metastases may occur in the liver, lung, bone, and brain. Treatment options for metastatic squamous cell carcinoma are limited and of modest benefit. Mortality is high with a 5-year survival rate of about 30%.

MELANOMA

The treatment for all lesions suspicious for melanoma is excisional biopsy down to fat. Narrow margins of 1–2 cm are adequate. Staging is based on tumor thickness, and prognosis depends on degree of spread. Five year survival rates approach 100% if the tumor thickness is less than 0.76 mm and fall to 65% if greater than 1.51 mm. Other poor prognostic indicators include anatomic site (scalp, hand, and foot lesions have poorer prognosis), older age, male sex, classification (superficial spreading and lentigo maligna melanoma have better prognosis), and histologic factors, including high mitotic activity, satellite lesions, ulceration, and high tumor volume.

Rates of local recurrences and metastases depend on tumor thickness. Palpation of regional lymph nodes indicates lymphatic spread, although hematogenous spread can occur in the absence of lymphangitic spread. Metastases can occur 10 or 15 years after removal of the primary tumor. Common sites of metastatic spread include lung, liver, gastrointestinal tract, spleen, bone, and brain. Many modalities have been employed in the treatment of metastatic melanoma but none have shown particular promise. Metastatic melanoma is a fatal disease, with death usually secondary to central nervous system involvement. The potential benefit of early detection and treatment cannot be overstated.

ILLUSTRATIVE CASES WITH SELF-ASSESSMENT QUESTIONS AND ANSWERS

Case 1

A 54-year-old man presents to you because he needs a new physician. His only medical problem is mild hypertension. He is a business executive who spends most of his free time playing golf, a hobby he began 25 years ago. His review of systems is negative. On examination you notice an 8 x 10 mm flat pigmented lesion at the back of his neck. When you question him about this, he states he cannot see it, but his wife has noticed that it has gotten somewhat larger but lighter in color.

QUESTIONS: *What is his likely diagnosis? What*

should you do now? What is the appropriate management?

ANSWERS: *This gentleman probably has melanoma more likely a superficial spreading or lentigo maligna variety. You should now examine his entire skin, including the scalp, perianal and genital areas, and palms and soles. All lesions found should be examined using the ABCD rule. You should palpate for lymph node enlargement. He should undergo excisional biopsy of any suspicious lesion.*

Case 2

A 62-year-old woman presents to you complaining of "chapped" lower lips for many months, not responsive to topical creams and lotions. She is a fair-skinned womsn in excellent physical health. She swims daily and in her younger days worked summers as a life guard. On examination she has actinic changes of her forehead, cheeks, and arms. Her lower lip is erythematous with some blisters and ulcerations.

QUESTION: *What is the cause of her "chapped" lips? What should you do now? What is the appropriate management?*

ANSWERS: *This patient has actinic chelitis secondary to chronic sun exposure. The upper lip is spared since it is shaded by the nose. This lesion may develop into squamous cell carcinoma. You should look for other lesions suspicious for squamous cell or basal cell carcinoma. Any suspicious lesion should be biopsied. This patient should be examined regularly for development of nonmelanoma skin cancer. She should be strongly advised to avoid sun exposure and to use sunscreen regularly.*

REFERENCES

Rash

1. Nelson C, McLemore T. The national ambulatory medical care survey 1975–1981 and 1985. Vital Health Stat 1988;93:1.
2. Johnson ML, Roberts J. Skin conditions and related needs for medical care among persons 1–74 years, U.S. 1971–1974. US Dept of Health, Education, and Welfare Publication 79–1660. Hyattsville, MD, National Center for Health Statistics, December 1978.
3. Hanifin JM. Atopic dermatitis: new therapeutic considerations. J Am Acad Dermatol 1991;24:1097.
4. Sampson HA, Jolie PL. Increased plasma histamine concentrations after food challenges in children with atopic dermatitis. N Engl J Med 1974;311:372.
5. Champion RJ. Abnormal vascular reactions in atopic eczema. Br J Dermatol 1963;75:12.
6. Ginsburg IO, Prystowsky JH, Kornfeld DS, et al. Role of emotional factors in adults with atopic dermatitis. Int J Dermatol 1993;32:656.
7. Fisher AA. Contact dermatitis, 3rd ed. Philadelphia: Lea & Febiger, 1986.
8. Parish WE, Welbourn E, Champion RH. Hypersensitivity to bacteria in eczema. Br J Dermatol 1976;95:493.
9. Farber EM, Nall ML. The natural history of psoriasis in 5,600 patients. Dermatologica 1974;148:1.
10. Straus SE, Ostrove JM, Inchausp G, et al. Varicella-zoster virus infections: biology, natural history, treatment, and prevention. Ann Intern Med 1988;108:221.
11. Recommendations of the immunization practices advisory committee (ACIP). Varicella-zoster immune globulin for the prevention of chickenpox. MMWR 1984;33:84.
12. Dunkle LM, Arvin AM, Whitley RJ, et al. A controlled trial of acyclovir for chickenpox in normal children. N Engl J Med 1991;325:1539.
13. Shepp DH, Dandliker PS, Meyers JD. Treatment of varicella-zoster virus infection in severely immunocompromised patients: a randomized comparison of acyclovir and vidarabine. N Engl J Med 1986; 314:208.
14. Esmann V, Geil JP, Kroon S, et al. Prednisolone does not prevent post-herpetic neuralgia. Lancet 1987;2:126.

Hair Loss

15. Bertolino AP. Clinical hair loss: diagnosis and treatment. J Dermatol 1993;20:604–610.
16. Habif TP. Clinical dermatology: a color guide to diagnosis and therapy. St. Louis: C.V. Mosby Co., 1990.
17. Rushton D H. Management of hair loss in women. Dermatol Ther 1993;11:47–53.

Skin Cancer

18. Preston DS, Stern RS. Nonmelanoma cancers of the skin. N Engl J Med 1992;327:23:1649–1662.

SUGGESTED READINGS

Rash

Farber EM, Nall ML. The natural history of psoriasis in 5,600 patients. Dermatologica 1974;148:1.

Fisher AA. Contact dermatitis, 3rd ed. Philadelphia: Lea & Febiger, 1986.

Hanifin JM. Atopic dermatitis: new therapeutic considerations. J Am Acad Dermatol 1991; 24:1097.

Hair Loss

Habif TP. Clinical dermatology: a color guide to diagnosis and therapy. 2nd ed. St. Louis: C.V. Mosby Co., 1990: chapter 24.

Sauer GC, Hall JC. Manual of skin diseases. 7th ed. Philadelphia: Lippincott-Raven, 1996: chapter 27.

Skin Cancer

Habif TP. Clinical dermatology: a color guide to diagnosis and therapy. 2nd ed. St. Louis: C.V. Mosby Co., 1990: chapters 21, 22.

Sauer GC, Hall JC. Manual of skin diseases. 7th ed. Philadelphia: Lippincott-Raven, 1996: chapter 32.

chapter 22

ORTHOPAEDICS

Leanne Forman

JOINT PAIN

Joint pain may be caused by a wide variety of disorders and, therefore, must be evaluated in a systematic way. Most people will at one point seek medical attention for joint pain. Because joint pain is so common, but may be caused by a serious underlying illness such as malignancy or infection, health care providers must be well versed in its evaluation. The clinical presentation, pathogenesis, and management of the disorders most common to each joint will be discussed in that chapter.

Osteoarthritis (OA) is the number one cause of disability in patients older than age 65 and therefore will be discussed first. Eighty-five percent of people older than age 65 have radiographic evidence of osteoarthritis and approximately half of those have symptoms. Three million Americans are unable to perform their major activities due to OA and half of those are completely disabled (confined to a wheelchair or bed). At this time, it is not possible to predict which of the patients with radiologic evidence of OA will develop symptoms.

Pathophysiologic Correlation

Before evaluating joint pain one must be familiar with the anatomy of the joint. Each joint has different components but includes osseous structures, cartilage, synovium, synovial cavity and a rich neurovascular supply. The joint is surrounded by fibrotendinous and muscular structures which support and protect the joint. Any of these components may be involved in the painful process.

NEURAL MECHANISMS OF PAIN

The neural mechanisms of joint pain are not well understood. There are sensory afferent fibers in the nociceptors of the joints and periarticular bone that have cell bodies in the dorsal ganglia. The

ligaments, capsule and to a lesser degree the synovium are innervated by these fibers. There are several inflammatory mediators that modulate the afferent nerves' response to painful stimuli and their functions differ in normal and inflamed synovium.

Serotonin, bradykinin, and possibly prostaglandins enhance the sensation of pain by the afferent nerves. Substance P has been present in increased amounts in the afferent nerves of patients with inflammatory arthritis and stimulates synovial cell proliferation and promotes neutrophil activation. It can facilitate pain transmission at the synapses of the nerves and be downmodulated by the opiate receptors.

The sympathetic nervous system may also play a role in regulating sensation of pain independent of inflammatory mediators. Catecholamines can induce hyperalgesia in patients who have undergone trauma but not in normal joints. Some investigation has been done using sympathetic blockade as a treatment for pain and initial trials of guanethidine have been promising.

The role of the central nervous system in the sensation of pain is the least well understood. The dorsal ganglia communicate with the substantia gelatinosa in the spinal cord but the higher pathways are not known. The argument used for a role of the CNS being involved in the regulation of pain is that when anesthetics are used prior to surgical intervention there is less post operative pain. This phenomenon is called "central sensitization." There may be pain pathways that can be avoided by pretreatment.

PATHOPHYSIOLOGY OF OA

Pathologically, OA is characterized by loss of cartilage, sclerosis of subchondral bone with the development of subchondral cysts, osteophyte formation, and varying degrees of synovial inflammation. The most widely held theory is that the cartilage loss is the primary process. Cartilage is unusual in that it lacks blood vessels, nerve supply, or lymphatics and is therefore dependent on the bathing synovial fluid and underlying chondrocytes for nutrients. Cartilage loss is usually irregular and not always correlated to degree of symptoms in patients with OA. Cartilage is composed of water, collagens, and proteoglycans. The proteoglycans function to draw water into the matrix. The alteration in the permeability leads to increased water and swelling and altered tensile properties. The chondrocytes produce collagen and proteoglycan that also change in OA. The chondrocytes are responsible for the repair of cartilage.

The pathophysiology of OA has been widely studied. The name osteoarthritis has been used interchangeably with degenerative joint disease and this is misleading as it implies that OA is simply a normal process of aging. Table 22.1 compares the differences between aging and osteoarthritis. Under normal circumstances, cartilage undergoes breakdown and repair which is under the influence of multiple growth factors. However, in OA that normal reparative process is disrupted. The synovium, cartilage, and subchondral bone microenvironments are interdependent. The mediators of matrix alteration gain access to the cartilage either through the synovial fluid or the chondrocytes themselves.

There are several theories about which substances are responsible for the degeneration of cartilage, but most implicate the metalloproteinases (collagenase, gelatinase, and stromelysin). In animal studies, OA was induced by trauma, but pretreatment with oral doxycycline precluded the development of OA. In theory, this result is a function of the ability of doxycycline to chelate metalloproteinases rather than the antibiotic property because non-antibiotic tetracyclines can prevent the development of OA. There are some reservations however because tetracyclines can increase the risk of osteoporosis. It is unusual for osteoporosis and OA to occur in the same individual. They seem to be opposing processes and may lead to some clues to the pathogenesis of both processes.

Clinical and Laboratory Evaluation

When evaluating joint pain, one must take into consideration the most likely processes to occur in that joint. For example, it is unusual for rheumatoid arthritis to be the cause of low back pain or for gout to affect only the shoulder. One must also consider the patient to determine which illnesses would most likely occur. For example, it would be highly unusual for idiopathic osteoporosis to occur in an individual under the age of 40. Historical and laboratory clues that are useful in evaluating joint pain are listed in Table 22.2. The evaluation of trauma is joint specific and therefore will be discussed in each chapter.

HISTORY

With a careful history, one may come to a differential diagnosis rather easily. Table 22.3 will help when evaluating joint pain. It is important to separate inflammatory from noninflammatory because the consequences of inflammatory arthritides tend to be more acute and severe and therefore the workup and treatment are very different.

PHYSICAL EXAMINATION

The examiner must attempt to localize the pain and determine whether it is periarticular or intraarticular. Other signs of a local inflammatory process include swelling, warmth and erythema, which may also occur with significant trauma. Many arthritides

Table 22.1.
Changes in Cartilage Associated with Aging and Osteoarthritis

Cartilaginous Factors	Aging	Osteoarthritis
Proteoglycan concentration	Normal or low normal	Decreased
Water content	Decreased	Increased
Synthesis of collagen and proteoglycanases	Decreased	Increased
Degradation enzymes such as proteoglycanases and colagenases	Normal or low normal	Increased
Degradation enzyme inhibitors	Normal	Decreased
Growth factors	Normal or low normal	Increased
Proteoglycan aggregation (proteoglycan interaction with hyaluronic acid)	Normal	Decreased

From Swedberg JA and Steinbauer JR. Osteoarthritis. American Family Physician 1992;45:563.

have prominent degrees of tendonitis associated with them such as calcium pyrophosphate disease, gout, rheumatoid arthritis (RA). One needs to determine the range of motion. It may be limited by soft tissue overgrowth in OA, pain or swelling. Range of motion may give some clue to the severity of the process or the etiology.

If there is evidence of trauma (abrasions or ecchymoses) but no history, beware of seizure disorders causing trauma or coagulopathies. Rashes may give a clue to the diagnosis of lupus, psoriatic arthritis, Lyme disease or gonococcal disease. Nodules may support the diagnosis of RA or gout depending on their quality and location.

LABORATORY EVALUATION

One needs to be judicious in the use of laboratory data to evaluate joint pain. Although serologic testing is very useful in differentiating inflammatory arthritides, it is important not to send a "battery" of tests but rather to aim the tests at a specific diagnosis. It is rarely important to know the diagnosis immediately except in the case of septic arthritis. If one suspects septic arthritis one is obliged to obtain synovial fluid both as a diagnostic and therapeutic maneuver. When evaluating whether an inflammatory process is occurring, a complete blood count (CBC) and erythrocyte sedimentation rate (ESR) are useful starting points. If these are normal and there is a low degree of suspicion, no further tests for inflammatory disorders should be ordered. A CBC is often helpful because it may reveal underlying disease (i.e., anemia or neutropenia), which may point towards a different diagnosis. Serum chemistries may also give helpful clues, e.g., if the liver function tests, uric acid or alkaline phosphatase are elevated (Table 22.4.)

In the synovial fluid of persons with OA, several body fluid markers have been shown to be elevated. The levels of specific cartilage breakdown products namely proteglycans and keratan sulfate are elevated. These may also be identified in the serum and urine of persons with OA, but in markedly reduced amounts. Synovial cartilage only accounts for 20% of the cartilage in the body and therefore serum levels may not reflect a process particular to a specific joint. There have been several studies demonstrating that one can obtain elevated levels in the vein draining the joint but these joints are often inaccessible. Elevated levels have been found in individuals prior to the development of OA and might eventually be used to identify people at risk

for developing OA. There are currently no reliable serum markers for OA.

Differential Diagnosis

Clinically, OA usually begins in one joint with chronic symptoms and then develops asymmetrically in other joints. Occasionally, it is inflammatory in nature and this may be a subset of patients who actually have pseudogout. It is not usually necessary to distinguish these patients clinically. The most common complaints are pain, decreased function and instability. Table 22.5 lists some of the criteria used to define OA. The greatest predictor of whether a patient will become disabled by OA is the presence of associated illnesses (e.g., coronary artery disease or congestive heart failure). Due to the tremendous impact on the health of society, more research effort is being focused on OA.

Several risk factors have been associated with OA. Advancing age is the single greatest risk factor. Others include female sex, obesity, trauma, crystal deposition disease, alcoholism, diabetes, and other types of arthritis. Some joints are predisposed to OA by the type of work a patient has done: heavy lifting in men increases the risk of hip OA and knee bending increases the risk of knee OA. The etiologic classification of joint pain is outlined.

Noninflammatory
  Osteoarthritis
  Metabolic bone disorders
    Osteoporosis
    Paget's disease
    Osteomalacia (hyperparathyroidism, renal
      osteodystrophy)
  Avascular necrosis
  Neuropathic arthropathies
  Musculotendinous injuries
Inflammatory
  Noninfectious
  Crystal deposition disease
    Gout
    Calcium pyrophosphate deposition
  Rheumatoid arthritis
  Systemic Lupus Erythematosis
  Psoriatic
  Reiter's syndrome
Infectious
  Gonococcal
  Lyme Disease
  Septic
  Tuberculous

Table 22.2.
Diagnostic Clues for the Evaluation of Joint Pain

Inflammatory	Age	Sex	Incidence	Duration	Mono vs. Polyarticular	Location	Extraarticular Manifestations	Associated Illnesses	Laboratory Findings	X-rays
Rheumatoid Arthritis	Bimodal	Female:male 2–3:1	0.3–1.5%	Intermittent then chronic	Poly	MCP/PIP Wrist Knee Cervical	Nodules Pulmonary Vasculitis		↑ESR RF	Subchondral erosions
Systemic Lupus Erythematosis	3rd–4th decade	Female:male 9:1	$\frac{2.9-400}{100,000}$	Flares	Poly	Hand Knee	Skin Renal Neuro Cardiac		+FANA ↑anti DNA ↓complement	None
GOUT	4–5th decade	Male:female 7:1	$\frac{275}{100,000}$	Initially acute then chronic	Mono	1st MCP Ankle Knee Wrist	Tophi Renal Tendonitis	Hyperlipidemia Obesity Diabetes	↑Uric Acid	Tophi
CPPD (Pseudogout)	>75	Male:female 1.4:1	$\frac{150}{100,000}$	Acute	Mono	Knee Hands Elbows Shoulders	Tendonitis	Hyperparathyroid Hemochromatosis		Calcified tendons
Psoriatic		Male:female	4.5% pts. with psoriasis	Varies	Poly	Spine Hands Knees	Conjunctivitis			Erosions
Septic	Infants or elderly			Acute	Mono	Knees	Fever	Underlying arthritis	WBC ESR +blood C&S	—
Lyme				3 stages	Poly	Knees	Neuro Skin Cardiac	—	+Lyme titer	—
Gonococcal	Young			Acute	Poly migratory	Knees Ankles	Oral Skin	—	+GC culture	—

	Age	Sex	Incidence	Onset	Pattern	Location	Clinical Features	Associated	Lab	X-ray
Reiter's	Young men	Male:female 5:1	27/100,000	Acute	Poly	Knees Ankles	Mucocutaneous Conjunctivitis Urethritis	—	—	—
Osteomyelitis	Infants or elderly			Acute or chronic	Mono	Tibia Feet Spine	Ulcer Sinus tract	Diabetes Alcoholism Trauma	CBC ESR +blood C&S	Periosted lifting
Infectious OA	>65	Male:female	40–50% over 65	Chronic	Mono or pauci	Hips Knees Hands Back	—	Obesity Other forms of arthritis	Biochemical markers—not available	Osteophytes
Osteoporosis	50–75	Women:men ~6:1	1/3 of women >65	Chronic	Pauci	Vertebrae Femoral Neck Radial Bones	—	Hypothyroidism	None	Bone density
Paget's	5–6th decade	Men:women slightly	10–15% elderly	Chronic	Pauci	Hips/femur Spine Skull	Rare CHF	—	AP	Sclerosis deformities
Avascular Necrosis	—	Women > men		Subacute or chronic	Mono	Femoral Neck Femoral Condyles Humeral Head	—	Steroids-SLE Diabetes Alcohol	—	
Neuropathic arthropathies	—	—	2% of diabetes	Chronic	Mono	Foot spine	Evidence of neuropathy and contractures	Diabetes Syphilis Leprosy	—	
Polymyalgia Rheumatica	>70	Women:men 2.5:1	—	Subacute	—	Muscles of shoulder Hips	Fatigue Weight loss Fevers	Temporal arteritis 15%	ESR >100 Anemia	None

Table 22.3.
Comparison of Inflammatory and Noninflammatory Arthritides

	Inflammatory	Non-Inflammatory
Duration	Acute or intermittent	Chronic
Age	Young or elderly	Elderly
Previous injuries	Unusual	Common
Number of joints involved	Polyarticular	Mono or pauciarticular
Type of joints	Often peripheral	Weight bearing
Diurnal pattern	Morning stiffness	Worse with use
Systemic symptoms	Fatigue, weight loss, fever	Not present
Rash	SLE-malar or discoid	Not present
	Lyme-ECM	
	Gonoccal	
	RA	
Exposures	Lyme—tick bite	AVN—steroids, alcohol
	Reiter's	Osteoporosis
	Septic	
	Tuberculosis	
Travel history	Rheumatic fever	Neuropathic arthropathy, i.e., leprosy
Family history	Rheumatoid arthritis	Pagets
	Systemic lupus erythematosus	?OA
	?Gout	

AVN (avascular necrosis); ECM (erythema chronicum migrans); RA (rheumatoid arthritis); SLE (systemic lupus erythematosis).

Management

The management of joint pain will depend on both the diagnosis and the joint involved. The lifestyle and general medical condition of the patient also play a large role in determining the treatment. The goals of treatment are symptomatic relief (pain, stiffness) and functional improvement in the most timely and cost effective manner. The side effects of all treatment must be considered before initiating therapy.

This section deals with the management of os-

teoarthritis. The major treatment objectives in osteoarthritis are pain relief and increased functional status. Non-pharmacologic intervention should be the initial step in treatment unless there is a significant degree of inflammation. Exercise increases

Table 22.4.
Implications of Abnormal CBC or Chemistry

CBC
Neutropenia—SLE, RA, AIDS associated arthritis
Neutrophilia—infectious e.g. septic, osteomyelitis
Anemia—infectious, RA, SLE
Thrombocytopenia—SLE, RA
Increased uric acid—gout
Hypercalcemia—malignancy (breast ca, multiple myeloma) hyperparathyroidism
Increased alkaline phosphatase—Pagets, malignancy
Hyperglycemia—infections, neuropathic, AVN
Renal insufficiency—renal osteodystrophy, gout, neuropathic, multiple myeloma

Table 22.5.
Diagnostic Clues for Osteoarthritis

History
    Joint pain for most days of previous month
    Morning stiffness <30 minutes
    Age >40
    No systemic symptoms
PE
    Crepitus on active motion
    Bony overgrowth
    Heberden's nodes
    Deformities c/w OA
    Decreased range of motion
Lab
    Normal WBC, ESR <20
    Synovial fluid <1000 WBC
X-rays
    Joint space narrowing
    Osteophyte formation
    Subchondral sclerosis

Adapted from Swedberg JA and Steinbauer JR. Osteoarthritis. American Family Physician 1992;45:564.

functional status as well as a sense of well being and possibly improves bloodflow to cartilage. The specific exercises prescribed for each joint and the rationale behind them will be discussed in each chapter. Weight loss seems prudent in terms of reducing the stress on affected joints. Weight reduction may reduce the likelihood of developing OA in unaffected joints, as obesity correlates with the development of OA in general. Local heat or cold may be helpful and the patient may experiment to decide which works best. If none of these measures are effective, then acetaminophen or NSAIDS should be considered.

There have been several large trials that have demonstrated the efficacy of acetaminophen for analgesia in OA. Some clinicians feel that nonsteroidal anti-inflammatory drugs (NSAIDs) play a small role in the treatment of OA except when acute inflammation is involved. This is in part because of the theoretical effects of prostaglandin inhibition on cartilage repair as well as the very serious side effects that may occur with chronic NSAID use. The side effect most frequently encountered is gastrointestinal bleeding, which is often asymptomatic and estimated to occur in 15–30% of chronic NSAID users. Other adverse effects of NSAIDs include exacerbation of hypertension, renal dysfunction, allergic reactions, and fluid retention (particularly important in patients with congestive heart failure or poor renal function). Often, inadequate doses are used. One may use up to 1 g of acetaminophen four times daily initially and then 1 g three times daily for maintenance therapy. The dosage of NSAID will depend on the agent used but the incidence of gastrointestinal hemorrhage is dose related and therefore the minimal dose which allows relief should be used. There are several other adjunctive measures that may be particularly helpful in patients who do not respond to any of the above measures. Antidepressants are often very helpful in relieving the chronic pain associated with OA as well as enabling patients to sleep. Sleep deprivation increases the pain experienced by patients and worsens their functional status. The tricyclics are the agents most commonly prescribed but need to be used cautiously in patients with a history of cardiac disease. One should begin with a low dose and have the patient return every 4 to 6 weeks to evaluate the response to pain and consider raising the dose. It should be explained to the patient that while he will immediately reap the benefits of enhanced sleep the analgesic effects take several weeks to reach their potential.

The use of opiates in OA is controversial. Many practitioners will use opiates, for example, tylenol with codeine, in patients who are unable to tolerate NSAIDs and are not candidates for other therapies. The use of opiates may not be appropriate in OA, but one must consider each patient individually and discuss the options and the side effects with each patient. A major concern is the addiction potential but the addiction potential is overrated by many in the health profession.

If pharmacologic agents have not worked, injections of long-acting corticosteroids, are often very helpful particularly in patients who have a significant degree of inflammation and are unable to tolerate NSAIDs. Corticosteroids may be injected only 2–3 times per year and the risk of infection is significant if proper technique is not followed. There is no role for systemic steroids in patients with OA. Ultimately, if patients are in significant pain or have reduced function, one must consider surgical options such as arthroscopic debridement, osteotomy or joint replacement. OA is the most common indication for joint replacement in the US and when done in the appropriate patient, improves the quality of life significantly.

ILLUSTRATIVE CASES WITH SELF-ASSESSMENT QUESTIONS AND ANSWERS

Case 1

A 23-year-old woman presents with 2 weeks of diffuse myalgias and arthralgias after an upper respiratory illness. On physical examination she has a low grade temperature, shotty adenopathy and diffuse muscle tenderness, but no effusions or erythema.

QUESTION: *What would the next step in evaluation be?*

a. ESR and CBC
b. Rheumatoid factor
c. X-rays of tender joints
d. Thyroid function tests

ANSWER: a. *There is no evidence of an inflammatory arthritis occuring, but one cannot entirely rule it out. A CBC and ESR would be reassuring if within normal limits and if abnormal, may point to diagnosis. It would be premature to test for rheumatoid factor. Her symptoms are not consistent with thyroid dysfunction. X-rays would have a very low yield in this patient.*

Case 2

A 75-year-old obese, hypertensive man presents with pain in the right knee. He has noticed the pain upon walking too much for the past year, but it is now starting to bother him even after he sits for too long. On physical examination, there is crepitance and soft tissue swelling, but no effusions or erythema. He is requesting medication for the pain because it prevents him from sleeping.

QUESTION: *What would the first choice for analgesia be?*

a. NSAIDs
b. Acetaminophen
c. Corticosteroids
d. Antidepressant

ANSWER: b. *In view of his history of hypertension and advanced age and without signs of inflammation tylenol would be the safest agent to choose. If used in appropriate doses, it should provide adequate analgesia. If insufficient relief occurs with tylenol and other nonpharmacologic therapies, you may want to prescribe a NSAID.*

BACK PAIN

Back pain is the most common joint pain for which patients seek medical attention. An estimated 80% of people will seek medical attention for back pain at some time with an annual cost of 24 billion dollars in the US. It is one of the leading causes of disability and due to the societal impact, all health care providers must be able to rationally evaluate back pain.

The evaluation and implications of acute and chronic back pain are vastly different. Acute back pain is defined as being present for less than 3 weeks and is usually mechanical in nature (i.e., brought on by movement). Although it may lead to significant acute loss of time from work, it is not as troublesome as chronic back pain. In the evaluation of

acute back pain, it is important to rule out any ominous causes such as cord compression due to a malignancy or infections (Table 22.6). It is not usually necessary to arrive at a definitive diagnosis when evaluating acute back pain if there are no ominous signs or symptoms.

Acute back pain may be caused by a variety of causes, which include acute processes such as muscular or ligamentous strain. It may also be due to exacerbation of a more chronic process such as degenerative arthritis or spondylosis. There may actually be an acute disc herniation or a nerve compression due to local strain. Sciatica implies that there is radiation of the pain into the buttocks or down the leg and that there is nerve involvement. It does not necessarily signify a worse prognosis, but more likely may become chronic. Patients with disc herniation often have a history of previous back injuries. Most acute back pain, regardless of whether a disc is involved, will resolve with conservative therapy.

Chronic back pain (symptoms lasting longer than 3 months) occurs in only 5% of the patients with back pain, but accounts for 85% of workman's compensation and lost time from work. The causes of chronic back pain are much the same as those for acute back pain, but tend to be less often simply muscular or ligamentous strain. The patients with chronic back pain are a different group of patients on psychological testing. They report low job satisfaction, and on personality testing, have a greater incidence of hysteria, substance abuse, depression, and anxiety. It is difficult to establish whether there is a causal relationship involved.

Pathophysiologic Correlation

In this section, the anatomy and function of the back as well as specific syndromes will be discussed. See Figure 22.1 for a review of the anatomy of the spine. The vertebral bodies provide the structure for the spine and protect the spinal cord. The spinal

Table 22.6.
Ominous Signs for Symptoms

Fever
Weight loss
Night pain
No relief from analgesics
History of malignancy
History of intravenous drug use
History of steroid use or immunodeficiency
Change in bowel or bladder habits

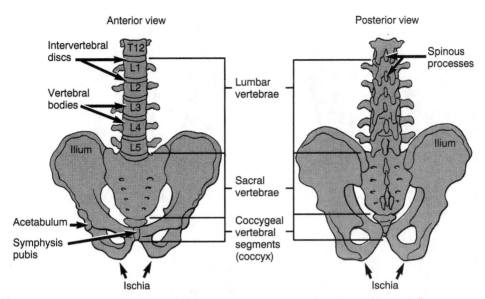

Figure 22.1. Bones and articulations of the lumbosacral spine and pelvis, shown schematically in anterior and posterior views. (From Willms JL, Schneiderman H, Algranati PS. Physical diagnosis: bedside evaluation of diagnosis and function. Baltimore: Williams & Wilkins. 1994:512.)

cord ends at approximately the third lumbar verte-brae and nerve roots exit laterally down into the cauda equina. There is limited articular movement due to the facets. There are ligaments that stabilize the articulation as well as the intervertebral discs which serve to cushion and protect. Any of these structures may be the culprit in back pain as well as the surrounding soft tissues.

One needs to be familiar with the dermatomes when evaluating back pain (Fig. 22.2). Many local processes may result in symptoms of nerve root compression, but there will not be motor weakness when only one nerve root is involved. If there is motor weakness, one should suspect either more than one nerve root is involved or that a peripheral nerve is compromised. As in other joints, local reactions to pain will greatly affect the outcome. Muscle spasm is particularly prominent with the large para-spinal muscles and due to the weight bearing nature even minimal use will exacerbate the muscle spasm.

Osteoporosis, the loss of bone density, is thought to be due to an imbalance in the control of bone formation and destruction which occurs in a well regulated fashion in healthy individuals. The most common form is the idiopathic form. Al-though osteoporosis is at least in part related to aging when osteoclastic activity is increased, there are many other factors involved, since not all elderly

patients exhibit osteoporosis. Table 22.7 lists the risk factors for osteoporosis. Another risk factor, estrogen deficiency, is well recognized. There are differences between the osteoporosis associated with aging and that of estrogen deficient states. The age associated osteoporosis is largely due to decreased osteoblastic activity whereas the estrogen deficient form is due to an imbalance between os-teoclastic activity and osteoblastic activity with an increase in both, but a greater increase in osteoclas-tic activity. Age-related osteoporosis occurs pri-marily in the cortical bone, whereas the estrogen deficient form affects mainly the trabecular bone.

Estrogen deficiency has a dramatic effect on osteoporosis and there are likely multiple factors involved (Table 22.8). There are cytokines that regulate the development and activity of the bone forming units (osteoblasts and osteoclasts) and the best recognized of these are interleukins 6, 11, and 1 in order of magnitude of effect. These in turn affect regulating proteins such as glycoprotein 130 which then affect the hormonal and electrolyte bal-ance. Age-related loss of bone mass begins in the fourth or fifth decade and accelerates with the loss of estrogen. Peak bone mass is achieved in the late teens and a wide variety of lifestyle factors affect the bone mass.

The pathogenesis of Paget's disease is not well

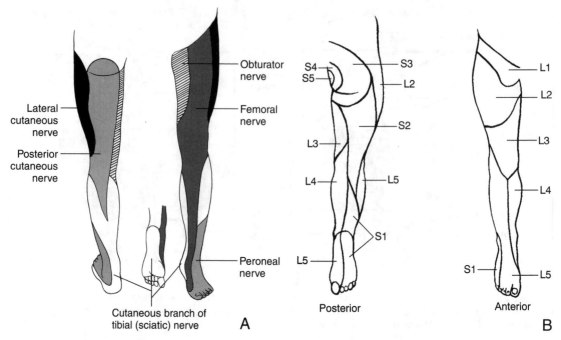

Figure 22.2. Sensory innervation of the lower extremity. (A) Peripheral nerve innervation. (B) Dermatomal (root) innvervation. (B: From Willms JL, Schneiderman H, Algranati PS. Physical diagnosis: bedside evaluation of diagnosis and function. Baltimore: Williams & Wilkins. 1994:527.)

understood. Pathologically focal areas of increased osteolysis and osteogenesis are found which result in structurally impaired bone. The new bone is often described as "woven" and is prone to fractures. There are many theories as to the etiopathogenesis. One which has gained some support is that there is a virus involved. This is because virus-

Table 22.8.
Effects of Estrogen Deficiency and Aging on Bone

Effects of estrogen deficiency
   Increased osteoblastic sensitivity to interleukin 6
   Decreased calcium absorption in the gut
   Increased calcium excretion in the urine
Effects of aging
   Decreased renal production of 1,25 dihydroxyvitamin D
   Decreased gut absorption of calcium

Table 22.7.
Risk Factors for Osteoporosis

Advancing age
Female sex
Premature menopause
Family history
White or Asian Race
Thin body habitus
Smoking
Alcohol abuse
Excessive caffeine intake
PMH: hyperthyroidism, diabetes, chronic renal failure, COPD, rheumatoid arthritis
Being bed bound
Meds: Corticosteroids, anticonvulsants, thyroid hormones, heparin, INH, aluminum containing antacids tetacycline

like particles have been found in the osteoclasts of Pagetic bone, but not in unaffected bone and because epidemics of Paget's have occurred. There are geographic variations as well, with the disease being common in Great Britain and continental Europe, but rare in Scandinavia, Africa and Asia.

Avascular necrosis (AVN) is found most often in association with corticosteroid use (Table 22.9). The pathogenesis of AVN is thought to be due to several contributing factors. The sinusoids in the bone marrow are believed to be the target with intravascular or extraosseous compression of the venules in the sinusoids leading to infarction and

Table 22.9.
Disorders Associated with AVN

Coricosteroid use (dose dependent)
Trauma (acute or chronic)
Alcohol abuse
Diabetes
Sickle cell anemia
Possible associations
    Cigarette smoking
    Pregnancy
    Hemodialysis
    Pancreatitis
    Antiphospholipid antibody syndrome

necrosis. Disorders such as sickle cell anemia or antiphospholipid disorders are believed to be examples of intravascular obstruction with the development of local fat hypertrophy occurring in patients taking corticosteroids or abusing alcohol. This, in turn, leads to high intraosseous pressures and infarction.

Clinical and Laboratory Evaluation

The causes, treatment, and prognosis of acute and chronic back pain differ greatly. When evaluating acute back pain, it is important to distinguish between mechanical and nonmechanical back pain. Mechanical back pain implies that the pain is brought on by movement and nonmechanical implies that the pain may be referred (e.g., from an aortic aneurysm). If one can determine that there is no evidence of ominous symptoms or signs on physical examination, then the evaluation and treatment of acute low back pain should be conservative and inexpensive. However, in chronic back pain there are often many other issues such as secondary gain and the effect of personality upon the painful experience.

HISTORY

When evaluating acute back pain, it will be helpful to know if there was a specific action which precipitated the pain. In herniated discs, fractures or ligamentous sprains the patient will remember the exact action which brought on the pain, whereas in muscular or ligamentous strains the patient may remember doing an excessive amount of work the day of the pain, but not a particular action. Patients with muscular strain are often unable to localize pain to a particular area whereas patients who have disc or nerve root involvement will often state that the pain radiates down the buttocks or leg. If pa-

tients give any symptoms of bowel or bladder dysfunction, it will be important to rule out cauda equina syndrome immediately.

It is important to distinguish sciatica from simple mechanical back pain because it is more likely for sciatica to become chronic and it will then require a different approach. Sciatica is defined as pain which radiates into the buttocks or down the legs (in the distribution of the sciatic nerve). It is frequently described as a burning or shooting pain which is worsened by actions which stretch the nerve, such as bending. It may occur because of nerve root compression or disc herniation. It is more likely to be due to disc herniation in young patients and spondylosis with nerve root involvement in elderly patients.

The ominous signs and symptoms that are often referred to in the evaluation of back pain or signs or symptoms which might lead one to suspect a more serious process occurring which would prompt a different evaluation of acute back pain (see Table 22.6).

When evaluating chronic back pain it is important to determine the mode of injury and treatment which has been administered. It is not uncommon for elderly patients to have chronic back pain due to arthritic or metabolic processes. It is, however, uncommon for mechanical back pain to become chronic; 50% of patients with acute low back pain will have a recurrence of back pain, but it is a recurrence rather than a chronic state. Depending on the age group, one may consider diagnoses such as ankylosing spondylitis in young men particularly, if there is a history of morning stiffness which resolves with walking and involvement of the sacroiliac joints.

PHYSICAL EXAMINATION

Begin the examination of the back by observing how the patient walks, stands, and sits. These will give clues to the severity of the pain and how the patient responds to it. Observe for loss of the normal lordosis; this may indicate muscle spasm in acute back pain or ankylosing spondylitis in chronic back pain. If the patient is able to sit with ease then the degree of injury is likely minimal, but if the patient needs to sit on the edge of the chair with legs extended, this is a way of alleviating stretch on the sciatic nerve and may be a clue. In acute trauma any swelling or ecchymoses may be helpful. Deformities such as scoliosis predispose to chronic back pain, but not to sciatica.

Localizing the pain is crucial. In muscular or

ligamentous injuries patients are often unable to localize the pain. However, many other disorders may be localized such as sacroiliitis, hip rather than back pain or sciatica. One should palpate for point tenderness and any dropoffs between the vertebrae, which would indicate spondylolisthesis. If one suspects simple muscular or ligamentous strain it is not necessary to categorize it further. If one suspects sciatica or any nerve pain, then it is necessary to perform a thorough neurologic examination. It will be important to examine for sensory, motor, and reflex abnormalities as well as for rectal tone and perineal sensation. If there is any evidence of bowel or bladder involvement, then immediate imaging of the spinal cord is indicated.

There are specific maneuvers that may be done to evaluate for sciatica. The most common one is the straight leg raise. The patient should be in a supine position and one leg should be passively raised at a time. If raising the leg between 30–60 degrees reproduces a sharp, burning pain in the sciatic distribution this is a positive straight leg raise. It is more specific for disc herniation if the crossed straight leg raise is positive, i.e., if passive lifting of the opposite leg reproduces the pain. If the pain is elicited at greater than 60 degrees or if the pain has a tight stretching quality, that is not a positive straight leg raise and is indicative of muscular strain. One may also check for a flip sign. The patient sits with knees dangling over the side of the examining table and when the clinician extends the knee to examine the feet he observes for change in position. This is another maneuver to induce nerve stretching and if the patient does not need to alter his or her position, it makes a positive straight leg raise suspicious.

Physical examination will not be helpful in diagnosing osteoporosis, although one may find evidence of vertebral compression fractures. Note that this is more likely to occur in thin white women. Patients with Paget's disease may have frontal bossing, bowing of the legs and warmth and erythema over the areas of tenderness. There also may be an accompanying effusion in joints near the affected bone. One may find evidence of neurologic involvement (e.g., deafness or peroneal nerve weakness) due to nerve entrapment by the diseased bone. It would be unusual to see signs of congestive heart failure.

In patients with AVN there will be a remarkable paucity of findings on physical exam and, therefore, this diagnosis will require clinical suspicion. The joints most likely to be involved are the hips and knees, when one finds a significant degree of pain

and limitation with few other findings in patients at risk (e.g., steroids, alcohol).

LABORATORY EVALUATION

It is rarely necessary to order laboratory tests to evaluate acute low back pain unless one suspects an ominous cause. In that situation some laboratory data which may be helpful include an erythrocyte sedimentation rate (ESR) which might be elevated in any inflammatory or malignant process. An elevated serum calcium would make one suspect either hyperparathyroidism or more commonly malignant bone disorders such as multiple myeloma or metastatic breast cancer. An elevated alkaline or acid phosphatase are nonspecific markers of increased bone remodeling and may be found in benign bone disorders such as Paget's disease or in metastatic processes such as prostate cancer. If one suspects multiple myeloma, a serum protein electropheresis may be helpful.

If one suspects an ominous cause or acute back pain does not resolve with appropriate therapy, then it would be wise to perform plain radiographs. If one suspects radicular involvement and the patient does not respond to conservative therapy or there is loss of motor function, one would consider performing a CAT scan or MRI to evaluate for possible surgical intervention. All findings on radiologic examinations must be correlated to the clinical picture. Up to 30% of normal individuals will be found to have disc abnormalities on MRI or CAT scanning and, therefore, it will be important to use these tools in the proper context.

Differential Diagnosis

Back pain is the most common presenting symptom in a large number of metabolic bone disorders with osteoporosis being by far the most common. It affects 15–20 million people in the US and cost 10 billion US dollars in 1991 and is projected to cost 60 billion by the year 2020. It leads to 1.5 million fractures each year − 250,000 of which are hip fractures with a 12–25% mortality; half of whom will never walk again. It is estimated that one out of every 3 women over the age of 65 will suffer a hip fracture. Idiopathic osteoporosis usually occurs in people aged 50–75. In the 50–55 year range, patients may present with vertebral compression fractures, then wrist fractures and by the 70–75 year range with femoral neck fractures. There is a marked predilection for women with a female male ratio of 6:1 (see Table 22.7). The differential diagnoses of back pain are listed in Table 22.10.

Table 22.10.
Differential Diagnoses of Back Pain

Acute back pain
  Simple mechanical
    Muscular or ligamentous strain
    Ligamentous sprain, disc herniation, fracture
  Radicular
    Disc herniation
    Spondylosis
  Referred
    Vascular
    Pelvic or retroperitoneal
  Ominous
    Infection
    Malignancy
Chronic back pain
  Mechanical
  Radicular
  Lesion
  Metabolic

Paget's disease is often incidentally discovered in patients when evaluating for other disorders — usually an incidentally elevated alkaline phosphatase (AP). It is the disease of people older than 40, with 3–4% of middle aged and 10–15% of the elderly being affected. Pain in the back, hips, femur, and skull is the most common symptom and is often described as deep and aching, worsened by weightbearing. There may also be local warmth over the tender area due to hypervascularity. Bony enlargement may lead to enlargement of features and nerve entrapment with resultant deafness or peripheral neuropathy. It is rare to see congestive heart failure and less than 1% of Pagetic lesions undergo malignant degeneration. Paget's disease is usually a slowly progressive disorder. If there is sudden acceleration of pain or increase in alkaline phosphate, malignant degeneration should be considered.

Avascular necrosis (AVN) usually occurs in patients with specific risk factors (see Table 22.9). It most commonly presents as pain in the hips, knees, or shoulders. It overwhelmingly occurs on the convex portion of the femoral head, condyle and humeral head which has lead to some theories regarding the etiology of AVN. It is defined as areas of infarction directly below the cartilage leading to pain, disablility and joint destruction. The most common association is with corticosteroid use, but it may be brought on by even minor trauma. It is an important diagnosis to make because it is often iatrogenic and will lead to serious pain and disability if not treated early.

The osteomalachic syndromes due to nutritional deficiencies such as Ricketts are now extremely rare. Due to the widespread screening of serum calcium, it is also rare to see bone disorders due to hyperparathyroidism. Renal osteodystrophy is, however, still common due to the increasing availability of dialysis and prolonged survival of these patients. There are certain therapeutic measures which may be taken to prevent the development of renal osteodystrophy, but it is beyond the scope of this chapter to go into detail about this disorder.

Management

The management of non-ominous acute low back pain will be the same regardless of whether there are signs of radicular involvement or the cause. Bedrest will be the first and most important therapy. Patients who comply with complete bedrest regardless of the degree or etiology of acute low back pain will recover more quickly. This means absolute bedrest except to go to the bathroom. There is debate as to the duration of bedrest, but for simple mechanical low back pain, 2 days is the standard recommendation and for radicular pain up to 2 weeks depending upon the degree of injury. However, very few patients comply with complete bedrest. A more typical recommendation is to resume activity as tolerated. Local measures such as ice for the first 24 hours and then heat or ice or local facients such as Ben-Gay are recommended.

An anti-inflammatory such as aspirin will also be of much help and should be used on a standing basis for the first few days rather than as needed to obtain its anti-inflammatory effects. If there is a significant amount of muscle spasm, a muscle relaxant such as flexeril or a benzodiazepine may be extremely helpful. One of the benefits of sedating the patient is improved compliance with complete bed rest. If the patient has pain that is not responding to conservative measures or the degree of injury appears severe on initial evaluation, a more potent analgesic such as a narcotic may be necessary. This should be prescribed for a limited period of time and if the patient requires more, one should reevaluate for a more serious cause or analgesic abuse.

Exercise is an important part of both treatment and prevention of back pain. It is important to teach patients methods of reducing strain upon the back and avoiding injury. The management of chronic back pain will be quite different and will rely more heavily upon exercises and anti-inflammatory agents. It is not wise to use narcotics in the treatment of chronic back pain unless there is an ominous cause or other methods have failed. Antidepressants such as the tricyclics have a role in chronic back pain as an adjunctive measure. They work by affecting the pain pathways as well as providing much needed assistance with sleep and treating the depression often associated with chronic pain. Diathermy (ultrasound) and TENS (transcutaneous electrical nerve stimulation) have not been shown to be helpful in osteoarthritis, but TENS may have a limited role in sciatica. It will be important to teach the patient preventative measures.

Hormone replacement therapy has become the mainstay of treatment for osteoporosis. It serves mainly to prevent further loss of bone mass in women who are post menopausal. Estrogen will increase bone mass by up to 11% in the first 18 months after menopause and thereafter, will reduce the subsequent loss of bone and reduce the number of fractures by 50%. Considering the large number of patients affected by osteoporotic fractures and the ensuing morbidity and mortality the prevention of osteoporosis is of great clinical significance. Patients who have had a hysterectomy may be given estrogen alone, but women with an intact uterus must receive progestational agents to offset the increased risk of endometrial cancer. With regular follow-up, although there is an increase in the incidence of endometrial cancer, the mortality in those women is not increased. This is likely due to the benign nature of the lesions and the fact that these patients are receiving regular care and the endometrial cancer is being detected at an early stage.

A more difficult question is whether there is an increase in the incidence of breast cancer. There is definitely an increased growth of estrogen dependent tumors, but these tend to have a more benign course and again the addition of a progestational agent may partially compensate for this. The reduction in coronary artery disease, osteoporosis and improved urogenital health make hormone replacement therapy seem beneficial in most patients except those with a personal history of breast cancer and possibly those with a strong family history (less than 5% of breast cancer is hereditary).

There are other options for treating osteoporosis which include calcitonin, calcium and vitamin D supplementation and the use of biphosphonates. Calcitonin decreases the lifespan and number of osteoclasts and has an analgesic affect on vertebral crush fractures. It retards the loss of bone mass in

the first 5 years after menopause and has very few side effects, none of which are dangerous. It must be administered subcutaneously, is very expensive, and does not have the additional benefits of cardiovascular protection or improved urogenital health, but may be a very good second choice in the treatment of osteoporosis particularly in those patients already suffering from vertebral fractures.

Calcium supplementation is superior to placebo in preserving bone mass and may be important in patients who have less than 400 mg/day calcium in their diet. Vitamin D supplementation may be particularly important in those patients who are homebound and do not have adequate dietary intake. Both of these should be considered as adjunctive measures. Fluoride has been widely used in Europe for many years, but is not approved for use in the US due to concerns over the quality of the new bone which is formed. The biphosphonates are endogenous inhibitors of osteoclast metabolic activity and maturation and have been shown to increase bone mass when used in a cyclical manner, but have not yet been shown to reduce fracture rate and are not FDA approved for the treatment of osteoporosis.

Weight bearing exercise reduces fracture rate both by increasing mass and by improving coordination and thus avoiding falls. All of the above measures must be considered in an individual patient. The prevention of osteoporosis has tremendous financial, social and medical benefits for our patients.

Paget's disease is often an asymptomatic process and, therefore, treatment will depend on the type of symptoms present and aims to prevent future complications. The management of pain would be the same as for other types of joint pain. There are specific medical therapies aimed at preventing further osteoclastic activity and bone absorption. The drugs most commonly prescribed include calcitonin, etidronate, and plicamycin. Calcitonin appears to directly inhibit the osteoclasts and results in acute improvement in bone pain and hyperemia in 80% of patients. It must be given subcutaneously at present, but forms of intranasal calcitonin are being investigated. Treatment is for 1–6 months and only results in a plateauing of symptoms and does not halt the disease progression. The most common side-effects are flushing and nausea which occur in 20–40%, but are usually only transient.

Etidronate is a biphosphonate and its mode of action in inhibiting bone resorption is not known. Etidronate may be given orally, but takes several weeks for the effects to be seen. It is continued for

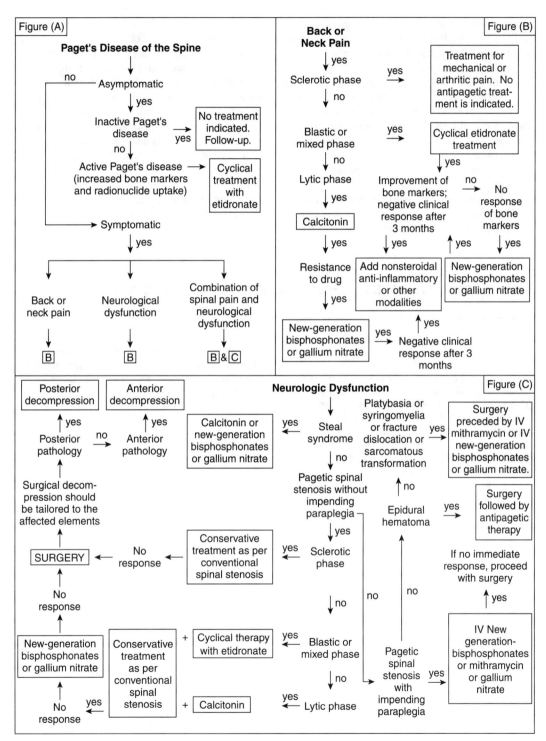

Figure 22.3. Algorithmic approach to the treatment of Paget's.

up to 6 months and one sees similar response rates as for calcitonin. It is better tolerated and easier to administer. Plicamycin inhibits osteoclast activity by inhibiting RNA synthesis. It must be given intermittently intravenously and has greater toxicity. It is not yet approved for the treatment of Paget's, but does result in rapid decreases in symptoms (within days). Surgical intervention is sometimes required for fractures (7% annual incidence) or deformities that occur due to bowing or bony overgrowth. Figure 22.3 outlines an algorithmic approach to the treatment of Paget's.

The treatment of avascular necrosis (AVN) needs to be focused on prevention. This can be accomplished by reducing the dose of corticoste-roids patients receive (it is dose dependant), counseling regarding alcohol abuse, and possibly avoiding cigarette smoking. The treatment in the early stages focuses largely on reducing further trauma and therefore, further degeneration of joints. This may be accomplished using four point crutch walking, which alleviates the degree of strain on bilateral joints. The treatment for later stages of AVN is surgical and may include decompression if the area of necrosis is small. However, if the area is significant joint replacement is usually required. These patients do very poorly with joint replacement and frequently need revision much earlier than patients with other indications for arthroplasty such as osteoarthritis.

ILLUSTRATIVE CASES WITH SELF-ASSESSMENT QUESTIONS AND ANSWERS

Case 1

A 45-year-old construction worker presents with acute back pain after lifting a heavy log at work. The patient describes the pain as occurring immediately and that he felt a popping sensation. He has injured his back previously at work, but has never needed to see a physician. This time the pain is much more severe and there is radiation of the pain down his left leg. He is requesting a pain medication and a note for his job. His exam is consistent with an L4-5 sensory radiculopathy.

QUESTION: *What would the next appropriate step be?*

a. Plain radiographs of the lumbar-sacral spine
b. CAT scan of L4–5 as you highly suspect disc herniation
c. Activity as tolerated for 2 weeks and local measures as well as anti-inflammatories
d. Referral to an orthopedic specialist

ANSWER: c. *Most likely he will improve with conservative management. Further investigation or referral is indicated if his pain continues.*

Case 2

A 70-year-old woman with no medical history presents to you with 1 week of excruciating back pain after falling when returning from the grocery store. She has tried various analgesics and even some of her friend's sleeping pills, but has not found any relief.

QUESTION: *All of the following are diagnostic possibilities except:*

a. Osteoperosis with a compression fracture on physical exam
b. Pathological fracture due to breast cancer
c. Avascular necrosis secondary to advanced age
d. Sciatica due to spondylosis

ANSWER: c *and* **d.** *Pain localized to the back would be unusual in avascular necrosis or sciatica.*

SHOULDER PAIN

The shoulder is the most mobile joint in the body and the most frequently used and is, therefore prone to injury. The shoulder is also affected by a variety of disorders not related to shoulder pathology such as cervical spine disorders or medical illnesses. The type of complaint pain, weakness, or abnormal range of motion (increased or decreased) and the age of the patient will allow the clinician to narrow the differential diagnoses.

Pathophysiologic Correlation

To review the anatomy of the shoulder please refer to Figure 22.4. The head of the humerus sits in the cup created by the glenoid process of the scapula, the labrum, and the surrounding musculotendinous structures. The four rotator cuff muscles may be thought of as one unit. They provide the majority of the support for the shoulder.

The rotator cuff is susceptible to impingement and inflammation due to the close proximity of the acromial arch and the humerus between which it passes and its poor blood supply (Fig. 22.5). Disorders of the rotator cuff include simple mechanical impingement and inflammation and irritation of the tendon or subacromial bursa. The inflammation leads to changes in the tendon including loss of the wavy pattern of collagen, hyalinization and microtears. If the degeneration progresses, it may lead to tears in the tendon, which are usually intraendinous rather than at the tendon insertion. Although some granulation and revascularization occurs after an acute tear, the vascular supply is usually insufficient for the tendon to heal.

The process occurs on a spectrum and is usually due to local factors except in the case of calcific tendinitis in which there is a more marked degree of inflammation. Corticosteroid injections will predispose the tendon to tearing as will the degenerative changes of aging which include loss of elasticity and thinning of the tendon.

Adhesive capsulitis is morphologically related to decreased intracapsular volume and increased intraarticular pressures. Experimentally, when the joint is immobilized, there is an increase in the synovial cellularity and vascular proliferation. After several weeks, adhesions develop involving the subcapsular bursa and the articular cartilage. In idiopathic adhesive capsulitis it is likely that capsular contracture is responsible, although the cause is unknown. However, in secondary causes of frozen shoulder, periarticular factors such as musculature and innervation serve a prominent role.

Shoulder instability may be thought of as acute, which is usually traumatic or chronic-recurrent, which may be either traumatic or atraumatic. Traumatic instability is felt to be due to detachment of the fibrous capsule of the joint from the glenoid-the "Bankart lesion." Atraumatic instability is likely due to laxity in the ligaments. The Bankart lesion occurs almost exclusively in football players or persons with a seizure disorder. Although simple acute shoulder dislocations usually occur from a fall on an outstretched arm, the Bankart results from direct force to the posterior aspect of the joint.

Cervical spine disorders may be due to disc herniation or nerve root compression due to hypertrophy of the facets. The interspaces most frequently involved are C5-C6, C6-C7 and then C4-C5. Processes such as rheumatoid arthritis are associated with an increased prevalence of cervical spine disorders. Table 22.11 helps determine which nerve is involved.

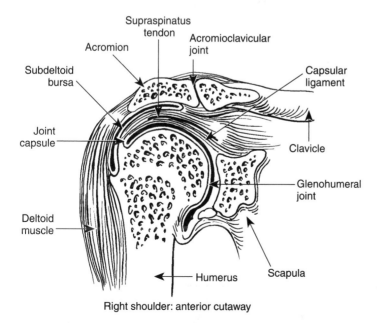

Right shoulder: anterior cutaway

Figure 22.4. Right shoulder: anterior cutaway. (From Willms JL, Schneiderman H, Algranati PS. Physical diagnosis: bedside evaluation of diagnosis and function. Baltimore: Williams & Wilkins. 1994:392.)

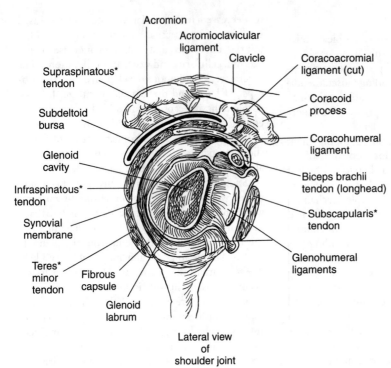

Figure 22.5. Shoulder joint, lateral view.
*tendons that form the rotator cuff.

The carpal tunnel is formed by the bones of the wrist and the overlying tendon sheath (Fig. 22.6). Tendons and the median nerve, which are responsible for the symptoms of carpal tunnel syndrome (CTS), run through the carpal tunnel. Because the carpal tunnel is a small space, any process such as swelling, bony enlargement or lipomas reduce the space and lead to symptoms of CTS. The most common associated processes are listed in Table 22.12.

The polymyositis/dermatomyositis syndromes are most likely immune-mediated and lead to inflammation and muscle atrophy. It is not known why there is an increased incidence of malignancy associated with these disorders. Polymyalgia rheumatica is also immune-mediated, but the etiology and pathology in fibromyalgia is unknown. Attempts to diagnose it histologically have been unsuccessful and it is thus far a clinical diagnosis.

Clinical and Laboratory Evaluation

The age of the patient and type of complaint are the two most important factors when evaluating

Table 22.11.
Cervical Nerve Root Compression Findings

Level	Root	Muscles Affected	Sensory Loss	Reflex
C3-C4	C4	Scapular	Lateral neck, shoulder	None
C4-C5	C5	Deltoid, biceps, rotator cuff	Lateral arm or none	Biceps
C5-C6*	C6	Wrist extensors, biceps, brachioradialis	Radial forearm or none	Brachioradialis
C6-C7*	C7	Triceps, wrist, flexors, finger extensors	Middle finger or none	Triceps
C7-C8	C8	Finger and wrist flexors, and extensors	Little finger	None
C8-T1	T1	Interossei	Ulnar forearm or none	None

*Most common.

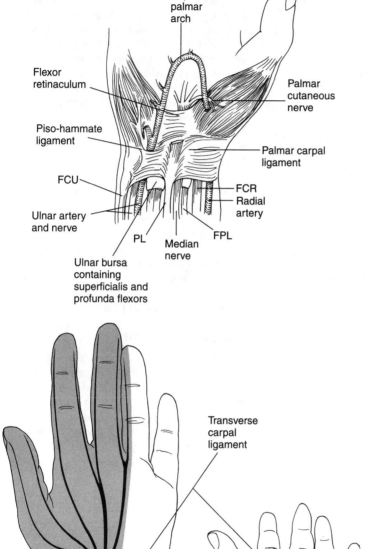

Figure 22.6. Carpal tunnel. (A) Diagram of carpal tunnel with its nine flexor tendons and the median nerve. FCR = flexor carpi radialis; FCU = flexor carpi ulnaris; PL = palmaris longus. (Redrawn from Goldner RD. Orthopaedic Surgery Update Series, Vol. 3, Lesson 28. Princeton, New Jersey, Continuing Professional Education Center, Inc.) (B) Diagram of carpal tunnel and its classic sensory distribution (stippled area). (Redrawn from American Society for Surgery of the Hand. The Hand: Examination and Diagnosis. 2nd edition. Edinburgh: Churchill Livingstone, 1983.)

shoulder disorders. The most common complaints are pain, weakness and instability and the workups should be distinct. When shoulder pain is unrelated to movement and there are other associated symptoms such as cough or nausea, suspect a medical condition causing referred pain and err on the side of caution when evaluating. It is, otherwise, unusual for laboratory data or x-rays to add much to what may be obtained by history and physical exam except in the case of trauma.

Table 22.12.
Conditions Associated with Carpal Tunnel Syndrome

Diabetes
Arthritis
Hypothyroidism
Pregnancy
Overuse syndromes

Table 22.13 lists differentials according to complaint.

HISTORY

Patients with rotator cuff disease often complain of pain over the deltoid region that worsens at night and with elevation of the arm. There may be some associated weakness or decreased range of motion. The weakness is usually in elevation or external rotation and may be elicited by asking the patient if he is able to comb his hair. Marked weakness may signify an acute rotator cuff tear and is more likely in the elderly or patients with a history of bursitis and corticosteroid injections.

Calcific tendonitis presents more acutely, with a greater degree of inflammation and pain which is more localized. Patients with arthritic processes such as rheumatoid arthritis usually have a previous diagnosis from other joints being involved. Osteoarthritis is the most common form of arthritis affecting the shoulder, but the shoulder is an unusual site for OA. Patients may even have significant limitation of motion if the arthritis has led to erosion and deformity.

In the case of shoulder instability it is important to separate acute traumatic instability which is most

Table 22.13.
Differential According to Complaint

Pain
   Tendonitis/bursitis
   Arthritis
   Cervical spine disorder
   Metabolic or infiltrative bone lesion
Weakness
   Rotator cuff pathology
   Cervical spine disorder
   Myopathic process
Decreased range of motion
   Adhesive capsulitis
   Rotator cuff tear
   Severe arthritic change

often anterior from chronic recurrent instability. The patient who has instability from hyperlax joints is often young and has evidence of increased joint mobility in other joints such as the knees and thumbs. He may only note pain in the shoulder and not be aware of the unstable joint. It is usually unstable in more than one direction.

Decreased range of motion may occur from adhesive capsulitis, rotator cuff tears or arthritic processes and usually the patient notes weakness. Adhesive capsulitis may be idiopathic or secondary to trauma or immobilization and therefore, it will be important to obtain a medical history from the patient.

Myopathic processes present as proximal muscle weakness that is diffuse, symmetrical and affects the shoulder and pelvic girdle muscles. There may be pain and systemic symptoms such as fever and fatigue. The age of the patient and accompanying symptoms will be helpful to distinguish the clinical syndromes which occur (Table 22.15). Rule out secondary causes of myopathies, the most common being alcohol ingestion (Table 22.14).

PHYSICAL EXAMINATION

The physical examination should begin with observing for gross deformities, differences in muscle bulk or dislocations. Look for signs of inflammation, swelling, warmth or erythema. If present, determine whether they involve the acromioclavicular or the shoulder joint. If a myopathic process is suspected, look for clues of systemic illness or classical dermatologic involvement.

Table 22.14.
Secondary Causes of Myopathic Processes

Drugs/alcohol
   Cocaine
   Heroin
Medications
   Lovastatin (all HMG reducers)
   Corticosteroids
   Immunosuppressants
   Colchicine
   Zidovidine
   Lopid
Medical conditions
   Endocrinopathies (hypothyroidism, hyperthyroidism, hyperparathyroidism)
   Viral infections (HIV, picornavirus)
   Electrolyte disturbances (hypokalemia, hypophosphatemia, hypomagnesemia, hypercalcemia)

Table 22.15.
Myopathic Processes

	Age	History	Diagnosis	Associated Illness	Treatment
Polymyalgia rheumatica	>70	Shoulder & girdle weakness Fatigue, fevers	ESR >100 Clinical picture	Temporal arteritis 15%	Steroids
Polymyositis Dermatolyositis	Bimodal 5–15 50–60	Weakness, proximal symptoms	Autoantibodies 80–90% EMG Muscle biopsy	Malignancy risk 1.8 to 3	Steroids Cyclophosphamide
Fibromyositis	Young women	Diffuse pain	Clinical "trigger points"	Sleep disorders Neuropsychiatric disorders	NSAIDS Physical therapy
Secondary myopathies drugs		Usually one month after starting the drug			Decrease drug
ETOH	Older	Dose dependent after years		Biopsy Vacular myopathy	Abstinence

All patients with shoulder pain must have a simple neurologic exam to rule out cervical spine disorders. If the cervical spine is involved, there is usually point tenderness over the back of the neck. Neurologic findings are often not present and therefore, diagnostic tests are often necessary if the patient has a suggestive history and physical examination.

Localization of the pain will also assist in limiting the diagnoses. Anterior shoulder pain is usually due to involvement of the acromioclavicular joint or bicipital etendonitis. Posterior shoulder pain, usually over the posterior humerus, suggests involvement of the glenohumeral joint. Pain over the trapezius, particularly if associated with neurologic symptoms, usually indicates cervical spondylosis. Pain over the deltoid region is often due to rotator cuff disorders.

When instability is suspected because of a history of weakness or "giving," instability can be elicited by placing anterior and posterior pressure on the glenohumeral joint in the abducted position. If there is a dislocation, it is usually apparent on gross examination. If the patient is able to voluntarily dislocate the shoulder by contracting muscles, a personality disorder is usually involved. Pain at extreme ranges of motion is usually periarticular.

Acromioclavicular (AC) joint involvement may be elicited by having the patient perform the "crossover test," which reduces the AC space increasing the pain in an inflamed joint. The patient crosses the affected arm across the body such that the elbow of the affected arm approximates the opposite shoulder and this should elicit pain. It can

be confirmed by injection of anesthetics such as lidocaine into the AC joint, which should relieve the pain. Separation of the AC joint will make the clavicle appear to ride up.

The impingement test confirms the suspicion of rotator cuff involvement by approximating the humerus and acromion and pinching the tendon that passes under the acromion. By injecting lidocaine and corticosteroids, one may both confirm the diagnosis and treat the disorder.

LABORATORY EVALUATION

Laboratory examinations will be helpful when an inflammatory or myopathic process is suspected. It is unusual for an infectious process to affect the shoulder and therefore, it will be rarely needed to perform an arthrocentesis. However, if there is fever, leukocytosis, and swelling of the joint, it will be necessary to perform an arthrocentesis.

If a myopathic process is suspected, it is necessary to rule out disorders that mimic myopathic processes such as hypothyroidism or electrolyte disorders such as hypokalemia (see Table 22.14). One can place the diagnostic suspicion depending on the age and clinical syndrome. If an elderly person presents with weakness and fatigue, a sedimentation rate over 100 will point to the diagnosis of PMR. In young women with symptoms of diffuse pain and point tenderness, collagen vascular diseases such as systemic lupus erythematosus must be ruled out.

Radiologic studies are indicated in some situations. In the setting of acute trauma, x-rays are necessary to rule out fractures or dislocations. Views with stress applied to the joint will reveal instability which is not evident on plain radiographs. Although calcifications may be present, they are not diagnostic of calcific tendonitis. A narrowing of the distance between the humeral head and the acromion is suggestive of rotator cuff tear. If there is a high degree of clinical suspicion, magnetic resonance imaging (MRI) may be helpful. MRI should be considered in only the appropriate clinical setting as there is a high rate of abnormal findings in people without complaints.

Electromyelographic (EMG) studies are indicated when trying to rule out a neuropathic process or polymyositis. The EMG is not very sensitive in cervical spine disorders, but is extremely useful in diagnosing CTS and should be done before surgery.

Differential Diagnosis

The differential diagnoses of shoulder pain includes disorders of the shoulder and periarticular structures predominantly (Table 22.16). However, referred pain and myositis syndromes should not be overlooked.

ROTATOR CUFF DISORDERS

Rotator cuff disorders include a spectrum of processes from tendonitis to bursal swelling to actual tendon tears. Tendonitis frequently precedes the development of tears and therefore, tears usually

Table 22.16.
Differential of Shoulder Pain

Rotator cuff disorders
  Tendonitis (simple or calcific)
  Tendon tears
Mobility disorders
  Adhesive capsulitis
  Instability
Arthritic processes
  Degenerative
  Rheumatoid
  Gout
Referred pain
  Cervical pathology
  Carpal tunnel syndrome
  Medical conditions
Myositis processes
  Polymyalgia rheumatica
  Polymyositis-dermatomyositis
  Fibromyositis

occur in patients older than age 50 with a history of previous episodes of tendonitis. Rotator cuff pain is usually described as a dull achy pain in the deltoid region often worsened at night especially if the patient tries to sleep on that side. The pain is brought on by movement and may be associated with limitation of elevation and external rotation.

Calcific tendonitis is an acute inflammatory process that may affect the muscles of the rotator cuff. The pain tends to be more severe, acute, and localized than that of simple tendonitis. It usually occurs in the 5th decade and is idiopathic. While there should be calcifications on x-ray, the x-ray is not diagnostic as calcifications may be present in the other processes as well. The diagnosis is usually made on clinical grounds.

MOBILITY DISORDERS

Adhesive capsulitis may be idiopathic or secondary to trauma or immobilization. The idiopathic form develops insidiously over weeks and usually takes up to 1–2 years to resolve. The secondary form may be seen in the case of trauma in which the patient was inappropriately immobilized, the shoulder is prone to "freezing" and will do so if immobilized for even as limited a time as one week especially in elderly patients. It may also occur in the setting of acute illnesses such as strokes or myocardial infarctions when the patient is not mobile. The patient will complain of pain and of being unable to use his shoulder.

Instability may be thought of as two groups classified using the acronyms TUBS (traumatic instability, unidirectional, with a Bankart lesion and responds to surgery) or AMBRI (atraumatic, multidirectional, bilateral shoulders, responds to rehabilitation). The TUBS form is usually seen in athletic men and the AMBRI is often seen in thin young women. Less frequently instability may also less frequently occur in the setting of rotator cuff tears.

ARTHRITIC PROCESSES

When arthritic processes affect the shoulder, the patient will complain of pain and have signs of inflammation at the shoulder joint. There may be decreased active range of motion, but normal passive range of motion unless there has been significant joint destruction. Osteoarthritis is the most common arthritic process affecting the shoulder followed by rheumatoid and gout. It is highly unusual for infectious processes to affect the joint except in the setting of injections or prosthesis.

Shoulder pain is frequently due to pathology in

other places. The most common causes include cervical disorders and medical conditions such as myocardial infarction. The medical conditions causing shoulder pain can usually be deduced by the lack of relation of shoulder movement to pain and the presence of signs of medical illness.

REFERRED PAIN

Cervical spine disorders are the most common cause of referred pain mistaken for shoulder pain. The neurologic quality of the pain, radiation down the arm and location over the trapezius are all clues to the cervical origin. The pain will also be able to be elicited by movement of the neck. Figure 22.7 compares the distribution of pain due to cervical disorders to that of shoulder pathology. There are

many causes of cervical pathology including arthritic and degenerative processes. It is crucial to rule out neurologic deficit, which would require more emergent intervention.

Carpal tunnel syndrome (CTS) is an extremely common orthopedic problem, but is an unusual cause of shoulder pain. When shoulder pain develops, it is usually in the setting of significant hand and arm pain and the patient is usually able to distinguish that the pain begins lower in the arm and radiates proximally. CTS is the result of compression of the median nerve as it passes through the narrow carpal tunnel (see Figure 22.6). The symptoms include numbness in the medial 3 and 1/2 digits and sharp radiating pains into the hand and arm. It is often worse at night or after overuse and has been associated with some jobs requiring

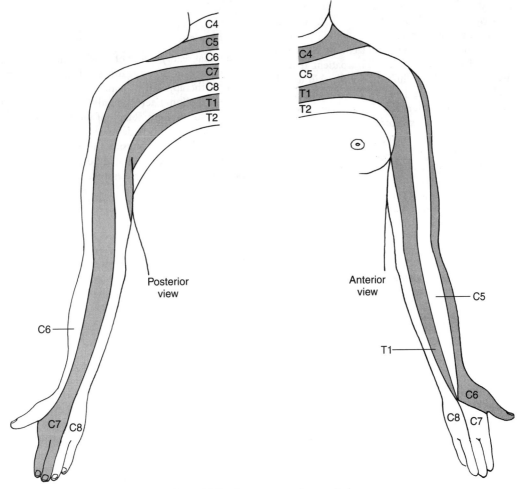

Figure 22.7. Dermatomes of upper limb.

repetitive motions. Table 22.12 lists possible causes.

MYOSITIS PROCESSES

Myositis processes often present in the shoulder and pelvic girdle muscles because they are large muscle groups. Clinicians frequently find an elevated creatinine phosphatase on routine screening and must know the proper evaluation of such. There are a variety of secondary causes that must be ruled out. These are often additive as in the example of gemfibrozil and lovastatin or HIV infection and zidorudine use. It will be important to try to determine a temporal relationship (see Table 22.17).

Polymyalgia rheumatica (PMR) is a disorder almost exclusively of patients older than age 70 and highly unlikely to occur in a patient younger than age 50. It typically consists of weakness in the shoulder and girdle muscles causing the patient to have difficulty with simple activities of daily living such as combing hair or rising from a sitting position. There may also be a significant component of fatigue and low grade fevers. The patient may be incapacitated. The sedimentation rate will usually be elevated to greater than l00. There is an association of temporal arteritis in l5% of patients with PMR. Recognize the symptoms of headaches, scalp tenderness, and visual complaints. Once there are visual disturbances progression to blindness may occur within days and is easily treated with high dose steroids.

The polymyositis syndromes have several pathological classifications, but most important clinically will be to determine if there is dermato-

logic involvement. Patients with dermatomyositis have a greater frequency of underlying malignancies which should be ruled out, but may occur up to several years after the dermatomyositis presents. The typical picture is of muscle pain, weakness and an elevated CPK. The treatment is not very effective and the course of the illness will be largely determined by the underlying cause.

The fibromyositis syndromes are the least understood and the most controversial. They occur most often in middle aged women with sleep and psychiatric disorders and present as chronic fatigue and muscle aching. There are trigger points that are frequently highly sensitive to even light touch. There have not been any pathologic correlations and many debate the existence of the disorder. It is recognized by the American College of Rheumatology who set the criteria and is estimated to occur in 5% of an internist's practice and 15% of a rheumatologist's.

Management

The initial management of shoulder disorders will largely be the same regardless of diagnosis. The goals of therapy will be pain relief and increasing range of motion. Exercises and NSAIDs will be the mainstay of therapy. Range of motion techniques are easily taught to patients and may be done in the patient's home if physical therapy is not readily available. The patient should begin with range of motion exercises that are not weight bearing such as the pendulum swing (Fig. 22.8). As the patient gains strength, he or she will be able to exercise against gravity, such as climbing the fingers up the wall. When the patient is able to use the shoulder against gravity and has increased the range of motion, weights may be added in small increments to the pendulum swing to increase strength.

In the case of calcific tendonitis or significant swelling in rotator cuff disorders, injection with corticosteroids may be helpful to allow the inflammation to decrease enough for the patient to perform these exercises. Occasionally, it is necessary to inject the calcium deposit itself in calcific tendonitis and even to surgically remove it if conservative therapy has not proved helpful. In the case of significant rotator cuff tears, it may also be necessary for surgical repair, but this is not a minor procedure for the elderly patients in whom rotator cuff tears occur. It will require months of intensive physical therapy for the patient to gain function and the patient needs to be aware.

The treatment of adhesive capsulitis begins with removing any aggravating or secondary factors fol-

---

Table 22.17.
Differential Diagnosis of Myositis in Adults

Myositis associated with autoantibodies
  Without other disease
  With connective tissue disease
Myositis associated with infection
  Viral infection—HIV, influenza and enterovirus (polio, coxsackie and echo virus)
  Protozoan infection—toxoplasma, trichinella
  Other infection—Lyme disease, mycoplasma
Myositis associated with medications
  Cholesterol lowering drugs—particularly gemfibrozil and HMG-COA reductase inhibitors
  L-tryptophan
  Zidovudine (AZT)
Other myositis
  Associated with malignancy
  Sarcoidosis

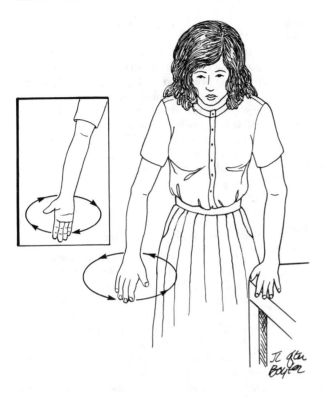

Figure 22.8. Pendulum swing. (Redrawn from Duralde et al. Frozen shoulder: Prevention, diagnosis and management. J Musculoskel Med 1994; 10:38–46.)

lowed by a regimen of range of motion exercises. If after several weeks, there is not a satisfactory increase in the range of motion, then corticosteroid injections or manipulation under anesthesia may be considered. It generally requires several months to years for adhesive capsulitis to fully resolve.

The treatment of CTS should begin with eliminating contributing factors such as repetitive motions. Nonsteroidal anti-inflammatory agents should be tried initially with splinting the wrist in

5–10 degrees of extension (dorsiflexion) to increase the size of the carpal tunnel. Injection with corticosteroids may be attempted if there is no improvement. Surgical decompression is often necessary when conservative treatment has failed or muscle atrophy has occurred.

Polymyalgia rheumatica responds rapidly to high-dose corticosteroids, which must be continued for at least 1 year because there is a high rate of relapse. An ESR will help guide clinical response.

ILLUSTRATIVE CASES WITH SELF-ASSESSMENT QUESTIONS AND ANSWERS

Case 1

Elaine is a 75-year-old with a history of rheumatoid arthritis and bursitis and at initial presentation can not raise her left arm. During the examination, she has no sign of inflammation and is unable to raise her arm above 90 degrees, but has normal passive range of motion.

QUESTION: *What is the most likely diagnosis?*

a. Osteoarthritis
b. Adhesive capsulitis
c. Bursitis
d. Rotator cuff tear

ANSWER: d. *The patient's normal passive range of motion rules out adhesive capsulitis and in the absence of inflammatory signs makes it unlikely for osteoarthritis or bursitis to be responsible for the limitation of movement. The fact that* *she is unable to raise the arm makes it more likely that there may be an actual tear of the rotator cuff rather than simple bursitis.*

Case 2

A 45-year-old man presents with shoulder weakness that has developed over the past 6 weeks. He has also experienced fatigue and some pain over both shoulders. Laboratory data reveals an elevated CPK.

QUESTION: *All of the following may be responsible except:*

a. Mevacor
b. Fibromyositis syndrome
c. Cocaine use
d. Hypothyroidism

ANSWER: b. *There are no laboratory abnormalities in the fibromyositis syndrome. The picture of a myopathic process may be caused by drugs and several medical conditions.*

KNEE PAIN

The knee is the largest weight-bearing joint in the body and has the most synovium, therefore many processes occur and in all age groups. The knee is affected by several inflammatory arthritides as well as osteoarthritis, infections, and trauma. The synovial fluid is easily accessible in a swollen knee and a helpful diagnostic tool. This chapter will discuss the evaluation of the acutely injured knee, common orthopedic problems, and the inflammatory rheumatologic disorders: rheumatoid arthritis (RA), systemic lupus erythematosus (SLE), and infectious arthritides.

Pathophysiologic Correlation

The knee can be considered to have three articulations: the patella in the patellofemoral groove, the femoral condoyles upon the tibial surfaces, and the interposing menisci (Fig. 22.9). The menisci function to cushion, lubricate, and stabilize the knee joint. The cruciate ligaments move the menisci backwards during flexion and stabilize the joint. The lateral ligaments support the knee and the surrounding bursae cushion and lubricate. The quadriceps and hamstrings also stabilize the joint and reduce the stress upon the knee joint.

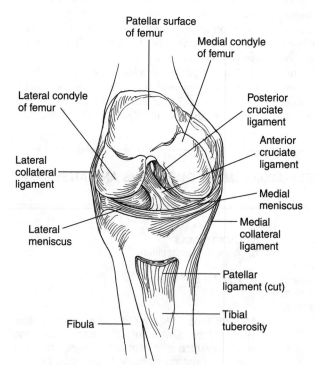

Patellar surface of femur
Medial condyle of femur
Lateral condyle of femur
Posterior cruciate ligament
Anterior cruciate ligament
Lateral collateral ligament
Medial meniscus
Lateral meniscus
Medial collateral ligament
Patellar ligament (cut)
Fibula
Tibial tuberosity

Figure 22.9. Knee joint, anterior view.

Due to the multiplicity of structures, several processes may occur and are often interrelated. The synovium is particularly prone to inflammatory processes which may lead to cartilage damage. No one process is unaffected by the rest of the structures. For example, trauma to the cruciate ligaments often results in meniscal injury as well due to anatomical connections.

The menisci cushion the articular cartilage, aid in joint lubrication, and stabilize the knee. The medial meniscus is attached to the medial collateral ligament, the posterior portion of the tibia, and the articular cartilage. The lateral meniscus is only loosely attached to the lateral collateral ligament. Therefore, the medial meniscus is unable to withstand significant degrees of distraction without tearing and is far more likely to be injured. The menisci are aneural and the pain produced is due to the torn meniscus rubbing against the cartilage. The menisci have a poor vascular supply, which is present in the peripheral portion. Therefore, only small peripheral tears have a chance of healing by themselves without surgical intervention. The patella sits in the patellofemoral groove and stabilizes the knee. It is affected by several processes: alignment, instability, and degeneration of the articular cartilage. Alignment with either the femur or the tibial condyles results in inordinate joint stress. A history of "giving way" does not indicate instability. Instability is characterized by documented patellar dislocation. Instability may be due to bone or ligament abnormalities. Chondromalacia is the idiopathic degeneration of articular cartilage resulting in deterioration of the collagen network.

Rheumatoid arthritis is an inflammatory process with systemic effects. Monocytes, macrophages, T and B cells, synoviocytes and endothelial cells have all been involved in the inflammatory process. The neuroendocrine system may also regulate the inflammatory process. The T cells are probably the initiating cells that release interleukin-2 and interferon-gamma. They stimulate macrophages to release cytokines such as interleukin-1 and 8 and tumor necrosis factor which in turn stimulate synoviocytes and endothelial cells. Endothelial cells and synoviocytes are probably the most important cells in the inflammatory process in RA. T cells may be the initiating cells because RA is strongly associated with HLA-DR4/1, which is responsible for the presentation of antigens to T cells. Also, therapies that inhibit T-cell function have been beneficial in the treatment of RA.

The evidence for the involvement of the hypothalamic-pituitary axis stems from the diurnal clinical pattern (early morning stiffness) which correlates with the pattern of cortisol secretion. Rheumatoid patients undergoing surgery do not have the same degree of cortisol response as patients with osteoarthritis or osteomyelitis. The comparison of patients with chronic osteomyelitis suggests that it is not inflammation alone that causes the suppression of cortisol. Some patients who have been treated with corticosteroids undergo clinical improvement. In animal models, the development of RA was prevented by giving corticosteroids concurrently with a stimulus that would normally cause the development of RA in rats. In order for this to be clinically relevant the initiating stimulus in the development of RA in humans must be identified.

Systemic lupus erythematosus (SLE) is characterized by the production of numerous autoantibodies. These antibodies result in renal immune complex deposition, vasculopathy due to coagulation with antibodies directed against anticoagulants, complement consumption and inflammation. The stimulus for antibody production is not known but theories include a viral precipitant or lack of normal down regulation. The circulating autoantibodies sometimes reflect disease activity as in the case of anti-DNA antibodies. The role of T cells is not as clear.

There is a genetic predisposition to SLE. One case in which it is particularly interesting is that of children with complement deficiencies. Although patients with SLE are susceptible to infections this seems to be independent of antibodies.

Clinical and Laboratory Evaluation

The knee is one of the joints most accessible to physical examination and the removal of synovial fluid. A thorough physical examination and evaluation of synovial fluid when indicated will establish a diagnosis most of the time. The knee should be thought of as having three compartments: anterior, posterior, and lateral.

HISTORY

Traumatic knee pain should be considered separately from a traumatic or chronic pain. The mechanism of trauma often determines the injury. A twisting injury in basketball would be more likely to result in a meniscal tear. A rapid deceleration injury such as a fall from a significant height would be likely to involve the cruciate ligaments. Immediate swelling implies intraarticular hemorrhage or more serious intraarticular damage.

Previous injuries may recur or cause stress resulting in present injury. If the patient felt or heard a pop at the time of injury, it may be a meniscal injury. A history of locking may clue one in to meniscal injury or patellar dislocation. If the patient complains of instability, this is a sign of ligamentous injury. The direction of force that occurred during the injury will help determine which structures are injured.

Patients with patellofemoral disorders (PFD) will complain of anterior knee pain worsened by stair climbing or sitting with knees flexed for prolonged periods (theater sign). They may also complain of "giving way" of the knee. Idiopathic chondromalacia is more common in tall young women whereas the degenerative forms are found in older patients.

The age and condition of the patient is helpful especially in chronic knee conditions. In an elderly patient even mild trauma may result in a tibial plateau fracture, which will usually present with swelling and some local tenderness although the patient may still be able to walk.

The most important step when evaluating an inflammatory process is to rule out infection. The most common infections are gonococcal, Lyme disease and septic arthritis. Obtain a travel and sexual activity history. If the patient has a prosthesis, he or she is susceptible to bacterial infection. A history of fever, weight loss, or systemic symptoms raises the suspicion. However, any inflammatory process may lead to these symptoms.

Once the possibility of infection has been ruled out, one should begin to think of processes such as RA, SLE, or psoriatic arthritis. The type of joints involved and the systemic symptoms will aid in making the diagnosis.

Rheumatoid arthritis (RA) is a symmetrical, polyarticular process involving the hands, wrists, knees, ankles, and cervical spine. It has a bimodal distribution with one peak occuring in young women and then again after the age of 50 at which time it increases in incidence with increasing age. Morning stiffness lasting greater than 1 hour is significant and patients will often have systemic complaints such as fatigue, malaise, and weight loss. The pattern of clinical activity varies and usually it takes several months to years for the patient to seek medical attention and obtain a diagnosis. In some cases there is a more rapid progression with early deformities due to bony erosions.

Systemic lupus erythematosis (SLE) is a migratory, oligoarticular process involving the knees, ankles, hands, and wrists. It does not affect the spine. There is often a disproportionate degree of pain compared with the physical findings. These patients often have systemic symptoms and frequently a family history. They may give a history of skin sensitivity to the sun.

The arthritis associated with psoriasis may precede the skin lesions by several years. There are several clinical patterns the most common being a seronegative RA pattern and one similar to sacroilitis. A rarer form known as arthritis mutilans is found in patients with pitting of the nails and is a more severe progressive form.

Physical Examination

When evaluating an injured knee, make the patient comfortable and relaxed so he or she will be able to comply with the examination. A systematic examination is necesssary beginning above the knee at the quadriceps and working down into the calf. The first part of the examination is inspection. Observe for swelling and its location. Look for ecchymoses which often point to where the damage is. Both knees must be examined at the same time for comparison — it is often difficult to detect swelling without looking at the opposite knee.

After inspection, have the patient try to localize the pain with one finger and palpate the landmarks to identify the point of tenderness. Palpate for lumps or disruptions in the tendons. Feel along the joint line for any tenderness, which infers meniscal or chondral injury. Palpate for crepitance, which suggests fluid or degenerative changes. Assess the mobility of the patella by trying to ballot the patella laterally with the knee extended and the muscles relaxed. Normally the patella should not be ballotable.

Specific maneuvers are done to assess ligamentous stability. To test the strength of the anterior cruciate ligament (ACL), the Lachman or anterior drawer test is done by holding the patient's knee in a 30 degree flexed position while applying pressure to the femur with one hand to stabilize it, and pull anteriorly on the calf with the other (Fig. 22.10). Test the uninjured knee first. If the injured knee has a softer endpoint or feels more lax, this is a sign of ACL injury. Apply posterior pressure to the tibia to test the posterior cruciate ligament. Assess the lateral collateral ligaments by applying pressure laterally and observing for any laxity in the joint.

The MacMurray maneuver tests the meniscii (Fig. 22.11). Place the patients leg in a frog leg position, which will allow the best exposure to the meniscii and then apply external and internal rotatory pressure. A pop or click over the joint line or pain elicited implies meniscal injury.

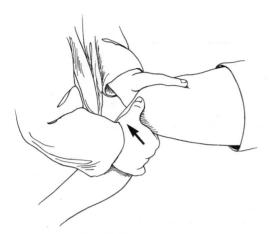

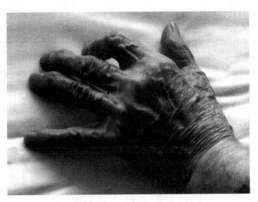

Figure 22.12. Rheumatoid arthritis.

Figure 22.10. Lachman test.

Patients with rheumatoid arthritis (RA) usually have a classical pattern of joints involved and effusions. The joints most commonly involved are the MCP and PIP and there may only be a bogginess. Classic deformities include subluxation of the MCP joints with ulnar deviation of the digits or "swan neck" deformities of the PIPs (Fig. 22.12). There may be synovitis or subcutaneous nodules. Nodules over the extensor surfaces (most often the elbow) are present in 25% of patients and are an indicator for extraarticular manifestations. There may be muscle atrophy or neurologic manifestations. Diffuse adenopathy or hepatomegaly may also be present.

In SLE, arthritis is oligoarticular and migratory. The pain is often disproportionate to the degree of physical findings. There may also be prominent tendonitis and even tendon rupture. The presence of a macuopapular rash over the neck and arms or less frequently a malar rash sparing the bridge of the nose may also be seen. A discoid rash may occur and is associated with less severe disease.

Dermatitis is present in 66% of patients with gonococcal arthritis. The classic form is that of multiple papules or macules which are frequently hemmorhagic and located on the palms and soles. There may also be a rash similar to erythema multiforme or nondescript macular rash.

LABORATORY EVALUATION

When evaluating traumatic injuries laboratory evaluation is not necessary except in the cases in which patients have had intraarticular hemorrhage and it is necessary to rule out a coagulopathy, such as VonWillebrands disease. However, when evaluating inflammatory processes laboratory data is very helpful. If the patient presents with an acute swelling of the joint in the absence of trauma, it is necessary to do an arthrocentesis. This is extremely important both diagnostically and therapeutically in the patient with septic arthritis and will often be the only way to come to a definitive diagnosis in disorders such as gout. Table 22.18 lists the abnormalities found in the synovial fluid of particular disorders.

X-rays are important in the evaluation of knee trauma. If there is significant swelling or the mechanism of injury appears severe, one should perform an x-ray to rule out fracture. The type of x-ray will depend on the suspected disorder. Skyline or Merchant's view x-rays are done to evaluate PFDs. If a meniscal tear is suspected, anteroposterior

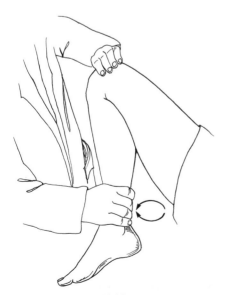

Figure 22.11. McMurray maneuver.

Table 22.18.
Synovial Fluid Analyses

Septic	Septic	Inflammatory	Noninflammatory
WBC	>50,000	3–50,000	<3,000
Protein	>3 g	>3 g	<3 g
Color	White	Yellow	Clear, pale yellow or bloody
Glucose	<30% of serum	10–20% decreased	NL–10% decreased

x-rays with the knees in 45 degrees of flexion are done to see if there is narrowing of the joint space. Tomograms are helpful in tibial plateau fractures to determine the degree of depression which correlates with neurovascular compromise.

With the widespread availability of magnetic resonance imaging (MRI) it is increasingly important to use this costly tool effectively. It is accurate 90% of the time when evaluating serious meniscal injuries and should be used if clinical signs do not clearly indicate meniscal injury. It does not replace the use of arthroscopy. It may lead credence to the need for arthroscopy, but will add expense often unnecessarily. CAT scans are not helpful if MRI is available.

When evaluating an inflammatory process, an erythrocyte sedimentation rate is helpful to confirm the presence of an inflammatory process. Rheumatoid factor is an antibody directed against IgG and is present in 85% of the cases. However, RF may be present in 5–10% of normal individuals and is

therefore only supportive of the clinical diagnosis. It may also be present in other collagen vascular disorders.

In SLE, the most common antibodies are the anti-nuclear antibodies (ANA), which are present in 95% of patients with SLE. Unfortunately ANA may be present in low titers in normal individuals and there is a very high rate of false positives and crossover with other collagen vascular diseases. Anti-DNA is more specific for SLE and is useful because it is also a marker for disease activity, correlating well with nephritis. Anti-Smith (Sm) is seen exclusively in SLE but is only present in 20% of patients. Other antibodies are associated with particular complications of SLE. See Table 22.19 for a summary of the antibodies. Complement levels are also helpful in determining disease activity and are more specific than an ESR. The antibody tests are very expensive and should be used for specific questions. It is reasonable to screen with the ANA and if that is positive to then perform and anti-

Table 22.19.
Antibodies in Systemic Lupus Erythematosis

Test	Reactions Against	% Present	Associations and Comments
ANA		95	Highly sensitive Variably specific Present in chronic inflammation
Anti-DNA	ds DNA	80	In high titer virtually diagnostic of SLE reflects disease activity.
Anti Smith (antigen)		10–20	Specific for SLE
Anti RNP	ENA antigen	50	Found in patients with mixed connective tissue disease (CTD)
Anti-Ro	RNA protein antigen	25	Sjogren's syndrome—congenital HB in fetuses
Anti-La	RNA protein antigen	20	Congenital heart block in fetus
Lupusanticoagulant antibodies		20	Associated with arterial and venous thromboses
		10–20	Mixed CTD

ANA: antinuclear antibodies; anti RNP: ribonuclear protein; RF: rheumatoid factor; CTD: connective tissue disease; SLE: systemic lupus erythematosis.
Adapted from Kaine JL and Kahl LE. Which laboratory tests are useful in diagnosing SLE? J Musculoskeletal Med 1992;9:17.

DNA and complement level if active disease is present.

Differential Diagnosis

Knee pain should be categorized as acute versus chronic and inflammatory versus noninflammatory (Table 22.20). This categorization will allow the clinician to limit the differential. The localization of the pain (anterior, posterior or lateral) is also useful.

TRAUMA

Meniscal tears may be due to acute significant trauma or degenerative changes with minimal trauma in patients older than age 40. The mechanism of injury is usually a twisting injury but there may be no clear history of trauma in the older patient. The tears are graded from 1 to 3 with the most severe tears being the ones that are usually clinically obvious and involving the articular cartilage. The knee usually swells within 24 hours and the patient may give a history of clicking, popping or "giving way." More immediate swelling is an indication of anterior cruciate ligament (ACL) injury or intraarticular hemorrhage.

Anterior cruciate ligament (ACL) injuries occur due to a rapid deceleration on an extended knee such as a fall from a significant height. There is usually immediate swelling and the patient is often

Table 22.20.
Differential Diagnoses

Noninflammatory processes
  Acute knee injury
    Meniscal damage
    Ligamentous injury
    Fracture
    Muscule injury
  Chronic knee disorders
    Patellar femoral disorders
    Osteoarthritis
Inflammatory
  Noninfectious
    Rheumatoid arthritis
    Systemic lupus erythematosis
    Crystal deposition disease
    Psoriatic arthritis
  Infectious
    Gonococcal
    Lyme disease
    Septic
    Reiter's syndrome

unable to walk. There is frequently associated meniscal injury. The medial and lateral collateral ligaments may be injured by excessive varus or valgus stress respectively. The pain and swelling are usually localized.

RHEUMATOID ARTHRITIS

Rheumatoid arthritis is symmetrical and polyarticular involving the metacarpophalangeal joints, wrists, knees, ankles, and cervical spine. It is three times as common in women and increases in incidence with age, most commonly beginning in the 4th or 5th decade. There is usually a prominent complaint of morning stiffness lasting for several hours and systemic symtpoms such as fatigue and malaise. It usually begins as an intermittent process but may then become progressive and destructive. Patients who have extraarticular manifestations especially subcutaneous nodules and pulmonary involvement are more likely to have severe disease. Unlike SLE, it does not present with extraarticular disease. Table 22.21 summarizes the criteria.

SYSTEMIC LUPUS ERYTHEMATOSIS

Systemic lupus erythematosis is an immune-mediated disorder involving the musculoskeletal system, skin, renal, neurologic and cardiac systems. There are strong genetic sexual and racial predispositions. There is an increased incidence of HLA DR4 in whites, and a 25% concordance rates in monozygotic twins. The typical patient is a young woman in her 3rd or 4th decade at which time there is a 5:1 female to male ratio. At extremes of age (10% occur in children and 10% older than age 50), there is a 2:1 female : male ratio. This supports the notion that the hormonal milieu contributes to the disorder. In the US, there is an increased prevalence in Blacks and Hispanics.

Arthritis is the most common complaint followed by rash and systemic symptoms. Table 22.22 reviews the criteria for diagnosis. Renal failure and infection are responsible for most of the morbidity and mortality and great effort has been spent trying to prognosticate and prevent the progression of renal failure. Although previously thought to have important prognostic importance, the pathologic classification of renal involvement is not as important as the degree of renal failure reflected by the creatinine level. The susceptibility to infection is due to both the underlying disease and the treatment with corticosteroids and immunosuppressive agents.

Neurologic involvement is also important and

Table 22.21.
1987 Revised Criteria for Classification of Rheumatoid Arthritis*

Criteria	Definition
1. Morning stiffness	In and around the joints, lasting at least 1 hour before maximal improvement
2. Arthritis of three or more joint areas	At least three joint areas simultaneously have had soft-tissue swelling or fluid (not bony overgrowth alone) observed by a physician. The 14 possible joint areas are (right or left) proximal interphalangeal, metacarpophalangeal, wrist, elbow, knee, ankle, and metatarsophalangeal joints
3. Arthritis of hand joints	At least one joint area swollen, as in criterion 2, in wrist, metacarpophalangeal, or proximal interphalangeal joint
4. Symmetric arthritis	Simultaneous involvement of the same joint areas as in criterion 2, on both sides of the body (Bilateral involvement of proximal interphalangeal, metacarpophalangeal, or metatarsophalangeal joints is acceptable without absolute symmetry)
5. Rheumatoid nodules	Subcutaneous nodules over bony prominences or extensor surfaces or in juxta-articular regions, observed by a physician
6. Serum rheumatoid factor	Demonstration of abnormal amounts of serum rheumatoid factor by any method that has been positive in fewer than 5% of normal control subjects
7. Roentgenographic findings	Changes typical of rheumatoid arthritis on posteroanterior hand and wrist x-ray studies, which must include erosions or unequivocal bony decalcification localized to or most marked adjacent to the involved joints (osteoarthritis changes alone do not qualify)

*For classification purposes, RA is said to be present if the patient has satisfied at least four of the above seven criteria. Criteria 1 through 4 must be present for a least 6 weeks. Patients with two clinical diagnoses are not excluded. Designation as classic, definite, or probable RA is not to be made.
Used with permission from Arnett FC, Edworthy SM, Block DA et al. The American rheumatism association of 1987. Revised criteria for the classification of Rheumatoid arthritis. Arthritis and Rheumatism 1988;31:319.

cognitive dysfunction is seen in up to 30% of patients. The majority of neurologic events are vascular in nature and felt to be due to the depletion of anti-coagulants in the blood by antibodies directed against them. Twenty percent of patients with SLE have anti-cardiolipin antibodies that result in arterial and venous thromboses, abnormal bleeding and recurrent spontaneous abortions.

PSORIATIC ARTHRITIS

The most common presentation of psoriatic arthritis is a nonerosive seronegative RA that affects the peripheral joints and correlates with disease activity. The sacroilitis presentation is usually more insidious and does not correlate with disease activity. The arthritis mutilans is rare and leads to severe erosions of cartilage and bone. It affects the hands of patients with nail pitting.

GONOCOCCAL ARTHRITIS

Gonococcal arthritis is by far the most common infectious arthritis in young sexually active patients

and presents as a migratory polyarthritis often with marked tenosynovitis accompanying the effusions. The patient does not usually appear systemically ill and the effusions resolve rapidly with or without antibiotic therapy. There often is no known history of gonococcal disease. Diagnosis relies upon culture of urogenital secretions, blood or joint fluid. However, none of these is very sensitive and presumptive diagnoses are frequently made based on the clinical picture.

LYME ARTHRITIS

Lyme arthritis is a late manifestation of Lyme disease, which is caused by *Borrelia burgdorferi* and is transmitted to humans by the deer tick. It is geographically limited to areas where deer live and is most common in the Northeastern US and upper Midwest. It affects large joints such as the knees and ankles and is preceded by erythema chronicum migrans, a rash with a bull's eye appearance. Only 50% of people remember the tick bite. If antibiotics are not initiated early in the course of disease it may lead to a chronic relapsing arthritis, which is very difficult to treat. The arthritis does not appear

Table 22.22.
Which Laboratory Tests Are Useful in Diagnosing SLE

1982 Revised Criteria for Classification of Systemic Lupus Erythematosus	
Criterion	Definition
Malar rash	Fixed erythema, flat or raised, over the malar eminences, tending to spare the nasolabial folds
Discoid rash	Erythematous raised patches with adherent keratotic scaling and follicular plugging; atrophic scarring may occur in older lesions
Photosensitivity	Rash, by patient history or physician observation, as a result of unusual reaction to sunlight
Oral ulcers	Oral or nasopharyngeal ulceration, usually painless, observed by physician
Arthritis	Nonerosive arthritis involving two or more peripheral joints, characterized by tenderness, swelling, or effusion
Serositis	Pleuritis: convincing history of pleuritic pain, or rub heard by a physician, or evidence of pleural effusion
	or
	Pericarditis documented by ECG, or rub, or evidence of pericardial effusion
Renal disorders	Persistent proteinuria greater than 0.5 g/d, or greater than 3+ if quantitation not performed
	or
	Cellular casts (may be red-cell, hemoglobin, granular, tubular, or mixed)
Neurologic disorder	Seizures in the absence of offending drugs or known metabolic derangements (uremia, ketoacidosis, electrolyte imbalance)
	or
	Psychosis in the absence of offending drugs or known metabolic derangements (uremia, ketoacidosis, electrolyte imbalance)
Hematologic disorder	Hemolytic anemia with reticulocytosis
	or
	Leukopenia, less than 4,000/μL total on two or more occasions
	or
	Lymphopenia, less than 1,500/μL on two or more occasions
	or
	Thrombocytopenia, less than 100,000/μL in the absence of offending drugs
Immunologic disorder	Positive LE cell preparation
	or
	Anti-DNA (antibody to native DNA in abnormal titer)
	or
	Anti-Sm (antibody to Sm nuclear antigen)
	or
	False-positive result on serologic test for syphilis; known to be positive for at least 6 months and confirmed by *Treponema pallidum* immobilization or fluorescent treponemal antibody absorption test
Antinuclear antibody	Abnormal titer of antinuclear antibody by immunofluorescence or equivalent assay at any time and in the absence of drugs known to be associated with drug-induced lupus syndrome

ECG, electrocardiogram; LE, lupus erythematosus; DNA, deoxyribonucleic acid.
From Tan EM, Cohen AS, Fries JF, et al: The 1982 revised criteria for the classification of systemic lupus erythematosus (SLE). Arthritis Rheum 1982;25:1274.

as inflammatory as septic arthritis and is not destructive.

SEPTIC ARTHRITIS

Septic arthritis occurs almost exclusively in the setting of an abnormal joint or bacteremia. Therefore it is important to suspect infection when a patient with arthritis presents with a severe flare or one that is not responding to usual measures. The most common organisms are *Staphylococcus aureus* and *Streptococci*. Gram-negative organisms found in synovial fluid imply sepsis. Septic arthritis is more common in the elderly and may occur with only a few systemic signs. Rheumatic fever, tuberculosis, and fungi are all rare causes of septic arthritis except in certain underdeveloped nations.

Management

TRAUMA

The management of acute knee injuries depends on the type and degree of injury sustained. If there is no fracture (the management of fractures is beyond the scope of this text), most acute knee injuries will be treated initially with immobilization and rest. If there is significant joint instability or there is neurovascular compromise then acute intervention may be indicated. The treatment will also depend upon the patient's health and lifestyle.

MENISCAL TEARS

The meniscii have very limited blood supply limited to the peripheral most region. Therefore, tears that are large or not peripherally located will not heal and require either surgical repair or removal of the torn piece. It is rare for nonsurgical intervention to be successful. Repair is done arthroscopically, which decreases the morbidity of the procedure and allows the patient to return to function earlier. Repair is followed by physical therapy to strengthen the quadriceps and hamstrings.

PATELLOFEMORAL DISORDERS

The patellofemoral disorders are managed by avoidance of aggravating circumstances, physical therapy to strengthen the quadriceps, which helps keep the joint aligned and relieves pressure. Surgical repair is rarely helpful even in patients with documented recurrent dislocations. Some advocate the use of taping for patients with recurrent dislocations for symptomatic relief.

RHEUMATOID ARTHRITIS

The goals of therapy for RA include prevention of disease progression, pain relief and increased function. If there is joint destruction, more aggressive intervention is warranted. Many clinicians now believe that disease modifying agents should be instituted early prior to the development of joint destruction. If the patient is elderly and there are indications of a mild course, it may be prudent to begin with antiinflammatory agents such as aspirin and non-steroidal anti-inflammatory agents (NSAIDs). No particular agent has been shown to

be more beneficial than another but disparities exist between the cost of older agents such as aspirin and ibuprofen and newer agents such as piroxicam. Interactions between NSAIDs and other drugs are summarized in Table 22.23.

When the decision has been made to begin a disease modifying agent the goals and side effects must be carefully considered. If the goal is immediate relief of inflammation, steroids may be helpful in reducing symptoms until other agents have time to work. The agents preventing disease progression include the anti-malarials, gold, and methotrexate. These all have significant side effects and should be instituted with the advice of a rheumatologist and close followup for side effects.

SYSTEMIC LUPUS ERYTHEMATOSIS

SLE leads to joint destruction by destruction of the surrounding tendons rather than bony erosions and therefore the disease modifying agents used in RA are not usually helpful. NSAIDS are used for pain relief and physical therapy may be helpful in strengthening the surrounding tissues. Steroids are used for progressive renal dysfunction and cerebral,

Table 22.23.
Major Interactions Between NSAIDs and Other Agents

Agent	Interaction
Aminoglycosides	Renal function decreased
Antacids	NSAID absorption reduced (in some cases)
Anticoagulants	Warfarin effect prolonged; risk of gastrointestinal bleeding increased
Antihypertensives	Therapeutic effect blunted
Barbiturates	NSAID metabolism accelerated
Cholestyramine	NSAID absorption inhibited
Cyclosporine	Cyclosporine level increased
Digoxin	Renal function decreased
Hypoglycemic	Hypoglycemic effect potentiates agents
Lithium	Renal excretion decreased
Phenytoin	Phenytoin metabolism inhibited
Potassium-sparing diuretics	Risk of hyperkalemia increased
Uricosuric drugs	Renal clearance and NSAID metabolism reduced
Valproate	Valproate metabolism inhibited

NSAIDs, nonsteroidal anti-inflammatory drugs.
From Hunder GG, Kaye RL, Williams RC. Therapies for rheumatoid arthritis: recent changes and future trends. J Musculoskeletal Med 1993;10:23.

pulmonary or cardiac manifestations. Immunosuppressants are usually reserved for renal disease.

INFECTIOUS ARTHRITIDES

Gonococcal arthritis resolves with or without antibiotics but antibiotics speed the resolution of arthritis. The regimen used will vary depending on the percentage of GC that is penicillin resistant in that geographic area. Lyme arthritis will require high dose intravenous third generation cephalosporins in order to eradicate the disease. Frequently the diagnosis is made at such a late stage that repeated courses of antibiotics are necessary and despite antibiotics a chronic relapsing arthritis develops.

Septic arthritis requires intravenous antibiotics, daily arthrocentesis, lavage and early immobilization. This should be followed by physical therapy. If antibiotics and drainage are not instituted early in the course of the infection, severe joint destruction may occur. Even with optimal management, only 60% of cases will resolve completely. Staphylococcal, gram negative and hip infections have a worse prognosis.

ILLUSTRATIVE CASES WITH SELF-ASSESSMENT QUESTIONS AND ANSWERS

Case 1

A 30-year-old woman presents with several months of knee pain and swelling worsened by walking long distances or climbing stairs. She had several sports related injuries but has not participated in sports recently. She initially got relief with Motrin but finds it is not working anymore. On physical examination, you localize the pain to the anterior knee and find no evidence of intraarticular damage or effusion. She also states that sometimes the knee seems to give out.

QUESTION: *Which of the following is not a reasonable next step?*

a. Skyline x-rays to rule out patellofemoral disorder
b. FANA to rule out SLE
c. Physical therapy to strengthen the quadriceps
d. Enteric-coated aspirin

ANSWER: b. *The clinical syndrome is suggestive but not diagnostic of a patellofemoral disorder such as chondromalacia. There is no evidence of patellar instability on physical exam and an x-ray may be helpful. The primary treatment would be strengthening the quadriceps and NSAIDs for pain relief as well as avoiding activities such as stair climbing, which exacerbate the problem. Only in rare instances would surgical intervention be recommended. There is nothing suggestive of SLE and a positive ANA would only create a diagnostic dilemma requiring more expensive tests.*

Case 2

A 52-year-old man presents with 3 weeks of diffuse joint pain, fever, and malaise. He denies recent change in sexual partners, travel, rash, or drug use. On physical he has swollen knees and wrists, is tender over the cervical spine, and is afebrile. Laboratory data reveal an ESR of 120 with a WBC of 15,000.

QUESTION: *What is the most likely diagnosis?*

a. Septic arthritis
b. Gonococcal arthritis
c. Reiter's syndrome
d. Rheumatoid arthritis

ANSWER: d. *Despite the elevated WBC count and history of fever it would be highly unlikely for a previously healthy man with no risk factors (prosthesis, intravenous drug use) and multiple joint involvement to have septic arthritis. The denial of a new sexual partner and lack of rash makes GC an unlikely diagnosis as well. Reiter's syndrome would be difficult to exclude but is usually associated with urethritis and eye involvement in a young man. The older age of onset makes it more likely statistically for a male to have RA and the signs and symptoms are classical except for the lack of complaint of morning stiffness, which is usually a prominent complaint. A rheumatoid factor and arthrocentesis would be reasonable diagnostic tools in this patient.*

FOOT PAIN

This section will discuss the evaluation of acute foot and ankle injuries and entities common in the foot. The topics to be discussed include crystal deposition diseases (gout and calcium pyrophosphate disease), neuropathic arthropathies, and tendonous problems such as plantar fasciitis and Achilles tendonitis. The management of hallux valgus and the lesser toe deformities will be discussed briefly because they affect many of our patients.

Pathophysiologic Correlation

To discuss the evaluation of the foot one needs to review the anatomy (Fig. 22.13). The foot may be thought of as having three compartments: the forefoot, midfoot, and hindfoot. The talus and the calcaneus are the bones of the hindfoot and articulate with the tibia and fibula and are supported by several ligaments. The talus and calcaneus then articulate respectively with the navicular and cuboid which distally articulate with the three cuneiforms forming the midfoot. Distally the metatarsals and phalanges make up the forefoot. The vascular supply to the foot is largely supplied by the posterior tibial artery which passes medially and has branches which pass dorsally and laterally. The venous system also runs medially and the nervous supply is more diffusely located.

Although the foot has several articulations, with the exception of the ankle joint there is not a great deal of mobility in these joints. The foot is designed to be able to withstand a great deal of force, which

is probably why there is not a great deal of flexibilty in the foot. Figure 22.14 depicts the normal range of motion of the foot.

Mechanical disorders of the foot are usually due to excessive strain or a structural abnormality. The ligaments and tendons in the foot may become strained and inflamed from overuse due to factors such as obesity, pes planus (flatfoot) or running. This may in turn lead to muscle spasm and actual articular swelling which will then form a vicious circle and enhance the inflammatory process. The ankle with its greater range of motion and reliance upon ligaments for structural support is more prone to acute injuries. The lateral ligaments are nine times more likely to be injured than the medial ligaments due to their greater length and less support. Figure 22.15 reviews the lateral ankle ligaments.

The pathogenesis of crystal deposition disorders is not well understood. Crystals may be found incidentally in joints which aren't inflamed (e.g., chronic renal insufficiency) and therefore there must be other inciting factors. Gout is usually due to underexcretion of urate rather than overproduction and the resultant crystals are likely proinflammatory. The crystals caused the release of lysosomal enzymes and the migration of neutrophils into the synovial fluid which in turn phagocytize the crystals.

Plantar fasciitis is histologically composed of collagen degeneration, matrix calcification and less commonly microtears in the fascia at its insertion. It has been associated with abnormal foot structures

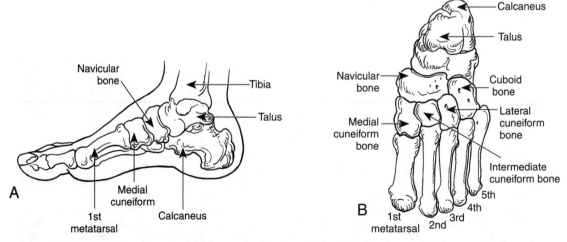

Figure 22.13. A, B. Bony anatomy of the foot and ankle. (From Willms JL, Schneiderman H, Algranati PS. Physical diagnosis: bedside evaluation of diagnosis and function. Baltimore: Williams & Wilkins. 1994:389.)

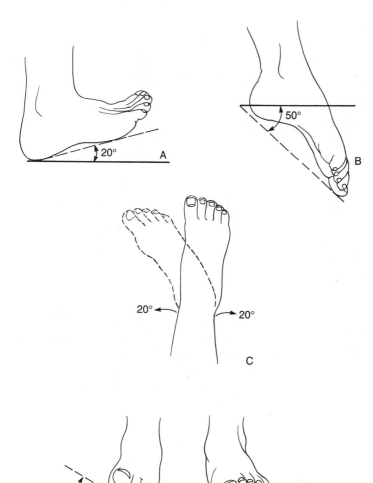

Figure 22.14. Range of motion of foot and ankle. (A) Tibiotalar motion—plantar flexion. (B) Dorsiflexion. (C) Axial subtalar motion. (D) Full range of subtalar motion. (Redrawn from Reilly B. Foot and ankle pain. In: Reilly B. ed. Practical strategies in outpatient medicine. 2nd ed. Philadelphia: W.B. Saunders, 1991:1239.)

such as pes planus and pes cavus (abnormally high arch) as well as heel pad atrophy and is therefore felt to be due to overload failure, inadequate healing and chronic inflammation. It is felt to be a syndrome with many possible etiologies and therefore when not responsive to usual therapies a cause should be sought. Possible causes include stress fractures, rheumatoid arthritis (RA) or osteomyelitis.

Neuropathic joints result from repetitive trauma which is inappropriately sensed by a joint, which does not have normal sensory mechanisms. This leads to swelling, loss of articular cartilage, fractures and eventual loss of joint mobility. Diabetes is the most common cause, but it may occur in any situation in which there is abnormal joint sensation.

The Achilles tendon is the largest tendon and is affected by many processes ranging from inflammatory disorders to infiltrative processes. It is a common place for deposits of cholesterol, tophi and other nodules such as rheumatoid nodules to be deposited. The tendon plantar flexes the foot. If tendonitis is recurrent and particularly if there is a history of steroid injection, the Achilles tendon may actually rupture.

Clinical and Laboratory Evaluation

Most foot disorders will be diagnosed by a simple history and physical exam. It is rare for a serious disorder such as malignancy to present as foot pain but the foot is a common site of osteomyelitis, which would be the only diagnosis that would require laboratory evaluation other than to determine the cause of a neuropathic arthropathy.

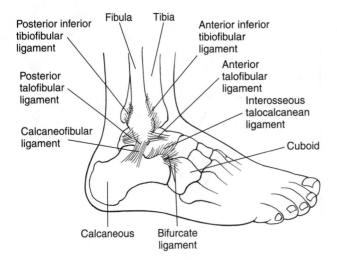

Figure 22.15. Ligaments of the ankle.

HISTORY

Begin by ascertaining the duration of pain and any preceding event. In most cases, foot pain is due to trauma or an underlying structural disorder such as pes planus or previous trauma. It is important to distinguish if the pain occurs with use which infers a musculotendinous cause or with rest as well which suggests a neuropathic or articular cause. Swelling is an important clue and particularly if it is localized.

Elicit clues as to the types of stress placed on the foot such as the type of shoes worn, if the patient stands or walks for prolonged portions of the day. Runners may have unusual types of stress on their feet. Obesity will also increase the load. Consider the patient's age. A young person is more likely to have a structural disorder such as pes planus or cavus. A middle-aged person is more likely to have overuse syndrome such as fasciitis, and an elderly person is more likely to have a degenerative process.

Certain illnesses will predispose to particular foot disorders. Diabetics are more likely to have a neuropathic or vascular process occurring. Patients with painful processes in other joints such as the hip or knees may be placing undue stress on the feet to avoid pain.

When assessing ankle trauma determine whether there was an inversion or eversion injury. Although inversion injuries with lateral ligament damage are far more common, an eversion injury may signify a more serious injury as it requires more force to cause injury to the medial ligaments with an eversion injury. Immediate swelling often

suggests hemarthroses and if there is a large amount of swelling this may be a clue to an underlying fracture. If the patient hears an audible pop at the time of injury this suggests tearing of the ligament. If the patient is unable to walk on the injury immediately after the trauma that also signifies significant trauma such as a fracture.

PHYSICAL EXAMINATION

One should examine the foot with the patient sitting with knees flexed at 90 degrees to allow for optimal examination. Begin by observing the shoes for signs of unusual stress and then the foot for deformities, swelling or callouses which may reveal unusual stresses placed upon the foot. Then have the patient point to where the pain is occuring. One should then palpate the structures in the area. It will be important to be familiar with the anatomy reviewed to localize the pain.

Then observe the gait. The normal gait should include the heel strike, then the transfer of weight along the lateral aspect of the foot and finally the liftoff from the ball of the foot. It is important to note the arch of the foot without weight bearing and again during ambulation. Some people have flexible pes planus, which may lead to chronic foot strain. It will be important to note if the patient favors an area of the foot, which may only be evident during ambulation.

In foot strain, the pain will often not be as localized as in plantar fasciitis. In plantar fasciitis the patient may have an area of point tenderness at the insertion of the plantar fascia at the calcaneum. Pain needs to be localized to the bone versus the soft tissue. Swelling denotes an inflammatory process or a more serious injury. Signs of local inflammation should raise a different list of diagnoses depending on the location of the findings.

Achilles tendonitis is usually obvious due to the location of the pain on the back of the heel and the localized tenderness. There may be associated pain and swelling in the calf. If there is a rupture of the Achilles tendon one may feel a space or dropoff in the tendon and the patient will be unable to plantar flex the foot. One may confirm the diagnosis by squeezing the gastrocnemius while the patient is lying facedown. The foot will not plantar flex due to the disruption of the tendon.

On physical examination in a patient suspected to have gout, tophi are often a helpful diagnostic clue. The most common places for tophi to be located are directly over the joint or on the auricular cartilage. Tophi do not appear until the patient has had gout for an average of 12 years and therefore usually the diagnosis of gout is already established. The gouty joint will be hot, swollen, and exquisitely sensitive to touch. In later stages of gout, there will be chronic swelling, joint destruction and in 25% of patients, tophi. Bursitis may also be a frequent accompaniment to gout. The places it is most likely to occur are the olecranon bursa and the prepatellar bursa.

Morton's neuroma is usually diagnosed on physical exam. The pain will be localized to the plantar aspect of the foot, will usually be a pinpoint localization and the most common location is in the 3rd webspace. One may best obtain this point tenderness if one feels a "Mulder's click" (Fig. 22.16). This is felt by holding the medial and lateral meta-

Table 22.24.
Indications for X-rays in Acute Ankle Injuries

History
    Immediate swelling
    Inability to walk
    Audible pop
    Severe mode of trauma
Physical exam
    Severe swelling
    Ecchymoses
    Instability

tarsals in one hand and applying transverse pressure and at the same time with the other hand applying pressure at the 3rd interspace. If one is uncertain of the diagnosis by history and physical exam, one may inject with anesthetic and cortisone. This will also prove therapeutic in approximately 20% of patients.

When examining the ankle it will be important to make the patient comfortable for the exam. If there is severe swelling, x-rays should be performed before examining the joint (Table 22.24 lists indications for x-rays in acute ankle injuries). One will need to palpate for the area of tenderness. One should palpate the tibulofibular joint and the bony prominences. There may be an avulsion fracture in severe sprains. Ecchymosis within the first few hours of injury may be an indicator of a more severe injury. If the swelling is not severe, then a "bulge sign" may be appreciated. This may be done by pressing behind the lateral malleolus and observing for a fluid wave anteriorly to the talofibular ligament. Asymmetric swelling usually indicates soft tissue rather than intraarticular damage.

One will need to assess the stability of the ankle. There are two ways in which this may be done. One is the drawer test in which the tibia is held in one hand while the other hand pulls forward on the heel. The joint is considered unstable if there is more than 2–3 mm movement on anterior pull. In order for the drawer test to be positive there must be disruption of both the anterior talofibular and calcaneofibular ligaments. The talar tilt test is the other and estimates the degree of distraction between the lateral malleolus and the talus.

LABORATORY EVALUATION

Laboratory information in mechanical disorders of the foot and ankle are not helpful. If one suspects a neuropathic process, osteomyelitis (elevated sedimentation rate or leukocytosis), or a systemic illness

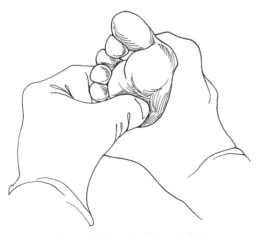

Figure 22.16. "Mulder's click."

(rheumatoid arthritis, diabetes), it is reasonable to perform these simple laboratory examinations. When one suspects gout, an elevated uric acid may lend credence to the diagnosis but 15% of patients with acute gout have normal serum uric acid. The other reason to obtain laboratory data when evaluating foot pain would be to guide the treatment decisions made.

If one suspects crystal deposition disease, it is crucial to obtain synovial fluid for the diagnosis. In gout, when using a light polarizing microscope, one will find needleshaped, negatively birefringent crystals, whereas in CPPD one will find rhomboidal, positively birefringent crystals. One will also usually find a moderate degree of inflammation as evidenced by a leukocytosis in the range of 50–100,000 with 50% polymorphonuclear cells. However, it would be unusual to find a low glucose or low PH and if these are present or if there are any organisms one must suspect a superimposed infectious process. Remember, most septic arthritides occur in joints that already are diseased and each flare needs to be carefully evaluated for signs of infection. The patient may have a moderate leukocytosis and a fever so it will be important to have a low degreee of suspicion and perform an arthrocentesis when there is a question. Ankle arthrocentesis is easiest done in the hollow between the extensor hallicus longus tendon and the medial malleolus. When blood is obtained one should suspect a ligamentous tear. Fat globules signify a fracture.

Differential Diagnosis

The differential diagnoses of foot pain are listed in Table 22.25. Common diagnoses will be discussed in this section.

GOUT

Gout has been recognized since early medicine when it was considered a disease of obese men prone to excesses of alcohol and food. It is difficult to estimate gout's true prevalence (estimated at 2.6/1,000) because it is often diagnosed presumptively. It usually occurs in the 5th to 6th decade and is more common in men. Although historically tied to alcohol consumption, the relation is not clear. It is, however, related to obesity and hyperlipidemia. The most common joints to be affected are in order: the first metatarsal, ankle, knee and less commonly the wrist. Initially it is an intermittent process with flares which over several years lead to a chronic arthritis. The flares are usually acute in onset lasting several days with severe pain and inflammation.

Table 22.25.
Differential Diagnosis of Foot Pain

Forefoot
    Crystal deposition disease
    Morton's neuroma
    Metatarsalgia
    Hallux valgus
Midfoot
    Plantar fasciitis
    Footstrain
    Neuropathic arthropathies
    Metatarsal stress fractures
    Tarsal tunnel syndrome
Hindfoot
    Achilles tendonitis
    Peroneal tendonitis
Ankle pain
    Acute sprain or strain
    Chronic ligamentous instability
    Inflammatory disorders
        Osteoarthritis
        Gout
        Osteomyelitis
        Rheumatoid arthritis

CALCIUM PYROPHOSPHATE DISEASE

Calcium pyrophosphate disease (CPPD) occurs with increasing incidence with advancing age. It is estimated to affect 15% of people older than 70 and 30% of people 80 years and older. It rarely occurs in the foot—the most common sites are the knees, wrists and elbows—however it may be confused with gout and expose the patient to potentially harmful treatment unecessarily and is therefore important to be aware of. It can only be distinguished from gout by synovial fluid analysis. It frequently occurs in patients with underlying OA and is simply thought to be an inflammatory phase of OA. Chondrocalcinosis is a frequent accompaniment and may be a helpful clue.

HALLUX VALGUS

Hallux valgus refers to lateral deviation of the first toe and is often referred to as a bunion when painful. It is extremely common in the elderly and may be related to foot deformities such as flatfoot or neuropathies. It may even lead to other foot deformities such as hammertoes and clawtoes if left untreated. It may also lead to a calcitrant callous on the plantar aspect of the second metatarsal, which may limit walking.

MORTON'S NEUROMA

Morton's neuroma (or interdigital neuroma) is due to entrapment of an interdigital nerve by fibrous tissue on the plantar aspect of the foot and is not a true neuroma. Most often it occurs in the 3rd webspace in middle-aged women, possibly related to wearing high-heeled shoes. It may, however, occur in any age or sex and is not consistently related to footwear. The patient usually describes a burning pain worsened by even minimal pressure such as from a stocking or shoe. The tenderness is between the metatarsal heads, which helps one distinguish it from metatarsalgia where the pain is directly over the metatarsal. If symptoms have been present for greater than 6 months then symptoms will respond to conservative measures (pads, injections) in less than 20% of the patients and surgical excision will be required for pain relief.

PLANTAR FASCIITIS

Plantar fasciitis occurs in approximately 10% of the population and is associated with excessive loading such as in running, obesity or jobs which require prolonged standing. It is a clinical syndrome of medial calcaneal pain made worse by weightbearing and is likely the result of several pathophysiologic processes. It usually occurs in persons over the age of 40 and may be associated with heel pad atrophy. It is typically described as worse in the morning with improvement in symptoms during walking until later in the day. It is usually a limited process, but if it persists despite therapy, one should consider an underlying inflammatory process such as RA or gout.

FOOT STRAIN

Foot strain, both the acute and the chronic forms, are also very common diagnoses in the foot. Acute foot strain is usually due to overuse such as excessive exercise whereas chronic foot strain may have several contributing factors such as pes planus, obesity, overuse or ill fitting shoes. Foot strain can usually be eliminated by avoiding exacerbating factors and changing footwear. Metatarsal stress fractures may be a cause of chronic foot strain and can occur without any discreet history of trauma especially in runners. X-rays may initially be negative and the diagnosis is sometimes confirmed by bone scan. Stress fractures are often misdiagnosed initially, leading to prolonged disability.

NEUROPATHIC ARTHROPATHY

Neuropathic arthropathies may occur due to any peripheral neuropathy but diabetes is the most common predisposing factor. It occurs in 1–2% of patients with diabetic neuropathy and therefore is

very uncommon but leads to significant disability. The joint is usually swollen and warm. The joint may be hypermobile due to joint destruction and often develops fractures. See Table 22.26.

OSTEOMYELITIS

Osteomyelitis occurs frequently in the feet of diabetic patients and is the cause of up to 25% of admissions for fevers in diabetic patients. It usually develops in patients with longstanding diabetes who have underlying peripheral neuropathies. The signs and symptoms may be very subtle—low grade fever, warmth, swelling, and tenderness. Usually it occurs at the site of a skin ulcer where the pathogen was likely introduced. One needs to maintain a high degreee of suspicion in any chronic foot ulcer or in the case of fever of unknown origin.

SPRAINS

Ankle sprains are the most common sports and recreational related musculoskeletal injury and may lead to chronic ligamentous instability in 30–40% of patients if inadequately treated. Ankle strains generally refer to stretching of the ligaments whereas as sprain denotes actual ligament tears. Ankle sprains are classified as mild or moderate to severe based upon whether there is significant ligamentous instability. Lateral ankle sprains are four to five times more common than medial sprains and are usually associated with inversion and plantar flexion forces. Fifteen percent of ankle trauma results in fracture and it is not always easy to distinguish between fracture and sprain by history and physical alone.

Management

The management of gout, plantar fasciitis, and sprains will be discussed in this section. The guiding recommendation is to reduce the patient's pain. The management of acute gout should be familiar to all practitioners. The initial therapy will be aimed at reducing inflammation and further accumulation of uric acid. Colchicine is the drug of choice if an

Table 22.26.
Causes of Neuropathic Arthropathies

Diabetes—by far most common cause
Trauma (acute or chronic)
Alcoholic neuropathy
Syphilis (previously the most common)
Vitamin B12 defiency
Hypothyroidism

attack is diagnosed within the first 24 hours but probably has no benefit after 48 hours. It should be given as 0.6 mg PO every 1–2 hours until diarrhea occurs or symptoms resolve up to 10 mg (less in the elderly or patients with impaired renal function). For patients in whom the flare has been ongoing for greater than 48 hours or who have bone marrow suppression, renal or hepatic failure, NSAIDs may cautiously be used. However, in these patients it may be wise to consider either intraarticular or oral steroids. Maintenance therapy with colchicine or allopurinol may be started after the acute flare has completely resolved. It will also be important to determine if there were any precipitating events such as surgery, diuretic use or dietary indiscretions. None of these can alone cause a flare but likely require other processes to be occurring such as renal insufficiency.

PLANTER FASCIITIS

The management of plantar fasciitis is through conservative and local measures. Initially one needs to begin by reducing the overload which is causing the inflammation. This will combine arch supports and avoiding precipitating activities. NSAIDs are important adjunctive measures as is local ice therapy especially prior to stretching exercises. If this approach does not work after 6 weeks one may consider injection with long-acting corticosteroids at the point of tenderness. This should not be done more than three times at weekly intervals or in patients who have heel pad atrophy as it may predispose to rupture of the fascia. Surgical release of the fascia would only be considered after 6 months if these therapies did not provide relief.

SPRAINS

The most important goal in managing ankle sprains is the reduction of swelling. Initially this will require immobilization, elevation, ice therapy and bandaging with tape or a lace up brace. It is important to emphasize to the patient that the bandaging will not prevent further injury and that it is necessary to avoid weight bearing until the swelling has resolved. If there is instability it will require immobilization for approximately 1–2 weeks until the swelling has resolved and then range of motion and eventually ligament strengthening exercises. It is crucial to treat the acute ankle sprain adequately to prevent the longterm complications. If the patient has a severe sprain with marked instability the patient should see an orthopedic surgeon who may consider casting or reconstructive surgery to prevent long-term instability.

ILLUSTRATIVE CASES WITH SELF-ASSESSMENT QUESTIONS AND ANSWERS

Case 1

Diana is a 45-year-old woman who comes to your office complaining of several weeks of worsening foot pain. It is painful standing and then again after prolonged standing. She has tried local soaks and facients without relief. She is no longer able to wear her shoes to her job as a secretary and has had to wear sneakers to work for the past several days. She points to her heel as being the most painful site but states that the entire bottom of her foot hurts by the end of the day.

QUESTION: *What is the most likely diagnosis?*

a. Chronic foot strain
b. Plantar fasciitis
c. Gout
d. Metatarsalgia

ANSWER: b. *Due to the location of the pain,*
the diagnoses you suspect include foot strain or plantar fasciitis. The symptoms of being worse on initial standing and the localization to the heel make plantar fasciitis the most likely diagnosis.

Case 2

John is a 56-year-old man with a history of hypertension who calls you in the middle of the night complaining of severe atraumatic foot pain. He has never had such a pain and has no family history of arthritis. He tells you the foot is hot and swollen and he is very worried. He asks you if he should go to the emergency room because he has a fever and does not think he can wait until the morning to see you.

QUESTION: *Which of the following is not an appropriate reply?*

a. Tell John he must go straight to the emergency room because you cannot rule out that he does not have a serious infection of his foot over the phone.

b. Tell John to take 2 aspirin and apply local ice and to call back if the pain worsens.

c. Tell John you know of a 24-hour pharmacy that delivers medications in emergencies and that you will call in a prescription for some indocin and allopurinol and he should see you first thing in the morning.

d. Tell John you will call in a prescription for a narcotic to the 24-hour pharmacy and he should call you if anything changes; otherwise, he should see you first thing in the morning.

ANSWER: c. *You highly suspect gout because John has no risks for a septic process occurring. The styles for managing patients vary greatly and any of the above may be appropriate depending on your knowledge of the patient, with the exception of prescribing allopurinol for an acute gouty flare. Allopurinol may actually precipitate worsening of the uric acid precipitation and it is not appropriate to prescribe any uricosuric reducing agent without a definitive diagnosis and serum electrolytes.*

Case 3

You are seeing a patient who has "sprained" his ankle in a soccer game.

QUESTION: *Which is not a sign of serious ankle injury?*

a. Ecchymosis
b. Swelling
c. Patient is unable to weight bear
d. Instability of the ankle

ANSWER: b. *Swelling is not an indication of a more serious ankle injury (i.e., a fracture or torn ligament). Swelling occurs in simple strains as well but needs to be treated aggressively to reduce pain and promote healing. Measures to reduce swelling in the immediate period include ice, elevation, and immobilization.*

SUGGESTED READINGS

Joint Pain

Bradley JD. Nonsurgical options for managing osteoarthritis of the knee. J Musculoskel Med 1994; 11:14–26.

Calin A. What causes osteoarthritis? J Musculoskel Med 1993;10:39–46.

Swedberg J, Steinbauer J. Osteoarthritis. Am Fam Physician 1992; 45:557–68.

Wong HY. Neural mechanisms of joint pain. Ann Academy Med 1993; 22:646–50.

Back Pain

Mankin HJ. Metabolic bone disease. J Bone Joint Surg 1994; 76:760–788.

Simkin PA, Gardner EC. Osteonecrosis: pathogenesis and practicalities. Hosp Pract 1994; 73–84.

Shoulder Pain

Burkholder JF. Inflammatory myopathies. Resident Staff Physician 1995; 39–45.

Fukuda M, Hamada K, Nakajima T, Tomonaga A. Pathology and pathogenesis of intratendinous tearing of the rotator cuff viewed from en bloc histologic sections. Clin Orthop 1994; 304:60–67.

Schollmeier G, Uhthoffmk, Sarkark, Fukuharak. Effects of immobilization on the capsule of the canine glenohumeral joint. Clin Orthop 1994; 304:37–42.

Knee Pain

Pincus T, Callahan LF. What is the natural history of rheumatoid arthritis? Rheumatic disease clinics of North America. 1993;19:123–151.

McNicholl JM, Glynn D, Mergey AB et al. A prospective study of neuropsychologic, neurologic and immunologic abnormalities in systemic lupus erythematosis. J Rheum 1994;21:1061–1066.

Cerrera R, Khamashta, Font J et al. Systemic lupus erythematosis: clinical and immunologic patterns of disease of 1000 patients. The European working party on systemic lupus erythematosis. Medicine 1993;72:113–124.

Foot Pain

Almekinders LC. Osteomyelitis: Essentials of diagnosis and treatment. J Musculoskel Med 1994;10:31–40.

Beutler, S Jr. Gout and "pseudogout"; When are arthritic symptoms caused by crystal deposition? Postgrad Med 1994; 95:103–116.

Kaye T. Watching for and managing musculoskeletal problems in diabetes. J Musculoskel Med 1994; 10:25–37.

Marder RA. Current methods for the evaluation of ankle ligament injuries. J Bone Joint Surg 1994; 76A: 1103–1111.

Teasdal RD, Saltzman CL, Johnson KA. A practical approach to Morton's neuroma. J Musculoskel Med 1993;9:41.

chapter 23

PSYCHIATRY

Andrew S. Lustbader[1]*, Carole Morgan, Rafael Pelayo, Luz S. Vasquez, Kin Yuen*

ANXIETY

Who has not experienced anxiety? Anxiety as an emotion is pervasive and an integral part of the vocabulary of human experience. Anxiety, however, can be more than a common emotion. It can become excessive and troublesome. Over the past decades, a concept of anxiety as a disease has emerged. As a consequence, anxiety — the universal emotional experience, and anxiety — the mental disorder have acquired different definitions. Varying theories have been proposed to explain the nature and function of anxiety in human experience. Some theorists view anxiety as a unitary concept and differences in intensity determine whether anxiety is normal or disordered. Others regard "disordered" anxiety as qualitatively different from common anxiety. In any case, clarifying the "exact" nature of the anxiety in question is often difficult. When conceptualized as an emotional response, anxiety can be defined as uneasiness, apprehension, dread, foreboding, a nameless fear. When anxiety is classified as a disorder, it is defined as symptoms of physiological arousal (e.g., palpitations, sweating) accompanied by a psychological mood of excessive worry that interferes with normal functioning and persists over time. Table 23.1 lists the symptoms associated with anxiety when it is diagnosed as a disorder.

Epidemiologic evidence suggests that anxiety disorders in adults are widespread. The most thorough data on incidence and prevalence of anxiety disorders comes from the Epidemiologic Catchment Area Study, an NIMH sponsored community survey done in the 1980s of the prevalence of psychiatric disorders in the U.S. Although the rates and risks for the different anxiety disorders in adults vary, an estimate of annual prevalence for all anxiety disorders is about 4–8 per 100 individuals (1). Panic disorder is one of the most highly prevalent types of anxiety and is often associated with other psychiatric conditions, primarily depression (2). Though women have higher rates of anxiety disorders than men, men still suffer from anxiety in large numbers.

The primary care clinician is often the first health care provider who sees the patient with anxiety. Issues of stigma may prevent a patient from seeking psychological help for anxiety, or the physical symptoms of anxiety may be dominant and suggest a physical problem to the patient. It is critically important for a primary care provider to be able to assess symptoms of anxiety in a patient and determine whether that patient is suffering from a primary anxiety disorder, a medical condition that mimics an anxiety disorder, anxiety caused by the response to a major stressor, a reaction to a medication or drug, or another condition entirely. The major challenge for the clinician confronted with an anxious patient lies in the differential diagnosis: is the patient suffering from a psychological problem or a physical one? Based on that diagnosis appropriate treatment decisions or referrals can be made. Though anxiety can be crippling, it can also be motivating and in some cases helpful for growth and learning. A key point to keep in mind is the distinction (first made by Freud) between anxiety as a signal – something else is wrong – or anxiety as the problem itself. This distinction is critical in how one approaches a patient with anxiety symptoms.

Pathophysiologic Correlation

There are several hypotheses about the pathophysiological processes involved in anxiety but at the

---

[1] I thank Elizabeth Prata for her advice and assistance.

Table 23.1.
Symptoms of Anxiety

Physiological
    Palpitations
    Shortness of breath
    Sweating or cold clammy hands
    Dry mouth
    Dizziness or light-headedness
    Gastrointestinal discomfort (diarrhea, nausea)
    Flushes or chills
    Frequent urination
    Trouble swallowing or lump in throat
    Trembling or feeling shaky
    Muscle tension, aches or soreness
    Restlessness
    Easy fatigability
Psychological
    Excessive worry
    Sleep disturbances
    Irritability
    Difficulty concentrating

present time they are incomplete understandings. Many systems are implicated in anxiety, both neuroanatomical structures (the limbic system including the amygdala and hippocampus, the thalamus, and the frontal cortex) and neurochemical systems (norepinephrine, serotonin, and GABA) (3). The same systems appear to be involved in "normal" and "dysfunctional" anxiety. Much of the understanding about the role of neurotransmitters and neurohormones in anxiety has come from observing the effects of pharmacologic agents which alleviate anxiety, notably the benzodiazepines. The partial understanding of the biology and pathophysiology of anxiety reflects the complexity of the pathways. The following are current active areas of research into the biological substate of anxiety.

GAMMA-AMINOBUTYRIC ACID (GABA)

Investigations into how and why benzodiazepines work to mitigate anxiety led to the discovery that they potentiate the action of GABA, the most prevalent inhibitory neurotransmitter in the CNS. The role of GABA in anxiety was further explicated by the discovery that benzodiazepine receptors exist in the brain and that they are coupled with receptors for GABA. Strong evidence implicates the GABA/benzodiazepine receptor in normal and pathologic anxiety (2).

BIOGENIC AMINES

The central noradrenergic system, especially norepinephrine-producing neurons located in the nu-

cleus locus ceruleus also play a significant role in anxiety-related phenomena. Specifically, panic anxiety may be related etiologically to abnormal regulation of central noradrenergic functioning. Reactions indistinguishable from panic have been elicited in monkeys whose locus ceruleus has been electrically stimulated.

Clinical and Laboratory Evaluation

A detailed interview is the central evaluative tool in the initial assessment of the nature, etiology, and extent of a patient's anxiety. A physical examination either to establish the presence of a medical condition or to reassure the patient is also always indicated. Laboratory tests are useful when drug-relaxed anxiety is suspected, or to confirm a specific physical diagnosis.

HISTORY

If a patient exhibits or reports anxiety symptoms, obtain a thorough history through interview. The interview is the first step in generating hypotheses about whether the patient is suffering from a primary anxiety disorder, an adjustment or situational reaction, or a medical condition with anxiety as a feature. Key pieces of information to gather include date of onset, nature, and duration of anxiety symptoms.

Each type of anxiety disorder, as well as anxieties associated with medical conditions, medications and stress, are associated with slightly different anxiety symptoms. Obtaining an accurate description of the symptoms enables the physician to make a diagnosis.

PHYSICAL EXAMINATION

A physical examination is always recommended, even if one suspects that the anxiety symptoms are related to a primary anxiety state and not caused by a medical condition or medications. When a primary medical condition (with accompanying anxiety symptoms) is suspected, a thorough physical examination appropriate to the suspected condition is indicated (Table 23.2). If one concludes that the anxiety is not due to a medical condition or medication but to a life circumstance or primary anxiety disorder, a physical examination is still useful in reassuring the patient that no serious physical disease is lurking.

LABORATORY EVALUATION

No laboratory findings have been identified that are diagnostic of primary anxiety disorders. However, a

Table 23.2.
Medical Conditions That May Cause Anxiety

Endocrine
  Hyper/hypothyroidism
  Hyperparathyroidism
  Pheochromocytoma
  Hypoglycemia
  Hyperadrenocorticism
  Cushing's syndrome
Cardiovascular
  Congestive heart failure
  Coronary Artery Disease
  Pulmonary embolism
  Mitral Valve Prolapse
  Arrhythmia
Respiratory conditions
  Chronic obstructive lung disease
  Asthma
  Pneumonia
  Hyperventilation
Metabolic conditions
  Vitamin B12 deficiency
  Porphyria
Neurological disorders
  Neoplasms
  Temporal Lobe epilepsy
  Vestibular dysfunction
  Encephalitis

Tomb DA. Psychiatry. Fourth ed, Philadelphia: Williams and Wilkins 1992:70.
Katon W. Panic disorder in the medical setting. National Institute of Mental Health.
DHHS Pub No (ADM) 89-1629, Washington, D.C.: Supt of Docs, US Gov't Printing Office, 1989.

variety of laboratory findings have been noted to be abnormal in certain individuals with panic disorder, e.g., some individuals show signs of compensated respiratory alkalosis (i.e., decreased carbon dioxide and decreased bicarbonate levels with an almost normal pH). With patients who present with somatic anxiety symptoms, a brief laboratory screen is helpful even when a primary anxiety disorder is suspected. These tests reassure patients that they are being taken seriously and that major problems are being ruled out (4). For patients suspected of having an anxiety disorder due to a medical condition, or anxiety as response to a medication or drug, appropriate laboratory tests (e.g., blood tests for drugs) should be performed.

Differential Diagnosis

Because anxiety as a symptom complex is prevalent and multidetermined, the heart of the approach to anxiety in the ambulatory care patient is to establish an accurate diagnosis. In classifying anxiety, this chapter will use the nomenclature and the diagnostic categories and criteria for Anxiety Disorders compiled by the American Psychiatric Association in the Diagnostic and Statistical Manual of Mental Disorders (DSM-IV) published in 1994 (5). However, this material will be organized in a way appropriate to a primary care clinician who must make a differential diagnosis within the context of seeing a medical patient in a medical clinic. A clinician examining a patient in an ambulatory care setting needs to identify the nature of the anxiety being presented and make quick judgments as to the etiology and severity of the anxiety. Most patients exhibiting anxiety will fit primarily into one of five categories. Treatment and management decisions will follow accordingly. These five categories are as follows:

1. Anxiety as a primary psychiatric disorder (anxiety disorders)
2. Anxiety as a response to psychosocial or physical stressors (adjustment disorder with anxious mood)
3. Anxiety associated with a medical condition (anxiety due to a medical condition)
4. Anxiety as a reaction to a drug or medication (substance-induced anxiety)
5. Anxiety as part of another psychiatric condition such as alcoholism, depression, or psychosis

ANXIETY AS A PRIMARY PSYCHIATRIC DISORDER—ANXIETY DISORDERS

Primary anxiety disorders are considered psychiatric disorders. DSM-IV lists nine primary anxiety disorders: panic disorder without agoraphobia; panic disorder with agoraphobia; agoraphobia without a history of panic disorder; specific phobia; social phobia; obsessive-compulsive disorder; posttraumatic stress disorder; acute stress disorder; generalized anxiety disorder. Several of them have been grouped together here for easier presentation.

Panic Attacks (With or Without Agoraphobia) and Agoraphobia. Panic attacks are characterized by the sudden onset of intense apprehension, fearfulness, or terror, often accompanied by feelings of impending doom. During these attacks, symptoms such as shortness of breath, palpitations, chest pain or discomfort, choking or smothering sensations, and fear of "going crazy" or losing control are present. To meet diagnostic criteria, a patient must have had four attacks within 4 weeks and have experienced at least four of the following symptoms during an attack (from DSM-IV):

- Shortness of breath (dyspnea) or smothering sensations
- Dizziness, unsteady feelings, or faintness
- Palpitations or accelerated heart rate (tachycardia)
- Trembling or shaking
- Sweating
- Choking
- Nausea or abdominal distress
- Depersonalization or derealization
- Numbness or tingling sensations
- Hot flashes or chills
- Chest pain or discomfort
- Fear of dying
- Fear of going crazy or doing something uncontrolled

Agoraphobia is anxiety about, or avoidance of, places or situations from which escape might be difficult (or embarrassing) or in which help may not be available in the event of having a panic attack or panic-like symptoms.

Phobias, Including Specific Phobias and Social Phobias. A specific phobia is an excessive and persistent fear of certain objects or situations. Being exposed to the phobic stimulus provokes an immediate anxiety response. Examples of phobic stimuli include dogs, spiders, and airplanes. The individual will try to avoid the feared object/situation or, if this is impossible, experience great anxiety while enduring it.

Social phobia is characterized by excessive anxiety provoked by exposure to certain types of performance or social situations. Examples include performing, giving a speech in public, or eating in public places. Because the person is afraid he will do something embarrassing he avoids engaging in the behavior. To meet diagnostic criteria, the avoidant behavior must interfere significantly with occupational functioning, social, and personal relationships.

Generalized Anxiety Disorder. This anxiety disorder is characterized by excessive worry and anxiety that occurs nearly every day and has persisted for at least 6 months. Three or more of the following six symptoms are predominant: restlessness or feeling keyed up or on edge; being easily fatigued; difficulty concentrating or mind going blank; irritability; muscle tension; sleep disturbance (difficulty falling or staying asleep, or restless unsatisfying sleep). The anxiety causes the person great distress or impairment in social or occupational areas of functioning. The worry

in generalized anxiety is distinguished from "obsessive" worry in that the excessive worry in generalized anxiety disorder centers about everyday problems while "obsessive" worry in obsessive-compulsive disorder takes the form of repugnant urges and impulses that are accompanied by compulsive behaviors that reduce the anxiety associated with the obsessions.

Obsessive-Compulsive Disorder. Obsessive-compulsive disorder is characterized by *obsessions,* which are recurrent or persistent thoughts, ideas, impulses, that are intrusive and repugnant to the individual experiencing them and cause the person a great deal of anxiety or distress, and *compulsions,* which are repetitive behaviors that a person performs in response to an obsession. The compulsions alleviate the anxiety. At some point during the course of the disorder, the patient has recognized that the obsessions or compulsions are excessive or unreasonable.

Posttraumatic Stress Disorders and Acute Stress Disorder. This disorder is characterized by re-experiencing a traumatic event, e.g., an accident, combat experience, rape. The event is re-experienced in the form of dreams, images, or feelings of reliving the event, often accompanied by intense psychological distress and physiological reactivity. Avoidance of stimuli associated with the trauma and numbing of general responsiveness are present. The duration of the disturbance must be more than 1 month to meet diagnostic criteria for this disorder. When anxiety, dissociative, and other symptoms occur within 1 month of the traumatic stressor, the disorder is called acute stress disorder.

ADJUSTMENT DISORDER WITH ANXIOUS MOOD

This type of anxiety can be highly prevalent among medical patients seen in outpatient settings and should be suspected in patients who are experiencing a major psychosocial stressor (e.g., a life crisis or serious physical illness) and do not meet the diagnostic criteria for a primary anxiety disorder. It is particularly important to be able to recognize this form of anxiety as distinct from primary anxiety disorders and anxiety due to medical conditions because "preventive" interventions to alleviate anxiety (e.g., supportive counseling, brief psychopharmacologic interventions) may prevent the development of generalized anxiety disorder or depression (6). For example, the clinician can prepare patients for serious procedures that naturally provoke anxiety and desensitize patients to threatening and terrifying situations.

ANXIETY DUE TO A MEDICAL CONDITION

The essential feature of anxiety due to a medical condition is severe anxiety judged to be a direct physiological effect of a general medical condition. Table 23.2 lists medical conditions that can produce anxiety symptoms. The anxiety symptoms experienced by patients can be generalized anxiety symptoms, panic attacks, obsessions, or compulsions. If a medical condition that produces anxiety as a symptom is suspected, complete history, physical examination and laboratory tests should be performed to determine the exact diagnosis.

SUBSTANCE-INDUCED ANXIETY

Anxiety also can be due to the direct physiological effects of certain medications, drugs or toxins (7). Medications reported to evoke anxiety symptoms include: anesthetics and analgesics; bronchodilators or other sympathomimetics; anticholinergics; insulin; thyroid preparations; oral contraceptives; antihistamines; antiparkinsonian medications; corticosteroids; antihypertensive and cardiovascular medications; anticonvulsants; lithium carbonate; antipsychotic medications; antidepressant medications.

Intoxication with the following classes of substances can cause anxiety symptoms: alcohol, amphetamine and related substances, caffeine, cannabis, cocaine, hallucinogens, inhalants, phencyclidine. Anxiety can also occur in association with withdrawal from the following classes of substances: alcohol, cocaine, sedatives, hypnotics, and anxiolytics. Heavy metals and toxins that may cause anxiety symptoms include: volatile substances such as gasoline and paint, organophosphate insecticides, nerve gases, carbon monoxide, carbon dioxide.

ANXIETY ASSOCIATED WITH OTHER PSYCHIATRIC DISORDERS

Prevalent psychiatric disorders such as depression or alcoholism can often present like anxiety disorders. Anxiety disorders also can co-exist with other psychiatric disorders. The condition diagnosed as the primary disorder usually should be treated first.

Depression. Discriminating between an anxiety disorder and a depressive illness can be difficult. Anxiety symptoms are common in many depressed patients and many anxious patients have symptoms of depression. The moods of anxiety and depression can overlap and a number of symptoms—sleep and appetite disturbances, difficulty concentrating, irritability, and fatigue—can be characteristic of both anxiety and depression. There are some distinguishing characteristics. For example, sleep problems present differently. Anxious patients tend to have difficulty falling asleep whereas depressed patients report early morning awakening (with inability to get back to sleep) and excessive sleeping.

Careful diagnosis is the key to appropriate treatment. See the section on depression in this chapter for a thorough discussion. If a depressive illness is suspected, the most appropriate action for the primary care provider is to consult with a mental health professional who can aid in the diagnosis and work in a coordinated manner with the provider and patient around treatment issues.

Alcoholism. All patients who present with anxiety-related symptoms should be screened for alcohol abuse. There is high comorbidity of alcohol and anxiety problems. Lifetime prevalence of anxiety disorders combined with alcohol disorders is 19.4%, substance abuse plus panic disorders is 35.8%, and substance abuse plus obsessive compulsive disorder is 32.8% (8). There is a high risk of suicide among these patients. The differential diagnosis of anxiety in patients with alcohol abuse and alcohol disorders in patients with anxiety disorders is very difficult because the symptoms overlap. The four-question CAGE questionnaire for alcoholism (9) is a good screen for alcoholism in the medical patient. If a diagnosis of alcoholism is suspected, the patient should be counselled to join a treatment recovery program.

Psychosis. Intense anxiety or agitation may be the presenting symptom for an acute attack of schizophrenia or other psychotic disorder. This can occur even when the person has no history of a previous psychotic disorder. The major diagnostic features to keep in mind when considering a diagnosis of psychosis are: thought disorganization, delusional thinking, paranoid ideation, marked fluctuations in affect and behavior. When a diagnosis of psychotic anxiety is suspected, the patient should be referred immediately to a psychiatrist.

Management

Management decisions should be based on an assessment of the causes of the anxiety. They should not reflect an effort to just treat the symptoms. A medical condition that causes anxiety always must be ruled out initially, as well as anxiety that arises from a withdrawal from drugs. In these cases, the primary medical condition must be treated. In cases in which the anxiety arises from a primary anxiety disorder or reaction to a stress or another psychiatric condition, combinations of pharmacologic and

Table 23.3.
Commonly Used Medications For Anxiety

Agent	Average Total Therapeutic Dosage Range (mg/day)[a]	Primary Uses
Benzodiazepines		
Alprazolam (Xanax)	.5–4	Generalized anxiety; short-term relief of anxiety symptoms; panic disorder with or without agoraphobia
Diazepam (Valium)	4–40	Generalized anxiety; alcohol withdrawal
Lorazepam (Ativan)	2–6	Generalized anxiety; anxiety associated with depressive symptoms
Oxazepam (Serax)	30–120	Anxiety and tension in older patients
Nonbenzodiazepine anxiolytics		
Buspirone (Buspar)	20–60	General anxiety and short term anxiety
Tricyclic antidepressants		
Imipramine (Tofranil)	75–300	Panic disorder
Amitriptyline (Elavil)	75–300	Panic disorder
Clomipramine (Anafranil)	100–250	Obsessive-compulsive disorder
MAO inhibitors		
Phenelzine (Nardil)	45–90	Panic disorders in those not responsive to tricyclic antidepressants
Beta blockers		
Propranolol (Inderal)	40–100	Panic disorders; performance anxiety

[a]Therapeutic dosage is influenced by patient characteristics such as age and individual metabolic differences as well as by concurrent use of other medicines. It is advisable to consult with a psychiatrist or psychopharmacologist to determine starting dose, incremental increases and therapeutic dosage.

psychological interventions are appropriate and available.

Several classes of medication are useful in the *pharmacologic* treatment of anxiety symptoms but different kinds of anxiety are responsive to different medications. All antianxiety drugs represent symptomatic treatments; they do not get rid of the underlying cause of the anxiety. Thus antianxiety agents always should be considered in the framework of other approaches.

Drug therapy should be initiated at low doses, with gradual increases as needed and tolerated. Each increment should be small, usually not exceeding 25 to 50% of the previous total daily dose. During the upward titration process, tolerance to side effects usually develops. The best approach is to continue raising the dose gradually until a balance is reached between side effects and benefits. In most cases an optimal dosage can be found at which side effects are absent or acceptably mild and therapeutic benefits become stable, without further need for dosage increments (6). Table 23.3 gives an overview of medications available for the treatment of anxiety. They include the following classes of drugs:

- Anxiolytics, benzodiazepines and nonbenzodiazepines (e.g., Buspirone, which does not seem to interact with benzodiazepine receptors but seems to interact with multiple neurotransmitter systems and does not interact with alcohol or other CNS system depressants)
- Tricyclic antidepressants
- Monoamine oxidase (MAO) inhibitors
- Beta adrenergic blockers

There are a variety of psychological treatments for anxiety depending on the type of anxiety. Table 23.4 gives an overview of these techniques. Psychological strategies usually work best in conjunction with drug therapies.

ANXIETY DISORDERS

Most primary anxiety disorders respond best to a combination of medication and psychological intervention. While the primary care provider can treat a patient with anxiety, in cases of primary anxiety disorders, referral is indicated. Most behavioral and psychological interventions for helping

Table 23.4.
Psychological Interventions for the Treatment Of Anxiety

Behavior Therapies (to change specific behaviors/responses)
  Systematic desensitization
  In vivo exposure to feared stimulus
  Progressive muscle relaxation training
  Biofeedback techniques
  Self-hypnosis
Cognitive methods (to change specific cognitions which influence behaviors and self esteem)
  Stress management (e.g. relaxation, meditation, guided imagery)
  Cognitive coping (e.g. distraction, self-statements, cognitive restructuring)
Psychoeducational approaches (to increase knowledge as means of alleviating anxiety and promoting compliance with treatment)
  Written material
  Group classes
Supportive counseling (to relieve anxiety symptoms)
  Crisis intervention
  Support groups
Psychotherapy (to uncover and eliminate source of anxiety symptoms)
  Individual, group and family interventions

patients manage anxiety require more time than the internist has available.

Panic Attacks and Agoraphobia. Of the pharmacologic treatments, three types of medication are effective: tricyclic antidepressants (e.g., imipramine); MAO inhibitors (e.g., phenelzine); benzodiazepines (e.g., alprazolam and clonazepam). All three classes of drugs are effective in the treatment of panic-related disorders. Basis of choice depends on side effects and individual response. A minimum 6-month trial of one of the drugs mentioned, with a tapered discontinuation over a 1- to 3-month period is recommended (4).

A major psychological approach used in panic disorder is in vivo exposure. This technique is used to treat phobic avoidance of situations or places which might trigger panic attacks. In vivo exposure involves actual (rather than imagined) immersion in the feared place or situation. General counseling or therapy is also useful.

Phobias. No specific pharmacologic treatments are recommended for phobias other than social phobias. For social phobias beta blockers, MAO inhibitors and benzodiazepines have been effective. For stage fright in particular, beta blockers are the drug of choice.

Psychologic approaches for treating simple phobias center on behavioral strategies like in vivo exposure to the feared situation. For social phobias, cognitive restructuring and behavioral strategies such as systematic desensitization, relaxation training and social skills training are helpful. Systematic desensitization, a technique in which relaxation exercises are used to counteract the anxiety aroused by imagining the phobic situation, is also effective.

Generalized Anxiety. Short-acting benzodiazepines (e.g., oxazepam, lorazepam, alprazolam) are a good first strategy for treating generalized anxiety. These medications often reduce distress to manageable levels so the patient's normal coping mechanisms will function again. Tricyclic antidepressants may be helpful for more chronic anxiety.

Among the psychologic approaches, supportive psychotherapy to provide reassurance and gain an understanding of the nature of the disorder, behavioral techniques for relaxation, and stress management are all helpful. Biofeedback sometimes works. Cognitive approaches which teach the patient how to change his appraisal of threatening situations coupled with teaching the relaxation response, with or without progressive muscle relaxation can be useful adjuncts to treating anxiety states.

Obsessive-Compulsive Disorder. Benzodiazepines may be helpful. Tricyclic antidepressants and MAO inhibitors are also effective, if depression is prominent. Clonipramine has been effective for those with obsessions.

Psychological approaches that use behavioral strategies, including in vivo exposure and systematic desensitization have shown some success. Psychotherapy is also useful.

Posttraumatic Stress Disorder. Tricyclic antidepressants, MAO inhibitors, and benzodiazepines have been used in acute and posttraumatic stress disorders with some success (6). Psychotherapy and support groups are important psychologic treatments for individuals with stress disorders. Relaxation training can also be helpful.

ADJUSTMENT DISORDER WITH ANXIOUS MOOD

A brief course of benzodiazepines is appropriate for individuals experiencing stress-related anxiety. A tricyclic antidepressant can be used in patients who have more chronic anxiety symptoms. The non-benzodiazepine, buspirone, is an alternative for a patient who requires more chronic use of anti-anxiety medication.

Situational or life-stress anxiety is often best managed psychologically with relaxation training and training in coping strategies. Supportive psychological counseling is also helpful. Brief pharmacologic interventions can augment psychological approaches.

ANXIETY DUE TO A MEDICAL CONDITION

If the patient's anxiety is part of a medical disorder, then the treatment of the primary medical condition should be the main approach to alleviating the anxiety. Psychological approaches for temporary symptom relief can include relaxation techniques, including self-hypnosis and progressive muscle relaxation. Benzodiazepines may be used for the short term.

SUBSTANCE-INDUCED ANXIETY

If the patient's anxiety is part of a response to a drug or medication, then the medication in question needs to be changed. For anxiety due to reactions to drugs of abuse, the patient should be referred to a drug detoxification program. Diazepam can be helpful in alcohol withdrawal.

OTHER PSYCHIATRIC DISORDERS

If a major psychiatric disorder other than anxiety is present, consultation with a psychiatrist, clinical psychologist, or psychiatric social worker is indicated. The treatment and management of psychiatric illness requires special expertise. The most helpful thing a primary care provider can do in these cases is make a good referral.

Alcoholism. When alcoholism is present with anxiety, the alcohol problem must be treated first.

Patients should firmly be told they need a treatment program. A combination of cognitive-behavioral, 12-step, and pharmacologic approaches is best. Anxiolytics should be used cautiously in the management of alcoholic patients with anxiety. The combination of benzodiazepines and alcohol can produce serious reactions. Referral to specialists in anxiety disorders or alcohol disorders or professionals skilled in treating both disorders is definitely indicated.

Depression. When anxiety is present along with depression, a combination of psychological

and pharmacologic treatment is indicated. Referral to a psychopharmacologist is recommended because of the complexity of medication issues. Psychotherapy is also important in the treatment of major depression.

Psychosis. Referral to a psychiatrist is imperative. Neuroleptic drugs are indicated. Hospitalization may be necessary.

SPECIAL POPULATIONS

A primary care clinician is often faced with a patient who is experiencing anxiety in response to a medical procedure. Anxiety management in these patients can make the procedure go more smoothly as well as reduce excessive distress. In addition, the treatment of anxiety symptoms in the elderly requires special tailoring.

Geriatric Populations. Managing anxiety in the elderly patient presents unique problems. Often anxiety is coexistent with depression, dementia, and physical illness, or it is a response to stressful life circumstances. Because the elderly usually run higher blood levels and show increased receptor responsiveness to psychoactive medications, they require lower doses of antianxiety medications. They are also more susceptible to side-effects and need to be monitored carefully. A final difficulty involves compliance with drug regimens. Many elderly individuals take multiple drugs and issues of forgetfulness, misunderstanding, fear of side effects, etc. can interfere with adherence. In episodes of acute anxiety among elderly patients who are experiencing life stressors, a limited course of short half-life benzodiazepines (e.g., oxazepam and lorazepam) can be very helpful. For Lorazepam, an initial dose of 1–2 mg/day in divided doses is recommended, to be adjusted as needed and tolerated. For Oxazepam, an initial dose of 10 mg, three times daily is recommended, with a gradual increase to 15 mg three or four times daily.

Surgical Patients. The anticipation of a medical procedure or surgery provokes anxiety in most patients. A number of psychological techniques are available which can diminish pre-procedure anxiety in some patients. These include provision of information about the procedure and its process, relaxation training (deep breathing exercises), self-hypnosis and guided imagery and cognitive techniques such as distraction and positive self-statements. Benzodiazepines are also effective in reducing anticipatory anxiety.

ILLUSTRATIVE CASES WITH SELF-ASSESSMENT QUESTIONS AND ANSWERS

Case 1

A 61-year-old white male comes to your office reporting daily episodes of palpitations, chest pain, shortness of breath and constant worry that he will have a heart attack. Four months ago he suffered a myocardial infarction, recovered well, and returned to work 2 months ago. In response to questioning, he reveals that he has been drinking more than usual lately to "make the worry go away."

QUESTION: *What is the most likely diagnosis?*

a. Alcoholism
b. Cardiovascular disease
c. Anxiety due to a medical condition

ANSWER: c. *Anxiety and depression after MI is common. However, it is very important to rule our further heart disease and to establish that alcohol intake is not excessive.*

QUESTION: *How would you manage the patient's anxiety symptoms?*

a. Reassure him that anxiety is natural and will disappear shortly
b. Refer him to a cardiac rehab counseling program
c. Prescribe a short course of benzodiazepine therapy

ANSWER: a, b, *and* c *(all of the above). Reassurance from the physician is useful but a formal counseling program that teaches skills to manage anxiety arising from adjustment to a heart condition is very helpful. A short course of anxiolytic medication can offer temporary symptom relief.*

Case 2

A 31-year-old white female comes to your office complaining of episodes of nausea and stomach cramps, dizziness, and feelings of depersonalization (as if her body were not real). These episodes often occur at work. She is a fashion designer.

They come on suddenly and for no apparent reason. They have been increasing. She is afraid she may be going crazy, and lately she almost can not go to work.

QUESTION: *What is the likely diagnosis?*

a. Malingering
b. Panic attacks
c. Stomach ulcer

ANSWER: b. *Panic disorder is the most likely diagnosis, though a complete physical examination and history are essential.*

QUESTION: *What is the most appropriate drug to begin with?*

a. Benzodiazepine
b. Tricyclic antidepressant
c. Beta-blocker

ANSWER: b. *Tofranil, a tricyclic antidepressant, is a good choice to treat panic attacks. It works best on the physical symptoms associated with panic. In addition, referral to a cognitive/behavioral therapist is important. The patient can learn techniques to cope with the symptoms and cognitions of panic, including relaxation training and restructuring of catastrophic thoughts.*

DEPRESSION

Depressive symptoms are a common human complaint and may be found in 9% to 20% of the general population (10). Depressive symptoms occur at various ages and stages of the adult life cycle. Therefore, the primary care provider will see adolescents through octogenarians presenting with a spectrum of depressive illness. Symptoms can range from mild somatic complaints with preserved functional status to a much more severe dysfunctional state with compromised functional capacity and risk for suicide and subsequent death. It is the responsibility of the primary care provider to identify patients with depressive disorders, to exclude medical illness as the cause of the episode, to evaluate the severity of the episode, and to initiate appropriate treatment and/or consultation. This section will define and review the epidemiology of the common mood disorders, assess the impact of depressive illness on the individual and society, review the pathophysiology of depression, and present guidelines for the diagnosis and treatment of depression in a primary care setting.

Defining Mood Disorders

Mood disorders can be broadly divided into two categories, unipolar and bipolar. The unipolar mood disorders are those in which depressive symptoms predominate, and thus are usually called "depressive disorders." In contrast, patients with bipolar disease will have a history of swings between depressive illness and episodes of abnormal persistent elevated mood known as mania or hypomania (11,12).

MAJOR DEPRESSION

The criteria for major depression demand that at least five of the depressive symptoms listed be present for at least 2 weeks and represent a change from the patient's baseline mood. At least one of the five qualifying symptoms must be depressed mood or loss of interest or pleasure (Table 23.5).

These symptoms must also cause significant compromise of the patient's social, occupational, or general functioning (11).

Table 23.5.
Symptoms of Depression

- Difficulty sleeping manifested as insomnia or hypersomnia.
- Changes in appetite resulting in more than a 5% weight gain or loss in a month (without dieting).
- Feelings of worthlessness or excessive guilt almost every day.
- Notable decreased interest or pleasure in all or mostly all activities for most of the day or all day.
- Feelings of constant fatigue or loss of energy.
- Feelings of worthlessness or excessive guilt (these feelings may be delusional in nature and can be reported by the patient or observed by others).
- Depressed mood (or irritability in adolescents) for most of the day, nearly every day.
- Difficulty with concentration, thought, or indecisiveness that occurs nearly daily.
- Frequent thoughts of death or suicide (both with and without clear-cut plan), or an actual attempt of suicide.
- Psychomotor retardation or agitation observed by others, not merely self-report.

DYSTHYMIA

Although major depressive episodes are the most common mood disorder the primary care provider will encounter, dysthymia is also prevalent in community-based studies. Most simply, dysthymia represents a low level depression, not meeting the criteria for major depression, and lasting for several years. The Diagnostic and Statistical Manual of Mental Disorders of the American Psychiatric Association (DSM IV) defines dysthymia as a depressed mood (or irritability in adolescents) which persists for most of the day, for more days than not, for at least 2 years. While the patient is depressed there must be at least two of the following criteria:

- Change in appetite, either hyper- or hypophagia
- Difficulty with sleep manifested by insomnia or hypersomnia
- Fatigue or low energy
- Diminished self esteem
- Indecisiveness or difficulty concentrating
- A sense of hopelessness

The dysthymic patient must not be free of the defining symptoms for more than 2 months and cannot have accompanying episodes of major depressive or bipolar illness. The symptoms must cause significant impairment in the patient's functioning, either social, occupational or both (11).

BIPOLAR ILLNESS

Bipolar illness is less common and is less likely to be managed independently by a primary care provider. Bipolar illness is sometimes difficult to diagnose. The treatment of bipolar illness is complicated. Therefore, it is preferable that a psychiatrist manage the bipolar patient (11). The definitions for mania and hypomania will be presented here mostly to enable the provider to distinguish these classes of mood disorder. Mania is defined in DSM IV as a period of abnormally and persistently elevated mood or irritable mood lasting at least a week (any duration if hospitalization is required). While this mood elevation is present, three or more of the following criteria must be present to a significant degree (if mood is irritable, then four criteria are required):

- Grandiosity (an overestimated sense of self-worth)
- Decreased need for sleep
- Pressured speech (the need to talk constantly,

even when the appropriate response is to be silent or pause)
- Racing thoughts or flight of ideas
- Distractibility, easily drawn to unimportant stimuli
- Psychomotor agitation or increase in goal-related activity
- Involvement in pleasurable activities that have high potential for unwanted or painful consequences (i.e., sexual indiscretion, spending sprees)

This mood alteration must not be causally related to an underlying medical condition or drug. The mood impairment must cause significant disruption in the individual's functioning, result in hospitalization to protect the patient from harming himself or others, or there must be psychotic features present. In hypomania, the same features must be present but the duration of mood change can be as brief as four days. The mood change in hypomania cannot result in the patient's hospitalization, must be noted as distinct from the patient's underlying nondepressed mood, must be notable to others, and must not substantially impair the patient's functioning (11).

Epidemiology of Depression/Dysthymia

The best information concerning mood disorders in the general population is reported in recent studies that benefit from the application of standardized definitions to large community samples. The lifetime prevalence of at least one mental disorder in the general population has been reported as 33%, with 6% having major depression (13). The onset of depression is most commonly between the ages of 18–44. The lifetime risk of major depression of 4.9–8.7% in women and 2.3–4.4% in men (14). Other studies report the prevalence rate of unipolar major depression to be as high as 4.7–25.8% for women and 2.1–12.3% for men (14). The higher frequency of depressive disease in women has been consistent across studies (15). The lifetime prevalence of dysthymia is approximately 3% in the United States. It is twice as common in adult women (14).

DEPRESSION IN THE ELDERLY

Several studies have examined the prevalence of depression in the elderly. Depressive symptoms are much more common than major depressive illness in the geriatric population. Of people older than 60 years, 27% reported depressive symptoms, most

commonly mild dysphoria (19%). Dysthymia occurred in 2% of the population, mixed anxiety and depression in 1.2 %, and major depression occurred in only 0.8 % (16). However, other elderly groups are at higher risk. In the institutionalized elderly, the prevalence of depression is about 23.7 % (16).

NATURAL HISTORY

The natural history of depression appears variable, ranging from a brief and self limited illness, to a significantly impairing disease with a high likelihood of recurrence. An untreated episode of major depression can typically last six months or longer. Five to 10% of individuals may meet the full criteria for major depression for 2 years or longer (11). At least one half of the individuals who experience a depressive episode will have a further attack and about 12% of these cases will go on to a more chronic course (17). Patients who have had three or more lifetime episodes of depression with a previous episode within 2 years have a 70–80% risk of recurrence without active treatment (17). The most severe outcome of undiagnosed depression is suicidal death. It is estimated that 10–15% of people with an affective disorder will end their lives by suicide (18). In the United States this amounts to 12–13 deaths from suicide per 100,000 (18).

IMPACT OF DEPRESSION ON THE INDIVIDUAL AND SOCIETY

The impact of depression on the daily functioning of individuals and society is profound.

Patients with depressive disorders and depressive symptoms were compared in terms of overall physical and social functioning to other chronic illnesses. Patients with depressive disorders and depressive symptoms had significantly more days in bed than six chronic medical conditions, including patients with current back problems, angina, and current arthritis. Depressed patients had worse general social and physical functioning as well as more bodily pain than patients with chronic medical disorders (19).

In a prospective study designed to assess the impact of both major and minor depression on disability days and days lost from work, patients were identified into various DSMIII categories of depression and followed for 1 year. When compared with the asymptomatic individuals, the risk of disability days and days lost from work was 4.78 times greater for people with major depression. People with minor depression with mood disturbance had a 1.55 times greater risk of disability.

Since people with minor depression are more prevalent than people with major depression, they were associated with 51% more disability days in the community than major depression. They were also at increased risk for developing major depression or anxiety disorder at 1 year (20).

DEPRESSION IN THE PRIMARY CARE SETTING

The estimates of the prevalence of depression in general medical practice range from 12% to 42% (21). Of those receiving treatment, more than 50% of people with mental illness receive their psychiatric care solely in the general medicine setting, while less than 20% receive care in mental health settings (13,21). Thus, depression is a common primary care problem.

Depressed patients have more vague complaints when presenting to their primary care provider, including vague musculoskeletal complaints, chest pain, headaches, gastrointestinal complaints, fatigue, and sleep disturbance (22,23). It is believed that this tendency toward somaticization may also result in more health visits and may impede the diagnosis of their underlying depressive disorders, since providers tend to focus on assessment of the somatic complaints (24). Patients with moderate to severe depression make more primary care ambulatory visits, make more telephone calls to their provider, and have more medical evaluations than nondepressed control patients. Patients with major depression take poorer care of their chronic medical illnesses. They are less likely to follow medical regimens. Studies with diabetics have shown that depressed diabetics were less likely to adhere to their diet, exercise, or blood and urine glucose checks (24). Maternal depression has been linked to an increased rate of academic problems, conduct disorders, and clinical depression in their children (15).

COMORBID PSYCHIATRIC AND MEDICAL DISORDERS

It is not uncommon for major depression and dysthymia to also be associated with comorbid psychiatric illness such as substance abuse and anxiety disorders. It is estimated that 65% of patients with dysthymia and 59% of major depressives have at least one additional psychiatric diagnosis (14). It is estimated that patients with major depression have an 18-fold increase in the risk of panic attacks. The risk of major depression in the alcoholic population has been estimated

at 18–25% (4). Thirty-two percent of all mood disorder patients are substance dependent in their lifetime.

The rates of depression reported in medically ill patients vary. There is a 19–29% depression prevalence in the first 3 years post-cerebrovascular accident, especially with left anterior brain lesions, dysphagia, cerebral atrophy, and living alone (25). Depression is also increased in Parkinson's disease. Depression is especially prevalent after myocardial infarction, with prevalence rates for major and minor depression as high as 45% initially and 33% at three months. Major depression has also been noted at increased rates in patients who have cancer, rheumatoid arthritis, chronic pain, chronic fatigue syndrome, and the HIV virus (24).

Pathophysiologic Correlation

Despite recent improvements in the diagnosis and treatment of depression, the etiology of depression and its pathophysiology are not well understood. There is a genetic predisposition to depression, however, the mode of genetic transmission has yet to be established. Twin studies done in patients with mood disorders note concordance rates between monozygotic twins ranging from 33 to 75%. Concordance ranges from 9 to 23% in dizygotic twins. Adopted twins reared apart have an incidence of affective illness consistent with their biologic parents as opposed to their adopted parents.

The proposed theories for mechanisms of depression have been developed in response to observations of the clinical action of antidepressant medications. Although it has not been proven, depression may occur as a result of depletion of the levels of serotonin and norepinephrine in the brain. This theory is known as the "biogenic amine hypothesis." There are other hypotheses that suggest that the two pathways may be interrelated in the ultimate development of depressive illness. Depression may result because of suprasensitive catecholamine receptors in response to decreased levels of catacholamines in the brain. This is an attractive theory because it rectifies the observations that antidepressant drugs cause blockade of uptake of neuroreceptors in a short time, but a clinical response often is delayed many weeks. The receptor suprasensitivity hypothesis is further bolstered by animal studies that have suggested that many different types of antidepressant drugs and electroconvulsive therapy cause either desensitization or downregulation of the catecholamine receptors with a time course that is similar to the clinical response to these drugs in humans.

Clinical and Laboratory Evaluation

Primary care providers diagnose depression in only 15–50% of patients but can improve sensitivity to 68% by using standardized screening tools (21). Beck has developed a screening scale that ambulatory patients can fill out in about 5 minutes. Depressed patients will present to primary care providers with varying chief complaints and symptom complexes. The reason the diagnosis is missed appears to be multifactorial, with some contributions more related to providers and others to patients.

Providers often will not consider depression in the differential diagnosis. This may be because primary care providers are not trained to think of depressive disorders as common mimickers of other disease processes. Therefore they get lost in the workup of physical complaints and symptoms and lose the overall view of the patient's presenting depressive disorder. They may also be confused by confounding medical or psychiatric illness like dementia, anxiety disorders, or sexual dysfunction. The patient's presentation may be early in the course of the disease or in a remitting stage making it difficult to diagnose. The provider must be open to the diagnosis of depression. As a primary provider, one must be aware that it may take multiple visits with a patient to establish enough rapport to allow him to disclose sensitive information. Providers more likely to diagnose depression ask more open-ended questions, are in less of a hurry, are good listeners, are more direct in asking questions of a psychological and social nature, are less likely to interrupt a patient and make more direct eye contact.

Patient-associated issues can also confound the diagnosis of depression. Patients can often medicate themselves with alcohol and other drugs that can complicate the presentation. Patients (and their primary care providers) may also erroneously attribute depressive symptoms to a negative life event and erroneously judge it sufficient to explain a major depressive episode. Patients may be reluctant to share depressive feelings with their provider due to feeling ashamed, guilty, or inadequate. They may stigmatize mental illness and resist responses to questions concerning depressive symptoms. Patients with depression may have problems with concentration and memory. If the clinician feels this is a possibility he or she must interview family members or people who live with the patient to get a better idea of the patient's history. There may be cultural and language barriers that lead to underdiagnosis or misdiagnosis (20).

HISTORY

When taking a medical history for depression, the primary care provider should have four goals in mind. First, the patient's symptomatology and other medical history should be assessed using criteria for the diagnosis of depression. Second, the history should be focused by the severity of the episode, including a clear discussion of suicidality. Third, there should be a careful assessment of any confounding medical and psychiatric illness which would influence the patient's treatment. Fourth, an assessment of the patient's risk factors and overall presentation should be organized in a manner that will allow an assessment for the choice of treatment.

Ideally, all patients should be screened for depressive symptoms either by use of a standardized scale or by a series of routine questions about their risk factors. Risk factors for depression include previous history of depression, dysthymia, family history of both bipolar and unipolar major depressive illness, history of substance abuse, medical illness, and stressful life events such as unemployment or marital conflict (24). Patients should be asked about their sleep patterns such as insomnia and early morning awakening. They should be questioned directly about their mood and energy level, with particular attention to tearfulness and feelings of hopelessness. Questioning should also address changes in appetite and weight, libido and changes in sex life. Life enjoyment should be pursued as depressed patients often report a loss of interest and a lack of joy in anything, even things they once enjoyed. It may also be important to interview a family member or someone who lives with the patient to assess how that patient has been doing at home or work. Have they changed substantially? Has the patient been confused or delusional? Depressed patients will often have mood congruent delusions that focus on their worthlessness, past or present failures, or their sinfulness or guilt (11). A detailed medication history should be obtained. The provider must also assess the patient's present and past illicit drug and alcohol history. Does the patient have systemic complaints that are incongruent with the diagnosis of depression? A search should be made for both confounding psychiatric and medical illness. Is the patient also experiencing panic attacks or extreme anxiety? Does the patient have either a present history or past history consistent with mania that would suggest bipolar illness? Is the patient currently suicidal? If the patient is suicidal, a detailed history of the patient's suicidal intent should be obtained (see Evaluation of the Suicidal Patient). What are the patients most debilitating symptoms? Does the patient have coexisting medical problems that would result in a preference for certain antidepressant drugs versus the use of psychotherapy? Has the patient responded well to a particular treatment in the past?

PHYSICAL EXAMINATION

A patient who presents with new onset of depression should have a detailed physical examination looking for other underlying illness which might be causative. The patient's weight should be documented and followed closely. Blood pressure should be checked in anticipation of starting antidepressant medication. Signs of thyroid disease should be searched for. This should include checking for tachycardia, tremor, thyroid enlargement or nodules, exophthalmos or lid lag, and "hung up" reflexes. In patients with weight loss, attention should be directed to finding masses, lymphadenopathy, or blood in the stool which would suggest an underlying carcinoma.

LABORATORY EVALUATION

There are no confirmatory laboratory tests for the diagnosis of depression. However, laboratory testing can occasionally uncover a medical illness in a "depressed" patient. Screen patients for electrolyte abnormalities including hypercalcemia and hyponatremia. Liver function tests and a complete blood count (CBC) may be useful to search for underlying infection or carcinoma. Thyroid disease may be subtle, especially in the elderly, therefore thyroid function tests may be of use in ruling out occult thyroid disease. If treatment with a tricyclic antidepressant drug is contemplated, a baseline electrocardiogram should be obtained. Assess the patient's renal and liver functions before drug treatment as reductions in drug clearance may potentiate side effects.

Differential Diagnosis

To correctly establish the diagnosis of major depression, symptoms cannot be caused by bereavement, adverse drug reaction, medical illness, or other psychiatric disorders. Uncomplicated bereavement acknowledges that the grieving individual may present with symptoms consistent with major depression including insomnia, decreased appetite, and weight loss. However, with bereavement, this symptom complex is directly related to a significant loss and occurs in a self-limited time frame. The diagnosis of major depression usually cannot be made until these symptoms have persisted beyond 2 months. However, one should consider the diagnosis of major depression if the grieving individual develops marked functional impairment, severe psychomotor retardation, an overwhelming sensation of worthlessness, excessive guilt, severe preoccupation with thoughts of death or suicide, or hallucinatory experiences beyond believing he or she hears the voice of or transiently sees the deceased loved one (11).

Medical illness presenting as depression needs to be considered. The literature estimates that 10–20% of patients with mood disorders have an undiagnosed medical condition or are taking medications that are causing the depression. However, the causal role of medical illness in depression may be overestimated. The clinician must be aware that certain drugs and many medical illnesses can cause depressive syndromes. Depression can be caused by many pharmaceuticals used in the outpatient setting, including beta blockers, corticosteroids, oral contraceptives and other hormonal preparations, anti-hypertensive drugs including reserpine, methyldopa, guanethidine, hydralazine and clonidine, and anti-Parkinsonian drugs, including amantadine and carbidopa. Benzodiazepines and antipsychotic drugs may cause depression. Alcohol may contribute to a depressive syndrome as does the use of amphetamines, opiates, and cocaine.

Some of the medical illnesses implicated as causative depression include the following:

- Metabolic/endocrine causes: hypothyroidism, hyperthyroidism, Cushing's syndrome, hypercalcemia, hyponatremia, B-12 deficiency
- Cancer: pancreatic, lung, renal, brain, gastrointestinal
- Neurologic: seizure disorder, Parkinson's disease, stroke, multiple sclerosis
- Autoimmune disease: lupus, rheumatoid arthritis, sarcoidosis
- Infections: hepatitis, pneumonia, HIV infection and others
- Toxins: lead, mercury

Table 23.6.
Issues in Prescribing Anti-Depressants

	Tricyclics	SSRIs
Common side effects	Orthostatic hypotension, sedation, constipation, dry mouth, blurred vision, urinary retention, weight gain, tremor, lowered seizure threshold, quinidine-like slowing of cardiac conduction.	Agitation, nausea, headaches, anorexia, loss or delay or orgasm, delayed ejaculation, weight loss, tremor, potential interactions with cytochrome P-450 metabolized drugs.
Drug levels to assess therapy	Yes	No
Cost	Less expensive	More expensive
Overdose potential	Lethal	Non-lethal
Other illnesses benefitted	Panic disorder, chronic pain syndromes, migraine headache.	Obsessive compulsive disorder, ? chronic pain syndromes, ? panic disorder, ? substance abuse.
Contraindications	Concomitant monoamine oxidase inhibitors (MAOIs), narrow angle glaucoma, myocardial infarction within two weeks, severe cardiac conduction abnormalities.	Concomitant MAOIs.

Because primary depression is a common illness, differentiating the less common secondary causes of depression requires a thorough clinical evaluation. Hints favoring a secondary cause of depression include: no prior personal or family history of depression, late onset of depression (i.e., age greater than 45), visual hallucinations, rapid weight loss, atypical course, non-response to adequate antidepressant treatment, or physical examination and laboratory abnormalities suggesting another disease process (19).

Differentiating depression from dementia or depression superimposed on dementia can be a particularly difficult task. Elderly patients with depression may be harder to diagnosis as they are more likely to have confounding medical illness or medical therapies that can confuse the diagnose. Misdiagnosis of depression as dementia occurs 10–15% of the time. About 17% of patients with dementia will develop major depression and about 15% of patients with major depression will show evidence of cognitive impairment. Depressed patients are also more likely to have an acute onset of symptoms and more depressive complaints than patients with dementia. Dementia is an illness that causes a patient to lose intellectual function with demonstrable deficits in short and long term memory. The ability to do tasks requiring higher cortical function (i.e., ability to name objects, follow three part commands, ability to write a sentence) can also be impaired (11). Formal mini-mental status testing and the use of neuropsychologic testing may help

distinguish dementia from depression. In cases in which it is unclear, a trial of antidepressant medication may be warranted to establish the diagnosis.

Schizophrenia with secondary depression may be confused with depression with delusional features. The time course of the illness may be helpful in differentiating the two. Patients with schizophrenia should have a history of auditory hallucinations, worsening psychosocial dysfunction and a thought disorder that precedes the onset of depressive symptoms. Ultimately differentiating the two may not be crucial at the onset, as the treatment may be the same for both entities. The long-term prognosis for schizophrenia is worse.

Management

Acute management of the depressed patient requires an evaluation of suicidality. Patients not requiring hospitalization can be managed with psychotherapy or pharmaceutical therapy. An overview of treatment is presented in this section.

EVALUATION OF THE SUICIDAL PATIENT

Often providers are concerned that if they bring up the issue of suicide, they may encourage a patient to have these thoughts or to follow through on these thoughts. This is not true. Approximately 50% of all people who commit suicide have seen their doctors in the weeks to months before suicide,

Table 23.7.
Differences Among Common Anti-Depressants

Drug	Benefits	Dose Range[a] (mg)	Side Effect Profile
Amitriptyline/Elavil	Can treat chronic pain and migraine, good for insomnia	75–300	Most anticholinergic and most sedating TCA
Nortriptyline/ Pamelor	Good cardiovascular profile, good for elderly patients as less orthostatic hypotension	50–150	Less anticholinergic than amitriptyline and not as activating as desipramine
Desipramine/ Norpramin	Good for patients that need a less sedating drug	75–300	Least anticholinergic and least sedating TCA
Fluoxetine/Prozac	Good cardiac profile, good overdose profile, treats obsessive compulsive disorder, may treat panic disorder, chronic pain syndromes, substance abuse	20–80	Activating drug, decreases appetite, can cause sexual dysfunction, nausea, headache, insomnia, agitation, long half life of drug and metabolites (2–3 days)
Sertraline/Zoloft	Shorter half life of drug than Fluoxetine (1 day versus 2 days)	50–200	Similar to Fluoxetine, may be less likely than Fluoxetine to cause psychomotor agitation

[a]Higher dose ranges are used for more severely depressed patients; Elderly dose ranges are one third to one half of the standard adult dosage.

and many of them use medications prescribed by their physicians to end their lives. The patient may be grateful to be "discovered" and direct questioning may reveal a plan that may have otherwise gone unmentioned. Risk factors for suicide include male sex (men complete suicide more but women attempt suicide more), a previous history of attempted suicide, debilitating medical illness such as cancer and HIV infection, family history of suicide, depression, psychosis, alcoholism and drug dependence, unemployment, and poor social support systems. If the patient reveals a history of suicidal thought it is essential to assess the extent. Does the patient have a clear plan? Does he or she have access to a firearm? Are there medications available to him that can easily be used for an overdose? Has she suddenly started to put her life in order? Has he had a sudden lift in his depressed mood (18,26)? The clinician must be aware that patients' ability to contemplate and plan suicide increases as they become less depressed and as their energy level lifts enough to allow them to successfully carry out a suicide plan (18). Does the patient have a support system or a belief system that will prevent action

on suicidal thoughts? Can the patient promise to contact someone if contemplating suicide or does she admit to impulsivity and an inability to avoid risk taking behavior? Is there loss of impulse control through the use of drugs or alcohol? Once a detailed history is obtained, it is the clinician's responsibility to evaluate the overall suicide risk. Suicidality should be handled as a psychiatric emergency. Individuals who are high risk (clear plan, low impulse control, psychosis, previous history of serious attempt) should be assessed psychiatrically for inpatient evaluation and treatment. Patients who remain outpatients should have frequent follow up and 24-hour call availability. If there is any concern about the patient's ability to remain an outpatient, psychiatric consultation should be obtained. There should be a low threshold for psychiatric consultation with suicidality. Ideally, family members or friends should be enlisted to help monitor the patient. They should also be instructed to remove firearms and medications from the patient's access. All medications prescribed during a suicidal time period should be kept to small quantities. Follow-up must be frequent.

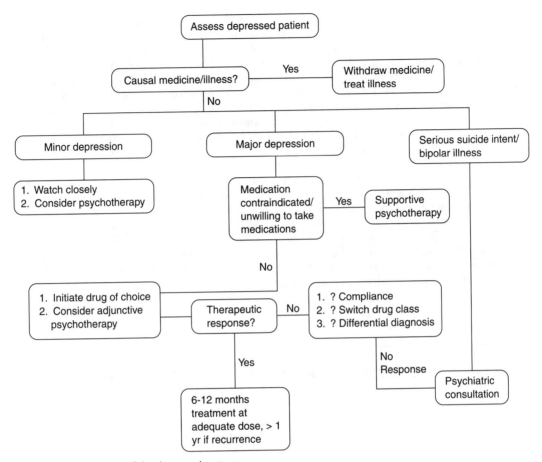

Figure 23.1. Treatment of the depressed patient.

TREATMENT STRATEGIES

Sufficient data exist to justify both the pharmacologic and psychotherapeutic treatment in certain categories of depression. The mainstay of treatment used by primary care providers is drug therapy. Most commonly, two classes of drugs, the tricyclic antidepressants (TCAs) and the selective serotonin reuptake inhibitors (SSRIs) will be selected. The primary care provider should also be aware of the efficacy of psychotherapy to adequately evaluate patients for referral.

Psychotherapy. The role of psychotherapy in the treatment of depression has not been established. The use of psychotherapy for the treatment of major depression has been evaluated in clinical trials.

Psychotherapy in the treatment of major depression is more efficacious than placebo and approaches the efficacy of drug treatment with tricyclic antidepressants. The literature also suggests

that the combination of psychotherapy with tricyclic antidepressant therapy may be a superior treatment modality to prevent recurrent depression. The studies cited looked at specific types of psychotherapy (interpersonal therapy and cognitive behavioral therapy) which makes it difficult to generalize these results to other types of psychotherapy.

Drug Therapy. The tricyclic antidepressant drugs have been in use for many years. They cause reuptake blockade of serotonin, norepinephrine and dopamine into the presynaptic neurons. They also cause blockade of the cholinergic, histaminergic and alpha-adrenergic receptors. Their degree of interaction with these various receptors causes them to have different side effect profiles. Clinical trials have well established the efficacy of tricyclic antidepressants in the treatment of major depression The SSRIs are potent inhibitors of the reuptake of serotonin. They are more selective for serotonin and have less interaction with norepinephrine and dopamine receptors, thus giving them a different side effect profile from the TCAs. SSRIs have been efficacious in the treatment of major depression. Long-term studies using these drugs for maintenance therapy are still pending. Current knowledge appears to indicate that for the majority of moderate to major depressions they may be interchangeable with TCAs. SSRIs for severe depression requiring hospitalization are less effective than the tricyclic drugs. Thus, in the severely depressed patient, TCAs may be the drug of choice. One advantage of the SSRIs is that the risk of lethal side effects with overdose is low as opposed to the tricyclic drugs that can have lethal effects in overdose. Table 23.6 compares the TCAs to the SSRIs. It is estimated that 60–70% of patients with acute major depression will respond to intensive drug treatment (27). Because no single drug has clear superiority, the choice of antidepressant drug becomes more

dependent on the patient's presentation, the potential interactions with the patient's current medical illnesses and medications, the desirable side effect profile of a particular drug, previous response to therapy, and cost. Table 23.7 compares three standard TCA therapies and two standard SSRI therapies. Three to six weeks may elapse before the antidepressant effect is appreciated. Patients need to be educated that it may take as long as a month before they note amelioration of their depressive symptoms. The need to be compliant with the drug despite the lack of early response needs to be emphasized. Patients must also be made aware that initially the side effects of the drug will often be most pronounced and, that with continued usage, many of their side effects will lessen or disappear. Figure 23.1 provides an algorithm for the evaluation of the depressed patient and treatment.

ILLUSTRATIVE CASES WITH SELF-ASSESSMENT QUESTIONS AND ANSWERS

Case 1

A 20-year-old college student comes to your office with complaints of fatigue, mild headaches, and an inability to concentrate on her work. These symptoms have been worsening over the last month and she often finds herself tearful over minor events.

QUESTION: *When taking her medical history, which of the following questions would be useful?*

a. Has she had a prior or family history of depression?
b. Is she currently sexually active?
c. Does she drink alcohol or take illicit drugs?
d. All of the above.

ANSWER: d. *The patient who presents with nonspecific complaints should raise the suspicion of undiagnosed depressive disease. History or family history of depression would increase this patient's risk. The use of illicit drugs and alcohol may be causal of the depressive symptoms and may also be self medication of an underlying de-*

pressive illness. Knowing the patient's sexual history may be helpful in confirming the diagnosis. A history of decreased libido would suggest depressive disease, while hypersexuality might hint at the diagnosis of bipolar illness. Contraception may also be a concern when the issue of treatment arises. A woman who is planning pregnancy may want to forgo drug therapy and use psychotherapy as the treatment of choice.

Case 2

A 68-year-old man is brought in to see you by his daughter. Since the death of his wife 6 months ago, he has not been himself. The daughter has noticed him to be tearful and often confused. She has been called by her father's landlord because he has not paid the rent in 2 months.

QUESTION: *What should you do next?*

a. Ask if his wife was managing their business affairs before her death?
b. Have the patient fill out a Beck's self-assessment depression questionnaire

c. Inform the daughter that her father is in a state of bereavement
d. Perform a mini-mental status exam on the patient
e. a, b, and d

ANSWER: e. *The differential diagnosis in this patient would be dementia versus depression or depression superimposed on previous dementia. It would be useful to find out if his wife was doing all the business transactions prior to her death. It may be helpful to have the patient do a Beck scale if he can cooperate with it: the inability to do one may indicate intellectual impairment seen in dementia. A mini mental status examination will also help quantify intellectual impairment and help to differentiate depression. This is not normal bereavement as it has continued for 6 months and presents with a prominent component of confusion.*

Case 3

A 37-year-old mother of two toddlers comes to your office distraught. She has a history of major depression in her 20s requiring hospitalization. She has been suicidal in the past. When questioned about suicide she initially admits she has been thinking of driving her car over a bridge. When you mention to her that these are worrisome thoughts she says, "I knew I shouldn't have come here, you can't help me. No one can!"

QUESTION: *What should you do?*

a. Allow her to go home and plan to call her tomorrow when she is feeling better
b. Seek psychiatric consultation immediately
c. Prescribe a mild tranquilizer to calm her nerves and help her get some sleep
d. Have her escorted to the psychiatric consultation area in the emergency room when she refuses to be evaluated voluntarily
e. b and d

ANSWER: e. *Suicidal ideation with a plan is a medical emergency especially in this high risk patient with a history of suicide attempt and severe major depression. It is inappropriate to prescribe tranquilizers to a potentially suicidal patient in this situation. If the patient is unwilling to present for psychiatric consultation or cannot be trusted to get there safely she should be escorted in a manner that will allow for her ultimate safety.*

MULTIPLE SOMATIC COMPLAINTS

Multiple somatic complaints are physical complaints out of proportion to or not attributable to what one would expect on the basis of objective medical findings. Somatizing patients are ubiquitous in health care settings worldwide, and make up the majority of patients who have multiple somatic complaints. Somatization may be defined as a tendency to experience physical distress in response to psychosocial difficulties and to seek medical help for this distress. Somatizers pose major medical, social, and economic problems because they often present with medical and diagnostic difficulties, and are major users of medical care, contributing to the increasing cost of health care.

For the purpose of understanding clinical pathology, most of the other chapters in this book deal with disease processes from which signs and symptoms are induced. The problems presented in this chapter, as well as in most of primary care clinical medicine, involve deductive reasoning; that is, a patient presents with certain signs and symptoms, the clinician creates a differential diagnosis, and then collects more data to make a definitive diagnosis on which treatment is based.

Unfortunately, when patients present with multiple somatic complaints, clinicians are often faced with patients who are difficult to treat. Some may have seen many physicians because they feel that no one seems to be able to diagnose their problem, or they feel they are not treated seriously by other health care providers. Some may be patients that many clinicians are thankful to be rid of because of frustration over the difficult relationship with these patients. In addition, most will have undergone many diagnostic tests and even "curative" procedures (e.g., hysterectomy), some of which may have been unnecessary (Table 23.8).

Pathophysiologic Correlation

Patients with somatic complaints force the clinician to enter the murky, but critical, area between internal medicine and neuropsychiatry. The body of literature regarding somatic symptoms is small in comparison to the large number of patients clinicians see with multiple somatic complaints. Knowledge of the brain and how it works lags substantially behind the body's other organ systems. With its hundreds of trillions of neuronal connections, the brain's complex physiology and pathophysiology is understood on a rudimentary level. Although modern science may not understand the pathophysiology of what these patients are suffering from,

Table 23.8.
Five Points to Remember Regarding Patients with Multiple Somatic Complaints

1. Multiple somatic complaints are extremely common in the primary care population.
2. Multiple somatic complaints have a high incidence of comorbidity with other psychiatric diagnoses, most notably, depression, panic, and substance abuse disorders.
3. The primary care clinician must employ his or her best deductive skills in reaching a diagnosis in this complex area; otherwise tests and procedures may be performed unnecessarily.
4. Often, negative countertransference (reaction) of physicians toward somatizing patients makes it difficult to engage these patients (and/or the physicians) in the treatment.
5. The problems these patients suffer are almost always very real to them, and are often treatable either by treating the underlying psychiatric disorder(s), or by treating the primary somatoform disorder.

they are, nonetheless, suffering from something that is most likely biologically based, is real to the patient, and is often treatable (with certain exceptions).

The pathophysiology of somatization disorder is unknown. Yet, other psychiatric diagnoses associated with somatization, mostly depression and panic disorders do have pathophysiological correlates but operate by mechanisms that are also largely unknown. Depression has been associated with a change in neuronal intracellular regulation in response to intrasynaptic decreases in monoamines such as serotonin and norepinephrine. Panic has also been associated with up and downregulation of various neurotransmitters including monoamines (especially norepinephrine), and GABA (gamma amino butyric acid).

EPIDEMIOLOGY

The few epidemiological studies that do exist indicate that a large percentage of the population (anywhere from 5 to 75%, depending on the study) visit primary care physicians because of psychosocial stress manifested by somatic complaints. Patients with psychiatric disorders have a very high incidence of somatic complaints (60 to 90%). Likewise, patients with somatization have a high lifetime prevalence of depression (approximately 50%).

Somatization disorder (Table 23.9), the most restrictive diagnosis among patients who somatize, has an incidence of 0.2 to 2.0% among women and less than 0.2% among men in the general population. In those patients who have somatization disorder found in a general primary care population, the prevalence of depression is as high as 90% among females, and a little more than 50% in all patients (both male and female).

There is a familial pattern to somatization disorder. It is observed in 10 to 20% of biological, first-degree female relatives of women with the disorder. The biological first degree male relatives of women with somatization disorder are at an increased risk for antisocial personality disorder and substance related disorders.

DEFINITION OF THE RELEVANT PSYCHIATRIC DISEASE STATES

The *Diagnostic and Statistical Manual of Mental Disorders*, Fourth Edition (better known as *DSM-IV*, the most recent version of the psychiatric diagnostic manual) lists the defining characteristics of each of the diagnoses considered in patients with multiple somatic complaints. There are four general groups for multiple somatic complaints.

The first category involves physical symptoms due to a general medical condition or due to drug use, or not in excess of such a medical condition or drug effect.

The term "general medical condition" literally refers to those diseases that fall under Axis III in the *International Classification of Diseases 9th Revision, Clinical Modification* (or ICD-9- CM). Axis III is one of five axes. Each axis refers to a different domain of information about a patient that may help the clinician plan treatment and predict outcome. A good example of a general medical condition causing a psychiatric problem (under Axis III) is HIV dementia, where the virus itself may cause all of the symptoms of full blown dementia.

DSM-IV gives an important caveat in noting that the term general medical condition is merely a shorthand among health care providers. It does not indicate that there are two unrelated realms of medicine and psychiatry; but rather that even though these two realms profoundly affect one another, treatment may be different depending on the problem. For example, the diagnoses of three patients who present with abdominal pain may be constipation, duodenal ulcer, or a somatoform disorder. Even though all of the patients may ultimately find the source of their problem to be due

Table 23.9.
Criteria for Diagnosis of Somatization Disorder

A. A history of many physical complaints beginning before age 30 years that occur over a period of several years and result in treatment being sought or significant impairment in social, occupational, or other important areas of functioning.

B. Each of the following criteria must have been met, with individual symptoms occurring at any time during the course of the disturbance:

1. *Four pain symptoms:* a history of pain related to at least four different sites or functions (e.g., head, abdomen, back, joints, extremities, chest, rectum, during menstruation, during sexual intercourse, or during urination)

2. *Two gastrointestinal symptoms:* a history of at least two gastrointestinal symptoms other than pain (e.g., nausea, bloating, vomiting other than during pregnancy, diarrhea, or intolerance of several different foods)

3. *One sexual symptom:* a history of at least one sexual or reproductive symptom other than pain (e.g., sexual indifference, erectile or ejaculatory dysfunction, irregular menses, excessive menstrual bleeding, vomiting throughout pregnancy)

4. *One pseudoneurological symptom:* a history of at least one symptom or deficit suggesting a neurological condition not limited to pain (conversion symptoms such as impaired coordination or balance, paralysis or localized weakness, difficulty swallowing or lump in throat, aphonia, urinary retention, hallucinations, loss of touch or pain sensation, double vision, blindness, deafness, seizures; dissociative symptoms such as amnesia; or loss of consciousness other than fainting)

C. Either 1 or 2:

1. After appropriate investigation, each of the symptoms in Criterion B cannot be fully expanded by a known general medical condition or the direct effects of a substance (e.g., a drug of abuse, a medication)

2. When there is a related general medical condition, the physical complaints or resulting social or occupational impairment are in excess of what would be expected from the history, physical examination, or laboratory findings

D. The symptoms are not intentionally produced or feigned (as in Factitious Disorder or Malingering).

From Diagnostic and Statistical Manual of Mental Health DSM-IV. 4th ed. Washington D.C.: American Psychiatric Association, 1994:349–450.

to psychosocial stressors, the way they are managed will be quite different.

The second of the four groupings for multiple somatic complaints involves physical symptoms that are self-induced. Self-induced physical symptoms fall into two diagnoses: factitious disorders and malingering. Factitious disorders are characterized by physical or psychological symptoms that are intentionally produced or feigned in order to assume the sick role. For example, an individual presenting with hematuria is found to have anticoagulants in his possession. The person denies having taken them, but blood studies are consistent with the ingestion of anticoagulants.

In malingering, the individual also produces the symptoms intentionally, but has a goal that is obviously recognizable when the environmental circumstances are known. For example, the intentional production of symptoms to avoid jury duty, standing trial, or conscription into the military would be classified as malingering.

Major psychiatric diagnoses, other than somatoform disorders, comprise the third diagnostic category of patients with multiple somatic complaints.

The most important psychiatric diagnoses that cause multiple symptoms include depression and anxiety disorders (Tables 23.10, 23.11, 23.12). Panic disorder is the most common of the anxiety disorders that cause multiple somatic complaints; although multiple symptoms may also be seen in obsessive-compulsive disorder (OCD).

Psychotic patients may also somatize. Schizophrenia is the major diagnosis within the group of pure psychotic disorders. Schizophrenia occurs in approximately one percent of the population. The lifetime prevalence of psychosis is much higher when one includes the mood disorders within this group of psychotic disorders, as patients with severe mood disorders may become psychotic. A patient can be diagnosed as psychotic if he or she has prominent hallucinations (of any sensory system) or has delusions (i.e., fixed, false beliefs).

Physical symptoms that are not part of the above three groupings are nearly all found under somatoform disorders. The common feature of the somatoform disorders is the presence of physical symptoms that suggest a general medical condition (hence, the term somatoform) and are not fully

Table 23.10.
Criteria for Diagnosis of Major Depression

A. Five (or more) of the following symptoms have been present during the same 2-week period and represent a change from previous functioning; at least one of the symptoms is either (1) depressed mood or (2) loss of interest or pleasure. Do not include symptoms that are clearly due to a general medical condition, or mood-incongruent delusions or hallucinations.
   1. Depressed mood most of the day, nearly every day, as indicated by either subjective report (e.g., feels sad or empty) or observation made by others (e.g., appear tearful). **Note:** In children and adolescents, can be irritable mood.
   2. Markedly diminished interest or pleasure in all, or almost all, activities most of the day, nearly every day (as indicated by either subjective account or observation made by others)
   3. Significant weight loss when not dieting or weight gain (e.g., a change of more than 5% of body weight in a month), or decrease or increase in appetite nearly every day. **Note:** in children, consider failure to make expected weight gains.
   4. Insomnia or hypersomnia nearly every day.
   5. Psychomotor agitation or retardation nearly every day (observable by others, not merely subjective feelings of restlessness or being slowed down).
   6. Fatigue or loss of energy nearly every day.
   7. Feelings of worthlessness or excessive or inappropriate guilt (which may be delusional) nearly every day (not merely self-reproach or guilt about being sick).
   8. Diminished ability to think or concentrate, or indecisiveness, nearly every day (either by subjective account or as observed by others).
   9. Recurrent thoughts of death (not just fear of dying), recurrent suicidal ideation without a specific plan, or suicide attempt or a specific plan for committing suicide.
B. The symptoms do not meet criteria for Mixed Episode.
C. The symptoms cause clinically significant distress or impairment in social, occupational, or other important areas of functioning.
D. The symptoms are not due to the direct physiological effects of a substance (e.g., a drug of abuse, a medication) or a general medical condition (e.g., hypothyroidism).
E. The symptoms are not better accounted for by Bereavement, i.e., after the loss of a loved one, the symptoms persist for longer than 2 months or are characterized by marked functional impairment, morbid preoccupation with worthlessness, suicidal ideation, psychotic symptoms, or psychomotor retardation.

From Diagnostic and Statistical Manual of Mental Health DSM-IV. 4th ed. Washington D.C.: American Psychiatric Association, 1994:327.

explained by a general medical condition, by the direct effects of a substance, or by another mental disorder (e.g., depression). The symptoms must cause clinically significant distress or impairment in social, occupational, or other areas of functioning. In contrast to factitious disorders and malingering, the physical symptoms are not intentional (i.e., under voluntary control). The grouping of these disorders in a single section is based on clinical utility (i.e., the need to exclude occult general medical conditions or substance-induced etiologies for the bodily symptoms) rather than on assumptions regarding shared etiology or mechanisms. These disorders are often encountered in general medical settings. DSM-IV defines them as follows:

Somatization Disorder (historically referred to as hysteria or Briquet's syndrome) is a polysymptomatic disorder that begins before age 30 years, extends over a period of years, and is characterized by a combination

of pain, gastrointestinal, sexual, and pseudo-neurological symptoms. (See Table 23.9).

Undifferentiated Somatoform Disorder is characterized by unexplained physical complaints, lasting at least 6 months, that are below the threshold for a diagnosis of somatization disorder.

Conversion Disorder involves unexplained symptoms or deficits affecting voluntary motor or sensory function that suggest a neurological or other general medical condition. Psychological factors are judged to be associated with the symptoms or deficits (e.g., an adolescent who loses the use of her leg the day before an important track meet)

Pain Disorder is characterized by pain as the predominant focus of clinical attention. In addition, psychological factors are judged to have an important role in its onset, severity, exacerbation, or maintenance.

Table 23.11.
Criteria for Diagnosis of Panic Disorder—Panic Attack

A panic attack is not a codable disorder. Code the specific diagnosis in which the panic attack occurs.

A discrete period of intense fear or discomfort, in which four (or more) of the following symptoms developed abruptly and reached a peak within 10 minutes.
1. palpitations, pounding heart, or accelerated heart rate
2. sweating
3. trembling or shaking
4. sensations or shortness of breath or smothering
5. feeling of choking
6. chest pain or discomfort
7. nausea or abdominal distress
8. derealization (feelings of unreality) or depersonalization (being detached from oneself)
9. fear of losing control or going crazy
10. fear of dying
11. paresthesias (numbness or tingling sensations)
12. chills or hot flushes

From Diagnostic and statistical manual of mental health DSM-IV. 4th ed. Washington D.C.: American Psychiatric Association, 1994:395.

Hypochondriasis is the preoccupation with the fear of having, or the idea that one has, a serious disease based on the person's misinterpretation of bodily symptoms or bodily functions.

Body Dysmorphic Disorder is the preoccupation with an imagined or exaggerated defect in physical appearance.

Somatoform Disorder Not Otherwise Specified is included for coding disorders with somatoform symptoms that do not meet the criteria for any of the specific Somatoform Disorders.

From Diagnostic and statistical manual of mental health DSM-IV. 4th ed. Washington D.C.: American Psychiatric Association, 1994:445.

Clinical and Laboratory Evaluation

Physical and laboratory evaluations are significantly unremarkable in patients with multiple somatic complaints. Their history, however, is most important in making a proper diagnosis.

HISTORY

Chief Complaint. Elicit a chief complaint (even if the patient is there for a physical). Why is the patient there? Why did he or she come in on this particular day? These may seem like obvious questions but all too often the patient gives an inadequate response to these questions and the clinician moves on without this valuable information. Often the clinician must repeat the question more than once until a clear response is obtained. Missing what is most important to the patient is a common error and can be a serious one.

Potentially, a somatizing patient may present with a list of mild or non-acute symptoms. The clinician has to prioritize which symptom she or he will deal with on each visit and may have to wait for subsequent visits to deal with other symptoms.

Table 23.12.
Criteria for Diagnosis of Panic Disorder Without Agoraphobia

A. Both 1 and 2:
   1. recurrent unexpected Panic Attacks
   2. at least one of the attacks has been followed by 1 month (or more) of one (or more) of the following:
      a. persistent concern about having additional attacks
      b. worry about the implications of the attack or its consequences (e.g., losing control, having a heart attack, "going crazy")
      c. a significant change in behavior related to the attacks
B. Absence of Agoraphobia
C. The Panic Attacks are not due to the direct physiological effects of a substance (e.g., a drug of abuse, a medication) or a general medical condition (e.g., hyperthyroidism).
D. The Panic Attacks are not better accounted for by another mental disorder, such as Social Phobia (e.g., occurring on exposure to feared social situations), Specific Phobia (e.g., on exposure to a specific phobic situation), Obsessive-Compulsive Disorder (e.g., on exposure to dirt in someone with an obsession about contamination), Posttraumatic Stress Disorder (e.g., in response to stimuli associated with a severe stressor), or Separation Anxiety Disorder (e.g., in response to being away from home or close relatives).

From Diagnostic and Statistical Manual of Mental Health DSM-IV. 4th ed. Washington D.C.: American Psychiatric Association, 1994:402.

Symptoms that are part of the chief complaint must be addressed in some fashion in the present visit.

History of Present Illness (HPI). Somatizers often describe their complaints in terms that are colorful and exaggerated; however, specific factual information may be lacking. The history may reveal visits to many physicians, use of multiple medications (prescribed and not prescribed), and multiple hospitalizations and procedures. In some cases, many of these medical treatments may be going on concurrently, leading to complicated and possibly hazardous therapy. Inherently, the treatments themselves may have morbidity associated with them.

As with all histories, one must illicit psychosocial stressors the patient may have in his or her life as well as if the patient is being seen in any type of mental health setting. Depression, anxiety, panic, and substance abuse disorders, in addition to histrionic, borderline and antisocial personality disorders are frequently associated with somatization disorder.

Past Medical History. Every surgery, procedure, hospitalization, medication, walk-in encounter with a clinician, and visits to other alternative types of healers, must be understood within the context of the patient's presenting symptoms, the diagnosis given, and the precise nature of each therapeutic intervention, if any. In somatizing patients, past diagnoses will be ambiguous and treatments will be few. The few treatments that were provided are usually difficult to understand from a medical standpoint.

Psychiatric History. In taking any history, the primary care clinician must devote at least one question to the patient's use of mental health services, as well as obtaining a substance abuse history. This is especially important when dealing with somatizing patients because of the high comorbidity with the psychiatric illnesses noted in the previous section.

Review of Systems (ROS). To make the proper diagnosis, a review of symptoms must be complete. In other chapters of this book, the approach to a patient's pain is reviewed. (The important points being: Duration of the pain, its exact location, quality of the pain [e.g., sharp, dull], etiologic associations [e.g., eating, exercise, stress], other associated symptoms [e.g., vomiting or dizziness with headaches], what makes the pain become worse and better [e.g., medications, food, change in body position]).

After each symptom is reviewed in this routine manner, one must then press on with questions that will help place the symptoms either in the realm of known medical illnesses or in the functional realm.

All symptoms are important, as noted in the present criteria for somatization disorder from DSM-IV in Table 23.9. The symptoms noted in the DSM-IV criteria are the more common symptoms for making the diagnosis of somatization disorder, but they are by no means all inclusive.

Again, the review of systems must be exhaustive in a patient presenting with multiple somatic complaints. (In other chapters, the systems that one reviews have been delineated.)

PHYSICAL EXAMINATION

The physical examination must also be extremely thorough for diagnostic as well as therapeutic purposes. One must be very cautious not to miss a medical problem that may not be related to a patient's symptomatology.

In addition, the therapeutic nature of a hands-on physical examination can be enormous. In fact, the anxiety often alleviated by a thorough physical exam is the backbone of current therapy for somatoform disorders.

LABORATORY EVALUATION

As with the physical examination and the history, the laboratory evaluation must be reasonably thorough. However, it becomes difficult to avoid wasting hundreds or thousands of dollars while still feeling satisfied as a clinician, as well as having the patient feel satisfied, that all significant medical diagnostic questions have been covered.

Again, it is therapeutic to the patient to know that his or her symptoms are being taken seriously. Indeed, a reasonably thorough evaluation truly reduces anxiety in all patients, not just somatizing patients.

Unfortunately, there is no absolute answer to the question of what is reasonably thorough. If one puts together a thorough history and physical, the clinician should have enough data to permit selective ordering of screening tests that are related to the data (noted in other chapters).

Differential Diagnosis

The symptomatology of patients with multiple somatic complaints usually presents a perplexing diagnostic dilemma for the primary care clinician. First of all, the symptoms can overlap with general (diagnosable) medical conditions. Often the general medical conditions or the medications given for these conditions have a large symptom profile.

GENERAL MEDICAL CONDITIONS AND PSYCHOLOGICAL PROBLEMS

If a general medical condition has been diagnosed, the clinician must be aware of how that condition is affected by the patient's psychological state. For example, psychological factors can play a significant etiological role in the development of common problems (Table 23.13). Grief, as a specific example, is known to cause a lowering of the immune system, allowing a patient to become prone to serious infection and even subsequent death. These illnesses are considered psychosomatic illnesses. Psychosomatic medicine emphasizes the mind/body unity and supports the conviction that all diseases have important psychological factors that can play a role in the initiation, the progression, the aggravation, the exacerbation, and the resolution of a disease.

There are many medical conditions which cause an alteration in a patient's psychological state. For a mild illness with a short course, other than the misery one may feel from the illness itself, there may be no long-lasting effects other than the anxiety the patient may have knowing he or she is behind when returning to school or work. If, however, a patient suffered many such short illnesses, the clinician would have to search for both medical and psychological etiological factors (the latter are detailed later).

Long-term illnesses are nearly always accompanied by significant psychological problems. Recovery time from cardiac surgery, for example, has been shown to be significantly reduced by treating the postoperative patient psychiatrically, as well as medically. Curable cancer patients, as well as terminal patients, have also been shown to benefit substantially from psychiatric help.

PSYCHIATRIC DIAGNOSES FOR MULTIPLE SOMATIC COMPLAINTS

Whether a patient has a diagnosable illness or not, the clinician must consider a psychiatric diagnosis (in addition to any medically diagnosed illness) if: (a) there is multiple organ system involvement; (b) symptoms have been chronically present for many years without historical evidence of physical signs, laboratory abnormalities, or structural abnormalities; or (c), symptoms are out of proportion to or not attributable to objective medical findings.

Two important points to remember before pursuing a psychiatric diagnosis are as follows:

(1) Rule out conditions such as hypothyroidism, hyperparathyroidism, multiple sclerosis, and systemic lupus erythematosus which can produce confusing, vague, multiple somatic complaints.

(2) Multiple physical symptoms presenting later in life (older than 40) are most often due to a general medical condition.

Self-Induced Disorders. The psychiatric differential diagnosis of a patient with multiple somatic symptoms begins with an assessment of whether the symptoms could be self-induced. A malingerer will feign physical or psychological symptoms for external secondary gain such as avoiding work, obtaining financial gain, evading criminal prosecution, or obtaining drugs. Malingering should be strongly suspected if an attorney refers the patient to the clinician and there is a lack of cooperation during the diagnostic evaluation or in complying with the prescribed regimen.

Factitious disorder is a bit more difficult to detect. The intentionally produced or feigned symptoms in this disorder provide the patient with internal rewards revolving around the psychological need for the patient to assume the sick role. Some clues that a patient may have factitious disorder include: Fabrication of subjective symptoms (e.g., complaining of pain that does not exist), self-

Table 23.13.
Some Psychosomatic Disorders

Acne	Mucous colitis
Allergic reactions	Nausea
Angina pectoris	Neurodermatitis
Angioneurotic edema	Obesity
Arrhythmia	Painful menstruation
Asthmatic wheezing	Pruritus ani
Cardiospasm	Pylorospasm
Chronic pain syndromes	Regional enteritis
Coronary heart disease	Rheumatoid arthritis
Diabetes mellitus	Sacroiliac pain
Duodenal ulcer	Skin disease, such as
Essential hypertension	psoriasis
Gastric ulcer	Spastic colitis
Headache	Tachycardia
Herpes	Tension headache
Hyperinsulinism	Tuberculosis
Hyperthyroidism	Ulcerative colitis
Hypoglycemia	Urticaria
Immune diseases	Vomiting
Irritable colon	Warts
Migraine	

From Kaplan HI, Sadock BJ, Grebb JA. Kaplan and Sadock's synopsis of psychiatry, 7th ed. Baltimore: Williams & Wilkins, 1994:754.

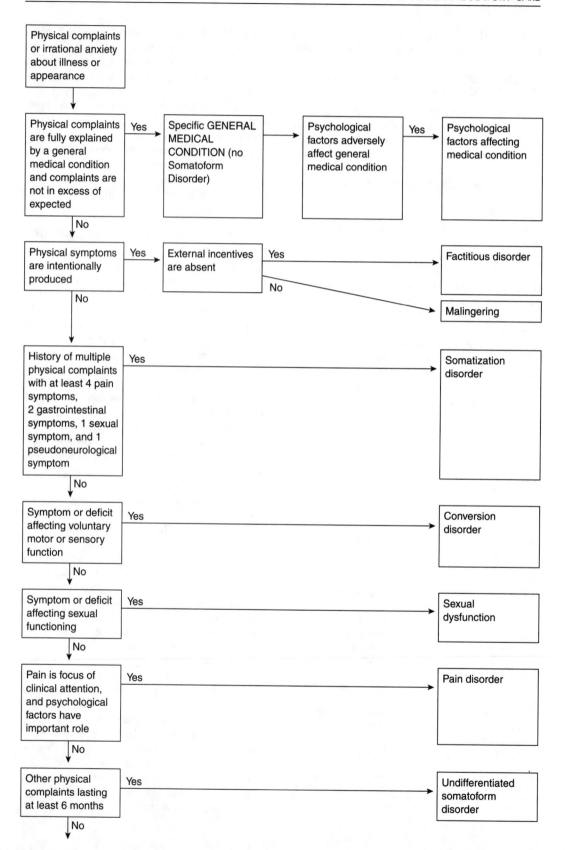

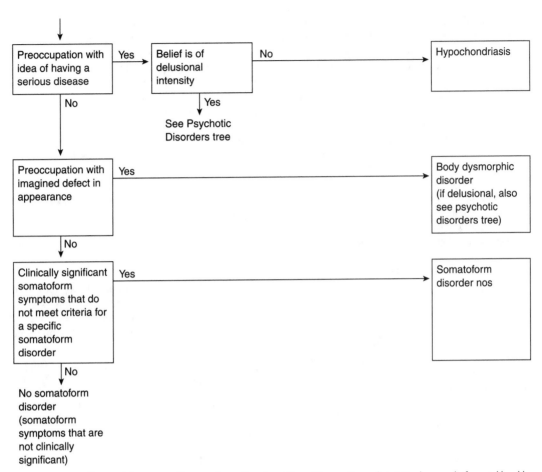

Figure 23.2. Differential diagnosis of somatoform disorders. (From Diagnostic and statistical manual of mental health DSM-IV. 4th ed. Washington D.C.: American Psychiatric Association, 1994:700–1.)

induced conditions (e.g., taking anticoagulants to produce hematuria), or exacerbation of preexisting medical problems (e.g., presenting with symptoms of a myocardial infarction but not having the MI, in a patient with known coronary artery disease), extremely vague and inconsistent histories, pathological lying, extensive knowledge of medical terminology and hospital routines, complaints of pain and requests for analysis, production of other symptoms when the initial work up is negative, and an eagerness to undergo procedures and surgery.

Often, these patients would not be discovered until someone recognizes a particular patient or a particular patient's story from another hospital. When the diagnosis of a factitious disorder is made, the patient will usually deny it and will then leave the hospital against medical advice, only to turn up in another hospital.

In almost all instances, feigned or intentionally produced symptoms will be ruled out early in the diagnostic process.

Psychotic, Affective, and Anxiety Disorders. The next important psychiatric group of illnesses to rule out are the psychotic disorders. When considering a psychiatric differential diagnosis, the clinician must inquire about past or present hallucinations. Delusions are difficult to identify, but they usually become evident in a history that allows the patients to talk about him or herself. Often this requires some open-ended personal questions, such as asking about a patient's family life. When a patient reports hallucinations or is noted to have delusions, it is less likely that a somatoform disorder exists although they rarely coexist as diagnoses in the same individual.

Psychotic patients may present with somatic delusions that focus on a few vague somatic symptoms (e.g., a belief that they have AIDS because they are feeling tired and have headaches, with the feared risk factor being the patient had kissed someone last year).

Mood disorders and anxiety disorders often co-exist with somatization disorder. As with psychosis, depression (which can present with psychosis), and panic disorder must be screened for in a patient in which a psychiatric diagnosis is being considered for multiple somatic complaints. If the somatic symptoms exist when the patient is not depressed or having panic attacks, then the patient is likely to have the additional diagnosis of a somatoform disorder as defined above. For example, if a depressed patient has somatic symptoms only while depressed (most commonly headaches, gastrointestinal disturbances or unexplained pain), he or she only needs to be treated for depression. The somatic symptoms will improve as the depression resolves.

Somatoform Disorders. If unexplained symptomatology still exists after general medical conditions, and psychosis, mood disorders, and anxiety disorders have all been considered, then the patient either has a somatoform disorder or has somatoform symptoms that are not clinically significant. Figure 23.2, from DSM-IV, provides an excellent algorithm for the differential diagnosis of somatoform disorders. Primary care clinicians should be able to distinguish between these diagnoses, as their involvement is instrumental in treating patients with somatoform disorders.

Among somatoform disorders, the most restrictive diagnosis is somatization disorder (See Table 23.9) that encompasses elements of all subsequent diagnoses. Note that if a patient has symptoms that fall under any one of the four criteria noted in section B (but none of the other criteria in section B), they would have either: (#1) pain disorder; (#3) sexual dysfunction; or (#4) conversion disorder, respectively. Patients who have multiple symptoms but do not meet criteria for somatization disorder, have either undifferentiated somatoform disorder if they have had the symptoms greater than 6 months; or somatoform disorder not otherwise specified (NOS), if it has been less than 6 months. Psychological factors must be judged to be associated with the symptoms for the diagnoses of conversion disorder and pain disorder to be made.

Hypochondriasis and body dysmorphic disorder both involve perceptual disturbances of how a patient's body functions or looks. In hypochondriasis,

a patient is preoccupied with the fear that they have a serious disease despite reassurance after medical evaluation that their symptoms are not due to serious illness. Body dysmorphic disorder is similar in that the patient's perceptions are distorted involving their physical appearance despite having either a minor or no physical anomaly present. In both disorders, the clinician must rule out delusional thinking and obsessive-compulsive disorder.

Once a patient has been diagnosed as having a psychiatric cause of her multiple symptoms, it is extremely important for her not to be labeled as a difficult patient. Labelling a patient in this negative way often interferes with treatment and may prevent the clinician from picking up other independent medical conditions.

Management

For the primary care clinician, the patient with unexplained multiple somatic complaints is often the most difficult and unrewarding patient to treat. These patients take a lot of office and phone time and rarely seem to get better.

PSYCHIATRIC MANAGEMENT OF PATIENTS WITH GENERAL MEDICAL CONDITIONS

It is much easier and more rewarding to treat patients with complicated medical problems because these patients have measurable changes in their physical health status. If the primary care clinician is attuned to the psychological factors affecting many common illnesses (see Table 23.13) he or she will be able to institute long-term preventive or maintenance therapy as well as addressing the immediate problems (e.g., stress reduction as well as pharmacotherapy after an MI).

In the past, psychotherapy and psychoanalysis had been the mainstays of psychiatric treatment for psychosomatic disorders (in addition to medical management). Over the last 20 years, many forms of behavioral modification (learning theory) have also proven to be effective treatment. Forms of behavioral therapy include biofeedback, hypnosis, controlled breathing, yoga, massage, and muscle relaxation therapy. From a psychiatric as well as a medical standpoint, regular exercise has also been an effective tool in improving psychosomatic illness. Psychological problems arising from long-term (or even short-term) medical illnesses usually respond to psychotherapy.

MANAGEMENT OF PSYCHIATRIC DISORDERS

Management for most psychiatric disorders should be instituted with psychiatric assistance. This does not necessarily mean that the primary care clinician will not be delivering the primary mode of management.

Self-Induced Symptoms. *Malingering* It is important to maintain the clinician-patient relationship in patients who are malingering. This requires the clinician not to divulge his or her suspicions. By maintaining the positive relationship without a confrontation, the patient is more apt to reveal the relevant issue, as he or she will not feel the need to be continuously on guard. It is usually best to use a psychotherapeutic intervention treatment approach, so when he gives up his symptoms, he can do so without losing face.

Factitious disorder The outcome in factitious disorders is not good. The disorders are often incapacitating to patients. Treatment is based on management as there is no cure. Most helpful, and probably most difficult, in managing these patients is early recognition of the disorder. This can forestall and possibly prevent useless and sometimes detrimental diagnostic tests and procedures.

Factitious disorder by proxy is most often found when a parent gives or does something to his or her child so that the parent can indirectly play the sick role. The primary care clinician must bring these cases to the attention of the child welfare services. They, in turn, will need to keep a presence in the home to protect at-risk children.

Treatment for people with factitious disorders is so difficult because once the patient's method of receiving attention is removed, they leave treatment and attempt to do the same thing at another facility. It is best to try and help the patient reframe their intentional illness as a cry for help, so that the patient does not see the clinician's actions as punitive.

For patients with factitious disorders, and even for malingerers, it is important for the primary care provider to work closely with a psychiatrist. It is also important to avoid showing the patient the anger often experienced by the patient's health care providers because of the patient's attempt to deceive them. Expressing this anger toward the patient only breaks an alliance that could otherwise be beneficial in treatment.

Psychotic, Affective, and Anxiety Disorders. Patients with psychotic, affective, and anxiety disorders can all present with multiple somatic complaints. The primary care provider must be able to recognize these disorders early, as nearly a quarter of all patients have a lifetime prevalence of one or more of these serious illnesses. Often these patients do not get diagnosed with a psychiatric problem until the patient's illness has progressed to a point where there is a substantial decline in one or more areas of the patient's life. Picking up these disorders early leads to more effective treatment, as well as less disruption in a patient's life.

Treatment for psychotic disorders should only be undertaken by psychiatrists; however, the primary care provider's role is critical in recognition and treatment. It is his or her role to help patients understand that they have a treatable illness and they need to be seen by a psychiatrist. The primary care clinician must still act as the liaison between the subspecialist (the psychiatrist) and the patient. Close contact with the primary care clinician while the patient is undergoing psychiatric treatment is seen as supportive and is likely to aid in recovery.

Psychosis For psychotic patients, the neuroleptic class of drugs are employed. Older, more sedating, drugs include chlorpromazine (Thorazine) and thioridazine (Mellaril). These drugs also tend to have a greater ability to induce seizures. They also tend to have more anticholinergic side effects which include dry mouth, urinary retention, constipation, blurry vision, flushing, and dementia (in overdoses). The more powerful drugs such as haloperidol (Haldol) and fluphenazine (Prolixin) tend to include more of the extra pyramidal side (EPS) effects, such as psychomotor retardation, increased muscle tone, rhythmic body movements, and cogwheeling rigidity. These drugs also tend to be less sedating and have less anticholinergic side effects. Perphenazine (Trilafon) is a drug that falls in between the extremes of side effects noted.

Two new, very expensive drugs, risperidone (Risperdal) and clozapine (Clozaril), are just beginning to show positive results in treating patients unresponsive to previous therapies or limited by side effect profiles of earlier drugs. Clozapine seems to be particularly effective in treating patients who have had negative sensitivity to other medications; however, there is a small risk of patients becoming neutropenic on clozapine. Therefore, patients presently on this medication need to have a CBC drawn every week.

With all neuroleptics, one must watch for neuroleptic malignant syndrome (NMS) noted most often by rigidity, fever, and an increase in CPK (creatine phosphokinase). One must also watch for the sometimes irreversible side effect of tardive dyskinesia — involuntary tic-like movements of the face and mouth.

Affective disorders For major affective disorders and anxiety disorders, there are different classes of drugs that can be effective. Severe depression is most effectively treated with tricyclic antidepressants (TCAs) such as desipramine, imipramine or nortriptyline. These drugs mostly have anticholinergic side effects noted in the previous section. As with the less powerful neuroleptics (e.g., chlorpromazine, thioridazine), orthostatic hypotension may develop with the tricyclics. Drug levels must be monitored regularly in patients on these medications.

Selective serotonin reuptake inhibitors (SSRIs) are also very effective antidepressant agents with excellent side effect profiles. Fluoxetine (Prozac), Paroxetine (Paxil), and Sertraline (Zoloft) presently are the major drugs in this class. Activation, headache, and weight loss are the most common side effects of these medications.

Monoamine oxidase inhibitors (MAOIs), such as phenelzine (Nardil) and tranylcypromine (Parnate), are another class of antidepressants most effective against atypical depression; however, with the advent of the SSRIs, these drugs are used far less than in the past. The decreased use of the MAOIs is due mostly to the food restrictions that are necessary because anyone taking the drug is likely to develop a hypertensive crisis if eating foods that contain tyramine (e.g., some cheeses, fruits, vegetables, meats, and alcohols, etc.)

Bupropion (Wellbutrin) and venlafaxine (Effexor) are new drugs that do not fall into any of the above classes of antidepressants. Their effectiveness as antidepressants is still to be tested and their side effect profile seems to be quite good.

Lithium is the mainstay of bipolar disorder therapy. It is often added to the regimen of patients with severe depression. Lithium has a small therapeutic index and drug levels must be monitored. Its side effects are many and include tremor, nausea and vomiting, diarrhea, thyroid dysfunction, diabetes insipidus, weight gain, cardiac arrhythmias, and EPS as noted above. Carbamazapine (Tegretol) and valproic acid (Depakene) are used also for emotionally labile patients if they cannot tolerate lithium.

Lithium and neuroleptics take 7 to 10 days to work effectively, while most of the antidepressants take 4 to 6 weeks to become effective. Overdoses of any of these medications can be quite serious. TCAs, MAOIs, and Lithium overdoses can be fatal in relatively small amounts. Although drugs from most different psychotropic classes can be used synergistically, MAOIs cannot be used safely with most other medications. Clinicians must be careful of the many interactions between psychotropic medications and other non-psychiatric medications.

Anxiety The class of drug most effective against anxiety is the benzodiazapines, which include lorazepam (Ativan), diazepam (Valium), alprazolam (Xanax), and chlordiazepoxide (Librium), to name but a few in this extensive class of medications. The major side effects noted with benzodiazapines are sedation and addiction. Tolerance to these medications is also a well-known phenomenon and therefore benzodiazapines are best used for individual episodes or for short periods of time.

Many of the antidepressants are used to prevent anxiety disorders. For example, anafranil (a TCA) is very effective against obsessive-compulsive disorder. Imipramine (a TCA), and MAOIs are known for their long-term success in treating panic disorders. The benzodiazapines work best for specific attacks or periods of anxiety. Though antidepressants are not effective during a panic attack, they are best used as an aid in prevention.

Somatoform Disorders. Treatment for somatoform disorders is a challenge. If the somatoform disorder exists only in the context of another psychiatric illness (e.g., if a person has multiple somatic symptoms only when depressed), treating the underlying illness is usually all that is necessary to resolve the somatoform disorder. If the primary disorder is a somatoform disorder, then a successful outcome is less likely. Most often, a good maintenance plan is the key to providing help to patients with somatoform disorders. Psychotherapy can be of value with these patients, but in somatoform disorders, as opposed to the psychotic, affective and anxiety disorders noted, the primary treatment is given by the primary care provider.

Somatization disorder Treatment for somatization disorder is the paradigm for the treatment of many of the other illnesses in this group of disorders. The treatment plan should essentially include:

1. The patient should have only one primary care provider.
2. The provider must be able to provide treatment with patience and care to this needy patient population.
3. Patients should be seen frequently — approximately once a month.
4. Visits should be brief and should focus on the specific symptom(s) the patient presents with at each visit.
5. A normal exam should be performed on any patient coming in with these specific presenting symptoms.
6. Be careful not to overlook objective signs. Maintaining suspicion of medical illness will not only prevent failure of catching some

unidentified problem, but will also be psychologically therapeutic as the patient will believe that the provider is taking the patient's symptoms seriously. This last point is most important because it is this belief in the patient's problems that creates the therapeutic alliance.

7. Order diagnostic tests and procedures only when medical illness is suspected.

8. Approach each of the patient's symptoms as expressions of emotional disturbance. Increase the patient's awareness that psychological factors may be playing a role in the patient's symptomatology. Assist the patient in obtaining psychiatric help.

Kaplan and Sadock note that individual and group psychotherapy decrease the health expenditures of patients with somatization disorder by 50%; the bulk of this is probably due to decreasing their rates of hospitalization. Psychotherapy helps patients develop alternate strategies for expression of their feelings.

In following the above treatment plan, patients will somatize less; however, if the provider sees that there are fewer symptoms and, therefore, decreases the frequency of visits beyond a certain point, it is likely that the symptoms will increase again.

Pain disorder Pain is a common symptom. In pain disorder, the pain begins suddenly and worsens over weeks to months. It can be completely disabling. When secondary gains are eliminated, patients often improve. The patients with the poorest prognosis are those who have underlying personality problems (especially passivity), could receive financial compensation, use addictive substances, and have long histories of pain.

Reducing the pain may not be possible. Psychological factors must be addressed. Patients need to understand that their psychological problems play an extremely important role in the cause of their physical pain (as well as their psychological pain).

Nonsteroidal anti-inflammatory medications (NSAIDs), sedatives and antianxiety medications are not helpful in treating pain disordered patients. These medications can, in fact, become problems in themselves because of their addictive qualities or in their side effects. With nerve blocks and surgical ablative procedures, the pain usually returns within months to a couple of years.

Antidepressants, biofeedback, hypnosis, acupuncture, transcutaneous nerve stimulation and dorsal column stimulation have all been helpful in reducing pain. Psychotherapy has been effective in

finding the root of the patient's psychological pain which is often associated with their physical pain. In-patient pain control programs with multi-modal treatment plans have also shown encouraging results.

Sexual dysfunctions There are many forms of sexual dysfunction. The nature of these dysfunctions and their treatments are beyond the scope of this text; however, primary care providers can help their patients significantly by asking about their sex lives. If the clinician makes such inquiries during routine examinations, he or she will be able to identify embarrassing, long-standing problems and be able to make an extremely important step toward their resolution.

Some of the more common treatments include: couples therapy, exercises, relaxation techniques, behavior therapy, group therapy, psychodynamic and psychoanalytic oriented therapy, as well as biological treatments. Each individual situation may be able to be treated by one or more of these therapies. The primary care provider must be able to help direct the patient to the proper therapy.

Conversion disorder Conversion disorder usually resolves spontaneously within a month. Over three quarters may never experience another episode. The prognosis is worse if the symptoms persist. One quarter to one half of patients with conversion disorder go on to have neurological problems; therefore, these patients require full medical and neurological workups. Resolution of the disorder is probably facilitated by supportive cognitive or behavior therapies.

Hypochondriases Hypochondriac episodes last from months to years and can have periods where there is no evidence of the disorder. Patients with hypochondriasis are usually resistant to psychiatric treatment. Treatment is similar to somatization disorder in that regularly scheduled visits with a single responsive primary care clinician can be helpful in reassuring these patients. The other somatization disorder treatment principles noted above generally apply to people who have hypochondriases.

Body dysmorphic disorder The onset of body dysmorphic disorder is gradual. A patient may be concerned about a specific body part for quite some time before functioning becomes compromised. Treatment with medical, surgical, or other procedures to address the alleged defects are almost always unsuccessful. The SSRI antidepressants have been found to reduce symptoms in about half of the patients with this disorder. Psychotherapy is also important in treating these patients.

ILLUSTRATIVE CASES WITH SELF-ASSESSMENT QUESTIONS AND ANSWERS

Case 1

A 30-year-old, thin, white female presents to an outpatient clinic with a chief complaint of difficulty breathing. She reports that she has had it for a couple of months and that it is getting worse, particularly at night. This is all the information she offers.

When asked if she has ever had difficulty breathing before, she responds that she had had the problem 2 to 3 years ago. She saw a physician at that time, who suggested she may have asthma and started her on medication which did not seem to help. The symptoms disappeared after a while on their own. When asked about other past medical problems, the patient reports a long history of abdominal pain while in her teens, which was diagnosed as irritable bowel syndrome. This problem also went away on its own, after a long time.

In trying to understand the nature of her complaint, she is asked to describe exactly what she feels when she has difficulty breathing. She reports that when she lays down at night, she senses pressure on her chest as she tries to breathe and feels short of breath. She says she often awakens in the middle of the night with the same symptoms. She says she thinks the shortness of breath is what causes her to awaken. She has no diaphoresis, left or right arm pain, no back pain, and reports the symptoms last an hour or longer. According to her, nothing she does seems to help.

Before doing a physical exam, the clinician asks her about her family history, particularly about heart and lung disease. The only thing she reports is that her father had a heart attack two years ago when he was 58 years old.

QUESTION: *What important questions have been omitted so far:*

a. Does she smoke cigarettes?
b. What was the reason she came in on this particular day?
c. Has she ever been treated for any psychological problems?
d. Is she taking any medication (including birth control pills)?
e. Is she in contact with anyone who may have TB or HIV disease?

ANSWER: *Although a, d, and e are important questions that must not be omitted, questions **b** and **c** will help you attain the diagnosis. When asked why she came in on this day, she replies that her symptoms were much worse over the past 24 hours. When asked if there is anything she can identify that has made it much worse, she replies that the only thing she can think of is that her boyfriend went away on a fishing trip yesterday and she is worried he might get into an accident. At some point in the exploration of the relationship between the boyfriend's trip and her breathing problem, she must be asked about her psychiatric history. (The clinician should have asked this earlier in the ROS.) Her response is to say that she has been treated for depression and obsessive-compulsive disorder (OCD) in the past.*

QUESTION: *What should the next steps be?*

a. Perform a complete physical exam.
b. Order a set of complete PFTs (pulmonary function tests) and refer to a pulmonologist.
c. Order an ECG, a chest radiograph, and consider referring to a cardiologist, depending on the outcome of these two studies.
d. Perform a modified physical exam as you would with any patient with cardio-respiratory symptoms, and obtain an office peak-flow measurement.
e. Inquire about possible current depressive and obsessive symptoms, and explore their nature, if present.
f. Refer to a psychiatrist.

ANSWER: d and e. *a, b, c, and f are not warranted at this time based on the present data. A modified physical exam must be performed, but further psychiatric history must be obtained first. In doing so, it is discovered that she has had an unexplained weight loss over the past several weeks, feels depressed and hopeless, is sleeping less (it is already known she has middle of the night awakenings), and has been obsessing about her breathing for months. Upon asking what she is most concerned about, she explains that her breathing may be normal but she is frightened that she may stop breathing at any time, because when she lays down to sleep at night* *she thinks her breathing becomes deeper, yet she feels she cannot catch her breath. At this point, a modified physical exam is performed. A thorough heart and lung exam shows no signs of any disease. The peak flow is normal for her size.*

The provider is now ready to give her an assessment of what he or she thinks is going on. First, she is told she does not appear to have any lung or heart disease but to prove it, she is lent a peak flow meter to use when she develops her breathing problem at night.

Next, the provider tells her that he or she believes the patient is depressed and probably has OCD, as well. She is then asked if there is a psychiatrist that she has seen in the past with whom she feels comfortable, or whether she would like to be referred to someone.

Lastly, the provider makes an appointment to see her sometime over the next few days. In that appointment, the patient will be assured again that she has no lung disease (with the normal overnight peak flow results), the provider will make sure the patient will be seeing the psychiatrist who was discussed during the last visit (and who has been called in the interim by the primary provider), and the patient will likely begin to feel that she has a medical alliance, allowing her to begin to feel helped.

INSOMNIA

"I cannot sleep" is a complaint every primary care provider is likely to hear. Insomnia is the subjective complaint of nonrestorative sleep due to difficulty initiating and or maintaining sleep (28). Sleep problems are common in the general population and they can contribute to impaired school and work performance. People can experience disturbances of mood and social adjustment, and decrease in marital satisfaction (29). A 1991 Gallup poll survey showed that 36% of the adult population had experienced trouble sleeping. A fourth of those surveyed have chronic problems (30). There are millions more with intermittent sleep problems. A third of the population has transient insomnia during the year. More than 40 million Americans suffer from chronic sleep disorders (31).

The National Commission on Sleep Disorders Research studied the impact of sleep disorders on society. The commission found the direct cost of sleep disorders in 1990 was $15.9 billion, and indirect cost was $60 billion (29). The true effect of poor sleep on the quality of life of millions of people in the United States and throughout the world is incalculable. Sleeping well improves the quality of life of people with poor sleep. However, only about 5% of chronic insomniacs see a health care provider. It is viewed as more of a nuisance than a medical problem. Even when patients do complain to their provider, he or she may not be trained in sleep disorders. Clinicians may use hypnotic medications inappropriately (31). Insomnia should be understood to be a symptom, and not a diagnosis. Diagnosis still requires generating a differential diagnoses based on a detailed history and physical examination with emphasis on sleep habits and patterns.

Pathophysiologic Correlation

To understand a patient's complaint of poor sleep, it is necessary to first review normal sleep physiology. Sleep is essential for a healthy life, but exactly why remains unknown. Sleep is a natural regular recurring state of reversible unresponsiveness that is restful for the body.

Sleep is an active neurological process with fluctuating states and dynamic cycles. Two separate states are recognized. The first state, Rapid Eye Movement Sleep (REM), comprises about 20% of the total sleep time. Dreaming is often recalled when an individual is awakened while in REM sleep. It is characterized by electroencephalographic activity similar to the awake state. Electrophysiologically, REM sleep is distinguished from wakefulness by the presence of active tonic inhibition of the majority of muscles. The extraocular muscles are a notable exception to the aforementioned muscle inhibition; their movements are used to identify patients in REM sleep. Deep tendon reflexes are absent in REM sleep.

The second state is non-rapid eye movement sleep (NREM), and it occupies approximately 80% of the sleep time. NREM is divided in four progressive stages. Stage I NREM sleep is the lightest form of sleep. Subjects in stage I often deny they are asleep. Fleeting dream mentation may be reported in the transition from the awake state to stage I. When these dream-like thoughts are vivid, they are called hypnogogic hallucinations. Hypnogogic hallucinations can occur in any REM sleep deprived person and are a feature of *narcolepsy*. There may also be myoclonic jerks at sleep onset that may startle the person, but are benign. More than 50% of sleep time is stage II. Stage II length is increased by most hypnotics. Stages III and IV, often collectively referred to as slow wave sleep, are the deepest form of sleep. The most difficult stages from which to awake a person are stages III and IV. The blood pressure, cerebral glucose metabolism, heart and respiratory rates are at their lowest in the 24-hour cycle. It is while in stage IV that events such as sleep walking and night terrors emerge. The electroencephalogram in slow wave sleep is characterized by high amplitude slow synchronous waves.

Sleep cycles are rhythmic fluctuations of REM and NREM sleep. REM alternates with NREM sleep with longer and more intense REM sleep as the night progresses. The first REM period is brief and occurs about 90 minutes after sleep onset, and occupies more than half of the total sleep time. The time to fall asleep and the first REM periods are defined as the *sleep latency* and *REM latency* respectively. The timing of the REM latency will depend on the person's age, health, emotional state, medication use or withdrawal, the prior amount of sleep, and time in bed. REM related events typically occur in the last third of the night. Slow wave sleep occurs mostly in the first third of the night. People will often have brief periods of arousal or awakening at the end of each 90 minute cycle. The total non-sleep time occupied by these periods is ideally 3–5% of the total time in bed. The ratio of the total sleep time to time in bed is the *sleep efficiency*.

Sleep is a circadian rhythm (happening at approximately the same time in each twenty-four hours) and the relationship between sleep cycles and stages is referred to as sleep architecture. Complaints of insomnia increase with age. It is therefore important to review how sleep architecture changes with aging.

At birth the time asleep is longer than the time awake. Newborns sleep 17–18 hours. The amount of sleep needed will progressively decrease until adulthood when the amount of total sleep time is about 8 hours with some variation. However, during adolescence there may be an increased need for sleep. Adolescents with insomnia often complain of trouble with sleep onset. Older people with insomnia typically complain of trouble with sleep maintenance or early awakening. As adults grow older, they may have decreased slow wave sleep and have increased night time awakening. There are changes in the circadian rhythm of sleep with aging. After retirement there is a greater tendency towards taking naps. Whether these changes are a part of normal aging, or the result of underlying pathology is unclear. A deterioration of the central nervous system circadian pacemaker is thought to play a role in the phenomenon of "sundowning." Sundowning is characterized by nocturnal wandering, disorientation, and confusion in the nighttime in patients with dementia (32).

Sleep is present throughout the animal kingdom. REM is practically ubiquitous among mammals and birds. When sleeping, animals are vulnerable to dangerous predators. They learn to sleep only when safe and comfortable. Anything that interferes with these feelings, physical or emotional, can disrupt sleep. To enhance adaptability to the environment and ultimately improve survival, the timing of sleep needs to be flexible. This flexibility also allows for adjustment of the sleep-wake cycle to the seasonal variations in the length of the day.

The need for sleep can be delayed or interrupted while attending other priorities such as taking care of a child. The ability to stay awake when needing sleep may be an adaptive response when one cannot sleep safely or comfortably. Children learn environmental associations that help them sleep by allowing them to feel safe and comfortable. Examples of these learned associations are being read a story, saying prayers or sleeping with a familiar toy such as teddy bear. When these associations are not present, insomnia may develop. Insomnia may result from either internal and external stimuli that interrupt sleep (e.g. anxiety, chronic pain).

Clinical and Laboratory Evaluation

The diagnosis of most sleep disorders is based on the patient's history. Physical examination is usually normal. Although laboratory evaluation is useful for some disorders, it is not always necessary.

HISTORY

The medical history in a patient complaining of insomnia needs to include a description of daytime and nighttime behavior. Specific questions to ask are listed in Table 23.14. The onset and evolution of the insomnia is important. A description of the sleep, including schedule and quality, is important.

Table 23.14.
Sleep History Questions

What time and shift does the patient work?
What time does the patient get home?
What are the living and sleeping arrangements?
What time does the patient eat and exercise?
What does the patient do if not able to sleep?
Who is the patient's bed-partner? Are there any pets, or loved ones to attend to?
How does the patient sleep while away from home?
What does the patient sleep on and in what position?
Are there any prescription, over the counter, or herbal substances used for sleep?
How does the patient decide the bedtime and get ready for bed?

The best historian is usually the bed partner who has been able to observe the patient sleeping. If the patient is able to fall asleep when not expecting to sleep (such as when watching television or during a conference) or is unable to sleep while at home in beds, environmental or psychophysiologic insomnia is suggested. Questions regarding sleep habits and quality should be included during the review of symptoms. Patients may not volunteer their sleep complaints at first. They may view them as a nuisance or as untreatable.

PHYSICAL EXAMINATION

The physical examination in patients complaining of insomnia is usually unremarkable. The physical examination should focus on possible medical, neurologic or psychiatric conditions. A thorough neurologic exam should be done on the initial visit. Physical signs of arthritis or back injury may help support a diagnosis of chronic pain causing sleep disturbance. Physical evidence of uremia will support a diagnosis of restless leg syndrome associated insomnia. Signs of rigidity and bradykinesia are typical features of Parkinson's disease which is associated with poor sleep. The mouth and pharynx merit special attention for signs of sleep disordered breathing such as retrognathia, dental crowding, large neck circumference, and a narrow airway with redundant tissue.

LABORATORY EVALUATION

A *sleep log* or diary of sleep is maintained by the patient. It can help determine the patient's sleep pattern. Having patients accurately chart their estimated hours in bed and asleep can be diagnostic. Sleep can vary from night to night. A sleep log of a minimum of 2 weeks should be recorded by the patient. The logs should include total time in bed and estimated time asleep, along with the time of exercise, eating, and medication use. The continued charting by the patients in therapy helps monitor progress. A sleep log is a simple pencil and paper test that a primary care provider can use to look for clues in determining the diagnoses and treatment progress of patients with insomnia.

Patients with sleep complaints often will have abnormal sleep architecture which reflects poor quality sleep. The best tool to evaluate the quality of sleep is the *polysomnogram*. The polysomnogram is the simultaneous and continuous recording of multiple physiological parameters. Staging sleep requires measurement of the eye movements, muscle tone and electroencephalogram (EEG). Other parameters that can be included in the polysomnogram are airflow at the nose and mouth, electrocardiogram (EKG), chest and abdominal excursion with respiration, oxygen saturation, and leg movements. Less detailed sleep studies may be obtained with portable machines that allow the patient to sleep at home. The polysomnogram is not part of the routine evaluation of insomnia. It should be reserved for difficult cases or for investigation of concomitant sleep disorders, such as sleep apnea and restless legs, which can complicate insomnia.

Activity monitors worn on the wrist can be a more accurate measure of sleep than the sleep log. These monitors detect motion which can distinguish sleep from waking activity. They can record the activity over several days. They can help evaluate the information recorded in sleep logs. The activity monitor is easy to use and a relatively inexpensive way to measure the efficacy of treatment interventions in insomniacs. It is an additional tool available to the primary care clinician managing patients with insomnia.

Differential Diagnosis

The insomnia types described are based on the International Classification of Sleep Disorders (28). There is a different, but comparable classification in the latest Diagnostic and Statistical Manual of Mental Disorders (DSM -IV). Although these insomnia types are listed as separate entries, there may be overlaps in individual patients. The initiating factors may be different from factors perpetuating the complaint of insomnia. The ICSD classifies sleep disorders as dyssomnias, parasomnias or sleep disorders associated with medical, neurologic or psychiatric disorder. *Dyssomnias* are primary disorders of initiating or maintaining sleep or of excessive sleepiness. The duration of the insomnia is diagnostically helpful. Transient insomnia is defined in the ICSD as less than one month's duration. Short-term duration is 1 to 6 months duration. These are the most common forms of insomnia, and they may affect a third of the population annually. Chronic insomnia is defined as insomnia lasting greater than 6 months. *Parasomnias* are disorders of arousal or sleep stage transition. Sleep walking is a type of parasomnia and may recur episodically. A decision tree for the most common forms of insomnia is included in Figure 23.3.

DYSSOMNIAS ASSOCIATED WITH TRANSIENT AND SHORT-TERM INSOMNIA

Environmental sleep disorder results in a complaint of insomnia due to a disturbing extrinsic factor

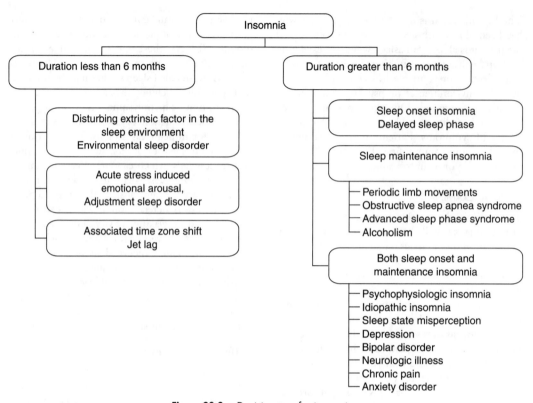

Figure 23.3. Decision tree for insomnia.

in the sleep environment. The onset, course, and termination of poor sleep is directly linked to the causative factor. Improving or removing the environmental condition will resolve the sleep problem. Causative factors include sleeping in an unfamiliar place (such as a hospital bed), or excessive heat, cold, noise, light or movements of bed partners. Other factors can be a need to stay vigilant in a situation of danger or a necessity to provide assistance to someone else such as an infant.

Adjustment sleep disorder is also referred to as stress-related transient insomnia. Any acute stress, conflict or environmental change may induce emotional arousal, and insomnia. Most adjustment sleep disorders are triggered by an emotional shock, or fear of threat to one's safety. Examples are the death of a loved one, divorce, a change in job or an upcoming examination. The sleep disturbance can also be related to intense positive emotions such as anticipating a vacation.

DYSSOMNIAS WITH CHRONIC INSOMNIA

Psychophysiologic insomnia is also referred to as conditioned or learned insomnia (28). It is charac-

terized by somatized tension and acquired sleep preventing associations that result in a complaint of difficulty initiating or maintaining sleep. For example, the patient may feel sleepy but when starting to get ready for bed, suddenly feels more awake. There can be an associated decrease in daytime function. Patients with this condition have a conditioned arousal at bedtime in their usual environment. They have an over concern with their inability to sleep. The patients are not consciously aware of their sleep-preventing associations, and thus may have no idea why they sleep so poorly. They can sleep better in places and at times when they normally do not expect to sleep: such as watching television in the living room. They sometimes sleep better when sleeping in a new place. Patients with this condition often have a prior history of bouts of insomnia and may view their condition as chronic. This insomnia may be exacerbated by the usual stresses: physical pain, shift work, family tragedy, pending job interviews or examinations. During the acute insomnia, the person may acquire maladaptive sleep habits and create associations at bed time that are alerting. For example, the person may insist on needing absolute silence to sleep. At bed time, that person then becomes hypervigilant for any noise and is easily alerted by minor sounds. Psychophysiologic insomnia will persist after the precipitating trigger has passed. These associations may be so strong that the thought of needing to sleep may cause anxiety and sleep onset difficulties. The patient may fear not being able to fall back asleep if awoken. The innate ability to fall asleep after brief arousals is diminished with resulting sleep maintenance problems. As sleep gradually deteriorates, the ability to sleep will cause an even greater concern to the patient. This concern itself may prevent sleep from occurring. The more the patient tries to sleep, the harder it becomes. A vicious circle is created. This frustration can lead to further maladaptive habits such as chronic hypnotic or alcohol use. There is an associated deterioration of mood and motivation. There can also be decreased attention, energy and concentration. Despite an increase in fatigue and malaise, there is no objective sleepiness. This condition is diagnosed in about 15% of all patients seen in sleep disorders centers. The true incidence in the general population is not known. Psychophysiologic insomnia typically starts in young adulthood and is more common in women. The course may gradually worsen with time and may last for decades without treatment.

Idiopathic insomnia is also referred to as childhood onset insomnia. It is a lifelong inability to obtain adequate sleep and is thought to be due to an abnormality of the control of the sleep-wake cycle (28). The neurologic control of the sleep cycle is complex and not completely understood. The lifelong poor sleep cannot be explained by either psychological trauma or known physical illness in childhood. Patients with idiopathic insomnia are distinguished from habitual short sleepers by their daytime function. Patients with idiopathic insomnia have a decreased feeling of well being when awake. They may adapt to the chronic sleep loss but depressive features may be present in severe cases. Idiopathic insomnia in the pure form is rare. A life time of chronic insomnia can lead to maladaptive behavior or psychiatric disturbances.

DYSSOMNIAS ASSOCIATED WITH CIRCADIAN RHYTHM SLEEP DISORDERS

Delayed sleep phase syndrome (DSP) is a circadian disorder. The major sleep period is delayed in relation to the desirable bed time; this results in symptoms of sleep onset insomnia and difficulty in awakening in the morning. Sleep is usually not disrupted once the person has fallen asleep. Although the sleep time and wake up time are later than desired, the actual sleep onset time occurs usually at the same time every night. When not forced to keep a strict sleep schedule, such as on vacation, the patient sleeps normally but at a delayed time. These patients characteristically feel more alert in the evening and may be referred to as "night owls." This condition may represent an extreme of a normal spectrum of behavior with "morning people" at the other end. The condition often becomes unmasked during adolescence. Teenagers may have a much later bed time on weekends compared to school nights. Teenagers that are susceptible will typically have great difficulty returning to their earlier bedtime on Sunday night. This will result in sleep onset insomnia. The person falls asleep at a later time similar to the previous night. There will be difficulty awakening in the morning due to lack of a full night of sleep. Adolescents with DSP have been reported to have more school difficulties and lower self esteem which can be mistaken for endogenous depression (33). As adults they will tend to try to find work that allows them to stay up late or provide flexible work hours.

Advanced sleep phase syndrome is a disorder in which the major sleep episode is advanced in relation to the desired clock time. Symptoms are comprised of compelling sleepiness, early sleep onset, and wakening earlier than desired. This is an apparently rare condition perhaps because these patients can be integrated into society more easily than those with DSP. The early morning arousal may be mistaken as a sign of depression. However unlike depressed patients, these patients have otherwise undisturbed sleep and have no major mood disturbance.

Jet lag is also called time zone change syndrome. It consists of difficulty initiating or maintaining sleep, decreased daytime alertness and performance, and malaise following rapid travel across multiple time zones. The insomnia is not due to jet travel per se, but rather the time zone shift that causes a misalignment of the body's underlying circadian rhythms with the new sleep schedule. The condition is usually self limited and an adjustment will be made to the new environment in about 1 week. The severity is dependent on the extent of the shift and the direction of travel. Adaptation on an eastward flight takes longer than a westward flight. Individuals who travel back and forth across time zones, such as flight personnel, may experience chronic symptoms of sleep disturbance, daytime malaise, irritability, and work impairment.

The need for 24 hour operations creates altered work schedules that can lead to *shift work sleep disorder* from cumulative sleep loss and circadian disruption. Shift workers may complain of disturbed and shortened sleep, chronic fatigue, gastrointestinal dysfunction, and high rates of job errors. These problems are felt to be secondary to the disruption of the body's circadian rhythm. There are individual differences in the ability to tolerate shift work. This ability may decrease in the fifth and sixth decade. The sleep difficulties of shift workers should improve with normalization of the work schedule. There is no clear evidence of long-term sequelae after stopping shift work. The sleep problems may be lessened if the worker avoids time shifts on days off, and continues on a schedule similar to work. The use of hypnotics for shift workers should be avoided because of problems with tolerance and dependence.

INSOMNIA ASSOCIATED WITH MENTAL DISORDERS

Most psychiatric disorders can have associated sleep disturbances. Patients with histories of mood disorders, anxiety disorders and substance abuse commonly present with sleep complaints. These conditions need to be considered in the differential diagnosis of patients complaining of insomnia. Treatment is focused on the primary psychiatric problem. Since these conditions are discussed in greater detail elsewhere in the text, only their sleep characteristics will be reviewed here.

Patients with major depression will complain of insomnia and non-refreshing sleep. They may have difficulty falling asleep, and frequent nocturnal and early morning awakening. Insomnia may herald an oncoming bout of depression. Patients with depression may also present with hypersomnia. These patients may complain of feeling tired but when given an opportunity to nap are unable to do so. Most effective antidepressants have REM sleep suppressant properties. An interesting observation is the remission of depression following acute sleep deprivation. This is an impractical treatment because the sleep deprivation is difficult to maintain.

Most patients with *bipolar disorder* also report insomnia when depressed, they may also develop symptoms of hypersomnia with difficulty awakening, and excessive daytime sleepiness. During manic episodes, patients often report a reduced amount of total sleep, and a subjective decreased need for sleep. Switches into manic episodes may be preceded by periods of sleeplessness.

The sleep of patients with *anxiety disorders* may

be characterized by sleep-onset or maintenance insomnia. The insomnia is due to excessive anxiety and apprehensive expectation. The patients may have ruminative thinking while lying in bed. Patients with *panic attacks* may have recurrent episodes during sleep. These attacks are associated with sudden awakening and symptoms of choking, palpitations, trembling, chest pain and sweating. The patient is subsequently hyperaroused and has difficulty returning to sleep. Some patients develop sedative or hypnotic abuse that can further complicate this condition.

Patients with *substance abuse problems* may also have difficulty sleeping. Alcohol is commonly self prescribed for insomnia. Acute alcohol use at bedtime initially produces increased sleepiness, however it may disrupt the latter part of the night with increased awakening. Alcohol at bed time is associated with bedwetting, sleepwalking, increased snoring and exacerbation of obstructive sleep apnea. Chronic excessive use of alcohol fragments sleep with short periods of deep sleep interrupted by brief arousals or periods of restlessness. Abstinence following chronic use may cause profound sleep disruption with insomnia. Nightmares may be pronounced.

Insomnia may be caused by dependence on hypnotics. Acute use of hypnotics for several days may result in sleeplessness upon withdrawal. This rebound insomnia leads to renewed use of the medication. Sustained use of hypnotics induces tolerance. When patients try to stop using the hypnotic, their insomnia will be acutely worse. The rebound insomnia may last 1–2 nights. This may be minimized if the hypnotics are withdrawn slowly. Long term hypnotic use is not effective in patients with chronic insomnia. The risk of rebound insomnia is greater with the benzodiazepines which have short half-lives than those with the long half-lives.

INSOMNIA ASSOCIATED WITH NEUROLOGICAL ILLNESS

Neurological conditions that are associated with insomnia are summarized in Table 23.15. Pain, fever, or pulmonary difficulty may cause the insomnia. Decreased sleep efficiency, REM and delta sleep are often reported.

Neurological illnesses provide insight to possible underlying mechanisms of insomnia and hypersomnia. Third ventricle and hypothalamus tumors may cause insomnia. Peripheral neuropathies and neuromuscular disease may also cause insomnia through involuntary movements, pain, dysautonomia, and breathing difficulty. In contrast, myotonic

Table 23.15.
Neurologic Conditions Associated with Insomnia

Movement disorder
Neuro muscular disease
Headache
Peripheral neuropathies
Oncologic illnesses
Trauma
Epilepsy
Cerebrovascular diseases
Degenerative conditions
Delirium

Table 23.16.
Medical Causes of Insomnia

Medical Category	Specific Conditions
Rheumatic disorders	Fibromyalgia, collagen vascular disease
Cardiovascular disease	Heart failure, coronary heart disease, angina
Pulmonary disorders	Asthma, alveolar hypo-ventilation, COPD
Gastrointestinal disorders	Peptic ulcer, GE reflex, hepatic failure
Renal disorders	Renal failure, polyuria & nocturia
Endocrine	Diabetes mellitus, thyroid disease

muscular dystrophy which is the most common muscular dystrophy in adults may present with hypersomnia. Most strokes occur within an hour of awakening. Insomnia may occur in stroke patients for a variable duration; strokes may be the trigger for a cycle of maladaptive sleep. Bilateral pontine lesions decrease REM sleep and disrupt sleep wake cycle organization. Insomnia may endure for months after head trauma recovery, and insomnia may be a symptom of a post-concussive syndrome. Delirium due to any toxic or metabolic problem is linked with insomnia. Degenerative conditions such as multiple sclerosis, amyotrophic lateral sclerosis, and Parkinson's disease have severe sleep disruptions. In Parkinson's disease the insomnia may be due to not only the central nervous system degeneration but may also be a side effect of the dopaminergic medications. The transition from either wakefulness or sleep is a vulnerable time for seizures.

INSOMNIA WITH MEDICAL CONDITIONS

Medical conditions that are associated with insomnia are summarized in Table 23.16. The insomnia caused by these disorders may be explained by several mechanisms. Patients with heart failure may have sleep disrupted by nocturia due to diuretics or paroxysmal nocturnal dyspnea. Respiratory conditions cause disrupted sleep secondary to oxygen desaturation and increased work of breathing. Diabetes can cause insomnia due to polyuria, hypoglycemia, peripheral and autonomic neuropathy.

Menstrual associated sleep disorder can manifest with either insomnia or hypersomnia. Menopausal insomnia is associated with typical menopausal changes. The insomnia may improve with hormonal therapy. Pregnancy may also be associated with disrupted sleep. Total sleep time increases

in the first trimester. An age matched controlled study of sleep in normal late pregnancy found that in accordance with their complaints, women in their third trimester demonstrated polysomnographic patterns of sleep maintenance insomnia. The most frequent sleep complaints in the pregnant group were restless sleep, low back pain, leg cramps and frightening dreams (34).

OTHER DIAGNOSES

When evaluating a new patient with a complaint of insomnia, the differential diagnoses should include the following three conditions which are not usually classified as insomnias: obstructive sleep apnea (OSA), periodic limb movements of sleep (PLMS) and restless legs syndrome (RSL). These conditions may be so common that if a practicing primary care provider has not diagnosed them at some time, they may have been overlooked. A conservative estimate of the prevalence of OSA in women and men ages 30–60 is 2–4% and may be as high as 9–24% respectively. OSA is a breathing disorder of sleep where collapse of the pharynx causes sleep fragmentation and oxygen desaturation. The typical features are nighttime snoring interrupted by apneic pauses and excessive daytime sleepiness. Sleep apnea may both cause and exacerbate prior insomnia.

Restless legs syndrome is common. It affects at least 5% of the general population, increases with age and is often associated with insomnia. Patients with restless legs report dyesthesias while at rest which are relieved by walking, cause significant discomfort and results in sleep disturbance. There is a circadian pattern with worse symptoms in the afternoon and evening with suppression in REM sleep and improvement in the morning. In some patients serum ferritin levels are inversely correlated with the severity of RLS symptoms. Improvement in symptoms of restless legs has been noted with iron repletion (35). PLMS, also called nocturnal myoclonus, are rhythmic brief leg movements with a frequency of 20–30 seconds. The resulting sleep disturbance is not apparent to the patient but may be reported by the bed partner. Patients with PLMS and RLS report better sleep and alertness on carbidopa/levodopa (36).

Management

Most cases of insomnia can be managed by a primary care clinician using behavioral techniques and occasional hypnotics. This section summarizes treatment recommendations under behavioral and pharmaceutical interventions. Referral to a sleep specialist should be reserved for chronic insomniacs with a history of treatment failure, or multiple sleep disorders. Insomnia associated with primary medical, neurologic or psychiatric diseases is best treated by addressing the underlying condition. However, it must be remembered that there may be multiple factors causing an individual case of insomnia. Therefore, the suggested therapies may be applied to a wide range of patients with insomnia.

DRUG THERAPY

Insomnia is a common complaint, and sleeping pills are among the most commonly prescribed drugs in medicine. The hypnotics should be used mainly for transient and short term insomnia complaints. They may be particularly useful for jet lag. On a west to east transcontinental overnight flight, the traveler will have a short night and an early morning. A hypnotic may allow the person to sleep better on the plane and avoid the characteristic traveler's "red eye" fatigued appearance. Hypnotics can be used effectively for insomnia during acute episodes of excitement or stress associated with starting a new job or school, marriage preparation or familial illness or death. The duration of therapy will be variable. Prescriptions should not be routinely refilled or given for large quantities. In a situation where poor sleep due to an unfamiliar or uncomfortable sleep environment can be anticipated, and optimal sleep is desired for the following day, medication can be considered. The commonly prescribed benzodiazepine hypnotics are relatively safe compared to the previously popular barbiturates.

Their side effects include daytime sedation, decrease in memory, anxiety, dizziness, and confusion. Choosing a hypnotic depends on the desired effect. All hypnotics shorten sleep-onset. A short-acting drug would avoid the next day hang over, but it is also more likely to induce rebound insomnia. A longer acting drug may help decrease arousals during the night and improve sleep efficiency.

BEHAVIORAL INTERVENTIONS

Successful treatment of chronic insomnia requires a lifestyle change. The clinician needs to identify which previous changes in the patient's sleeping environment and mind set are perpetuating the insomnia. Recommendations for healthy sleep habits are referred to as *sleep hygiene* and are given in Table 23.17. Like all conditions that demand a patient's involvement, motivation will determine outcome. Motivation may be enhanced with partial sleep deprivation by restricting the total hours in bed allowed per night to increase sleep efficiency. The patient should start to look forward to going to sleep and not fear an inability to sleep. Patients need to understand why they developed insomnia and how the body establishes a sleep rhythm.

Exposure to bright light helps re-establish a

Table 23.17.
Sleep Hygiene Recommendations

Establish a regular enjoyable bed time routine.
The sleeping environment should be dark, safe and comfortable.
Relaxation exercises, meditation, prayer or light conversation with the bed partner may be helpful to establish a pleasant feeling at bed time.
Establish a regular bed and awake time seven days a week. Set up wake up time first to help establish the sleep-onset time. Determine the total amount of hours of sleep needed to be refreshed. Restrict the time in bed to those hours.
Get regular exercise. Exercise increases the depth of sleep. Exercise in the evening prior to sleep may, however, be disruptive.
Get 30 minutes of sunlight or similar light exposure upon awakening. Avoid bright light if sleep is disrupted during the night.
Avoid heavy meals or drinking large amounts of liquid prior to bed time.
Schedule a "worry" time prior to getting ready to sleep. This helps control racing thoughts which are disruptive to sleep.
Use your bed and bed room for sleeping and sex only.

sleep rhythm; it is an effective behavioral therapy for insomnia. Light therapy trains the circadian pacemaker. It has been used for patients with sea- sonal affective syndrome. It is also effective for night-shift workers, transmeridian travelers, de- layed and advance sleep phase disorder (37).

ILLUSTRATIVE CASES WITH SELF-ASSESSMENT QUESTIONS AND ANSWERS

Case 1

A 26-year-old man comes to your office complaining of insomnia for 6 months. He reports that he has had intermittent trouble sleeping in the past. However since starting his new job and working the night shift, he had trouble falling asleep. He began drinking a shot of tequila before going to bed. He was then able to fall asleep but kept waking up at night. He has been waking up tired. He is worried that he may lose his job if he does not get enough sleep. Past medical history is unremarkable and he uses no medications. On physical examination he is overweight and has borderline hypertension. He sleeps alone and is not aware of any snoring. He is requesting that you help him sleep.

QUESTION: *The BEST diagnosis and initial management is which of the following?*

a. Diagnose the patient with insomnia induced by obstructive sleep apnea which was unmasked by the alcohol. Refer to an accredited sleep clinic for a polysomnogram.
b. Stop alcohol 6 hours prior to bedtime, and warn the patient of possible alcohol withdrawal. Modify the patient's sleep hygiene.
c. Prescribe a limited course of a short-acting hypnotic such as zolpidiem while weaning off alcohol.
d. Diagnose with shift work associated insomnia. Refer to psychiatry for suspected insomnia due to occult depression.

ANSWER: b. *The night time alcohol must be stopped because it is fragmenting the patient's sleep. Patients ought to be reminded that they need to change their lifestyles. The patient's prior history of insomnia and relapse with a new job suggest environmental and perhaps conditioned insomnia as possible etiologies. A review of sleep hygiene may identify maladaptive behaviors per-*

petuating the insomnia. Sleeping pills are not usually effective in chronic insomnia. A referral to a sleep disorder center may be necessary if the patient does not improve but would not be the initial management. Patients with sleep apnea are more likely to be sleepy than to have insomnia. Shift work may be part of the problem but there is not enough evidence of depression to warrant a referral to a psychiatrist.

QUESTION: *Hypnotics are helpful for which of the following situations?*

a. 1,2,3
b. 1,3
c. 2,4
d. only 4
e. all of the above:

1. Jet lag
2. shift work
3. Insomnia prior to marriage ceremony
4. Improvement of sleep efficiency of patients with insomnia associated with sleep apnea by decreasing the arousal threshold.

ANSWER: b. *Jet lag and transient insomnia are both situations in which short acting hypnotics are effective. Shift workers need to adapt their circadian rhythm on a long term basis and should avoid sleeping pills. All sedating and muscle relaxing drugs are contraindicated in obstructive sleep apnea.*

QUESTION: *Changes seen in sleep with normal aging include which of the following?:*

a. 1,2,3
b. 1,3
c. 2,4
d. only 4
e. all of the above:

1. Sleep maintenance insomnia is typical of adolescents.
2. Children have the most REM sleep at birth.
3. Unlike REM the amount of slow wave sleep remains constant as we grow older.
4. Deterioration of the circadian pacemaker may lead to nocturnal disorientation ("sundowning").

ANSWER: c. *REM is maximal at birth, and it decreases and plateaus eventually to about 20% of the total sleep time. Sundowning is felt to be associated to pacemaker degeneration. Adolescents typically complain of sleep-onset insomnia.*

REFERENCES

Anxiety

1. Weissman MM, Merikangas KR. The epidemiology of anxiety and panic disorders: an update. J Clin Psych 1986;47 (6 Suppl): 11–17.
2. Breier A. Panic disorder: clinical features, neurobiology and pharmacology. NYS J Med, 1991;91: 43S-46S.
3. Tomb DA. Psychiatry. Fourth ed. Philadelphia: Williams & Wilkins, 1992:70.
4. Katon W. Panic disorder in the medical setting. National Institutes of Mental Health. DHHS Pub No (ADM) 89–1629, Washington, D.C.: Supt of Docs, US Gov't Printing Office, 1989.
5. Diagnostic and statistical manual of mental disorders, 4th Edition (DSM-IV). Washington, D.C.: American Psychiatric Association, 1994.
6. McGlynn TJ, Metcalf HL, eds. Diagnosis and treatment of anxiety disorders: a physician's handbook. Washington, D.C.: American Psychiatric Press, Inc., 1989.
7. Derogatis LR, Wise TN. Anxiety and depresssion disorders in the medical patient. Washington, D.C.: American Psychiatric Press, Inc., 1989:189–93.
8. Frances RJ, Borg L. The treatment of anxiety in patients with alcoholism. J Clin Psych 1993;54 (5 Suppl): 37–43.
9. Ewing JA. Detecting alcoholism, the CAGE questionnaire. JAMA 1984;252, 1905–1907.

Depression

10. Horwath E, Johnson J, Klerman GL, et al. Depressive symptoms as relative and attributable risk factors for first-onset major depression. Arch Gen Psychiatr 1992; 49:817–823.
11. Diagnostic and Statistical manual of mental disorders. 4th ed. Washington D.C.: American Psychiatric Association, 1994.
12. Cassano GB, Musetti L, Soriani A, et al. The pharmacologic treatment of depression: drug selection criteria. Pharmacopsychiatry 1993; 26 (supplement): 17–23.
13. Michels R, Marzuk PM. Progress in psychiatry. N Engl J Med 1993;329/8: 552–560.
14. Pies RW, Shader RI. Approaches to the treatment of depression. In: Shader RI,ed. Manual of Psychiatric Therapeutics. 2nd ed. Boston/ New York/ Toronto/ London: Little, Brown and Company, 1993.
15. Coyne JC, Schwenk TL. Depression in the female patient. Female Patient 1994;19:59–71.
16. Small GW. Recognition and treatment of depression in the elderly. J Clin Psychiatr 1991; 56/6 (supplement): 11–22.
17. Thase ME. Relapse and recurrence in unipolar major depression: short-term and long-term approaches. J Clin Psychiatr 1990; 51/6 (supplement): 51–59.
18. Shader RI. Assessment and treatment of suicide risk. In: Shader RI, ed. Manual of Psychiatric Therapeutics. 2nd ed. Boston/ New York/ Toronto/ London: Little, Brown and Company, 1993.
19. Wells KB, Stewart A, Hays RD, et al. The functioning and well being of depressed patients. JAMA 1989;262/7:914–919.
20. Broadhead WE, Blazer DG, George LK, et al. Depression, disability days, and days lost from work in a prospective epidemiologic survey. JAMA 1990; 264/19:2524–2528.
21. Zung WWK, Magill M, Moore JT, et al. Recognition and treatment of depression in a family medicine practice. J Clin Psychiatr 1983;44/1:3–6.
22. Gerber PD, Barrett JE, Barrett JA, et al. The relationship of presenting physical complaints to depressive symptoms in primary care patients. J Gen Intern Med 1992;7:170–173.
23. Von Korff M, Le Resche L, Dworkin SF. First onset of common pain symptoms: a prospective study of depression as a risk factor. Pain1993; 55:251–258.
24. Katon W, Sullivan MD. Depression and chronic medical illness. J Clin Psychiatr 1990; 51/6 (supplement): 3–14.
25. Astrom M, Asolfsson R, Asplund K. Major depression in stroke patients a 3-year longitudinal study. Stroke 1993;24/7:976–982.
26. Blumenthal SJ. A guide to risk factors, assessment and treatment of suicidal patients. Med Clin North Am 1988; 72/4:937–970.
27. Klerman GL. Treatment of recurrent unipolar major depressive disorder. (Comment) Arch Gen Psychiatr 1990;47: 1158–1162.

Insomnia

28. Diagnostic Classification Steering Committee, Thorpy MJ, Chairman. International classification of sleep disorders: Diagnostic and coding manual. Rochester, Minnesota: American Sleep Disorders Association, 1990.
29. The National Commission on Sleep Disorders Research: Wake up America. Dement WC, chairman. National Institute of Health. Washington, D.C.1993.

30. The Gallup Organization: Sleep in America: a national survey of US adults. Princeton, NJ, 1991.
31. Shorr RI, Bauwens SF. Diagnosis and treatment of outpatient insomnia by psychiatric and nonpsychiatric physicians. Am J Med 1992; 93(1):78–82.
32. Bliwise DL. What is sundowning? J Am Geriatr Soc 1994;42(9):1009–11.
33. Thorpy MJ, Korman E, Spielman AJ, et al. Delayed sleep phase syndrome among adolescents. J Adolec Med 1988; 9:22–27.
34. Hertz G, Fast A, Feinsilver SH, et al. Sleep in normal late pregnancy. Sleep Disorders Center, Winthrop University Hospital, SUNY, Stony Brook, Mineola ll50l. Sleep l992;15(3):246–5L.
35. O'Keefe ST, Gavin K, Lavan JN. Iron status and restless legs syndrome in the elderly. Department of Geriatric Medicine, Beaumont Hospital, Dublin. Age Ageing 1994;23(3):200–3.
36. Kaplan PW, Allen RP, Buchholz DW, et al. A double-blind, placebo-controlled study of the treatment of periodic limb movements in sleep using carbiodopa/levodopa and propoxphene. Department of Neurology, Francis Scott Key Medical Center, Baltimore, Maryland. Sleep 1993;16(8):717–23.
37. Czeisler CA, Allan JS, Stogatz, et al. Bright light resets the human circadian pacemaker independent of the sleep-wake cycle. Science 1986;233:667–671.

SUGGESTED READINGS

Anxiety

Kandel ER. From metapsychology to molecular biology: explorations into the nature of anxiety. Am J Psychol 1983;140:1277–1293.

Spielberger CD, Diaz-Guerrero R. Cross-Cultural anxiety. Hemisphere Publishing Company: New York, 1986.

Depression

Goodwin F. A 47-year-old man with chronic depression. JAMA 1996; 275: 479–485.

Pakel ES, Priest RG. Recognition and management of depression in general practice: consensus statement. BMJ 1992; 305:1198–202.

Blumenthal SJ. A guide to risk factors, assessment and treatment of suicidal patients. Med Clin North Am 1988;72/4:937–970.

Small GW. Recognition and treatment of depression in the elderly. J Clin Psychiatr 1991; 56/6 (supplement): 11–22.

Multiple Somatic Complaints

Diagnostic and statistical manual of mental health DSM-IV, 4th ed. Washington D.C.: American Psychiatric Association, 1994.

Kaplan HI, Sadock BJ, Grebb JA. Kaplan and Sadock's synopsis of psychiatry, 7th ed. Baltimore: Williams & Wilkins, 1994.

Goldman HH. Review of general psychiatry. Los Altos, CA: Lange Medical Publications, 1984.

Katon W, Ries RK, Kleinman A. The prevalence of somatization in primary care. Comp Psych 1984;25: 208–215.

Smith RG. The epidemiology and treatment of depression when it coexists with somatoform disorders, somatization or pain. Gen Hosp Psych 1992;14:265–272.

Insomnia

Wake Up America: a national sleep alert: report of the National Commission on Sleep Disorders Research / submitted to the United States Congress and to the Secretary, U.S. Dept. of Health and Human Services. 1993. *If you have any interest in sleep disorders, this is "must" reading. The commission chair was W.C. Dement. Paid for by U.S. taxpayers and should be available for a nominal fee.*

Meir H. Kryger, Thomas Roth, William C. Dement, eds. Principles and practice of sleep medicine. 2nd ed. Philadelphia: WB Saunders, 1994.

Sleep. *The official journal of the American Sleep Disorders Association, European Sleep Disorders Association, Latin American Sleep Disorders Association, and Japanese Sleep Disorders Association. Christian Guilleminault, editor-in-chief.*

INDEX

Page numbers in *italics* denote figures; those followed by "t" denote tables.

HIV-associated thrombocytopenia, 218
HIV-infected patients, 55–66. *See also* AIDS/HIV
HMG CoA reductase inhibitors, 381–382. *See also*
Cholesterol-lowering drugs
Home health care, 39–43
case illustration: congestive heart failure, 42–43
for chronic conditions, 40t
conditions effectively treated by, 40t
goals for primary care provider, 41–42
historical perspective on, 39–40
professionals involved in, 40t
rationale for, 40–41
Homophobia, 34
Homosexuals, 34
urinary tract infections in, 316, 317
"Honeymoon" cystitis, 316
Hormone replacement therapy, 493–495. *See also*
Estrogen therapy
Hospice, 41
Hospitalization, hazards of, *41*
Hot/cold balance concept of health, 35
Human chorionic gonadotrophin (HCG) test,
457–458, 476
Human immunodeficiency virus (HIV). *See* AIDS/
HIV
Hydralazine, 469
Hydrocephalus, 154
Hyperadrenocorticism (Cushing's disease), 185, 187,
344, 387, 388
Hyperbilirubinemia, 304. *See also* Jaundice
differential diagnosis, 311t
Hypercalciuria, idiopathic, 337
Hypercholesterolemia, 372–384. *See also*
Hyperlipidemia
Hyperfunctioning thyroid adenoma, 367, 370
Hyperglycemia, 343. *See also* Diabetes mellitus
reactive (Somogyi phenomenon), 355
Hyperlipidemia, 372–384
case illustrations, 383–384
clinical and laboratory evaluation, 376–378, 378t
cholesterol measurement, 377–378
differential diagnosis, 378
genetic factors in, 376
management, 378–382
in coronary artery disease, 382
diet, 378–379, 379t
in elderly, 382
pharmacologic treatment, 379–392, 380t
in women, 382
pathophysiologic correlation, 372–376
atherosclerosis and hypercholesterolemia,
375–376, *376, 377*
lipid metabolism, 372–375, *373,* 373t, *374*
as risk factor for renal disease, 332t
Hyperopia, 97, 99
Hyperparathyroidism, 331. *See also* Renal insufficiency
Hypersensitivity
to drugs, 399
edema in, 198

Hypertension, 147, 183–194, 266
case illustrations, 192–194, *193–194*
CHAOS syndrome (syndrome X), 358
clinical and laboratory evaluation, 185–187, 187t
clinical trials, 183–185
in diabetes mellitus, 358–360, *359*
differential diagnosis, 187
epidemiology, 183
headache in, 121, 126–127
malignant, 194
management, 187–192, *190*
in African-Americans, 190–191
in diabetes, 191
in elderly, 191
follow-up recommendations, 188t
goals of treatment, 191–192
nonpharmacologic therapy, 187–188
pharmacologic therapy, 188–189, 189t
in pregnancy, 191
in special populations, 191t
in women, 189–190
myocardial infarction and, *192*
pathophysiologic correlation, 183–184
in pregnancy, 463, 467, 469
as risk factor for renal disease, 330–331
screening for, 16
in stroke/TIAs, 138, 139
target-organ manifestations, 185t
white coat, 186
Hypertension Detection and Follow-up Program
(HDFP), 184
Hyperthyroidism, 186, 365t, 367, 369–370, 388–389.
See also Thyroid disorders; Thyroid function tests
in pregnancy, 469–470
Hyperuricemia, 336
Hyperuricosuria, 337
Hypnotics, 612, 615
Hypocalcemia, 147
Hypochondriasis, 596, 605
Hypoglycemia
reactive, 355
seizures in, 147
versus stroke, 140
Hypoglycemic agents
insulin, 352–355, 353t, 354t
oral, 355–357, 356t
Hyponatremia, 147
Hypothalamic disease, 388
Hypothyroidism, 121, 186, 358–371, 365t, 388, 389.
See also Thyroid disorders; Thyroid function tests
in pregnancy, 469–470
Hypoxemia, 147

I
Icterus (jaundice), 303–312. *See also* Jaundice
IDDM (insulin-dependent diabetes mellitus, type 2),
341, 344. *See also* Diabetes mellitus

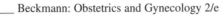
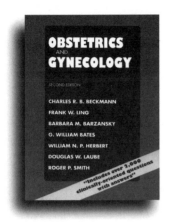